The Blood-Brain Barrier in Health and Disease

The Blood-Brain Barrier in Health and Disease

Editor: Kason Benson

AMERICAN
MEDICAL PUBLISHERS
www.americanmedicalpublishers.com

AMERICAN
MEDICAL PUBLISHERS
www.americanmedicalpublishers.com

Cataloging-in-Publication Data

The blood-brain barrier in health and disease / edited by Kason Benson.
p. cm.
Includes bibliographical references and index.
ISBN 979-8-88740-493-6
1. Blood-brain barrier. 2. Blood-brain barrier disorders. 3. Brain--Diseases--Treatment.
4. Brain--Blood-vessels--Innervation. 5. Cerebral circulation. I. Benson, Kason.
QP375.5 .B56 2023
612.824--dc23

American Medical Publishers,
41 Flatbush Avenue,
1st Floor, New York,
NY 11217, USA

ISBN 979-8-88740-493-6 (Hardback)

Contents

Preface

This book has been a concerted effort by a group of academicians, researchers and scientists, who have contributed their research works for the realization of the book. This book has materialized in the wake of emerging advancements and innovations in this field. Therefore, the need of the hour was to compile all the required researches and disseminate the knowledge to a broad spectrum of people comprising of students, researchers and specialists of the field.

The blood-brain barrier (BBB) is responsible for the movement of ions, molecules, and cells between the blood and the CNS. This barrier is essential for providing the right environment for healthy neuronal function and also for protecting the CNS from injury and disease. The BBB is made up of three biological components of the brain microvasculature: brain endothelial cells (BECs), astrocyte end-feet, and pericytes (PCs). BECs are essential components of the BBB, responsible for protecting the brain from pathogens while also limiting the flow of circulatory factors. Astrocytes, which are five times the number of neurons in the CNS, provide simple structural and nutritional support for neurons and also contribute to the composition of the BBB. Pericytes play an essential role in angiogenesis, vascular remodeling, vascular tone, and BBB development. Several neurologic diseases such as stroke and neuroinflammatory disorders are affected by the BBB dysfunction. This book presents researches and studies performed by internationally acclaimed experts on the role of blood-brain barrier. It will serve as a valuable source of reference for graduate and post graduate students.

At the end of the preface, I would like to thank the authors for their brilliant chapters and the publisher for guiding us all-through the making of the book till its final stage. Also, I would like to thank my family for providing the support and encouragement throughout my academic career and research projects.

Editor

1

Barrier mechanisms in neonatal stroke

***Ingrid Kratzer*[†]*, Sophorn Chip*[†] *and Zinaida S. Vexler**

Department of Neurology, University of California San Francisco, San Francisco, CA, USA

Correspondence:
Zinaida S. Vexler, Department of Neurology, University of California San Francisco, 675 Nelson Rising Lane, San Francisco, CA 94158-0663, USA
e-mail: zena.vexler@ucsf.edu

[†]*These authors have contributed equally to this work.*

Clinical data continue to reveal that the incidence of perinatal stroke is high, similar to that in the elderly. Perinatal stroke leads to significant morbidity and severe long-term neurological and cognitive deficits, including cerebral palsy. Experimental models of cerebral ischemia in neonatal rodents have shown that the pathophysiology of perinatal brain damage is multifactorial. Cerebral vasculature undergoes substantial structural and functional changes during early postnatal brain development. Thus, the state of the vasculature could affect susceptibility of the neonatal brain to cerebral ischemia. In this review, we discuss some of the most recent findings regarding the neurovascular responses of the immature brain to focal arterial stroke in relation to neuroinflammation. We also discuss a possible role of the neonatal blood-CSF barrier in modulating inflammation and the long-term effects of early neurovascular integrity after neonatal stroke on angiogenesis and neurogenesis.

Keywords: vascular permeability, microglia, leukocyte, inflammation, CSF-brain barrier, neonatal ischemia

INTRODUCTION

The blood-brain barrier (BBB) protects the central nervous system (CNS) and prevents non-specific leakage of molecules and cells from the blood into the brain. Stroke can disintegrate the BBB in many ways by disrupting cell-cell communication between endothelial cells (ECs), pericytes, and astrocytes, cumulatively referred to as the "neurovascular unit" (NVU), and by affecting neurons and microglial cells, thereby enhancing injury. Reperfusion and re-oxygenation of previously ischemic brain regions further affect BBB function, restoring or disrupting, depending on various factors such as the extent, length of initial cerebral blood flow (CBF) disruption, genetic background, sex, age, and the presence of other confounding factors.

The timing of injury during brain development has a major impact on determining the pathophysiology of ischemic brain damage. Maturation of individual cell types, individual components of the NVU and of the extracellular matrix (ECM), and of individual brain regions is not synchronized, contributing to the existence of "windows of susceptibility" to ischemia during particular fetal and postnatal periods. Here we discuss some of the most recent findings regarding the neurovascular responses of the immature brain to focal arterial stroke in relation to neuroinflammation and long-term effects on repair.

AGE AT THE TIME OF CEREBRAL ISCHEMIA AS A DETERMINANT OF THE PATHOPHYSIOLOGY OF BRAIN DAMAGE: PRETERM vs. TERM

In preterm human babies (23–32-weeks of gestation) intracerebral hemorrhage (ICH), intraventricular hemorrhage (IVH), and periventricular white matter injury (PWMI) are the most common types of ischemia-related injuries (Volpe, 2009). Clinical aspects of perinatal stroke have been extensively discussed (Ferriero, 2004; Nelson and Lynch, 2004). Vulnerability of oligodendrocyte progenitor cells (OPCs) to ischemia and hypoxia including a concomitant loss of subplate neurons, a transient neuronal subpopulation important in corticogenesis and proper wiring of the developing brain, contribute to PWMI (McQuillen et al., 2003; Volpe, 2009). The germinal matrix with its weak, leaky vasculature, high local production of vascular endothelial growth factor (VEGF), angiopoietin-2 (Angpt2), and matrix metalloproteinases (MMPs) also make the preterm brain prone to ICH and IVH (Ballabh, 2010). Low pericyte coverage and ensheathement of astrocytic endfeets along blood vessels, together with immaturity of the basal membrane (BM), also make the preterm brain susceptible to ischemia-related injury (El-Khoury et al., 2006; Braun et al., 2007). At term (between birth and 28 days of life), ischemia-related white matter injury does occur (Rothstein and Levison, 2005; Van Den Broeck et al., 2008), but injury predominantly affects gray matter (Ferriero, 2004).

Several models were developed to understand the pathophysiological mechanisms of hypoxic-ischemic encephalopathy (HIE) and focal arterial stroke at term (Yager and Ashwal, 2009). A model of hypoxia-ischemia (HI) consists of a unilateral ligation of the common carotid artery (CCA) followed by a variable duration of exposure to 8% O_2 in postnatal day 7 (P7) rats (Rice et al., 1981), and P9 mice and mimics HIE, whereas transient middle cerebral artery occlusion (tMCAO) model in P7 rats (Derugin et al., 1998), P10 rats (Mu et al., 2003), and P9 mice (Woo et al., 2012), and a combined permanent MCAO and transient CCA occlusion in P7 rats (Renolleau et al., 1998) mimic focal arterial stroke. The HI is associated with increased CBF during systemic hypoxia whereas CBF is disrupted after MCAO. Models of HI were also developed in rabbit and sheep (Marks et al., 1999; Derrick et al., 2007).

Studies in these age-appropriate ischemic models revealed several features unique to neonatal brain injury. First, excitotoxicity-induced neuronal death is a significant injury component (Ikonomidou et al., 1989). Second, neonatal brain is prone to reactive oxygen species (ROS) after HI (Sheldon et al., 2004). Third, apoptosis, a major neuronal cell death mode during this period, coexists with necrosis and necroptosis, creating a "*continuum*" with features of both cell death types (Blomgren et al., 2007; Northington et al., 2011). Finally, inflammation associated with failure to complete apoptosis is pivotal to ischemia-induced injury (Vexler and Yenari, 2009). **Figure 1** outlines identified differences in ischemic injury mechanisms between adults and neonates.

BRAIN MATURATION-DEPENDENT SUSCEPTIBILITY OF THE BBB AFTER STROKE

The BBB undergoes major disruption early after adult stroke. Depending on initial stroke severity BBB opening can be biphasic or gradual (Knowland et al., 2014). The timing, extent of leukocyte-mediated BBB disturbances and redistribution of tight junctions (TJs) can vary. Degradation of TJ proteins occludin, claudin-5, and of a TJ-associated protein, zonula occludens 1 (ZO-1), is increased after stroke in part due to activation and/or *de novo* synthesis of MMPs (Yang et al., 2007a; Liu et al., 2012). TJ proteins can also internalize into the cytosol by caveolin-1-mediated endocytosis or redistribute to other membrane domains after cerebral ischemia, coinciding with the early post-ischemic BBB opening. Adherens junction proteins support BBB properties (Petty and Lo, 2002) and their altered composition after stroke changes TJ stability, affecting BBB permeability (Dejana and Giampietro, 2012; Wacker et al., 2012).

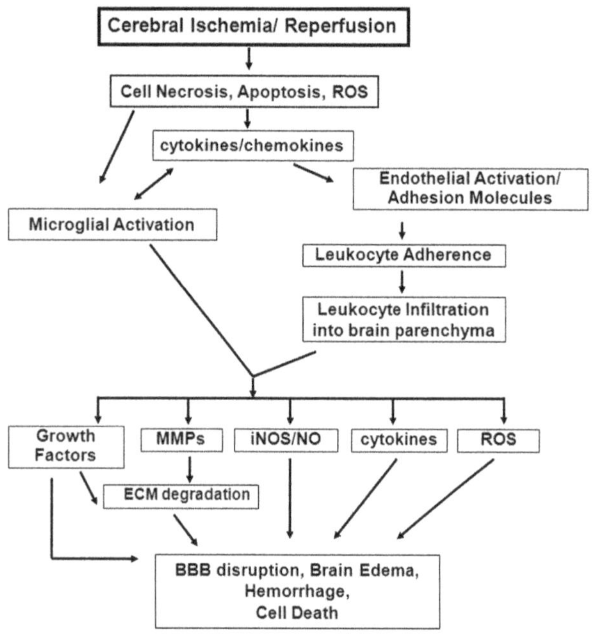

FIGURE 1 | Inflammatory mechanisms following acute cerebral ischemia-reperfusion injury. There are both common and distinct features of the inflammatory response to cerebral ischemia between adults and neonates. However, neonatal brain is more susceptible to excitotoxic-damage and oxidative injury by ROS, resulting in necrosis and apoptosis *continuum*. The induction of cytokine/chemokine production, activation of microglial cells, and the systemic inflammatory response lead to neuroinflammation. Differences of adhesion molecule expression on ECs and on peripheral leukocytes exist between the injured adult and neonatal brain. Among the inflammatory mediators, activated matrix metalloproteinases (MMPs), inducible nitric oxide synthase (iNOS), and further cytokine and ROS accumulation also contribute to the variance in magnitude and spatial distribution of BBB disruption, brain edema and injury between neonatal and adult stroke. (modified from Vexler et al., 2006).

Surprisingly little is known about BBB function after neonatal ischemic injury. Major differences in functional BBB response to acute ischemia-reperfusion between neonates and adults have been recently identified (Fernandez-Lopez et al., 2012). While BBB permeability to albumin or intravascular tracers of a similar size is significantly increased after acute tMCAO in adult rats, BBB permeability remains low in injured neonatal rats. Gene and protein expression of occludin, claudin-5 and ZO-1 are better preserved in injured neonatal brain than in injured adult brain, whereas gene expression of the efflux transporters ATP-binding cassette, subfamily G2 (Abcg2) and P-glycoprotein (P-gp) is reduced in both ages 24 h after reperfusion (Fernandez-Lopez et al., 2012). Transcript levels of several adhesion molecules and ECM components are differentially affected by injury in immature and adult brain, including E-selectin and P-selectin. Gene expression of Mmp-9 is significantly upregulated in injured adults and, while high transcript levels of collagen type IV α1 (Col4a1), and Col4a2 remain unaltered in neonates, a significant increase of these two genes is evident in injured adult rats. Interestingly, transcripts of angiogenic regulators Vegfr-2, and Angpt2 are increased after stroke in adults but not in neonates (Fernandez-Lopez et al., 2012). **Figure 2** summarizes these findings. In contrast, a transient leakage of much smaller tracers, sucrose and inulin, was observed in a mouse HI model, with the peak at 6 h and normalization by 24 h (D'Angelo et al., 2012), conveying that size and chemical structure of molecules affect leakage and highlighting the need for future BBB studies in injured immature brain.

The ECM proteins and their corresponding receptors on ECs and astrocytes provide both physical and biochemical glial-vascular "scaffolding" while BM components laminin, collagen IV (Col-IV), fibronectin, and perlecan provide proper cell-cell interactions. Endothelial-ECM interaction via β1 integrins regulates the expression of claudin-5 and BBB tightness whereas other ECM proteins, like galectin-3 mediate integrin-induced stabilization of focal adhesions, and activate cytokine receptors to enhance actions of growth factors (Goetz et al., 2008). Homozygous mutations in Col-IV are lethal in mid-gestation due to blockage of capillary bed development, and mutations in the COL4A1 gene cause ICH both in newborn mouse and human (Gould et al., 2005; Labelle-Dumais et al., 2011). Laminin degradation after focal stroke in adults causes detachment of astrocytic endfeet, disrupts BBB and induces ICH (Fukuda et al., 2004), while in neonates expression of this ECM protein is not reduced acutely (Fernandez-Lopez et al., 2012). The role of other ECM proteins in injured neonates is less studied but opposite effects of galectin-3 in adult stroke and HI has been demonstrated (Doverhag et al., 2010; Lalancette-Hebert et al., 2012).

PARENCHYMAL BRAIN CELLS AS MODULATORS OF BBB INTEGRITY AFTER NEONATAL STROKE

Neuroinflammation is a characteristic feature of stroke progression and a major contributor to brain injury (Iadecola and Anrather, 2011). Multiple cell types (i.e. neurons,

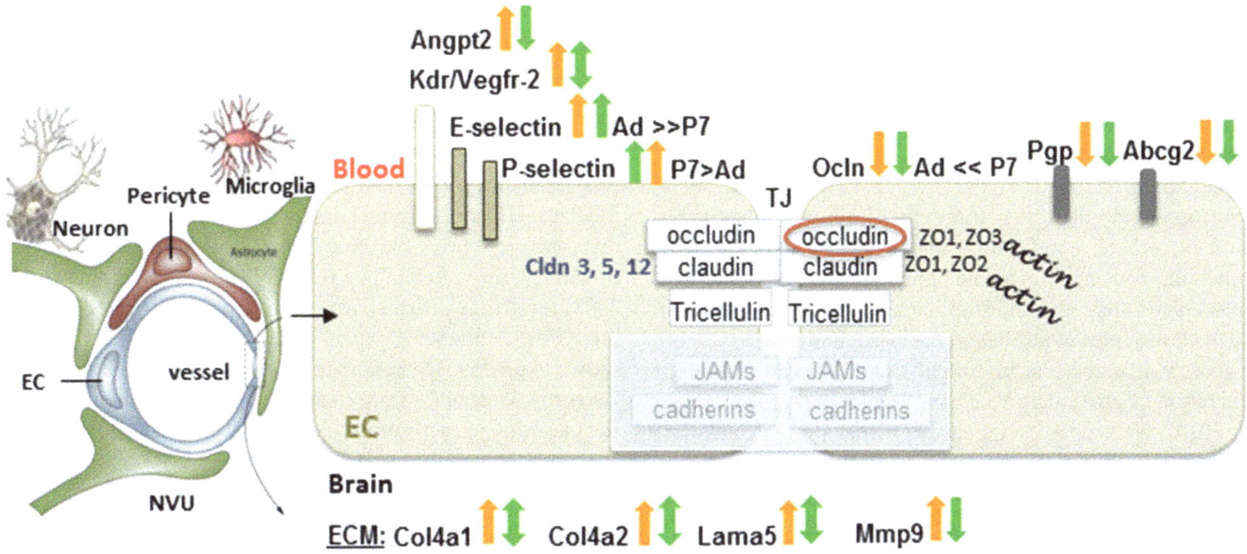

FIGURE 2 | Differences in the gene expression of the BBB components between adults and neonates 24 h after tMCAO. On a diagram of the NVU, arrows demarcate the gene expression changes in injured vs. matching contralateral region (ratio, ipsilateral/contralateral) in adult (orange arrows), and neonatal rats (green arrows) subjected to 3 h of MCAO followed by 24 h of reperfusion. Arrows pointing upwards demarcate increased gene expression in injured regions vs. matching contralateral regions (statistically significant > 2-fold change). Downward arrows show reduced expression in injured regions vs. matching contralateral regions (statistically significant > 2-fold change). Double-sided arrows indicate no changes between injured and contralateral regions. Abbreviations: Ad: adult, P7: postnatal 7-days-old, EC, endothelial cell; angiopoetin 2, Angpt2; Kdr, Vegfr-2; Cldn, claudin; Ocln, occludin; ZO, zonula occludens; JAM, junctional adhesion molecules; TJ, tight junction; Pgp, P-glycoprotein; Abcg2, ATP-binding cassette transporter, subfamily G 2; Col4a1, collagen, type IV, alpha 1; Col4a2, collagen, type IV, alpha 2; Lama5, laminin, alpha 5; Mmp-9, matrix metalloproteinase 9. Original data are published in Fernandez-Lopez et al. (2012). The NVU contains fragments from Eichler et al. (2011).

astrocytes, ECs, and microglia) increase production of inflammatory mediators post-ischemia, which can adversely affect BBB integrity and propagate injury.

ECs are sensitive to oxidative stress (Freeman and Keller, 2012). Excessive ROS accumulation generated by ischemia/reperfusion contributes to damage of TJs and other EC components, and promotes activation of cell death pathways (Rizzo and Leaver, 2010). Although less sensitive to cerebral ischemia than neurons, ECs also undergo cell death via several mechanisms (Rizzo and Leaver, 2010). Our comparison of gene expression in ECs from injured and contralateral cortex in neonatal and adult rats after tMCAO (endothelial transcriptome) revealed a markedly distinct signature of up-regulated and down-regulated transcripts in injured regions between two ages (Fernandez-Lopez et al., 2012).

Astrocytes are rather resistant to ischemic injury but impairment of water fluxes through astrocytic swelling and increased expression of aquaporin 4 (AQP4) leads to edema after adult focal ischemia (Loreto and Reggio, 2010). No edema was observed in injured P10 pups in brain regions with greatest AQP4 expression (Badaut et al., 2007), suggesting that enhanced water clearance at border regions can protect.

Microglial cells have been considered toxic after cerebral ischemia due to production of inflammatory mediators. However, phagocytotic ability and production of growth factors by microglia can be beneficial via several mechanisms, including support of neuronal and endothelial survival (Baburamani et al., 2012; Luo and Chen, 2012). Microglial cells have several direct modulatory effects on the vasculature. During brain development they mediate vasculogenesis (Arnold and Betsholtz, 2013), and act as a physical bridge that guides vascular anastomosis, facilitating normal angiogenesis, and vascular sprouting. Microglia patrol the vasculature in the naïve brain (Davalos et al., 2012) and, upon BBB disruption, rapidly extend their processes, shielding injured sites (Nimmerjahn et al., 2005). Depletion of microglia worsens parenchymal injury in neonatal rats after tMCAO, increases levels of inflammatory mediators in acutely injured regions, and induces hemorrhagic transformation (Faustino et al., 2011; Fernandez Lopez et al., 2014) perhaps due to differing cell phenotypes in the immature brain.

Pericytes are important regulators of vessel contractility. Pericyte loss or dissociation from vessels lead to edema (Peppiatt et al., 2006) and impaired reflow (Yemisci et al., 2009). Lower than in adult pericyte coverage in the neonatal brain (Daneman et al., 2010) may differentially affect CBF regulation and BBB function after injury but this is yet to be demonstrated.

OPCs support EC survival but they are sensitive to ROS and can adversely affect BBB integrity via release of inflammatory mediators. Mast cells contribute to early ischemic brain swelling, BBB leakage and neutrophil infiltration (Strbian et al., 2006). Their stabilization protects and reduces hemorrhage formation (Strbian et al., 2007). Degranulation of mast cells is injurious in neonatal HI (Jin et al., 2007) and stroke (Biran et al., 2008) but direct effects on BBB have not been studied.

SYSTEMIC INFLAMMATION ALTERS BBB PERMEABILITY AFTER NEONATAL STROKE

Parenchymal, perivascular and peripheral circulating cells independently and in concert contribute to stroke-induced production of inflammatory mediators, upregulation of integrins and adhesion molecules on ECs and leukocytes (Iadecola and Anrather, 2011).

Neutrophils rapidly, often transiently infiltrate ischemic tissue and exacerbate reperfusion injury in adults by priming the endothelium, causing "no-reflow" phenomenon, releasing ROS and proteolytic enzymes, and stimulating cytokine release (Mori et al., 1992; Amantea et al., 2009; Engelhardt and Liebner, 2014). Both loosely attached and infiltrated leukocytes can contribute to generation of pro-inflammatory molecules in the CNS (Denes et al., 2010). Neutropenia or treatments that prevent leukocyte adhesion and infiltration are neuroprotective (Kochanek and Hallenbeck, 1992; Yamasaki et al., 1995). Compared to adults, in neonates neutrophil infiltration is markedly lower in response to HI (Hudome et al., 1997; Bona et al., 1999), and tMCAO (Fernandez-Lopez et al., 2012). Neutralization of cytokine-induced neutrophil chemoattractant 1 protein (CINC-1) following tMCAO in adults holts neutrophil transmigration, reduces brain edema and protects (Yamasaki et al., 1997) whereas it promotes neutrophil infiltration following tMCAO and disrupts the BBB in neonates (Fernandez-Lopez et al., 2012).

Monocytes have been recently shown to have a dual role, elicit both inflammatory effects and maintain NVU integrity following cerebral ischemia. Monocyte depletion, chemokine (C-C motif) receptor 2 (CCR2) knockout, and bone marrow chimeric approach in murine stroke models demonstrated that CCR2 in bone marrow-derived cells alters injury and hemorrhagic transformation (Gliem et al., 2012). The stabilizing effects of monocytes are transforming growth factor beta 1 (TGF-β1)-dependent (Gliem et al., 2012). Compared to adult stroke, infiltration of circulating monocytes across the BBB is relatively low during the acute injury phase in neonates (Denker et al., 2007). It remains poorly understood whether leukocyte immaturity at the time of insult or a distinct gene expression pattern of selectins, and cytokines/chemokines account for the difference.

T and B cell infiltration may be less profound (Bona et al., 1999) or transient (Benjelloun et al., 1999) in injured neonates than in adults (Catania and Lipton, 1998; Chu et al., 2014).

INDIVIDUAL INFLAMMATORY SIGNALING MECHANISMS

Evidence is growing that the inflammatory responses after stroke are different in neonates and adults (Vexler and Yenari, 2009). Genetic deletion of various inflammatory mediators, including NADPH oxidase (Doverhag et al., 2008), or interleukin 1 (IL-1) β, IL-1α, or both αβ (Hedtjarn et al., 2005) are not neuroprotective in the neonatal brain compared to adults. Some mediators that are upregulated and injurious during the acute injury phase, such as nitric oxide (NO), MMPs, macrophage inflammatory protein 1 alpha (MIP-1α), monocyte chemoattractant protein 1 (MCP-1), and complement, may be beneficial and mediate repair (Fernandez-Lopez et al., 2014).

MMPs degrade TJ and BM proteins, including collagen, laminin and fibronectin, thereby leading to brain edema, BBB leakage and leukocyte infiltration. MMP upregulation after stroke contributes to ECM breakdown and acute brain damage (Rosenberg et al., 1998; Asahi et al., 2000). MMP-2 and MMP-9, the two most studied MMPs in stroke, play different roles in BBB disruption (Asahi et al., 2001). MMP-3 targets several ECM components, including laminin and proteoglycans, and propagates injury by mediating BBB opening by inflammatory mediators (Cunningham et al., 2005). While activated microglia, macrophages and infiltrating leukocytes are the major sources of MMPs early after injury (Gidday et al., 2005; McColl et al., 2008), over time activated astrocytes and neurons begin producing MMPs, enhancing repair (Zhao et al., 2006). MMP-9 was shown to predict HIE in human newborns (Bednarek et al., 2012). Cerebrovascular ECs from neonates in culture contain more tissue plasminogen activator (t-PA) and gelatinases upon glutamate challenge than adult cells (Omouendze et al., 2013). MMP inhibition is protective after HI (Chen et al., 2009) but long-term MMP inhibition may holt ECM remodeling, as shown in adult stroke (Zhao et al., 2006).

The patterns of monocyte and neutrophil recruitment are cytokine- and chemokine-specific. The multifaceted roles for α, β, and δ classes of chemokines were shown in adult stroke models (Yamasaki et al., 1995). Integrins are central for cell communication within the NVU and for leukocyte recruitment after stroke (Iadecola and Anrather, 2011) but information on the role of integrins in neonatal stroke is scant.

BLOOD-CSF BARRIER (BCSFB)

The choroid plexuses (CPs), forming the BCSFB, are involved in immune cell entry after brain injury (Shechter et al., 2013). CPs express chemokines and support transepithelial trafficking of neutrophils, monocytes and T cells (Szmydynger-Chodobska et al., 2009, 2012; Kunis et al., 2013). Engraftment of CPs in adult stroke models reduced infarct size and improved neurological function, in part via secretion of glial cell line-derived neurotrophic factor (GDNF), brain-derived neurotrophic factor (BDNF), and nerve growth factor (NGF) (Borlongan et al., 2004). CPs have unique functions in the developing brain (Dziegielewska et al., 2001) but their role in protection of the immature brain after stroke is unknown.

NEUROVASCULAR RESPONSES AND REPAIR AFTER NEONATAL STROKE

Long-term neural repair is less studied after neonatal stroke than after adult stroke. Cell proliferation in the subventricular zone (SVZ) after ischemia is triggered in both adults (Ohab et al., 2006), and neonates (Plane et al., 2004; Yang et al., 2007b). The dynamic changes within the SVZ neurogenic niche permit neuroblast migration into the ischemic striatum (Young et al., 2011) in the adult, where they express phenotypic region-specific mature neuronal markers (Parent et al., 2002), and into peri-infarct striatum after neonatal HI (Plane et al., 2004; Yang et al., 2007b). Niche astrocytes and SVZ microglia are also involved in neuroblast migration (Young et al., 2011). The newborn SVZ contains numerous cell types, including unipotential astrocytes and OPCs as well as bipotential glial progenitors (Levison and Goldman, 1997).

Given the dynamic nature of postnatal brain development one would expect robust repair processes in neonatal stroke but a 1–2 week delay in induction of angiogenesis was shown after tMCAO in P7 and P10 rats (Shimotake et al., 2010; Dzietko et al., 2013; Fernandez-Lopez et al., 2013) despite induction of VEGF (Mu et al., 2003). Another obstacle for endogenous repair is that proliferating cells in the postnatal SVZ differentiate into astrocytes, rather than neurons or oligodendrocytes, and astrogliosis holts the repair (Spadafora et al., 2010; Gonzalez et al., 2013). Changing the neural stem cell fate to route the differentiation into neurons and oligodendrocytes after stroke, for example, with erythropoietin, enhances the repair (Iwai et al., 2010; Gonzalez et al., 2013). Cell based therapies, including mesenchymal stem cells, improve functional outcomes after neonatal HI (Van Velthoven et al., 2010) and arterial stroke (Van Velthoven et al., 2013) by changing the microenvironment and stimulating Angpt1 and VEGF signaling, which amplify angiogenesis and "loosen" the barrier, allowing vessel remodeling and neuroblast migration.

TRANSLATIONAL ASPECTS AND FUTURE DIRECTIONS

A broad range of therapeutic agents was used in neonatal ischemic brain injury models to target the excitotoxic, oxidative, and inflammatory injury components, but, as in adult stroke, studies revealed limits in protection. To date, hypothermia is the only neuroprotective treatment for perinatal HIE with efficacy limited to moderate injury (Azzopardi et al., 2009; Edwards et al., 2010).

Importantly, recent studies have improved our understanding of the events at the BBB after neonatal ischemia by revealing that the developmental stage of the BBB at the time of ischemic insult is of prime importance and that careful consideration should be given to whether the BBB is in fact disrupted or it limits therapies from reaching an injured neonatal brain. The role of local parenchymal cells, microglia, as modulators of neurovascular integrity after neonatal stroke was also uncovered. Future studies should shed light on relationships between neurovascular integrity and interaction with neuroprogenitors, endogenous, or engrafted, including the migration and differentiation of neural progenitors during stroke-induced neurogenesis.

AUTHOR CONTRIBUTIONS

Ingrid Kratzer and Sophorn Chip wrote individual parts of the review and contributed equally. Together with Zinaida S. Vexler who provided conceptual framework and wrote parts of the review, they contributed to revisions and prepared artwork.

ACKNOWLEDGMENTS

The following grants NS080015 (Zinaida S. Vexler), NS44025 (Zinaida S. Vexler), and NS76726 (Zinaida S. Vexler) were used as principal sources of funding.

REFERENCES

Amantea, D., Nappi, G., Bernardi, G., Bagetta, G., and Corasaniti, M. T. (2009). Post-ischemic brain damage: pathophysiology and role of inflammatory mediators. *FEBS J.* 276, 13–26. doi: 10.1111/j.1742-4658.2008.06766.x

Arnold, T., and Betsholtz, C. (2013). The importance of microglia in the development of the vasculature in the central nervous system. *Vasc. Cell* 5, 4. doi: 10.1186/2045-824X-5-4

Asahi, M., Asahi, K., Jung, J. C., Del Zoppo, G. J., Fini, M. E., and Lo, E. H. (2000). Role for matrix metalloproteinase 9 after focal cerebral ischemia: effects of gene knockout and enzyme inhibition with BB-94. *J. Cereb. Blood Flow Metab.* 20, 1681–1689. doi: 10.1097/00004647-200012000-00007

Asahi, M., Sumii, T., Fini, M. E., Itohara, S., and Lo, E. H. (2001). Matrix metalloproteinase 2 gene knockout has no effect on acute brain injury after focal ischemia. *Neuroreport* 12, 3003–3007. doi: 10.1097/00001756-200109170-00050

Azzopardi, D. V., Strohm, B., Edwards, A. D., Dyet, L., Halliday, H. L., Juszczak, E., et al. (2009). Moderate hypothermia to treat perinatal asphyxial encephalopathy. *N. Engl. J. Med.* 361, 1349–1358. doi: 10.1056/NEJMoa0900854

Baburamani, A. A., Ek, C. J., Walker, D. W., and Castillo-Melendez, M. (2012). Vulnerability of the developing brain to hypoxic-ischemic damage: contribution of the cerebral vasculature to injury and repair? *Front. Physiol.* 3:424. doi: 10.3389/fphys.2012.00424

Badaut, J., Ashwal, S., Tone, B., Regli, L., Tian, H. R., and Obenaus, A. (2007). Temporal and regional evolution of aquaporin-4 expression and magnetic resonance imaging in a rat pup model of neonatal stroke. *Pediatr. Res.* 62, 248–254. doi: 10.1203/PDR.0b013e3180db291b

Ballabh, P. (2010). Intraventricular hemorrhage in premature infants: mechanism of disease. *Pediatr. Res.* 67, 1–8. doi: 10.1203/PDR.0b013e3181c1b176

Bednarek, N., Svedin, P., Garnotel, R., Favrais, G., Loron, G., Schwendiman, L., et al. (2012). Increased MMP-9 and TIMP-1 in mouse neonatal brain and plasma and in human neonatal plasma after hypoxia-ischemia: a potential marker of neonatal encephalopathy. *Pediatr. Res.* 71, 63–70. doi: 10.1038/pr.2011.3

Benjelloun, N., Renolleau, S., Represa, A., Ben-Ari, Y., and Charriaut-Marlangue, C. (1999). Inflammatory responses in the cerebral cortex after ischemia in the P7 neonatal Rat. *Stroke 30*, 1916–1923. discussion 1923-4.

Biran, V., Cochois, V., Karroubi, A., Arrang, J. M., Charriaut-Marlangue, C., and Heron, A. (2008). Stroke induces histamine accumulation and mast cell degranulation in the neonatal rat brain. *Brain Pathol.* 18, 1–9. doi: 10.1111/j.1750-3639.2007.00092.x

Blomgren, K., Leist, M., and Groc, L. (2007). Pathological apoptosis in the developing brain. *Apoptosis* 12, 993–1010. doi: 10.1007/s10495-007-0754-4

Bona, E., Andersson, A. L., Blomgren, K., Gilland, E., Puka-Sundvall, M., Gustafson, K., et al. (1999). Chemokine and inflammatory cell response to hypoxia-ischemia in immature rats. *Pediatr. Res.* 45, 500–509. doi: 10.1203/00006450-199904010-00008

Borlongan, C. V., Skinner, S. J., Geaney, M., Vasconcellos, A. V., Elliott, R. B., and Emerich, D. F. (2004). Intracerebral transplantation of porcine choroid plexus provides structural and functional neuroprotection in a rodent model of stroke. *Stroke* 35, 2206–2210. doi: 10.1161/01.STR.0000138954.25825.0b

Braun, A., Xu, H., Hu, F., Kocherlakota, P., Siegel, D., Chander, P., et al. (2007). Paucity of pericytes in germinal matrix vasculature of premature infants. *J. Neurosci.* 27, 12012–12024. doi: 10.1523/JNEUROSCI.3281-07.2007

Catania, A., and Lipton, J. M. (1998). Peptide modulation of fever and inflammation within the brain. *Ann. N.Y. Acad. Sci.* 856, 62–68. doi: 10.1111/j.1749-6632.1998.tb08313.x

Chen, W., Hartman, R., Ayer, R., Marcantonio, S., Kamper, J., Tang, J., et al. (2009). Matrix metalloproteinases inhibition provides neuroprotection against hypoxia-ischemia in the developing brain. *J. Neurochem.* 111, 726–736. doi: 10.1111/j.1471-4159.2009.06362.x

Chu, H. X., Kim, H. A., Lee, S., Moore, J. P., Chan, C. T., Vinh, A., et al. (2014). Immune cell infiltration in malignant middle cerebral artery infarction: comparison with transient cerebral ischemia. *J. Cereb. Blood Flow Metab.* 34, 450–459. doi: 10.1038/jcbfm.2013.217

Cunningham, L. A., Wetzel, M., and Rosenberg, G. A. (2005). Multiple roles for MMPs and TIMPs in cerebral ischemia. *Glia* 50, 329–339. doi: 10.1002/glia.20169

D'Angelo, B. D., Baburamani, A., Hagberg, H., and Mallard, C. (2012). "Role of blood-brain barrier in perinatal brain injury," in *Abstract Presented at the SfN in a Nanosymposium, New Orleans, LA, USA. Abstract 831.0399.* Available online at: http://am2012.sfn.org/am2012/pdf/ final_program/final_program_b6.pdf

Daneman, R., Zhou, L., Kebede, A. A., and Barres, B. A. (2010). Pericytes are required for blood-brain barrier integrity during embryogenesis. *Nature* 468, 562–566. doi: 10.1038/nature09513

Davalos, D., Ryu, J. K., Merlini, M., Baeten, K. M., Le Moan, N., Petersen, M. A., et al. (2012). Fibrinogen-induced perivascular microglial clustering is required for the development of axonal damage in neuroinflammation. *Nat. Commun.* 3, 1227. doi: 10.1038/ncomms2230

Dejana, E., and Giampietro, C. (2012). Vascular endothelial-cadherin and vascular stability. *Curr. Opin. Hematol.* 19, 218–223. doi: 10.1097/MOH.0b013e3283523e1c

Denes, A., Thornton, P., Rothwell, N. J., and Allan, S. M. (2010). Inflammation and brain injury: acute cerebral ischaemia, peripheral and central inflammation. *Brain Behav. Immun.* 24, 708–723. doi: 10.1016/j.bbi.2009.09.010

Denker, S., Ji, S., Lee, S. Y., Dingman, A., Derugin, N., Wendland, M., et al. (2007). Macrophages are comprised of resident brain microglia not infiltrating peripheral monocytes acutely after neonatal stroke. *J. Neurochem.* 100, 893–904. doi: 10.1111/j.1471-4159.2006.04162.x

Derrick, M., Drobyshevsky, A., Ji, X., and Tan, S. (2007). A model of cerebral palsy from fetal hypoxia-ischemia. *Stroke* 38, 731–735. doi: 10.1161/01.STR.0000251445.94697.64

Derugin, N., Ferriero, D. M., and Vexler, Z. S. (1998). Neonatal reversible focal cerebral ischemia: a new model. *Neurosci. Res.* 32, 349–353. doi: 10.1016/S0168-0102(98)00096-0

Doverhag, C., Hedtjarn, M., Poirier, F., Mallard, C., Hagberg, H., Karlsson, A., et al. (2010). Galectin-3 contributes to neonatal hypoxic-ischemic brain injury. *Neurobiol. Dis.* 38, 36–46. doi: 10.1016/j.nbd.2009.12.024

Doverhag, C., Keller, M., Karlsson, A., Hedtjarn, M., Nilsson, U., Kapeller, E., et al. (2008). Pharmacological and genetic inhibition of NADPH oxidase does not reduce brain damage in different models of perinatal brain injury in newborn mice. *Neurobiol. Dis.* 31, 133–144. doi: 10.1016/j.nbd.2008.04.003

Dziegielewska, K. M., Ek, J., Habgood, M. D., and Saunders, N. R. (2001). Development of the choroid plexus. *Microsc. Res. Tech.* 52, 5–20. doi: 10.1002/1097-0029(20010101)52:1<5::AID-JEMT3>3.0.CO;2-J

Dzietko, M., Derugin, N., Wendland, M. F., Vexler, Z. S., and Ferriero, D. M. (2013). Delayed VEGF treatment enhances angiogenesis and recovery after neonatal focal rodent stroke. *Transl. Stroke Res.* 4, 189–200. doi: 10.1007/s12975-012-0221-6

Edwards, A. D., Brocklehurst, P., Gunn, A. J., Halliday, H., Juszczak, E., Levene, M., et al. (2010). Neurological outcomes at 18 months of age after moderate hypothermia for perinatal hypoxic ischaemic encephalopathy: synthesis and meta-analysis of trial data. *BMJ* 340, c363. doi: 10.1136/bmj.c363

Eichler, A. F., Chung, E., Kodack, D. P., Loeffler, J. S., Fukumura, D., and Jain, R. K. (2011). The biology of brain metastases-translation to new therapies. *Nat. Rev. Clin. Oncol.* 8, 344–356. doi: 10.1038/nrclinonc.2011.58

El-Khoury, N., Braun, A., Hu, F., Pandey, M., Nedergaard, M., Lagamma, E. F., et al. (2006). Astrocyte end-feet in germinal matrix, cerebral cortex, and white matter in developing infants. *Pediatr. Res.* 59, 673–679. doi: 10.1203/01.pdr.0000214975.85311.9c

Engelhardt, B., and Liebner, S. (2014). Novel insights into the development and maintenance of the blood-brain barrier. *Cell Tissue Res.* 355, 687–699. doi: 10.1007/s00441-014-1811-2

Faustino, J., Wang, X., Jonhson, C., Klibanov, A., Derugin, N., Wendland, M., et al. (2011). Microglial cells contribute to endogenous brain defenses after acute neonatal focal stroke. *J. Neurosci.* 31, 12992–13001. doi: 10.1523/JNEUROSCI.2102-11.2011

Fernandez-Lopez, D., Faustino, J., Daneman, R., Zhou, L., Lee, S. Y., Derugin, N., et al. (2012). Blood-brain barrier permeability is increased after acute adult stroke but not neonatal stroke. *J. Neurosci.* 32, 9588–9600. doi: 10.1523/JNEUROSCI.5977-11.2012

Fernandez-Lopez, D., Faustino, J., Derugin, N., and Vexler, Z. S. (2013). Acute and chronic vascular responses to experimental focal arterial stroke in the neonate rat. *Transl. Stroke Res.* 4, 179–188. doi: 10.1007/s12975-012-0214-5

Fernandez Lopez, D., Faustino, J., Klibanov, A., Derugin, N., Akassoglou, K., and Vexler, Z. S., (2014). "Activated microglia contribute to neurovascular integrity and limit brain injury after acute neonatal focal stroke," in *International Stroke Meeting* (San Diego, CA).

Fernandez-Lopez, D., Natarajan, N., Ashwal, S., and Vexler, Z. S. (2014). Mechanisms of perinatal arterial ischemic stroke. *J. Cereb. Blood Flow Metab.* 34, 921–932. doi: 10.1038/jcbfm.2014.41

Ferriero, D. M. (2004). Neonatal brain injury. *N. Engl. J. Med.* 351, 1985–1995. doi: 10.1056/NEJMra041996

Freeman, L. R., and Keller, J. N. (2012). Oxidative stress and cerebral endothelial cells: regulation of the blood-brain-barrier and antioxidant based interventions. *Biochim. Biophys. Acta* 1822, 822–829. doi: 10.1016/j.bbadis.2011.12.009

Fukuda, S., Fini, C. A., Mabuchi, T., Koziol, J. A., Eggleston, L. L. Jr., and Del Zoppo, G. J. (2004). Focal cerebral ischemia induces active proteases that degrade microvascular matrix. *Stroke* 35, 998–1004. doi: 10.1161/01.STR.0000119383.76447.05

Gidday, J. M., Gasche, Y. G., Copin, J. C., Shah, A. R., Perez, R. S., Shapiro, S. D., et al. (2005). Leukocyte-derived matrix metalloproteinase-9 mediates blood-brain barrier breakdown and is proinflammatory after transient focal cerebral ischemia. *Am. J. Physiol. Heart Circ. Physiol.* 289, H558–H568. doi: 10.1152/ajpheart.01275.2004

Gliem, M., Mausberg, A. K., Lee, J. I., Simiantonakis, I., Van Rooijen, N., Hartung, H. P., et al. (2012). Macrophages prevent hemorrhagic infarct transformation in murine stroke models. *Ann. Neurol.* 71, 743–752. doi: 10.1002/ana.23529

Goetz, J. G., Joshi, B., Lajoie, P., Strugnell, S. S., Scudamore, T., Kojic, L. D., et al. (2008). Concerted regulation of focal adhesion dynamics by galectin-3 and tyrosine-phosphorylated caveolin-1. *J. Cell Biol.* 180, 1261–1275. doi: 10.1083/jcb.200709019

Gonzalez, F. F., Larpthaveesarp, A., McQuillen, P., Derugin, N., Wendland, M., Spadafora, R., et al. (2013). Erythropoietin increases neurogenesis and oligodendrogliosis of subventricular zone precursor cells after neonatal stroke. *Stroke* 44, 753–758. doi: 10.1161/STROKEAHA.111.000104

Gould, D. B., Phalan, F. C., Breedveld, G. J., Van Mil, S. E., Smith, R. S., Schimenti, J. C., et al. (2005). Mutations in Col4a1 cause perinatal cerebral hemorrhage and porencephaly. *Science* 308, 1167–1171. doi: 10.1126/science.1109418

Hedtjarn, M., Mallard, C., Iwakura, Y., and Hagberg, H. (2005). Combined deficiency of IL-1beta18, but not IL-1alphabeta, reduces susceptibility to hypoxia-ischemia in the immature brain. *Dev. Neurosci.* 27, 143–148. doi: 10.1159/000085986

Hudome, S., Palmer, C., Roberts, R. L., Mauger, D., Housman, C., and Towfighi, J. (1997). The role of neutrophils in the production of hypoxic-ischemic brain injury in the neonatal rat. *Pediatr. Res.* 41, 607–616. doi: 10.1203/00006450-199705000-00002

Iadecola, C., and Anrather, J. (2011). The immunology of stroke: from mechanisms to translation. *Nat. Med.* 17, 796–808. doi: 10.1038/nm.2399

Ikonomidou, C., Mosinger, J. L., Salles, K. S., Labruyere, J., and Olney, J. W. (1989). Sensitivity of the developing rat brain to hypobaric/ischemic damage parallels sensitivity to N-methyl-aspartate neurotoxicity. *J. Neurosci.* 9, 2809–2818.

Iwai, M., Stetler, R. A., Xing, J., Hu, X., Gao, Y., Zhang, W., et al. (2010). Enhanced oligodendrogenesis and recovery of neurological function by erythropoietin after neonatal hypoxic/ischemic brain injury. *Stroke* 41, 1032–1037. doi: 10.1161/STROKEAHA.109.570325

Jin, Y., Silverman, A. J., and Vannucci, S. J. (2007). Mast cell stabilization limits hypoxic-ischemic brain damage in the immature rat. *Dev. Neurosci.* 29, 373–384. doi: 10.1159/000105478

Knowland, D., Arac, A., Sekiguchi, K. J., Hsu, M., Lutz, S. E., Perrino, J., et al. (2014). Stepwise recruitment of transcellular and paracellular pathways underlies blood-brain barrier breakdown in stroke. *Neuron* 82, 603–617. doi: 10.1016/j.neuron.2014.03.003

Kochanek, P. M., and Hallenbeck, J. M. (1992). Polymorphonuclear leukocytes and monocytes/macrophages in the pathogenesis of cerebral ischemia and stroke. *Stroke* 23, 1367–1379. doi: 10.1161/01.STR.23.9.1367

Kunis, G., Baruch, K., Rosenzweig, N., Kertser, A., Miller, O., Berkutzki, T., et al. (2013). IFN-gamma-dependent activation of the brain's choroid plexus for CNS immune surveillance and repair. *Brain* 136, 3427–3440. doi: 10.1093/brain/awt259

Labelle-Dumais, C., Dilworth, D. J., Harrington, E. P., De Leau, M., Lyons, D., Kabaeva, Z., et al. (2011). COL4A1 mutations cause ocular dysgenesis, neuronal localization defects, and myopathy in mice and Walker-Warburg syndrome in humans. *PLoS Genet.* 7, e1002062. doi: 10.1371/journal.pgen.1002062

Lalancette-Hebert, M., Swarup, V., Beaulieu, J. M., Bohacek, I., Abdelhamid, E., Weng, Y. C., et al. (2012). Galectin-3 is required for resident microglia activation and proliferation in response to ischemic injury. *J. Neurosci.* 32, 10383–10395. doi: 10.1523/JNEUROSCI.1498-12.2012

Levison, S. W., and Goldman, J. E. (1997). Multipotential and lineage restricted precursors coexist in the mammalian perinatal subventricular zone. *J. Neurosci. Res.* 48, 83–94.

Liu, J., Jin, X., Liu, K. J., and Liu, W. (2012). Matrix metalloproteinase-2-mediated occludin degradation and caveolin-1-mediated claudin-5 redistribution contribute to blood-brain barrier damage in early ischemic stroke stage. *J. Neurosci.* 32, 3044–3057. doi: 10.1523/JNEUROSCI.6409-11.2012

Loreto, C., and Reggio, E. (2010). Aquaporin and vascular diseases. *Curr. Neuropharmacol.* 8, 105–111. doi: 10.2174/157015910791233196

Luo, X. G., and Chen, S. D. (2012). The changing phenotype of microglia from homeostasis to disease. *Transl. Neurodegener.* 1, 9. doi: 10.1186/2047-9158-1-9

Marks, K. A., Mallard, C. E., Roberts, I., Williams, C. E., Gluckman, P. D., and Edwards, A. D. (1999). Nitric oxide synthase inhibition and delayed cerebral injury after severe cerebral ischemia in fetal sheep. *Pediatr. Res.* 46, 8–13. doi: 10.1203/00006450-199907000-00002

McColl, B. W., Rothwell, N. J., and Allan, S. M. (2008). Systemic inflammation alters the kinetics of cerebrovascular tight junction disruption after experimental stroke in mice. *J. Neurosci.* 28, 9451–9462. doi: 10.1523/JNEUROSCI.2674-08.2008

McQuillen, P. S., Sheldon, R. A., Shatz, C. J., and Ferriero, D. M. (2003). Selective vulnerability of subplate neurons after early neonatal hypoxia-ischemia. *J. Neurosci.* 23, 3308–3315.

Mori, E., Del Zoppo, G. J., Chambers, J. D., Copeland, B. R., and Arfors, K. E. (1992). Inhibition of polymorphonuclear leukocyte adherence suppresses no-reflow after focal cerebral ischemia in baboons. *Stroke* 23, 712–718. doi: 10.1161/01.STR.23.5.712

Mu, D., Jiang, X., Sheldon, R. A., Fox, C. K., Hamrick, S. E., Vexler, Z. S., et al. (2003). Regulation of hypoxia-inducible factor 1alpha and induction of vascular endothelial growth factor in a rat neonatal stroke model. *Neurobiol. Dis.* 14, 524–534. doi: 10.1016/j.nbd.2003.08.020

Nelson, K. B., and Lynch, J. K. (2004). Stroke in newborn infants. *Lancet Neurol.* 3, 150–158. doi: 10.1016/S1474-4422(04)00679-9

Nimmerjahn, A., Kirchhoff, F., and Helmchen, F. (2005). Resting microglial cells are highly dynamic surveillants of brain parenchyma *in vivo*. *Science* 308, 1314–1318. doi: 10.1126/science.1110647

Northington, F. J., Chavez-Valdez, R., and Martin, L. J. (2011). Neuronal cell death in neonatal hypoxia-ischemia. *Ann. Neurol.* 69, 743–758. doi: 10.1002/ana.22419

Ohab, J. J., Fleming, S., Blesch, A., and Carmichael, S. T. (2006). A neurovascular niche for neurogenesis after stroke. *J. Neurosci.* 26, 13007–13016. doi: 10.1523/JNEUROSCI.4323-06.2006

Omouendze, P. L., Henry, V. J., Porte, B., Dupre, N., Carmeliet, P., Gonzalez, B. J., et al. (2013). Hypoxia-ischemia or excitotoxin-induced tissue plasminogen activator- dependent gelatinase activation in mice neonate brain microvessels. *PLoS ONE* 8:e71263. doi: 10.1371/journal.pone.0071263

Parent, J. M., Vexler, Z. S., Gong, C., Derugin, N., and Ferriero, D. M. (2002). Rat forebrain neurogenesis and striatal neuron replacement after focal stroke. *Ann. Neurol.* 52, 802–813. doi: 10.1002/ana.10393

Peppiatt, C. M., Howarth, C., Mobbs, P., and Attwell, D. (2006). Bidirectional control of CNS capillary diameter by pericytes. *Nature* 443, 700–704. doi: 10.1038/nature05193

Petty, M. A., and Lo, E. H. (2002). Junctional complexes of the blood-brain barrier: permeability changes in neuroinflammation. *Prog. Neurobiol.* 68, 311–323. doi: 10.1016/S0301-0082(02)00128-4

Plane, J. M., Liu, R., Wang, T. W., Silverstein, F. S., and Parent, J. M. (2004). Neonatal hypoxic-ischemic injury increases forebrain subventricular zone neurogenesis in the mouse. *Neurobiol. Dis.* 16, 585–595. doi: 10.1016/j.nbd.2004.04.003

Renolleau, S., Aggoun-Zouaoui, D., Ben-Ari, Y., and Charriaut-Marlangue, C. (1998). A model of transient unilateral focal ischemia with reperfusion in the P7 neonatal rat: morphological changes indicative of apoptosis. *Stroke* 29, 1454–1460. discussion: 1461. doi: 10.1161/01.STR.29.7.1454

Rice, J. E. D., Vannucci, R. C., and Brierley, J. B. (1981). The influence of immaturity on hypoxic-ischemic brain damage in the rat. *Ann. Neurol.* 9, 131–141. doi: 10.1002/ana.410090206

Rizzo, M. T., and Leaver, H. A. (2010). Brain endothelial cell death: modes, signaling pathways, and relevance to neural development, homeostasis, and disease. *Mol. Neurobiol.* 42, 52–63. doi: 10.1007/s12035-010-8132-6

Rosenberg, G. A., Estrada, E. Y., and Dencoff, J. E. (1998). Matrix metalloproteinases and TIMPs are associated with blood-brain barrier opening after reperfusion in rat brain. *Stroke* 29, 2189–2195. doi: 10.1161/01.STR.29.10.2189

Rothstein, R. P., and Levison, S. W. (2005). Gray matter oligodendrocyte progenitors and neurons die caspase-3 mediated deaths subsequent to mild perinatal hypoxic/ischemic insults. *Dev. Neurosci.* 27, 149–159. doi: 10.1159/000085987

Shechter, R., Miller, O., Yovel, G., Rosenzweig, N., London, A., Ruckh, J., et al. (2013). Recruitment of beneficial M2 macrophages to injured spinal cord is orchestrated by remote brain choroid plexus. *Immunity* 38, 555–569. doi: 10.1016/j.immuni.2013.02.012

Sheldon, R. A., Jiang, X., Francisco, C., Christen, S., Vexler, Z. S., Tauber, M. G., et al. (2004). Manipulation of antioxidant pathways in neonatal murine brain. *Pediatr. Res.* 56, 656–662. doi: 10.1203/01.PDR.0000139413.27864.50

Shimotake, J., Derugin, N., Wendland, M., Vexler, Z. S., and Ferriero, D. M. (2010). Vascular endothelial growth factor receptor-2 inhibition promotes cell death and limits endothelial cell proliferation in a neonatal rodent model of stroke. *Stroke* 41, 343–349. doi: 10.1161/STROKEAHA.109.564229

Spadafora, R., Gonzalez, F. F., Derugin, N., Wendland, M., Ferriero, D., and McQuillen, P. (2010). Altered fate of subventricular zone progenitor cells and reduced neurogenesis following neonatal stroke. *Dev. Neurosci.* 32, 101–113. doi: 10.1159/000279654

Strbian, D., Karjalainen-Lindsberg, M. L., Kovanen, P. T., Tatlisumak, T., and Lindsberg, P. J. (2007). Mast cell stabilization reduces hemorrhage formation and mortality after administration of thrombolytics in experimental ischemic stroke. *Circulation* 116, 411–418. doi: 10.1161/CIRCULATIONAHA.106.655423

Strbian, D., Karjalainen-Lindsberg, M. L., Tatlisumak, T., and Lindsberg, P. J. (2006). Cerebral mast cells regulate early ischemic brain swelling and neutrophil accumulation. *J. Cereb. Blood Flow Metab.* 26, 605–612. doi: 10.1038/sj.jcbfm.9600228

Szmydynger-Chodobska, J., Strazielle, N., Gandy, J. R., Keefe, T. H., Zink, B. J., Ghersi-Egea, J. F., et al. (2012). Posttraumatic invasion of monocytes across the blood-cerebrospinal fluid barrier. *J. Cereb. Blood Flow Metab.* 32, 93–104. doi: 10.1038/jcbfm.2011.111

Szmydynger-Chodobska, J., Strazielle, N., Zink, B. J., Ghersi-Egea, J. F., and Chodobski, A. (2009). The role of the choroid plexus in neutrophil invasion after traumatic brain injury. *J. Cereb. Blood Flow Metab.* 29, 1503–1516. doi: 10.1038/jcbfm.2009.71

Van Den Broeck, C., Himpens, E., Vanhaesebrouck, P., Calders, P., and Oostra, A. (2008). Influence of gestational age on the type of brain injury and neuromotor outcome in high-risk neonates. *Eur. J. Pediatr.* 167, 1005–1009. doi: 10.1007/s00431-007-0629-2

Van Velthoven, C. T., Kavelaars, A., Van Bel, F., and Heijnen, C. J. (2010). Mesenchymal stem cell treatment after neonatal hypoxic-ischemic brain injury improves behavioral outcome and induces neuronal and oligodendrocyte regeneration. *Brain Behav. Immun.* 24, 387–393. doi: 10.1016/j.bbi.2009.10.017

Van Velthoven, C. T., Sheldon, R. A., Kavelaars, A., Derugin, N., Vexler, Z. S., Willemen, H. L., et al. (2013). Mesenchymal stem cell transplantation attenuates brain injury after neonatal stroke. *Stroke* 44, 1426–1432. doi: 10.1161/STROKEAHA.111.000326

Vexler, Z. S., and Yenari, M. A. (2009). Does inflammation after stroke affect the developing brain differently than adult brain? *Dev. Neurosci.* 31, 378–393. doi: 10.1159/000232556

Vexler, Z. S., Tang, X. N., and Yenari, M. A. (2006). Inflammation in adult and neonatal stroke. *Clin. Neurosci. Res.* 6, 293–313. doi: 10.1016/j.cnr.2006.09.008

Volpe, J. J. (2009). The encephalopathy of prematurity–brain injury and impaired brain development inextricably intertwined. *Semin. Pediatr. Neurol.* 16, 167–178. doi: 10.1016/j.spen.2009.09.005

Wacker, B. K., Freie, A. B., Perfater, J. L., and Gidday, J. M. (2012). Junctional protein regulation by sphingosine kinase 2 contributes to blood-brain barrier protection in hypoxic preconditioning-induced cerebral ischemic tolerance. *J. Cereb. Blood Flow Metab.* 32, 1014–1023. doi: 10.1038/jcbfm.2012.3

Woo, M. S., Wang, X., Faustino, J., Derugin, N., Wendland, M. F., Zhou, P., et al. (2012). Genetic deletion of CD36 enhances injury after acute neonatal stroke. *Ann. Neurol.* 72, 961–970. doi: 10.1002/ana.23727

Yager, J. Y., and Ashwal, S. (2009). Animal models of perinatal hypoxic-ischemic brain damage. *Pediatr. Neurol.* 40, 156–167. doi: 10.1016/j.pediatrneurol.2008.10.025

Yamasaki, Y., Matsuo, Y., Matsuura, N., Onodera, H., Itoyama, Y., and Kogure, K. (1995). Transient increase of cytokine-induced neutrophil chemoattractant, a member of the interleukin-8 family, in ischemic brain areas after focal ischemia in rats. *Stroke 26*, 318–22; discussion 322-3. doi: 10.1161/01.STR.26.2.318

Yamasaki, Y., Matsuo, Y., Zagorski, J., Matsuura, N., Onodera, H., Itoyama, Y., et al. (1997). New therapeutic possibility of blocking cytokine-induced neutrophil chemoattractant on transient ischemic brain damage in rats. *Brain Res.* 759, 103–111. doi: 10.1016/S0006-8993(97)00251-5

Yang, Y., Estrada, E. Y., Thompson, J. F., Liu, W., and Rosenberg, G. A. (2007a). Matrix metalloproteinase-mediated disruption of tight junction proteins in cerebral vessels is reversed by synthetic matrix metalloproteinase inhibitor in focal ischemia in rat. *J. Cereb. Blood Flow Metab.* 27, 697–709. doi: 10.1038/sj.jcbfm.9600375

Yang, Z., Covey, M. V., Bitel, C. L., Ni, L., Jonakait, G. M., and Levison, S. W. (2007b). Sustained neocortical neurogenesis after neonatal hypoxic/ischemic injury. *Ann. Neurol.* 61, 199–208. doi: 10.1002/ana.21068

Yemisci, M., Gursoy-Ozdemir, Y., Vural, A., Can, A., Topalkara, K., and Dalkara, T. (2009). Pericyte contraction induced by oxidative-nitrative stress impairs capillary reflow despite successful opening of an occluded cerebral artery. *Nat. Med.* 15, 1031–1037. doi: 10.1038/nm.2022

Young, C. C., Brooks, K. J., Buchan, A. M., and Szele, F. G. (2011). Cellular and molecular determinants of stroke-induced changes in subventricular zone cell migration. *Antioxid. Redox Signal.* 14, 1877–1888. doi: 10.1089/ars.2010.3435

Zhao, B. Q., Wang, S., Kim, H. Y., Storrie, H., Rosen, B. R., Mooney, D. J., et al. (2006). Role of matrix metalloproteinases in delayed cortical responses after stroke. *Nat. Med.* 12, 441–445. doi: 10.1038/nm1387

2

Efflux transporters in blood-brain interfaces of the developing brain

Nathalie Strazielle[1,2] and Jean-François Ghersi-Egea[2,3]*

[1] Brain-i, Lyon, France
[2] Oncoflam Team, Lyon Neuroscience Research Center, INSERM, U1028, CNRS, UMR5292, Université Lyon 1, Lyon, France
[3] BIP Platform, Lyon Neuroscience Research Center, INSERM, U1028, CNRS, UMR5292, Université Lyon 1, Lyon, France

Correspondence:
Jean-François Ghersi-Egea, Blood-Brain Interface Group, Oncoflam Team, INSERM U 1028, CNRS UMR5292, Lyon Neuroscience Research Center, Oncoflam Team, Faculté de Médecine RTH Laennec, Rue Guillaume Paradin, 69372 Lyon, France
e-mail: jean-francois.ghersi-egea@inserm.fr

The cerebral microvessel endothelium forming the blood-brain barrier (BBB) and the epithelium of the choroid plexuses forming the blood-CSF barrier (BCSFB) operate as gatekeepers for the central nervous system. Exposure of the vulnerable developing brain to chemical insults can have dramatic consequences for brain maturation and lead to life-long neurological diseases. The ability of blood-brain interfaces to efficiently protect the immature brain is therefore an important pathophysiological issue. This is also key to our understanding of drug entry into the brain of neonatal and pediatric patients. Non-specific paracellular diffusion through barriers is restricted early during development, but other neuroprotective properties of these interfaces differ between the developing and adult brains. This review focuses on the developmental expression and function of various classes of efflux transporters. These include the multispecific transporters of the ATP-binding cassette transporter families ABCB, ABCC, ABCG, the organic anion and cation transporters of the solute carrier families SLC21/SLCO and SLC22, and the peptide transporters of the SLC15 family. These transporters play a key role in preventing brain entry of blood-borne molecules such as drugs, environmental toxicants, and endogenous metabolites, or else in increasing the clearance of potentially harmful organic ions from the brain. The limited data available for laboratory animals and human highlight transporter-specific developmental patterns of expression and function, which differ between blood-brain interfaces. The BCSFB achieves an adult phenotype earlier than BBB. Efflux transporters at the BBB appear to be regulated by various factors subsequently secreted by neural progenitors and astrocytes during development. Their expression is also modulated by oxidative stress, inflammation, and exposure to xenobiotic inducers. A better understanding of these regulatory pathways during development, in particular the signaling pathways triggered by oxidative stress and xenobiotics, may open new opportunities to therapeutic manipulation in view to improve or restore neuroprotective functions of the blood-brain interfaces in the context of perinatal injuries.

Keywords: blood-brain barrier, choroid plexus, development, ABC transporter, SLC transporter, perinatal injury, hypoxia, xenobiotic

INTRODUCTION

Blood-brain interfaces comprise the cerebral microvessel endothelium forming the blood-brain barrier (BBB) and the epithelium of the choroid plexuses forming the blood-CSF barrier (BCSFB). These interfaces operate as gatekeepers for the central nervous system, hence providing the cerebral homeostasis necessary for normal neuronal growth and activity.

During brain development, these CNS barriers display stage specific properties. For instance, in rat, the activity of gamma-glutamyl-transferase, an enzymatic marker of brain microvessels, continuously increases from birth to adulthood (Betz and Goldstein, 1981; Gazzin et al., 2008). Conversely, the metabolic barrier to DOPA mediated by DOPA-decarboxylase is most effective in young animals (Betz and Goldstein, 1981). Blood to brain influx of pyruvate, lactate and β-hydroxybutyrate, as well as large neutral amino acids is greater in suckling rats compared to adult animals, while active efflux of amino acids across the BBB may not occur before 21 days of age (review in Betz and Goldstein, 1981). In the choroid plexus epithelium, the composition in tight junction proteins changes during brain development. Notably, expression of the pore-forming claudin-2 is upregulated and that of the tightening claudin-3 is downregulated, probably reflecting perinatal changes in inorganic anion transport and related CSF secretion rate at the BCSFB (Kratzer et al., 2012). These various examples illustrate changes in barrier functions that occur

Abbreviations: BBB, blood-brain barrier; BCSFB, blood-CSF barrier; ABC, ATP-Binding Cassette; OATP, organic anion transport polypeptide; HNF-4 α, hepatic nuclear factor 4α; Nrf2, nuclear factor erythroid 2-related factor 2; AhR, aryl hydrocarbon receptor; CAR, constitutive androstane receptor; PXR, pregnane X receptor.

to face specific needs of the brain at different developmental stages.

The vulnerability of the developing brain to chemical insults, especially during the late prenatal/early postnatal period (herein referred to as perinatal period) can have dramatic consequences for brain maturation, leading to life-long neurological diseases (Kaindl et al., 2009; Landrigan and Goldman, 2011; Miodovnik, 2011). The ability of blood-brain interfaces to efficiently protect the immature brain is therefore a major pathophysiological issue. It is also key to our understanding of therapeutic drug entry into the brain of neonate and pediatric patients. Little is known about the mechanisms protecting the developing brain from harmful compounds and regulating the cerebral entry of pharmacologically active compounds. The cerebral interstitial fluid concentration of xenobiotics is set by their ability to cross the brain endothelium and the choroidal epithelium, as well as a number of other parameters. These include protein binding, local cerebral capillary density and cerebral blood flow, intraparenchymal diffusion rate, movement by fluid flow along perivascular spaces and within ventricular and cisternal spaces, and CSF turnover (reviewed in Ghersi-Egea et al., 2009; Westerhout et al., 2011). These parameters change during development. Plasma protein concentration is lower during development than in adult, so are cerebral blood flow and capillary density (Caley and Maxwell, 1970; Nehlig et al., 1989). Intracerebral fluid dynamic differs between adult and developing brain. CSF turnover increases at birth, and the total CSF (cisternal, subarachnoid, and ventricular) to brain volume ratio is largely higher in perinatal brain (unpublished data). Taken together, these observations indicate that the impact of blood-CSF exchanges on the overall cerebral bioavailability of drugs or toxic compounds is likely to be more important in young than in adult individuals. At the level of the BBBs proper, the neuroprotective functions result from intercellular tight junctions sealing the barrier cell layers, as well as detoxification enzymes and efflux transporters located in the barrier cells (Strazielle and Ghersi-Egea, 2013). It is now clearly established that non-specific paracellular diffusion through the cerebral endothelium and the choroidal epithelium is efficiently restricted by the tight junctions early during development (Liddelow et al., 2013).

This review focuses on efflux transporters and analyses the data relative to their developmental pattern of localization, expression and function. These multispecific transport systems play a key role in preventing the entry into the brain and CSF of numerous blood-borne xenobiotics, including drugs, or in increasing the clearance of potentially harmful organic ions from the brain. They include ATP-Binding Cassette (ABC) transporters of the ABCB, ABCC, and ABCG families, solute carriers for organic anions and cations of the SLC21/SLCO and SLC22 families, and peptide transporters of the SLC15 family[1] (**Figure 1**). These efflux transporters also recognize biologically active endogenous compounds, including steroid hormones and eicosanoids (leukotrienes, prostaglandins), thus protecting the brain from a potentially deleterious overproduction of these compounds.

[1]Capitalized characters are used when referring to human transporters or to transporters listed in a general context. Minor characters are used when specifically referring to rodent transporters.

ATP-BINDING CASSETTE TRANSPORTERS

Multispecific efflux transporters that belong to the ABC transporter superfamily and are found in blood-brain interfaces include ABCB1 (P-glycoprotein), ABCG2 (breast cancer resistance protein, Bcrp), and several ABCCs (multidrug-related resistance proteins, Mrp) (Schinkel et al., 1996; Nishino et al., 1999; Wijnholds et al., 2000; Cooray et al., 2002; Strazielle and Ghersi-Egea, 2013). Located at the blood-facing membranes they prevent brain penetration of their substrates by an energy-dependent, unidirectional, outwardly directed transport mechanism. They are responsible for the efflux of many structurally unrelated lipophilic and amphiphilic environmental toxic compounds or drugs, including anti-inflammatory, immunosuppressive, anti-infectious, and antineoplastic drugs, some antiepileptic, antidepressant and psychotropic agents, and drug conjugates in the case of ABCCs (Schinkel and Jonker, 2003; Leslie et al., 2005; Staud and Pavek, 2005; Strazielle and Ghersi-Egea, 2005). These ABC transporters are differentially localized between the two main blood-brain interfaces (**Figure 1**). ABCB1 and ABCG2 are highly expressed at the BBB, while ABCC1 is a landmark of the BCSFB (Daood et al., 2008; Gazzin et al., 2008). Abcc2 has been described in the rodent BBB (e.g., Wang et al., 2014), and Abcc4 expression and function have been described in both interfaces in mice (Leggas et al., 2004). Species differences are found, namely for ABCG2 which is likely to play a more important protective function in human than in rodent (Shawahna et al., 2011), and ABCB1, which is encoded by a single gene in human and 2 genes in rat and mouse. Species difference may also exist for ABCC2 whose expression at the BBB in normal human brain is still an open question (Kubota et al., 2006; Dauchy et al., 2008).

Several studies suggest that ABC transporters are already functional at the blood-brain interfaces in neonates, but that their expression is developmentally regulated in a protein- and barrier-specific manner.

Developmental pattern of ABCB localization, expression and activity at blood-brain interfaces

In mouse and rat, the Abcb1-dependent phenotype of multidrug resistance is associated with 2 genes Abcb1a and Abcb1b, both homologs to the human ABCB1 transporter gene. Abcb1a and Abcb1b are expressed in a tissue-specific manner, and also differ to some extent in their transport properties. Abcb1a is closer to the human transporter in terms of amino acid primary sequence and gene regulatory region, and is the predominant gene expressed at the BBB. Its expression is already detectable in endothelial cells in the neural tube of 10.5-day-old mouse embryos (Qin and Sato, 1995). Immunohistochemical analysis performed with different antibodies on human tissues showed that Abcb1 protein consistently localizes at the membrane of brain microvessels by mid-gestation. Before this stage, the signal is heterogeneous and displays regional differences (Schumacher and Mollgard, 1997; Virgintino et al., 2008). Accordingly, Gazzin and coll. reported that this transporter is present in rat brain

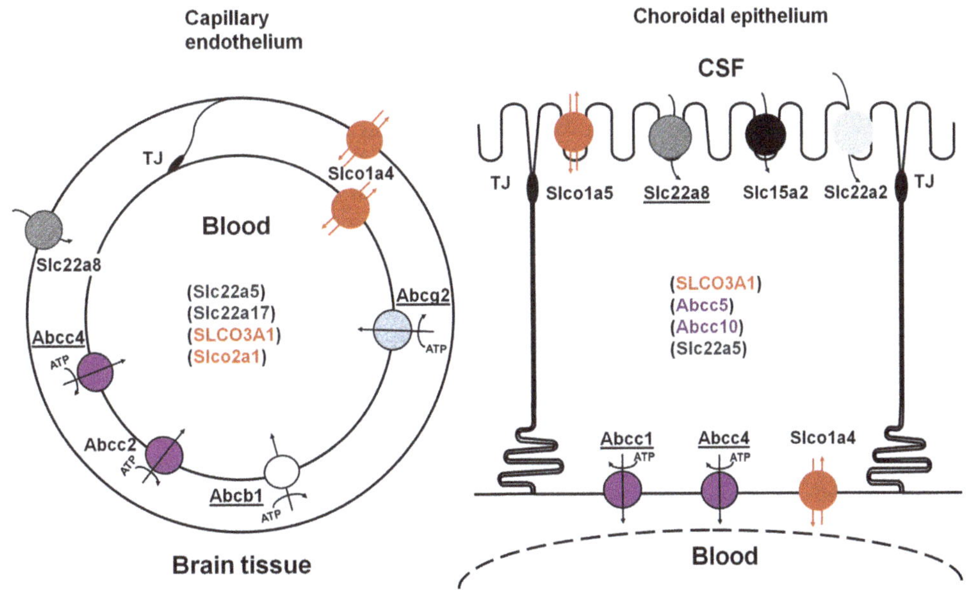

FIGURE 1 | Schematic representation of the main multispecific transporters involved in neuroprotective efflux at the blood-brain (left) and blood-CSF (right) barriers. Underlined names represent transporters for which evidence has also been reported in human. The ATP-dependency is shown only for primary ATP-dependent transporters. Transporters in parenthesis are carriers for which evidence of their involvement in CNS-blood efflux processes is still limited. See text for references. TJ, tight junction.

microvessels at birth, a developmental stage which corresponds to preterm development in human (Gazzin et al., 2008). As would be required for its neuroprotective efflux function, Abcb1 immunoreactivity was found at the luminal membrane of the endothelial wall. Because the cerebral capillary density increases greatly during development, the amount of Abcb1 protein at the BBB cannot be compared between stages using total brain homogenates. A standard curve-based quantitative Western blot analysis performed on isolated microvessels showed that the amount of Abcb1 in the BBB in 9- and 17-day-old rats was only one-fifth of that found in microvessels isolated from adult animals (Gazzin et al., 2008, 2011). This is in agreement with the more intense immunohistochemical signal observed in brain microvessels from adult as compared to perinatal or postnatal developmental stages in human, rat or mouse (Matsuoka et al., 1999; Tsai et al., 2002; Daood et al., 2008; Gazzin et al., 2011). It is also consistent with the 3-to-4-fold increase in Abcb1a mRNA levels measured in endothelial cells from adult mice or rats compared to levels in endothelial cells of developing animals (2- to 8-day-old mouse, 14-day-old rat) (Daneman et al., 2010a; Harati et al., 2012a). The low expression and protein level of Abcb1 observed at the BBB in different species at late prenatal and early postnatal developmental stages may therefore result in a weaker protection of the brain against circulating compounds that are handled by this transporter. Accordingly, a 80–90% lower brain accumulation of cyclosporin A and digoxin, assessed as brain-blood/plasma ratio 2 h following administration, was observed in adult mice compared with 1-day-old mice, a difference which was abolished in Abcb1a deficient animals (Goralski et al., 2006). A number of other functional studies have been conducted using digoxine as Abcb1 substrate. A greater accumulation of this molecule was observed in the brain of 15.5-day-old embryonic mice compared to the brain of 18.5-day-old embryonic mice (Petropoulos et al., 2010). In rat, the unbound brain-to-plasma concentration ratio of the molecule measured at steady-state was not different between 3-week- and 12-week-old animals (Harati et al., 2012a). A positron emission tomography study conducted in rhesus monkeys showed a significantly higher clearance value for verapamil uptake in 9-month-old animals than in 2- and 4-year-old animals (Takashima et al., 2011). With the reservation that substrate specificities for Abcb1 are not absolute, in particular for digoxin which can be recognized by other transporters such as Slco1a4/oatp2, overall, these partial data suggest that ABCB1 functional activity parallels gene expression levels, both increasing from prenatal to pre-adult stages in various animal species, including non-human primates.

The amount of ABCB1 protein in rat and human choroid plexus is low by comparison to the levels measured in brain microvessels (Gazzin et al., 2008), and its cellular and subcellular localization within the choroidal tissue is subject to conflictual results. Its implication in the regulation of exchanges across the BCSFB is likely limited. In contrast to the BBB, Abcb1a mRNAs are not detected by RT-PCR in the BCSFB. The gene expressed in rat choroid plexus is Abcb1b. The level of expression, very low in adult rat tissue, is 4–8 times higher during the perinatal period of development, with a peak on postnatal day 2 (Kratzer et al., 2013). The actual functional activity of the transporter and the significance of this perinatal upregulation of choroidal Abcb1b expression are not known.

Developmental pattern of ABCG2 localization, expression and activity at blood-brain interfaces

There are few data available on the developmental expression of ABCG2, but there is a general agreement that the transporter is associated with the brain vasculature and localizes at the luminal membrane of brain endothelium early during development, specifically by week 22 of gestation in human (Daood et al., 2008), embryonic day 12.5 in mouse and in rat (Tachikawa et al., 2005; Orford et al., 2009; Ek et al., 2010). No apparent difference in signal intensity was observed throughout development in these studies. Only a moderate (2-fold or less) increase in Abcg2 mRNA levels was observed in endothelial cells isolated from adult vs. postnatal mouse brain (Daneman et al., 2010a) or between cerebral capillary preparations of comparable purity isolated from 14-day-old rats vs. adult animals (Harati et al., 2012a). In the latter study no difference in Abcg2 protein level was observed by Western blot between the two stages. Functional studies on Abcg2 mediated transport during development have been performed only in rat on postnatal day 21. At that stage, blood-to-brain prazosin transport was not different from that measured in adult rats (Harati et al., 2012a). Overall, ABCG2 seems to reach high levels of expression at the BBB early during development. It may compensate for the lack of Abcb1-dependent protection at a period of high brain vulnerability.

Studies on the expression and function of Abcg2 in choroid plexus generated apparently conflicting results, possibly linked to species differences, or due to difficulties in achieving specific immunolabeling in this tissue. The level of protein assessed by Western blot is clearly much lower in choroidal tissue than in brain capillaries, as illustrated in the work performed by Reichel and colleagues in rat (Reichel et al., 2011). They loaded 10 times more proteins from choroidal tissue than from microvessels to be able to detect Abcg2 in the former sample, while the capillary fraction yielded an intense signal. In line with that report, an immunohistochemical study conducted on human tissue failed to detect ABCG2 in the choroid plexus at any developmental stage (extending from 22 weeks of gestation to adult), while the transporter was clearly detected in the microvasculature (Daood et al., 2008). Using transgenic mice expressing GFP under the control of Abcg2 promoter/enhancer sequences, Orford and colleagues showed that the transporter is associated with choroidal vessels from early on during development but not with the choroidal epithelium (Orford et al., 2009). By contrast, the protein was detected at the apical membrane of the choroidal epithelium in adult mouse, a signal that was not seen in Abcg2 knock-out animals (Tachikawa et al., 2005; Zhuang et al., 2006). No developmental data was provided in these studies. Other studies failed to detect the protein in choroid plexus epithelium of the adult rat (Roberts et al., 2008; Ek et al., 2010). One of the latter studies reported Abcg2 immunoreactivity at the basolateral membrane of the choroidal epithelium only at early developmental stages (embryonic day 15 and postnatal day 1) (Ek et al., 2010). This pattern of Abcg2 protein expression in rat parallels the temporal profile of choroidal Abcg2 mRNA levels which are also higher in pre- and perinatal stages than in adult (Ek et al., 2010; Kratzer et al., 2013). It has to be noted that mRNA levels are low in choroid plexus in both rat and mouse (Tachikawa et al., 2005; Kratzer et al., 2013). Overall, if Abcg2 has any significant transport function at the BCSFB, it should be especially relevant to the developing period.

Developmental localization, expression and activity of efflux transporters of the ABCC family at blood-brain interfaces

An immunohistochemical signal for ABCC1 was consistently observed in human choroid plexus epithelium early in gestation, from week 22 onwards (Daood et al., 2008). In rat, Abcc1 protein was detected in choroid plexus epithelial cells as early as embryonic day 15, with a basolateral localization consistent with its efflux transporter activity and a neuroprotective function (Gazzin et al., 2008; Ek et al., 2010). Choroidal mRNA levels were 2- to 3-fold lower in 15-day-old embryos and 7-day-old rat pups than in adult (Ek et al., 2010; Kratzer et al., 2013), but at birth, protein levels measured by quantitative Western blot are similar to those in adult (Gazzin et al., 2008), suggesting that Abcc1-mediated efflux at the BCSFB is active early during development. Protein and mRNA levels of Abcc1 are low in both the rodent and human microvasculature in comparison to choroidal levels, and the actual localization and efflux activity of the protein at the BBB proper remains controversial (reviewed in Gazzin et al., 2008). One study investigated ABCC1 protein in the human BBB during development and failed to detect the transporter at any developmental stage (Daood et al., 2008). Only rat mRNA expression data are available concerning the developmental pattern of other Abcc transporters. In the choroid plexus, the temporal expression profile for Abcc4, for which functional evidence of transport has been provided *in vivo* in adult mice (Leggas et al., 2004), follows a developmental pattern similar to that of Abcc1, with a limited increase in mRNA level in adult tissue compared to tissue from embryonic day 19. As in choroid plexus, mRNA levels in brain endothelial cells are moderately (3.3 times) lower in young mice (postnatal day 2–8) than in adult animals (Daneman et al., 2010a). The concurrent expression of this transporter in the BCSFB and the BBB from early stages on, and its polarized localization at blood-facing membranes in both barriers suggest that it plays an important role in the clearance of endogenous substrates in young and adult individuals.

Abcc5, Abcc9, and Abcc10 genes investigated in rat choroid plexus are expressed at a similar or higher level in developing animals compared to adults (Kratzer et al., 2013). Functionally, an Abcc-dependent basolateral efflux of intracellularly formed drug conjugates has been demonstrated in freshly isolated choroid plexuses or in choroid plexus epithelial cells, both obtained from 2-day-old rats (Strazielle and Ghersi-Egea, 1999; Ghersi-Egea et al., 2006). These *ex vivo/in vitro* studies indicated that one or several Abcc proteins are efficiently participating to a neuroprotective enzymatic BCSFB during development.

SOLUTE CARRIER PROTEINS

The SLC superfamily comprises virtually all transporters that do not belong to the ABC family. Multispecific SLC transporters responsible for the neuroprotective efflux of exogenous and endogenous toxic molecules from brain or CSF to blood belong mainly to three subfamilies. The SLC22 subfamily includes organic anion and cation efflux transporters also referred to as OAT, OCT, and OCTN proteins. SLCO transporters, previously known as SLC21 form another subfamily of organic anion transport polypeptides (OATPs). Of note, several SLCO rodent genes have no homologs in human, and vice-versa. SLCO and SLC22 transporters accept as substrates a broad range of cationic and anionic compounds, including environmental pollutants, and various drugs such as antibiotics and nucleosidic antiviral drugs, non-steroidal anti-inflammatory agents, and some antiepileptic drugs. They also transport steroid or drug conjugates, and lipid mediators (Strazielle et al., 2003; Hagenbuch and Stieger, 2013; Koepsell, 2013). Finally, members of the SLC15 family, known as peptide/proton cotransporters, transport in addition to endogenous di- and tripeptides, some peptidomimetic drugs, e.g., β-lactam antibiotics, antiviral nucleoside prodrugs or angiotensin converting enzymes (Daniel and Rubio-Aliaga, 2003).

Some of these solute carriers are bidirectional. Others function as unidirectional inwardly-directed multispecific transport systems and exchange their substrates with specific intracellular divalent organic anions by a coupled secondary energy-dependent mechanism. SLC transporters that are involved in brain efflux localize at the abluminal (BBB) or apical (BCSFB) membrane of barrier cells, where they remove drugs and toxic compounds from brain extracellular and CSF spaces. The most documented SLC efflux transporters at blood-brain interfaces are the following. SLC22A8/OAT3 is present at both brain endothelial cells and choroidal epithelial cells in rodents, and is also detected in human choroid plexus (Nagata et al., 2002; Alebouyeh et al., 2003; Kikuchi et al., 2003; Mori et al., 2003; Ose et al., 2009). Slco1a5/Oatp3, Slc15a2/Pept2, and possibly Slc22a2/Oct2 are restricted to choroid plexus (Kusuhara et al., 2003; Ohtsuki et al., 2003). Other organic anion transporters are found at blood-brain interfaces, but their possible involvement in brain efflux rather than influx processes remaining to be established (**Figure 1**). Slco1a4/oatp2 is found at both luminal and abluminal membranes of brain endothelial cells, and only at the basolateral membrane of the choroidal epithelium in rat (Gao et al., 1999). In human, two SLCO3A1 variants v1 and v2, of similar and broad substrate specificity, are respectively located on the basolateral and apical membranes of the choroidal epithelium, suggesting that SLCO3A1 may function both as an influx and an efflux transporter (Huber et al., 2007). SLCO1A2 and SLCO2B1, also expressed at the human BBB, are likely to mediate brain influx rather than brain efflux, on the basis of their localization at the luminal membrane of the endothelium (Gao et al., 2000; Bronger et al., 2005).

Developmental localization, expression and activity of SLC22 and SLCO efflux transporters at blood-brain interfaces

Data on the developmental expression of efflux transporters that belong to the SLC22 and SLCO gene families are scarce and obtained only from rat and mouse studies. Transcriptomic analysis of endothelial cells isolated from adult vs. postnatal mouse brains suggests that developmental profiles are heterogeneous among genes (Daneman et al., 2010a). While mRNA levels for Slc22a5 (octn2) and Slco1a4 were 2-to 5-fold lower in endothelial cells from developing animals compared to adults, Slc22a8 expression was similar at both stages. Slc22a17 and Slco2b1, whose precise functions are currently unknown at brain barriers, did not display developmental changes either. Of note in this study, the mRNA levels of Slco2a1, the prostaglandin transporter with an unknown directionality of transport, were much higher at the BBB from developing vs. adult mice. This suggests a developmentally regulated mechanism for blood-brain exchange of prostaglandins, possibly related to the function of these lipid mediators in brain maturation. In rat, a lower expression was reported for Slco1a4 between developing and adult animal, while there was no change for Slc22a8 (Harati et al., 2012a). This was assessed by quantitative PCR and Western blot on isolated capillaries and confirms the mouse transcriptomic observations.

The analysis of transcriptomic profiles established in rat choroid plexus for 14 Slco and Slc22 members showed that most genes, including Slc22a5, Slco1a4, and Slco1a5 are expressed at similar or higher levels during the perinatal period than at the adult stage. One exception is Slc22a8, for which expression levels are respectively 4-fold and 2-fold lower in 19-day-old embryos and 2-day-old rats than in adults. At an earlier stage, in 15-day-old embryos, gene expression levels relative to adult were more heterogeneous (Kratzer et al., 2013). A functional analysis showed that *ex vivo* uptake of bromosulfophthalein, a typical Slco substrate, was 3-fold higher in choroid plexuses isolated from newborn rat compared to adult rat (Angeletti et al., 1998). Western blot and immunohistochemical localization of Slco were also performed in this study, but are difficult to interpret as, at that time, Slco1a5 was mistakenly identified as Slco1a1 in this tissue. As further evidence of organic anion transport maturity at the BCSFB, choroidal epithelial cells isolated from newborn rats efficiently mediate the transport of Slc22 and Slco substrates such as 2,4-dichlorophenoxyacetic acid, benzylpenicillin, zidovudine or taurocholate in an unidirectional CSF-to-blood direction (Strazielle et al., 2003).

Developmental localization and expression of SLC15 efflux transporters at the choroid plexus

Among members of the SLC15 family, Slc15a2 is well expressed in the brain, with the highest level in the choroid plexus (Shen et al., 2004). Both mRNA levels and immunohistochemical signals for Slc15a2 were similar in rat choroid plexuses at perinatal and adult stages (Shen et al., 2004; Kratzer et al., 2013). The apical localization of this choroidal transporter suggests its efficacy in exporting neuropeptides, peptide fragments, and peptide-like drugs out of CSF from early on during brain development.

The overall developmental profiles of all ABC and SLC efflux transporters reviewed above are summarized in **Table 1**. It shows that regarding the expression of efflux transporters, an overall adult-like phenotype is reached earlier at the BCSFB than at the BBB.

REGULATION OF EFFLUX TRANSPORTER ASSOCIATED BARRIER PROPERTIES DURING DEVELOPMENT

Signaling pathways involved in the early specification of brain barrier cells have been identified in the last decade, pointing out a few molecular cues that specifically regulate the developmental expression of efflux transporters. In addition, these transport systems are modulated in disease and by various xenobiotics via mechanisms that may bear developmental specificities.

Table 1 | Comparative analysis of the developmental expression pattern of efflux transporters between the blood-brain- and blood-CSF barriers.

Blood-brain barrier			Blood-CSF barrier		
Major efflux transporters	**Developmental pattern**		**Major efflux transporters**	**Developmental pattern**	
ABCB1/Abcb1a	↗	mRNA, Prot, Fc	Abcc	=	Fc
ABCG2/Abcg2	=	mRNA, (Prot)	Abcc1	=	mRNA, Prot
Abcc4	↗	mRNA	Abcc4	≤	mRNA
Slc22a8	=	mRNA, Prot	Slc22a8	↗	mRNA
			Slco	↘	Fc
			Slco1a5	=	mRNA
			Pept2/Slc15	=	mRNA (Prot)
Other multispecific transporters	**Developmental pattern**		**Other multispecific transporters**	**Developmental pattern**	
Slc22a5	↗	mRNA	Abcb1b	↘	mRNA
Slco1a4	↗	mRNA, Prot	Abcg2	↘	mRNA (Prot)
Slc22a17	=	mRNA	Abcc5	=	mRNA
Slco2b1	=	mRNA	Abcc9	↘	mRNA
Slco2a1→	↘	mRNA	Abcc10	=	mRNA
			Slc22a5	=	mRNA
			Slco1a4	=	mRNA

↗, ↘, = increased, decreased, similar expression in adult as compared to neonatal stages, respectively. mRNA, assessed by qRTPCR or gene array. Prot, assessed by quantitative western blot. (Prot), assessed by immunohistochemical signal intensity. Fc, assessed by functional studies, using specific substrates. For references, see text.

Pathways involved in the developmental regulation of efflux transporters at blood-brain interfaces

The unique phenotype of brain microvessel endothelial cells compared to other endothelia in the body has long ago raised the hypothesis that surrounding neural cells were responsible for inducing BBB characteristics. A series of grafting experiments generated controversial results regarding this theory (reviewed in Bauer and Bauer, 2000). Arguments in favor of a role for adjacent cells, notably astrocytes emerged from many *in vitro* studies. It was thought for example, that the BBB hallmark transporter Abcb1 was under astrocytic regulation on the basis that its expression and functionality, which are partially lost in brain microvessel endothelial cells in culture were reinduced in endothelial cells co-cultured with glial cells. However, because of the temporal pattern of neural cell differentiation and the late apparition of mature astrocytes which in rat and mouse occurs only around birth, these cells obviously cannot impart the inducing signals that trigger BBB formation in neovessels. Astrocytes nonetheless are essential later for further maturation of the BBB (see infra), or for maintenance of its properties as suggested by the link between some astrocyte diseases and BBB dysfunction (Keller, 2013).

A large number of studies have recently been directed toward identifying the molecules, pathways, and cells responsible for CNS specific vascular differentiation. The Wnt/β-catenin canonical pathway has emerged as a prominent signaling mechanism, promoting angiogenesis and concurrently inducing hallmark features of the BBB, such as the expression of the glucose transporter Slc2a1 (reviewed in Liebner et al., 2011). Wnt factors are secreted as early as embryonic day 9 by neural progenitors. The various studies dedicated to this topic did not examine the direct effects of Wnt signaling on the expression of ABC and SLC efflux transporters at the BBB. DNA binding sites for T cell factor/lymphoid enhancer-binding factor TCF/LEF, the transcriptional activating factor downstream of the Wnt/β-catenin pathway, are present in the human ABCB1 gene promoter (Yamada et al., 2000). Functional evidence linking β-catenin accumulation with intestinal expression of the human ABCB1 gene or the mouse Abcb1a gene has been reported in intestinal cells (Scotto, 2003). Regarding the BBB, activation of β-catenin signaling by GSK-3 inhibition in the human brain endothelial cell line hMEC/D3 as well as in rat brain endothelial cells in primary culture similarly increased ABCB1 expression and function (Lim et al., 2008). The expression of ABCC4 and ABCG2 genes was also modulated in the hMEC/D3 cells in response to β-catenin signaling activation or inhibition, suggesting that the early embryonic expression of Abcg2 described in rat and mouse could depend on the same regulatory pathway. Although direct evidence in the embryonic brain is lacking, these data support the idea that the range of genes associated with the BBB phenotype and induced by the canonical Wnt pathway in newly formed cerebral vessels include efflux transporters. Other regulatory mechanisms are expected to add on this triggering mechanism to explain the different profiles observed among efflux transporters, such as between Abcb1 and Abcg2 for example (see supra).

Retinoic acid, a potent morphogen directing the development of the nervous system, has been proposed as another signaling cue contributing to the induction of the specific BBB phenotype at an early stage of angiogenesis. In human fetal brain, radial glial cells express the final enzyme involved in retinoic acid biosynthesis, while endothelial cells express one of the receptors for this signaling factor (Mizee et al., 2013). Treatment of mice from day 10.5 to day 16.5 of gestation with a retinoic acid receptor antagonist led to the downregulation of several BBB distinct properties in embryos, in particular to a decrease in the expression level of Abcg2 gene. One limitation of this result was that RNA levels were measured on the whole brain including a priori the choroid plexus as well as the subventricular zone, both regions of the brain that express the Abcg2 gene at substantial levels during this period. It is possible that the decrease observed in treated embryos on day 16.5 may not reflect changes at the BBB *per se*, but rather in either one or both of these regions (Orford et al., 2009). Immunostaining of Abcg2 in these animals should clarify this point.

In addition to neural progenitors and radial glial cells, pericytes are present in the early phase of cerebral angiogenesis, and are recruited by the nascent vessels invading the neuroectoderm. A major role of pericytes in influencing the endothelial phenotype has been clearly demonstrated *in vivo* for a number of features, including the loss of transcytotic vesicles, or the induction of the glucose transporter Slc2a1 (Armulik et al., 2010; Daneman et al., 2010b). By contrast, transcript levels for Abcb1a and Abcg2 in endothelial cells of 18-day-old mouse embryos did not differ between pericyte deficient Pdgfrb-/- animals and littermate controls (Daneman et al., 2010b), suggesting that initial induction of these efflux transporters is not under pericyte control.

Because similar deletion of astrocytes *in vivo* is not possible, current evidence for the influence of these cells on the differentiated status of BBB endothelial cells has been gathered using culture systems. One bias in these *in vitro* studies arises from the fact that endothelial cells are isolated from adult brain, thus with an already mature phenotype, and they downregulate some of their BBB-specific properties. For that reason, astrocytic effects observed *in vitro* may reflect not only maturation processes occurring when these cells appear, but also repair mechanisms triggered under pathological conditions. With regard to efflux transporters, the focus has been mainly on ABCB1. Its protein level and function are increased in endothelial cells cocultured with astrocytes, compared to endothelial cells alone (see for example Fenart et al., 1998; Gaillard et al., 2000). This reinduction occurs in the absence of any direct contact between the two cell populations, inferring the role of astrocytic soluble factors. Some of these astrocyte-derived molecules that act on endothelial receptors to promote BBB-specific properties have been identified (Abbott et al., 2006; Alvarez et al., 2011, for a review). They include sonic hedgehog ligands, angiopoietin 1 which is a ligand for the endothelial Tie2 tyrosine kinase receptor, or TGF-β1.Their role on the expression and function of ABC and SLC efflux transporters still need to be evaluated *in vivo*, using animals deficient for these pathways or pharmacological inhibition approaches. Evidence for the role of these signaling molecules in regulating the expression and activity of efflux transporters has been provided in other cell types. For example, activation of the sonic hedgehog pathway associates with elevated therapeutic resistance in cancer cells, in part due to increased protein level and activity of both ABCB1 and ABCG2 (Sims-Mourtada et al., 2007). Consistently, the promoter region of the ABCG2 gene contains a binding site for the downstream transcription factor Gli and is a direct target of sonic hedgehog signaling (Singh et al., 2011). Tie2 activation also promotes a chemoresistance phenotype in gliomas by inducing ABCB1 expression level and activity (Martin et al., 2009), and TGF-β1-mediated increase in Abcb1 expression and activity has been demonstrated in guinea pig brain endothelial cells in culture (Baello et al., 2014).

If significant progress has been achieved in the understanding of how the BBB gains its distinct phenotype, the signaling pathways responsible for the early specification of the choroidal epithelium vs. ependyma remain obscure, in particular concerning the regulation of expression of Slc and Abcc genes. The hepatic nuclear factor 4α (HNF-4α) is a key regulator of differentiation in the liver or the intestine, where it stimulates in particular the transcription of drug metabolizing enzymes and efflux transporters. HNF-4α is expressed in choroid plexus epithelial cells in rat and human at the adult stage, and can bind to regulatory sites in the ABCC1 gene promoter (Niehof and Borlak, 2009). Further work is needed to confirm its potential role in controlling the early choroidal-specific transcription of Abcc1.

Modulation of efflux transporters in response to injury and environmental insults during development

The pathogenesis of perinatal injuries most frequently involves hypoxia/ischemia, maternal-fetal infection or inflammation (Aden et al., 2010). These insults are associated with the secretion of proinflammatory cytokines, as well as oxidative/electrophilic stress for which the neonatal brain shows a selectively high susceptibility (Ferriero, 2001). Neuroprotective genes including anti-oxidant genes and efflux transporter genes of the ABC and SLC families are known to be regulated by these stress signals as part of the coordinated defense mechanisms implemented by the cells in response to oxidative stress. The regulatory pathways involve transcription factors that generally act as sensors in the cytoplasm and translocate to the nucleus to increase the transcription of target genes. Oxidative species and the lack of oxygen can be sensed by the nuclear factor erythroid 2-related factor 2 (Nrf2) and the hypoxia inducible factor 1alpha HIF-1α, respectively. There is mounting evidence that these stress sensing factors are expressed and functional in cells of the blood-brain-interfaces. Nrf2-dependent signaling increases Abcb1, Abcg2, and Abcc2 expression levels in rat brain microvessels, and accordingly decreases brain uptake of verapamil, a substrate of Abcb1 (Wang et al., 2014). The efficacy of Nrf2 signaling in improving neuroprotection at the microvasculature during brain development has not been explored. The functionality of the Nrf2-dependent pathway at the BCSFB was assessed *in vitro*, in choroidal epithelial cells, through Nrf2 translocation in the nucleus upon isothiocyanate treatment and transcriptional upregulation of downstream genes (e.g., heme oxygenase, Xiang et al., 2012). It is notable that in rat choroid plexus, Nrf2, HIF-1α, and HIF-1β display a strikingly steady expression from embryonic day 15 to the adult stage (Kratzer et al., 2013). We can therefore speculate that the choroid plexus will react to oxidative/electrophilic and hypoxic stresses at least, by increasing neuroprotective genes at the BCSFB early during development. Yet, this needs further investigation, since hypoxia/ischemia in 9-day-old mice did not change the level of expression of Abcc1 in the choroid plexus, although other target genes for Nrf2, such as heme oxygenase or glutathione-S-transferase a1 were strongly upregulated (D'Angelo et al., 2013). This suggests that Nrf2 signaling is functional in the choroid plexus of young animals, but that not all target genes are equally sensitive at that stage, or share the same kinetic of induction.

Regarding the consequences of inflammatory challenges on efflux transporters, Abcb1 regulation has been investigated in details in freshly isolated rat capillaries (reviewed in Hartz and Bauer, 2010). Its expression and functional activity in adult is differently modulated by short term and long term exposure to pro-inflammatory stimulus. The extent and direction of change in ABCB1 expression is also disease-specific (reviewed in Stolp et al., 2013). During development, inflammation-associated changes in BBB efflux transporters can be stage-dependent. For instance, Abcb1 and Abcg2 efflux function at the BBB increase in response to endothelin-1 in adult, but not in juvenile (21-day-old) rats. This difference may be related to the lower cytokinic response of the BBB to endothelin-1 treatment in juvenile compared to adult animals (Harati et al., 2012b). More work is needed to delineate the role of inflammation in the regulation of efflux transporters at the BBB during development, and the actual window of susceptibility. The choroid plexus is very sensitive to inflammatory challenges, rapidly responding through increased secretion of inflammatory mediators including chemoattractants and pro-inflammatory cytokines. Exposure of the choroidal epithelium *in vitro* to activated immune cells or cytokines leads to a decrease in CSF-to-blood efflux of prostaglandin E_2, a transport process which is likely mediated by SLC and ABC efflux transporters (Khuth et al., 2005; Batisson et al., 2006). Little is known so far on the regulation of efflux transporters *in vivo* at the BCSFB in the context of perinatal inflammation. Changes in such transport mechanisms that set the CSF levels of different biologically active endogenous organic anions including prostanoids may have dramatic consequences for brain development and maturation, and deserves further exploration.

In different peripheral organs such as the liver, exposure to environmental toxicants or food components can activate additional transcription factors belonging to the nuclear factor family, which in turn trigger the induction of protective genes including efflux transporter genes. Among these xenosensors, the aryl hydrocarbon receptor (AhR), the constitutive androstane receptor (CAR), or the pregnane X receptor (PXR) have efflux transporters among their target genes (see Scotto, 2003 for a review of the mechanisms involved). Current knowledge about these nuclear receptors indicates that they are expressed in cells of the blood-brain interfaces in animals and human. AhR is expressed in human brain microvessels, while additional expression of PXR and CAR genes has been reported for the rodent BBB (Dauchy et al., 2008; Hartz and Bauer, 2010). Upon ligand activation, these nuclear factors were shown to induce the expression and/or function of Abcb1, Abcc2, or Abcg2 (reviewed in Hartz and Bauer, 2010). It is still unknown whether nuclear receptors are expressed and modulate efflux transporters at the BBB during development.

In choroid plexus, gene expression can be detected for a wide range of these transcription factors in prenatal, postnatal, and adult stages of rat development, and their role in the coordinated induction of detoxifying enzymes and transporters at the BCSFB has been suggested (Kratzer et al., 2013).

CONCLUSION

The current limited data available in the literature reveal transporter-dependent developmental profiles of expression in blood-brain interfaces both in laboratory animals and in human. The developmental pattern of a given transporter can also differ between the BBB and the BCSFB (**Table 1**). The BCSFB achieves an "adult-like" phenotype earlier than the BBB. For instance, in the latter, Abcb1 displays a major increase in expression postnatally. On the basis of recent studies on early BBB differentiation, we can speculate that neural progenitors and radial glial cells have a major role in triggering the endothelial expression of certain efflux transporters via Wnt and retinoic acid signaling. This would provide some degree of protection against deleterious compounds to the developing brain. Once vascular networks have formed, newly generated astrocytes induce further differentiation of the BBB, through the sonic hedgehog pathway. The concept of barrier immaturity during brain development may therefore hold for selected efflux transporters at the BBB. This novel view of a restricted barrier capacity of the developing brain endothelium is independent from the efficacy of its tight junctions sealing the paracellular pathway, which is established early during prenatal development. It needs to be taken into account when neonatal and pediatric treatments are discussed. The developmental regulation of efflux transporters at the choroid plexus remains obscure. Further work is needed on the signaling cues responsible for specifying the choroidal phenotype of the neuroepithelium and in particular for governing the expression of efflux transporter genes.

A number of choroidal ABC transporters, as well as choroidal and endothelial SLCO transporters display a higher expression or activity in developing animals than in adults. Additional studies, tackling especially the functionality and substrate specificity of these transporters, are necessary to better appreciate the significance of their stage-specific expression.

In the context of developmental diseases, aberrations in one of the signaling pathways that induce efflux transporter-dependent protective functions in blood-brain interfaces may lead to substantial changes in fetal/neonatal brain exposure to undesired substrates, and subsequently alter normal brain development.

Choroid plexus studies suggest that from early on during development, brain efflux may be enhanced following exposure to xenobiotic inducers including drugs and environmental toxins. The modulation of efflux transporter expression and function by oxidative stress and inflammation often associated with perinatal injuries deserves further investigation. A better understanding of the regulatory pathways, in particular the relative contribution of the different transcription factors sensing oxidative stress or xenobiotics during development, is clinically relevant. It may open new opportunities for therapeutic manipulation designed to improve or restore blood-brain interface neuroprotective functions in the context of perinatal injuries.

ACKNOWLEDGMENTS

This work was supported by ANR-10-IBHU-0003 Cesame grant and by the European Union Seventh Framework Program under grant agreement No. HEALTH-F2-2009-241778 Neurobid

REFERENCES

Abbott, N. J., Ronnback, L., and Hansson, E. (2006). Astrocyte-endothelial interactions at the blood-brain barrier. *Nat. Rev. Neurosci.* 7, 41–53. doi: 10.1038/nrn1824

Aden, U., Favrais, G., Plaisant, F., Winerdal, M., Felderhoff-Mueser, U., Lampa, J., et al. (2010). Systemic inflammation sensitizes the neonatal brain to excitotoxicity through a pro-/anti-inflammatory imbalance: key role of TNFalpha pathway and protection by etanercept. *Brain. Behav. Immun.* 24, 747–758. doi: 10.1016/j.bbi.2009.10.010

Alebouyeh, M., Takeda, M., Onozato, M. L., Tojo, A., Noshiro, R., Hasannejad, H., et al. (2003). Expression of human organic anion transporters in the choroid plexus and their interactions with neurotransmitter metabolites. *J. Pharmacol. Sci.* 93, 430–436. doi: 10.1254/jphs.93.430

Alvarez, J. I., Dodelet-Devillers, A., Kebir, H., Ifergan, I., Fabre, P. J., Terouz, S., et al. (2011). The Hedgehog pathway promotes blood-brain barrier integrity and CNS immune quiescence. *Science* 334, 1727–1731. doi: 10.1126/science.1206936

Angeletti, R. H., Bergwerk, A. J., Novikoff, P. M., and Wolkoff, A. W. (1998). Dichotomous development of the organic anion transport protein in liver and choroid plexus. *Am. J. Physiol.* 275, C882–C887.

Armulik, A., Genove, G., Mae, M., Nisancioglu, M. H., Wallgard, E., Niaudet, C., et al. (2010). Pericytes regulate the blood-brain barrier. *Nature* 468, 557–561. doi: 10.1038/nature09522

Baello, S., Iqbal, M., Bloise, E., Javam, M., Gibb, W., and Matthews, S. G. (2014). TGF-beta1 regulation of multidrug resistance P-glycoprotein in the developing male blood-brain barrier. *Endocrinology* 155, 475–484. doi: 10.1210/en.2013-1472

Batisson, M., Strazielle, N., Hejmadi, M., Thomas, D., Ghersi-Egea, J. F., Etienne, J., et al. (2006). Toxic shock syndrome toxin-1 challenges the neuroprotective functions of the choroidal epithelium and induces neurotoxicity. *J. Infect. Dis.* 194, 341–349. doi: 10.1086/505428

Bauer, H. C., and Bauer, H. (2000). Neural induction of the blood-brain barrier: still an enigma. *Cell. Mol. Neurobiol.* 20, 13–28. doi: 10.1023/A:1006939825857

Betz, A. L., and Goldstein, G. W. (1981). Developmental changes in metabolism and transport properties of capillaries isolated from rat brain. *J. Physiol.* 312, 365–376. doi: 10.1113/jphysiol.1981.sp013633

Bronger, H., Konig, J., Kopplow, K., Steiner, H. H., Ahmadi, R., Herold-Mende, C., et al. (2005). ABCC drug efflux pumps and organic anion uptake transporters in human gliomas and the blood-tumor barrier. *Cancer Res.* 65, 11419–11428. doi: 10.1158/0008-5472.CAN-05-1271

Caley, D. W., and Maxwell, D. S. (1970). Development of the blood vessels and extracellular spaces during postnatal maturation of rat cerebral cortex. *J. Comp. Neurol.* 138, 31–47. doi: 10.1002/cne.901380104

Cooray, H. C., Blackmore, C. G., Maskell, L., and Barrand, M. A. (2002). Localisation of breast cancer resistance protein in microvessel endothelium of human brain. *Neuroreport* 13, 2059–2063. doi: 10.1097/00001756-200211150-00014

Daneman, R., Zhou, L., Agalliu, D., Cahoy, J. D., Kaushal, A., and Barres, B. A. (2010a). The mouse blood-brain barrier transcriptome: a new resource for understanding the development and function of brain endothelial cells. *PLoS ONE* 5:e13741. doi: 10.1371/journal.pone.0013741

Daneman, R., Zhou, L., Kebede, A. A., and Barres, B. A. (2010b). Pericytes are required for blood-brain barrier integrity during embryogenesis. *Nature* 468, 562–566. doi: 10.1038/nature09513

D'Angelo, B., Ek, C. J., Sandberg, M., and Mallard, C. (2013). Expression of the Nrf2-system at the blood-CSF barrier is modulated by neonatal inflammation and hypoxia-ischemia. *J. Inherit. Metab. Dis.* 36, 479–490. doi: 10.1007/s10545-012-9551-5

Daniel, H., and Rubio-Aliaga, I. (2003). An update on renal peptide transporters. *Am. J. Physiol. Renal Physiol.* 284, F885–F892. doi: 10.1152/ajprenal.00123.2002

Daood, M., Tsai, C., Ahdab-Barmada, M., and Watchko, J. F. (2008). ABC transporter (P-gp/ABCB1, MRP1/ABCC1, BCRP/ABCG2) expression in the developing human CNS. *Neuropediatrics* 39, 211–218. doi: 10.1055/s-0028-1103272

Dauchy, S., Dutheil, F., Weaver, R. J., Chassoux, F., Daumas-Duport, C., Couraud, P. O., et al. (2008). ABC transporters, cytochromes P450 and their main transcription factors: expression at the human blood-brain barrier. *J. Neurochem.* 107, 1518–1528. doi: 10.1111/j.1471-4159.2008.05720.x

Ek, C. J., Wong, A., Liddelow, S. A., Johansson, P. A., Dziegielewska, K. M., and Saunders, N. R. (2010). Efflux mechanisms at the developing brain barriers: ABC-transporters in the fetal and postnatal rat. *Toxicol. Lett.* 197, 51–59. doi: 10.1016/j.toxlet.2010.04.025

Fenart, L., Buee-Scherrer, V., Descamps, L., Duhem, C., Poullain, M. G., Cecchelli, R., et al. (1998). Inhibition of P-glycoprotein: rapid assessment of its implication in blood-brain barrier integrity and drug transport to the brain by an *in vitro* model of the blood-brain barrier. *Pharm. Res.* 15, 993–1000. doi: 10.1023/A:1011913723928

Ferriero, D. M. (2001). Oxidant mechanisms in neonatal hypoxia-ischemia. *Dev. Neurosci.* 23, 198–202. doi: 10.1159/000046143

Gaillard, P. J., Van Der Sandt, I. C., Voorwinden, L. H., Vu, D., Nielsen, J. L., De Boer, A. G., et al. (2000). Astrocytes increase the functional expression of P-glycoprotein in an *in vitro* model of the blood-brain barrier. *Pharm. Res.* 17, 1198–1205. doi: 10.1023/A:1026406528530

Gao, B., Hagenbuch, B., Kullak-Ublick, G. A., Benke, D., Aguzzi, A., and Meier, P. J. (2000). Organic anion-transporting polypeptides mediate transport of opioid peptides across blood-brain barrier. *J. Pharmacol. Exp. Ther.* 294, 73–79.

Gao, B., Stieger, B., Noe, B., Fritschy, J. M., and Meier, P. J. (1999). Localization of the organic anion transporting polypeptide 2 (Oatp2) in capillary endothelium and choroid plexus epithelium of rat brain. *J. Histochem. Cytochem.* 47, 1255–1264. doi: 10.1177/002215549904701005

Gazzin, S., Berengeno, A. L., Strazielle, N., Fazzari, F., Raseni, A., Ostrow, J. D., et al. (2011). Modulation of Mrp1 (ABCc1) and Pgp (ABCb1) by bilirubin at the blood-CSF and blood-brain barriers in the Gunn rat. *PLoS ONE* 6:e16165. doi: 10.1371/journal.pone.0016165

Gazzin, S., Strazielle, N., Schmitt, C., Fevre-Montange, M., Ostrow, J. D., Tiribelli, C., et al. (2008). Differential expression of the multidrug resistance-related proteins ABCb1 and ABCc1 between blood-brain interfaces. *J. Comp. Neurol.* 510, 497–507. doi: 10.1002/cne.21808

Ghersi-Egea, J. F., Monkkonen, K. S., Schmitt, C., Honnorat, J., Fevre-Montange, M., and Strazielle, N. (2009). Blood-brain interfaces and cerebral drug bioavailability. *Rev. Neurol. (Paris)* 165, 1029–1038. doi: 10.1016/j.neurol.2009.09.011

Ghersi-Egea, J. F., Strazielle, N., Murat, A., Jouvet, A., Buenerd, A., and Belin, M. F. (2006). Brain protection at the blood-cerebrospinal fluid interface involves a glutathione-dependent metabolic barrier mechanism. *J. Cereb. Blood Flow Metab.* 26, 1165–1175. doi: 10.1038/sj.jcbfm.9600267

Goralski, K. B., Acott, P. D., Fraser, A. D., Worth, D., and Sinal, C. J. (2006). Brain cyclosporin A levels are determined by ontogenic regulation of mdr1a expression. *Drug. Metab. Dispos.* 34, 288–295. doi: 10.1124/dmd.105.007427

Hagenbuch, B., and Stieger, B. (2013). The SLCO (former SLC21) superfamily of transporters. *Mol. Aspects Med.* 34, 396–412. doi: 10.1016/j.mam.2012.10.009

Harati, R., Benech, H., Villegier, A. S., and Mabondzo, A. (2012a). P-glycoprotein, breast cancer resistance protein, Organic Anion Transporter 3, and Transporting Peptide 1a4 during blood-brain barrier maturation: involvement of Wnt/beta-catenin and endothelin-1 signaling. *Mol. Pharm.* 10, 1566–1580. doi: 10.1021/mp300334r

Harati, R., Villegier, A. S., Banks, W. A., and Mabondzo, A. (2012b). Susceptibility of juvenile and adult blood-brain barrier to endothelin-1: regulation of P-glycoprotein and breast cancer resistance protein expression and transport activity. *J. Neuroinflammation* 9, 273. doi: 10.1186/1742-2094-9-273

Hartz, A. M., and Bauer, B. (2010). Regulation of ABC transporters at the blood-brain barrier: new targets for CNS therapy. *Mol. Interv.* 10, 293–304. doi: 10.1124/mi.10.5.6

Huber, R. D., Gao, B., Sidler Pfandler, M. A., Zhang-Fu, W., Leuthold, S., Hagenbuch, B., et al. (2007). Characterization of two splice variants of human organic anion transporting polypeptide 3A1 isolated from human brain. *Am. J. Physiol. Cell Physiol.* 292, C795–C806. doi: 10.1152/ajpcell.00597.2005

Kaindl, A. M., Favrais, G., and Gressens, P. (2009). Molecular mechanisms involved in injury to the preterm brain. *J. Child Neurol.* 24, 1112–1118. doi: 10.1177/0883073809337920

Keller, A. (2013). Breaking and building the wall: the biology of the blood-brain barrier in health and disease. *Swiss Med. Wkly* 143:w13892. doi: 10.4414/smw.2013.13892

Khuth, S. T., Strazielle, N., Giraudon, P., Belin, M. F., and Ghersi-Egea, J. F. (2005). Impairment of blood-cerebrospinal fluid barrier properties by retrovirus-activated T lymphocytes: reduction in cerebrospinal fluid-to-blood efflux of prostaglandin E2. *J. Neurochem.* 94, 1580–1593. doi: 10.1111/j.1471-4159.2005.03309.x

Kikuchi, R., Kusuhara, H., Sugiyama, D., and Sugiyama, Y. (2003). Contribution of organic anion transporter 3 (Slc22a8) to the elimination of p-aminohippuric acid and benzylpenicillin across the blood-brain barrier. *J. Pharmacol. Exp. Ther.* 306, 51–58. doi: 10.1124/jpet.103.049197

Koepsell, H. (2013). The SLC22 family with transporters of organic cations, anions and zwitterions. *Mol. Aspects Med.* 34, 413–435. doi: 10.1016/j.mam.2012.10.010

Kratzer, I., Liddelow, S. A., Saunders, N. R., Dziegielewska, K. M., Strazielle, N., and Ghersi-Egea, J. F. (2013). Developmental changes in the transcriptome of the rat choroid plexus in relation to neuroprotection. *Fluids Barriers CNS* 10:25. doi: 10.1186/2045-8118-10-25

Kratzer, I., Vasiljevic, A., Rey, C., Fevre-Montange, M., Saunders, N., Strazielle, N., et al. (2012). Complexity and developmental changes in the expression pattern of claudins at the blood-CSF barrier. *Histochem. Cell. Biol.* 138, 861–879. doi: 10.1007/s00418-012-1001-9

Kubota, H., Ishihara, H., Langmann, T., Schmitz, G., Stieger, B., Wieser, H. G., et al. (2006). Distribution and functional activity of P-glycoprotein and multidrug resistance-associated proteins in human brain microvascular endothelial cells in hippocampal sclerosis. *Epilepsy Res.* 68, 213–228. doi: 10.1016/j.eplepsyres.2005.11.011

Kusuhara, H., He, Z., Nagata, Y., Nozaki, Y., Ito, T., Masuda, H., et al. (2003). Expression and functional involvement of organic anion transporting polypeptide subtype 3 (Slc21a7) in rat choroid plexus. *Pharm. Res.* 20, 720–727. doi: 10.1023/A:1023473216759

Landrigan, P. J., and Goldman, L. R. (2011). Children's vulnerability to toxic chemicals: a challenge and opportunity to strengthen health and environmental policy. *Health Aff. (Millwood)* 30, 842–850. doi: 10.1377/hlthaff.2011.0151

Leggas, M., Adachi, M., Scheffer, G. L., Sun, D., Wielinga, P., Du, G., et al. (2004). Mrp4 confers resistance to topotecan and protects the brain from chemotherapy. *Mol. Cell Biol.* 24, 7612–7621. doi: 10.1128/MCB.24.17.7612-7621.2004

Leslie, E. M., Deeley, R. G., and Cole, S. P. (2005). Multidrug resistance proteins: role of P-glycoprotein, MRP1, MRP2, and BCRP (ABCG2) in tissue defense. *Toxicol. Appl. Pharmacol.* 204, 216–237. doi: 10.1016/j.taap.2004.10.012

Liddelow, S. A., Dziegielewska, K. M., Ek, C. J., Habgood, M. D., Bauer, H., Bauer, H. C., et al. (2013). Mechanisms that determine the internal environment of the developing brain: a transcriptomic, functional and ultrastructural approach. *PLoS ONE* 8:e65629. doi: 10.1371/journal.pone.0065629

Liebner, S., Czupalla, C. J., and Wolburg, H. (2011). Current concepts of blood-brain barrier development. *Int. J. Dev. Biol.* 55, 467–476. doi: 10.1387/ijdb.103224sl

Lim, J. C., Kania, K. D., Wijesuriya, H., Chawla, S., Sethi, J. K., Pulaski, L., et al. (2008). Activation of beta-catenin signalling by GSK-3 inhibition increases p-glycoprotein expression in brain endothelial cells. *J. Neurochem.* 106, 1855–1865. doi: 10.1111/j.1471-4159.2008.05537.x

Martin, V., Xu, J., Pabbisetty, S. K., Alonso, M. M., Liu, D., Lee, O. H., et al. (2009). Tie2-mediated multidrug resistance in malignant gliomas is associated with upregulation of ABC transporters. *Oncogene* 28, 2358–2363. doi: 10.1038/onc.2009.103

Matsuoka, Y., Okazaki, M., Kitamura, Y., and Taniguchi, T. (1999). Developmental expression of P-glycoprotein (multidrug resistance gene product) in the rat brain. *J. Neurobiol.* 39, 383–392.

Miodovnik, A. (2011). Environmental neurotoxicants and developing brain. *Mt. Sinai J. Med.* 78, 58–77. doi: 10.1002/msj.20237

Mizee, M. R., Wooldrik, D., Lakeman, K. A., Van Het Hof, B., Drexhage, J. A., Geerts, D., et al. (2013). Retinoic acid induces blood-brain barrier development. *J. Neurosci.* 33, 1660–1671. doi: 10.1523/JNEUROSCI.1338-12.2013

Mori, S., Takanaga, H., Ohtsuki, S., Deguchi, T., Kang, Y. S., Hosoya, K., et al. (2003). Rat organic anion transporter 3 (rOAT3) is responsible for brain-to-blood efflux of homovanillic acid at the abluminal membrane of brain capillary endothelial cells. *J. Cereb. Blood Flow Metab.* 23, 432–440. doi: 10.1097/00004647-200304000-00007

Nagata, Y., Kusuhara, H., Endou, H., and Sugiyama, Y. (2002). Expression and functional characterization of rat organic anion transporter 3 (rOat3) in the choroid plexus. *Mol. Pharmacol.* 61, 982–988. doi: 10.1124/mol.61.5.982

Nehlig, A., Pereira De Vasconcelos, A., and Boyet, S. (1989). Postnatal changes in local cerebral blood flow measured by the quantitative autoradiographic [14C]iodoantipyrine technique in freely moving rats. *J. Cereb. Blood Flow. Metab.* 9, 579–588. doi: 10.1038/jcbfm.1989.83

Niehof, M., and Borlak, J. (2009). Expression of HNF4alpha in the human and rat choroid plexus: implications for drug transport across the blood-cerebrospinal-fluid (CSF) barrier. *BMC Mol. Biol.* 10:68. doi: 10.1186/1471-2199-10-68

Nishino, J., Suzuki, H., Sugiyama, D., Kitazawa, T., Ito, K., Hanano, M., et al. (1999). Transepithelial transport of organic anions across the choroid plexus: possible involvement of organic anion transporter and multidrug resistance-associated protein. *J. Pharmacol. Exp. Ther.* 290, 289–294.

Ohtsuki, S., Takizawa, T., Takanaga, H., Terasaki, N., Kitazawa, T., Sasaki, M., et al. (2003). *In vitro* study of the functional expression of organic anion transporting polypeptide 3 at rat choroid plexus epithelial cells and its involvement in the cerebrospinal fluid-to-blood transport of estrone-3-sulfate. *Mol. Pharmacol.* 63, 532–537. doi: 10.1124/mol.63.3.532

Orford, M., Mean, R., Lapathitis, G., Genethliou, N., Panayiotou, E., Panayi, H., et al. (2009). Generation of an ABCG2(GFPn-puro) transgenic line–a tool to study ABCG2 expression in mice. *Biochem. Biophys. Res. Commun.* 384, 199–203. doi: 10.1016/j.bbrc.2009.04.089

Ose, A., Ito, M., Kusuhara, H., Yamatsugu, K., Kanai, M., Shibasaki, M., et al. (2009). Limited brain distribution of [3R,4R,5S]-4-acetamido-5-amino-3-(1-ethylpropoxy)-1-cyclohexene-1-carboxylate phosphate (Ro 64-0802), a pharmacologically active form of oseltamivir, by active efflux across the blood-brain barrier mediated by organic anion transporter 3 (Oat3/Slc22a8) and multidrug resistance-associated protein 4 (Mrp4/Abcc4). *Drug Metab. Dispos.* 37, 315–321. doi: 10.1124/dmd.108.024018

Petropoulos, S., Gibb, W., and Matthews, S. G. (2010). Developmental expression of multidrug resistance phosphoglycoprotein (P-gp) in the mouse fetal brain and glucocorticoid regulation. *Brain Res.* 1357, 9–18. doi: 10.1016/j.brainres.2010.08.016

Qin, Y., and Sato, T. N. (1995). Mouse multidrug resistance 1a/3 gene is the earliest known endothelial cell differentiation marker during blood-brain barrier development. *Dev. Dyn.* 202, 172–180. doi: 10.1002/aja.1002020209

Reichel, V., Burghard, S., John, I., and Huber, O. (2011). P-glycoprotein and breast cancer resistance protein expression and function at the blood-brain barrier and blood-cerebrospinal fluid barrier (choroid plexus) in streptozotocin-induced diabetes in rats. *Brain Res.* 1370, 238–245. doi: 10.1016/j.brainres.2010.11.012

Roberts, L. M., Black, D. S., Raman, C., Woodford, K., Zhou, M., Haggerty, J. E., et al. (2008). Subcellular localization of transporters along the rat blood-brain barrier and blood-cerebral-spinal fluid barrier by *in vivo* biotinylation. *Neuroscience* 155, 423–438. doi: 10.1016/j.neuroscience.2008.06.015

Schinkel, A. H., and Jonker, J. W. (2003). Mammalian drug efflux transporters of the ATP binding cassette (ABC) family: an overview. *Adv. Drug Deliv. Rev.* 55, 3–29. doi: 10.1016/S0169-409X(02)00169-2

Schinkel, A. H., Wagenaar, E., Mol, C. A., and Van Deemter, L. (1996). P-glycoprotein in the blood-brain barrier of mice influences the brain penetration and pharmacological activity of many drugs. *J. Clin. Invest.* 97, 2517–2524. doi: 10.1172/JCI118699

Schumacher, U., and Mollgard, K. (1997). The multidrug-resistance P-glycoprotein (Pgp, MDR1) is an early marker of blood-brain barrier development in the microvessels of the developing human brain. *Histochem. Cell Biol.* 108, 179–182. doi: 10.1007/s004180050159

Scotto, K. W. (2003). Transcriptional regulation of ABC drug transporters. *Oncogene* 22, 7496–7511. doi: 10.1038/sj.onc.1206950

Shawahna, R., Uchida, Y., Decleves, X., Ohtsuki, S., Yousif, S., Dauchy, S., et al. (2011). Transcriptomic and quantitative proteomic analysis of transporters and drug metabolizing enzymes in freshly isolated human brain microvessels. *Mol. Pharm.* 8, 1332–1341. doi: 10.1021/mp200129p

Shen, H., Smith, D. E., Keep, R. F., and Brosius, F. C. III. (2004). Immunolocalization of the proton-coupled oligopeptide transporter PEPT2 in developing rat brain. *Mol. Pharm.* 1, 248–256. doi: 10.1021/mp049944b

Sims-Mourtada, J., Izzo, J. G., Ajani, J., and Chao, K. S. (2007). Sonic Hedgehog promotes multiple drug resistance by regulation of drug transport. *Oncogene* 26, 5674–5679. doi: 10.1038/sj.onc.1210356

Singh, R. R., Kunkalla, K., Qu, C., Schlette, E., Neelapu, S. S., Samaniego, F., et al. (2011). ABCG2 is a direct transcriptional target of hedgehog signaling and involved in stroma-induced drug tolerance in diffuse large B-cell lymphoma. *Oncogene* 30, 4874–4886. doi: 10.1038/onc.2011.195

Staud, F., and Pavek, P. (2005). Breast cancer resistance protein (BCRP/ABCG2). *Int. J. Biochem. Cell Biol.* 37, 720–725. doi: 10.1016/j.biocel.2004.11.004

Stolp, H. B., Liddelow, S. A., Sa-Pereira, I., Dziegielewska, K. M., and Saunders, N. R. (2013). Immune responses at brain barriers and implications for brain development and neurological function in later life. *Front. Integr. Neurosci.* 7:61. doi: 10.3389/fnint.2013.00061

Strazielle, N., Belin, M. F., and Ghersi-Egea, J. F. (2003). Choroid plexus controls brain availability of anti-HIV nucleoside analogs via pharmacologically inhibitable organic anion transporters. *AIDS* 17, 1473–1485. doi: 10.1097/00002030-200307040-00008

Strazielle, N., and Ghersi-Egea, J. F. (1999). Demonstration of a coupled metabolism-efflux process at the choroid plexus as a mechanism of brain protection toward xenobiotics. *J. Neurosci.* 19, 6275–6289.

Strazielle, N., and Ghersi-Egea, J. F. (2005). Factors affecting delivery of antiviral drugs to the brain. *Rev. Med. Virol.* 15, 105–133. doi: 10.1002/rmv.454

Strazielle, N., and Ghersi-Egea, J. F. (2013). Physiology of blood-brain interfaces in relation to brain disposition of small compounds and macromolecules. *Mol. Pharm.* 10, 1473–1491. doi: 10.1021/mp300518e

Tachikawa, M., Watanabe, M., Hori, S., Fukaya, M., Ohtsuki, S., Asashima, T., et al. (2005). Distinct spatio-temporal expression of ABCA and ABCG transporters in the developing and adult mouse brain. *J. Neurochem.* 95, 294–304. doi: 10.1111/j.1471-4159.2005.03369.x

Takashima, T., Yokoyama, C., Mizuma, H., Yamanaka, H., Wada, Y., Onoe, K., et al. (2011). Developmental changes in P-glycoprotein function in the blood-brain barrier of nonhuman primates: PET study with R-11C-verapamil and 11C-oseltamivir. *J. Nucl. Med.* 52, 950–957. doi: 10.2967/jnumed.110.083949

Tsai, C. E., Daood, M. J., Lane, R. H., Hansen, T. W., Gruetzmacher, E. M., and Watchko, J. F. (2002). P-glycoprotein expression in mouse brain increases with maturation. *Biol. Neonate* 81, 58–64. doi: 10.1159/000047185

Virgintino, D., Errede, M., Girolamo, F., Capobianco, C., Robertson, D., Vimercati, A., et al. (2008). Fetal blood-brain barrier P-glycoprotein contributes to brain protection during human development. *J. Neuropathol. Exp. Neurol.* 67, 50–61. doi: 10.1097/nen.0b013e31815f65d9

Wang, X., Campos, C. R., Peart, J. C., Smith, L. K., Boni, J. L., Cannon, R. E., et al. (2014). Nrf2 upregulates ATP binding cassette transporter expression and activity at the blood-brain and blood-spinal cord barriers. *J. Neurosci.* 34, 8585–8593. doi: 10.1523/JNEUROSCI.2935-13.2014

Westerhout, J., Danhof, M., and De Lange, E. C. (2011). Preclinical prediction of human brain target site concentrations: considerations in extrapolating to the clinical setting. *J. Pharm. Sci.* 100, 3577–3593. doi: 10.1002/jps.22604

Wijnholds, J., Delange, E. C., Scheffer, G. L., Van Den Berg, D. J., Mol, C. A., Van Der Valk, M., et al. (2000). Multidrug resistance protein 1 protects the choroid plexus epithelium and contributes to the blood-cerebrospinal fluid barrier. *J. Clin. Invest.* 105, 279–285. doi: 10.1172/JCI8267

Xiang, J., Alesi, G. N., Zhou, N., and Keep, R. F. (2012). Protective effects of isothiocyanates on blood-CSF barrier disruption induced by oxidative stress. *Am. J. Physiol. Regul. Integr. Comp. Physiol.* 303, R1–R7. doi: 10.1152/ajpregu.00518.2011

Yamada, T., Takaoka, A. S., Naishiro, Y., Hayashi, R., Maruyama, K., Maesawa, C., et al. (2000). Transactivation of the multidrug resistance 1 gene by T-cell factor 4/beta-catenin complex in early colorectal carcinogenesis. *Cancer Res.* 60, 4761–4766.

Zhuang, Y., Fraga, C. H., Hubbard, K. E., Hagedorn, N., Panetta, J. C., Waters, C. M., et al. (2006). Topotecan central nervous system penetration is altered by a tyrosine kinase inhibitor. *Cancer Res.* 66, 11305–11313. doi: 10.1158/0008-5472.CAN-06-0929

3

Neurogenic niches in the brain: help and hindrance of the barrier systems

Helen B. Stolp[1]* and Zoltán Molnár[2]

[1] Division of Biomedical Engineering and Health Sciences, Department of Perinatal Imaging and Health, King's College London, London, UK
[2] Department of Physiology, Anatomy and Genetics, University of Oxford, Oxford, UK

Correspondence:
Helen B. Stolp, Department of Perinatal Imaging and Health, Level 1, 1st Floor, South Wing, St Thomas' Hospital, King's College London, London, SE1 7EH, UK
e-mail: helen.stolp@kcl.ac.uk

In the developing central nervous system, most neurogenesis occurs in the ventricular and subventricular proliferative zones. In the adult telencephalon, neurogenesis contracts to the subependyma zone and the dentate gyrus (subgranular zone) of the hippocampus. These restricted niches containing progenitor cells which divide to produce neurons or glia, depending on the intrinsic and environmental cues. Neurogenic niches are characterized by a comparatively high vascular density and, in many cases, interaction with the cerebrospinal fluid (CSF). Both the vasculature and the CSF represent a source of signaling molecules, which can be relatively rapidly modulated by external factors and circulated through the central nervous system. As the brain develops, there is vascular remodeling and a compartmentalization and dynamic modification of the ventricular surface which may be responsible for the change in the proliferative properties. This review will explore the relationship between progenitor cells and the developing vascular and ventricular space. In particular the signaling systems employed to control proliferation, and the consequence of abnormal vascular or ventricular development on growth of the telencephalon. It will also discuss the potential significance of the barriers at the vascular and ventricular junctions in the influence of the proliferative niches.

Keywords: neurogenesis, neuronal progenitors, neurogenic niche, blood-brain barrier, cerebrovasculature, cerebrospinal fluid, choroid plexus

INTRODUCTION

It is essential that an organ and its blood supply should develop together in synchrony to allow optimal conditions for the different stages of growth, differentiation and changing functional requirements. This co-dependence is particularly evident in the brain, where the vascular network originates from the peri-neural vascular plexus in early embryonic development and undergoes multiple stages of remodeling to meet the changing needs of the complex developing environment (Bautch and James, 2009). Barrier functions of the neurovasculature start from the earliest stages of development and are coupled with other aspects of vascular and neuro development (Ruhrberg and Bautch, 2013).

Close examination of developing brain has led to the hypothesis that signals from the brain parenchyma itself regulate the sites of penetrance by the pioneering vascular branches from the peri-neural plexus, and there is now increasing evidence that variations in normal brain growth can alter the vasculature (Vasudevan et al., 2008) in the same way that altered vascular development affects neural patterning (Javaherian and Kriegstein, 2009). This is, at least partly, due to the presence of a variety of co-signaling systems, e.g., vascular endothelial growth factor (VEGF), Notch, Sonic Hedgehog (Shh) and their receptors, which clearly have a role in both the developing neural system as well as the developing vascular system. The involvement of signaling molecules in the neural and vascular systems, while implying close interaction between vascular and neural development, also makes independent manipulation of the systems difficult, and therefore determination of cause and effect in vascular and neural developmental processes is an intractable issue.

During development, the primary regions of proliferation are the ventricular and subventricular zones (VZ and SVZ, respectively, see **Figure 1**). These are substantive pools of progenitor cells which over time gradually become restricted in their differentiation capacity, and which ultimately produce the diverse neuronal populations of the brain as well as most of the glial cells. In the adult brain (see **Figure 2**), the proliferative zones are confined to two main areas of the brain, the subependymal zone (SEZ, also called the adult SVZ) and the subgranular zone (SGZ), and the progenitor cells have a more restricted potential fate.

The relationship between neural progenitors and the vasculature has been extensively described, for both the adult SEZ (Shen et al., 2008), and SGZ (Palmer et al., 2000), as well as for the SVZ in the developing cerebral cortex (Stubbs et al., 2009) and developing rostral migratory stream (Nie et al., 2010). In all cases, a clustering of progenitor cells in close proximity with the cerebral endothelial cells was found to occur to at a greater frequency that expected by chance. This observation has led to the hypothesis that the endothelial cells provide a support for the neural progenitors, either structural or chemical, a concept that is

Abbreviations: CSF, cerebrospinal fluid; SEZ, subependymal zone/also called the adult SVZ; SGZ, subgranular zone; Shh, sonic hedgehog; Smo, smoothened receptor; SVZ, subventricular zone; VCAM, vascular cell adhesion molecule; VEGF, vascular endothelial growth factor; VZ, ventricular zone.

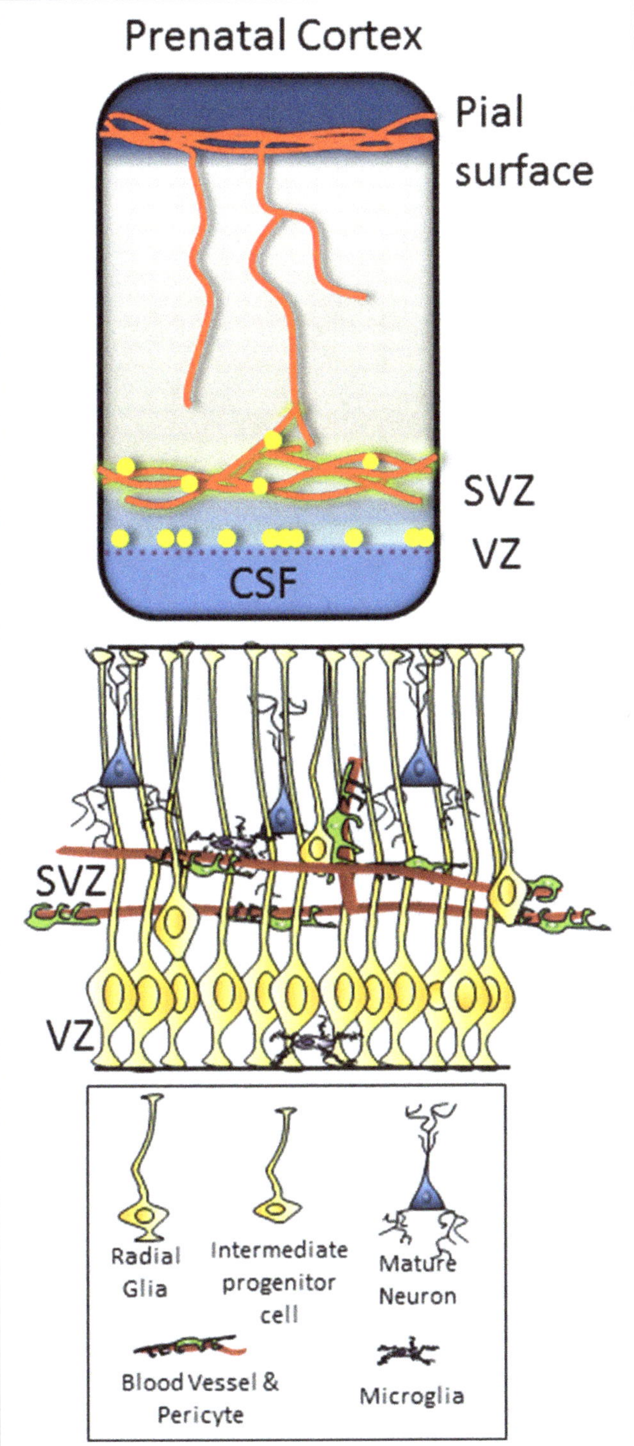

FIGURE 1 | Dorsal telencephalon in the fetus, showing pial and ventricular vascular plexi and the location of the VZ and SVZ progenitor zones. Microstructure and cellular component of the VZ and SVZ illustrated below, with VZ progenitors contacting the ventricular surface of the brain and SVZ progenitors in close contact with the vascular plexus.

now supported by substantial evidence and is discussed in detail below.

The structure and location of the proliferative zones suggest a second regulator of the neurogenic niche, the cerebrospinal fluid (CSF). Both the VZ in the developing brain and the SEZ in the adult have close association with the ventricular surface and the CSF. Therefore, in addition to proliferative support from the cerebrovasculature, trophic regulation/modulation is thought to come from the CSF (Dziegielewska et al., 2000).

The vasculature in the brain is specialized compared to that of the rest of the body. The presence of the blood-brain barrier means there is a tighter control of brain microenvironment as there is limited paracellular transport and reduced vesicular transport of molecules from the blood into the brain. The composition of the CSF is also tightly controlled, in this case by the choroid plexus. The presence of a structural and functional barrier at the epithelial interface of the choroid plexus with the CSF is an essential element of this control. During development, the composition of the CSF is very dynamic, and is considered to be an important for the regulation of a number of neurodevelopmental processed. The specifics of CSF composition regulation and the role of the blood-CSF barrier is beyond the scope of this work, readers are directed to recent reviews by Bueno et al. (2014) and Johansson (2014).

Very few studies have assessed whether the brain barriers actively control progenitor proliferation in neurogenic niches within the brain, but it is likely that at the least the presence of these barriers make an important contribution to the signaling environment of the neurovascular niches. In the case of the VZ, the developmental barrier between the brain and the CSF (Mollgard et al., 1987) may also contribute directly to the proliferative environment.

In this review we will explore the intertwined development of the vasculature and the progenitor pools in the developing brain, the signaling systems common to all neurogenic niches and whether the brain- barrier systems at the endothelial cell and ventricular surface contribute to the control of these specialized brain regions.

REGULATION OF VASCULAR GROWTH AND BARRIER FORMATION IN THE BRAIN

The blood vessel ingrowth from the peri-neural plexus (as shown in **Figure 1**) to the brain parenchyma is regulated by a number of signaling cues from the parenchyma itself. VEGF signaling is of particular importance, with James et al. (2009) showing that the stereotypical pattern of vascular ingrowth into the neural tube can be disrupted by local over expression of VEGF isotypes (causing ectopic vessel ingrowth) or the VEGF receptor Flt1 (which reduces angiogenesis).

Vasudevan et al. (2008) have shown that the formation of the vascular plexus in the cortex is guided by the neural transcription factors that regulate the proliferation in the pallium and subpallium (e.g., Pax6, Nkx2.1, Dlx1/2). They also put forward the idea that vascular plexi of different origin (e.g., ventral pallium or peri-neural plexus) are differentially controlled by the local proliferative transcription factors. This interplay between neural cells and the vasculature does not stop at proliferative stages of brain growth. The radial migration of vessels from the vascular plexus through the cortex in the human brain appears to be regulated by cxcl12/cxcr4/cxcr7 signaling between the vessels, the radial glial and the perivascular astrocytes (Virgintino et al., 2013). The cxcl12 signaling system appears to be key in regulating

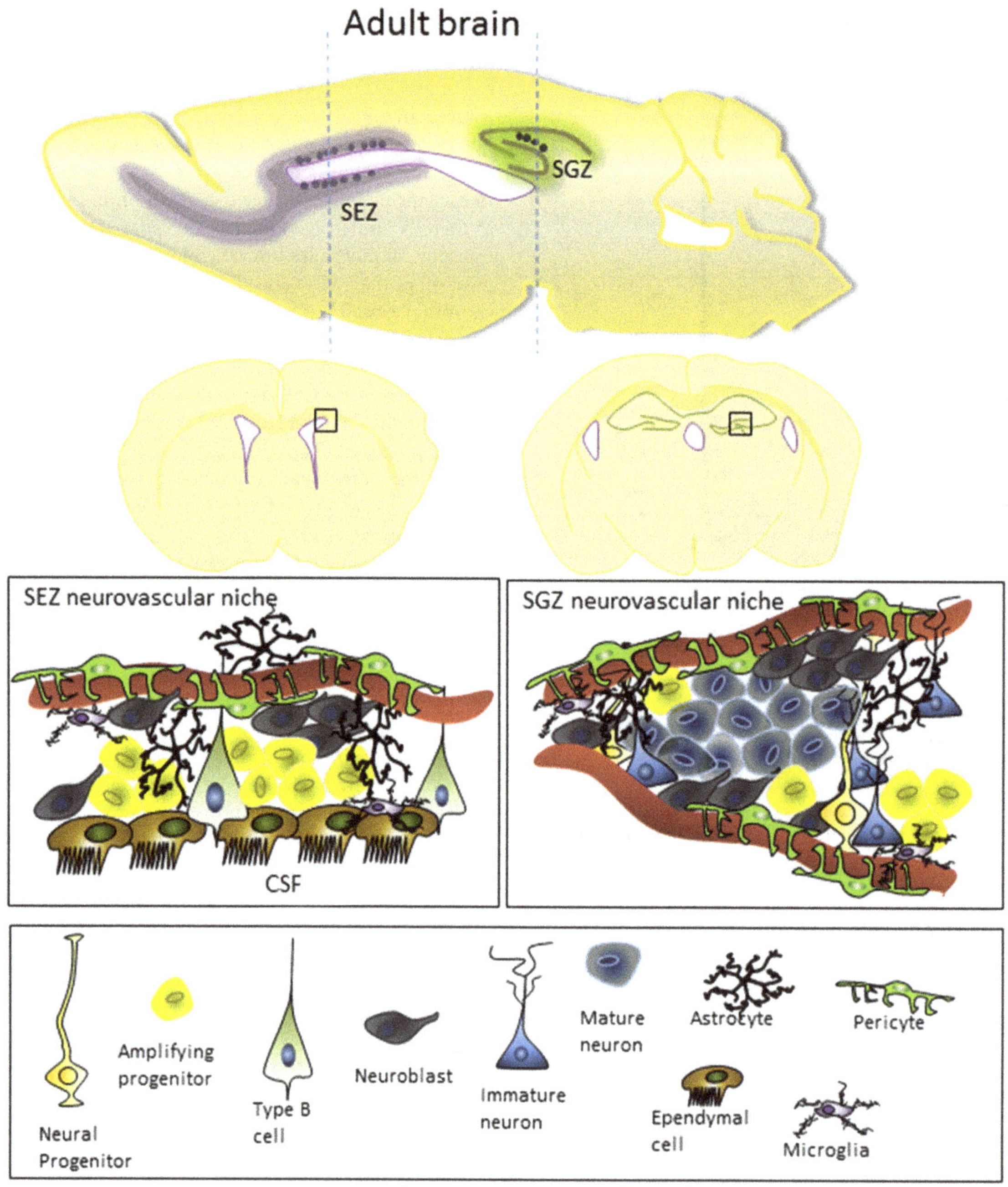

FIGURE 2 | Adult cortex in the mouse, shown from both sagittal and coronal views, indicating the location of the SEZ and SGZ neurovascular niches. The microstructure and cellular component of the SEZ and SGZ are shown underneath. In the SEZ, progenitor cells are in close contact with the CSF and ventricular ependymal cells as well as the vasculature, while the SGZ is restricted to influences from the vasculature. For details on the cell types involved and the molecular characteristics of these cells see the recent review from Fuentealba et al. (2012).

many migratory processes in the developing brain, and is probably also involved in controlling progenitor differentiation and migration (discussed below).

Sonic hedgehog (Shh) is a major signaling molecule that regulates both vascular and neural development and may be important in the establishment of the neurovascular niche. Shh has a clear role in regulating neural development, and in the dorsal cortex conditional knockout of Shh or its receptor Smoothened (Smo) results in reduced cell division, and a smaller cortex (Komada et al., 2008). There is also recent evidence that Shh regulates vascular development and blood-brain barrier formation (Alvarez et al., 2011). *In vitro*, Shh in astrocytes conditioned media interacts with receptors on endothelial cells facilitating formation of barrier type properties. Vascular specific knockout of Smo results in impaired blood-brain barrier formation and disrupted extracellular matrix, detectable as early as E14 (Alvarez et al., 2011). It is important to remember that astrocytes are not a major constituent of the brain during very early stages of neurovascular development and therefore more work is required to determine (a) if neural progenitors may be an additional source of Shh, contributing to the control of vascular development in the embryo, and (b) whether vascular Shh contributes a proliferative signal to the neural progenitors.

β-catenin and the Wnt signaling pathway also affect vessel ingrowth from the peri-neural plexus and the structure of the developing vessels. Endothelial specific modifications of β-catenin expression, Wnt7 knockout or delivery of the soluble frizzled-8 receptor to bind extracellular Wnt ligand all cause a disruption in the vascular ingrowth into the parenchyma and malformation of the vessel beds, characterized by enlarged vascular space and thickening of the vascular wall with multiple layers of endothelial cells (Stenman et al., 2008; Daneman et al., 2009). In addition, Wnt signaling has also been shown to affect the barrier properties of the developing parenchymal vessels. Knockout of Wnt7 was associated with reduced GLUT1 expression (Stenman et al., 2008; Daneman et al., 2009), although there was no change in the expression of tight junction proteins. In contrast, endothelial specific β-catenin knockout showed an increased GLUT1 expression (Daneman et al., 2009), indicating that regulation of GLUT and barrier properties by the Wnt pathway is not a clear cut mechanism, and instead is likely to respond to numerous conflicting regulatory signals. However, in general the canonical Wnt signaling has been shown to affect blood-brain barrier permeability and the presence of tight junction proteins at the endothelial cells, where β-catenin gain-of-function stabilizes barrier properties, in response to other changes in Wnt signaling (Liebner et al., 2008). It is possible that the mechanism for this variation is a change in the polarity of the endothelial cells, mediated by Wnt signaling (Artus et al., 2014), which inhibits the formation of tight junctions. The polarity of progenitor cells in the VZ is of clear importance for the formation of junctions and regulating neurogenesis (discussed in more detail below), which provides support for a similar mechanism in the vasculature.

Contact-dependent signaling is another local environmental regulator of growth. McCarty et al. (2002) have shown that deletion of av-integrin causes abnormal vascular ingrowth and alignment into the ganglionic eminence from as early as E10.5. These ultimately led to enlarged vascular space, thinning of the endothelial lining and hemorrhage, and are associated with disruption of the neuroepithelial cells in the surrounding tissue. These disruptions appear to be due to the lack of adhesion with the perivascular basement membrane, rather than endothelial specific signaling or pericyte localization with the vasculature (McCarty et al., 2002), and highlights the importance of all components of the brain microenvironment for the establishment of the neurovascular and neurogenic niche.

VASCULAR CONTROL OF NEURAL PROLIFERATION

In turn, vascular development can control proliferation and brain development. For example, ectopic vascular development, induced by *in utero* injection of VEGF into the dorsal cortex, causes a change in distribution of the Tbr2 positive SVZ progenitor cells in conjunction with the new vascular network, and a disruption of radial fibers and axonal ingrowth into the surrounding tissue (Javaherian and Kriegstein, 2009). One of the first studies confirming that cerebral endothelial cells produce neurotophic factors was performed by Leventhal et al. (1999), where co-culture of cells from the adult SEZ with endothelial cells was found to enhance cell survival *in vitro*. These studies confirmed that BDNF produced by the endothelial cells was in fact secreted to affect the neurogenic precursors. Further co-culture studies confirmed that secretions from endothelial cells increased proliferation of precursors and ultimately facilitated the production of a larger number of neurons, of all neuronal classes (Shen et al., 2004). Early work from Tavazoie et al. (2008) suggests that elements of the blood-brain barrier may be different in the SEZ neurovascular niche. They specifically showed that progenitor cells contact blood vessels in place of some of the normal astrocytic endfeet contacts and that this appears to correlate with patches of reduced presence of tight junction proteins and increased permeability. Thus, they hypothesize that cells within the SEZ have an altered exposure to secreted proteins due to changed blood-brain barrier function.

There are certainly many studies showing both secreted protein from endothelial cells, and progenitor-endothelial cell contact is important for maintain proliferation in the SEZ. Transplant studies of neural precursor cells into the SEZ have shown that the chemokine cxcl12, which is produced by endothelial cells, is important for the localization of these cells to the vasculature. Cxcl12 appears to act through the activation of integrin that allows cell binding to the endothelial cell wall, and support migration of differentiating cells out of the SEZ (Kokovay et al., 2010).

Vascular production of VEGF is likely to be due to HIF activation in response to the low oxygen environment of the developing brain. HIF knockout in neural crest cells leads to reduced vascular density in the developing brain, and gross abnormalities in cellular migration (Tomita et al., 2003). There is also substantial hydrocephaly in these animals, possibly suggesting altered neural proliferation and/or the over production of CSF. Tamoxifen-induced knockout of HIF-1α in neural stem cells in the SEZ confirms a constitutive role for this molecule in maintenance of the progenitor population as well as vascular development (Li et al., 2014). As well as altering VEGF production, HIF activation can induce nitric oxide synthesis. Endogenous production of nitric oxide has been shown to negatively regulate progenitor production (Moreno-Lopez et al., 2004), and may act through one of a number of signaling pathways [reviewed by Goldman and Chen (2011)]. Neurotrophin-3 is another molecule released by endothelial cells and found in the CSF that appears to maintain progenitor quiescence/self-renewal through nitric oxide signaling (Delgado et al., 2014). Endothelial-derived pigment epithelium derived factor (PEDF) is another trophic factor that has been show to maintain stem cell renewal in the SEZ, in this case acting through notch signaling (Ramirez-Castillejo et al., 2006; Andreu-Agullo et al., 2009). Local purinergic signaling has also recently be suggested to contribute to self-renewal of progenitors in the SEZ, though it is currently unclear whether these come from the endothelial cells, or other components of the neurogenic niche (see Goldman and Chen, 2011).

Recent work has provided evidence in support of a further neurogenic niche in the adult brain, that of perivascular stem cells that do not proliferate in control conditions, but are upregulated following injury, such as ischemia (Ohira et al., 2010; Nakagomi et al., 2011). The nature of the neurogenic niche for this proliferative population is still not clear, though the recovery of the cortex after ischemia has been shown to be improved by cotransplantation of endothelial cells and neural stem cells (Nakagomi et al., 2009). However, the cells produced from the perivascular progenitors activated by ischemia appear to be more gliogenic than neurogenic (Nakagomi et al., 2011), and may, therefore, have a different relationship with the vasculature. As an extension to this, it has recently been suggested that signaling from the meninges call also regulate proliferative/differentiation decisions made in the VZ and SVZ of the developing brain [discussed by Sockanathan and Gaiano (2009)].

ROLE OF CELL-TO-CELL CONTACTS IN REGULATION OF PROLIFERATION

In addition to secreted signaling to neural precursors, the endothelial cells may also support the progenitor population in a contact-dependent manner (contact between type B and endothelial cells in the SEZ is shown in **Figure 2**). Ephrin and notch signaling have both been shown to be activated by contact between type B progenitors and endothelial cells (Ottone et al., 2014). Notch signaling pathways were up-regulated in cells co-cultured with endothelial cells, and Shen et al. (2004) hypothesized that the expansion of the progenitor population in connected sheets co-cultured with endothelial cells might also induce β-catenin signaling, another indication that junctions between progenitor cells may be essential for proliferation. This is certainly the case in the VZ, where the junctions between the neuroepithelial cells at the CSF-brain barrier appear to be essential for normal proliferation. β-catenin and N-cadherin are important components of these junctions, and disruption of β-catenin in the apical endfeet of the projector cells results in reduced proliferation, increased cell death and cortical malformation (Junghans et al., 2005). Hatakeyama et al. (2014) have also clearly shown that disruption of junctions at the ventricular surface affect proliferation. Electroporation with a dominant-negative form of cadherin, which lack the extracellular domain and disrupts the adherens junctions, resulted in a retraction of apical foot process followed by the production of ectopic neurons within the VZ and a clear abolishment of immunoreactivity of the junctional protein ZO-1 in the adjacent area of the ventricular surface. The upshot of this process was an increased differentiation of neurons over production of progenitors within the electroporated region of the brain. Further work from these researchers suggest that in this experimental paradigm canonical β-caterinin/Wnt signaling was not affected, but that Notch signaling was down-regulated (Hatakeyama et al., 2014). In both endothelial cells and neuroepithelial cell progenitors, the production of delta-like ligand from selected cells in the population appear to regulate Notch signaling in the juxtaposed neighboring cells, and this may facilitate selective population changes like initiating vessel sprouting (e.g., Hellstrom et al., 2007) or selective neuronal differentiation. Further work is required to determine whether this sort of interaction between juxtaposed neural stem cells and endothelial cells is part of the signaling system in the neurovascular niche.

While the ventricular zone in the developing brain is characterized by specialized junctions between the neuroepithelial cells, there are no such junctions between the ependymal cells that make the border with the CSF in the adult SEZ. The absence of these junctions between the ependymal cells appears to be very important for the structure of the SEZ, as progenitor cells are intercalated between the ependymal cells (Shen et al., 2008) and the ependymal cells of the ventricular wall form a rosette like arrangement where projections from the progenitor cells protrude through the center of the rosette to make direct contact with the CSF (Mirzadeh et al., 2008). However, it has been hypothesized that while traditional junctions don't exist between ependymal cells, the maintenance of apical adhesions between cells at the ventricular surface is essential for the formation of this specialized proliferative zone (Mirzadeh et al., 2008). The finding that there is close association of the cell adhesion molecule VCAM1 with the type B1 cells at the center of the pinwheels/rosettes, and that rosette formation is disrupted when VCAM is knocked out (Kokovay et al., 2012), supports this hypothesis.

CSF-NEUROGENIC NICHE

Both the VZ in the developing brain and the SEZ in the adult brain have clear connections with the CSF (see **Figures 1, 2**), and it has been shown that the CSF contains many trophic factors important for regulating proliferation in these zones (Johansson et al., 2010; Falcao et al., 2012; Stolp, 2013). Johansson et al. (2013) showed that knockout of the 4th ventricle choroid plexus by selective Otx2 deletion was sufficient to change the composition of the CSF and proliferation in the cortical VZ. These changes were likely, at least in part, to be mediated by Wnt signaling, which was found to be modulated in the CSF of transgenic animals (Johansson et al., 2013). Insulin-like growth factor (Igf) 2 is another molecule that has been shown to be produced by the choroid plexus to circulate in the CSF during early development. It is then able to interact with the Igf receptors on the ventricular surface and regulate proliferation within the VZ in an age dependent manner (Lehtinen et al., 2011).

The possibility that systemic signaling may directly alter the neurogenic niche has been explored by a number of authors, and it is clear that signaling through inflammatory pathways can cause short- and long-term changes in proliferation in the brain (Stolp et al., 2012; Stolp, 2013). In the developing brain, a systemic inflammatory challenge resulted in decreased proliferation in the VZ, which was associated with local changes in β-catenin immunoreactivity and the integrity of the junctions at the ventricular surface (Stolp et al., 2011). Prenatal inflammation produces a long-term reduction in proliferation, as shown in the SGZ by Graciarena et al. (2013), which is equivalent to that produced by an adult systemic inflammatory response. In this case, the SGZ was affected, rather than the SVZ, implying a tissue specific alteration, which may be more related to the vasculature or local microglia than changes in CSF signaling. Chronic inflammation, such as in models of Multiple Sclerosis, has also been found to result in reduced neurogenesis within the brain, though the mechanisms of this have not been fully explored (Pluchino et al., 2008; Tepavcevic et al., 2011). One potential mediator of this response is IL-1β. The IL-1 receptor is found on the type B cell in the SEZ. IL-1 is produced by the choroid plexus cells and released into the CSF (Kokovay et al., 2012), and is upregulated by peripheral inflammation (Marques et al., 2007). Injection of IL-1β into the lateral ventricles increased VCAM-1 expression in the SEZ and reduced the proliferation of type B cells (Kokovay et al., 2012). Cxcl12 is another typically inflammatory mediator that appears to play an important role in the regulation of the SEZ. As well as being produced by endothelia cells (as described above), it is highly expressed by the ependymal cells of the SEZ, and helps to maintain progenitors in their proliferative state (Kokovay et al., 2010). The contribution of cxcl12 to the neurogenic niches is a clear example of the dual influence of the CSF/ependymal and the microvasculature in neurogenesis, and the stage specific mobilization of progenitors through to differentiated neurons or glia which is essential in the brain [discussed by Kokovay et al. (2010); reviewed by Goldman and Chen (2011)].

CONCLUSION

Both the CSF and the vasculature of the brain provide regulatory niches for neurogenesis in the developing and adult brain. Variation in angiogenesis and CSF production clearly affect proliferation in the neurogenic niches as a result of cross-talk between these regions, which appears to be dependent both on secreted tropic factors and contact-dependent signaling pathways. The brain barriers, which regulate the internal environment and contribute to the contact between cells in the neurogenic niches are part of this complex system that can be altered both in systemic and central injury. The localization of neurogenic niches makes them sensitive to circulating soluble factors. Recent work from Villeda et al. (2011) highlights this point, showing that the chemokine CCL11 in the plasma and CSF during aging can regulate neurogenesis in the SGZ, which in turn affects learning and memory. The local and systemic control of the neurogenic niches therefore has significant impact on brain function throughout life. Disruption of neurovascular/CSF signaling in early development is likely to contribute to long-term disruption of neural organization and may be a contributor to neurodevelopmental disorders such as autism, schizophrenia and epilepsy. As such, it is essential that we increase our understanding of the control of neurogenic niches and how local and systemic injury/inflammation affect proliferative and differentiation cues in these regions.

REFERENCES

Alvarez, J. I., Dodelet-Devillers, A., Kebir, H., Ifergan, I., Fabre, P. J., Terouz, S., et al. (2011). The Hedgehog pathway promotes blood-brain barrier integrity and CNS immune quiescence. *Science* 334, 1727–1731. doi: 10.1126/science.1206936

Andreu-Agullo, C., Morante-Redolat, J. M., Delgado, A. C., and Farinas, I. (2009). Vascular niche factor PEDF modulates Notch-dependent stemness in the adult subependymal zone. *Nat. Neurosci.* 12, 1514–1523. doi: 10.1038/nn.2437

Artus, C., Glacial, F., Ganeshamoorthy, K., Ziegler, N., Godet, M., Guilbert, T., et al. (2014). The Wnt/planar cell polarity signaling pathway contributes to the integrity of tight junctions in brain endothelial cells. *J. Cereb. Blood Flow Metab.* 34, 433–440. doi: 10.1038/jcbfm.2013.213

Bautch, V. L., and James, J. M. (2009). Neurovascular development: the beginning of a beautiful friendship. *Cell Adh. Migr.* 3, 199–204. doi: 10.4161/cam.3.2.8397

Bueno, D., Parvas, M., Hermelo, I., and Garcia-Fernandez, J. (2014). Embryonic blood-cerebrospinal fluid barrier formation and function. *Front. Neurosci.* 8:343. doi: 10.3389/fnins.2014.00343

Daneman, R., Agalliu, D., Zhou, L., Kuhnert, F., Kuo, C. J., and Barres, B. A. (2009). Wnt/beta-catenin signaling is required for CNS, but not non-CNS, angiogenesis. *Proc. Natl. Acad. Sci. U.S.A.* 106, 641–646. doi: 10.1073/pnas.0805165106

Delgado, A. C., Ferron, S. R., Vicente, D., Porlan, E., Perez-Villalba, A., Trujillo, C. M., et al. (2014). Endothelial NT-3 delivered by vasculature and CSF promotes quiescence of subependymal neural stem cells through nitric oxide induction. *Neuron* 83, 572–585. doi: 10.1016/j.neuron.2014.06.015

Dziegielewska, K. M., Knott, G. W., and Saunders, N. R. (2000). The nature and composition of the internal environment of the developing brain. *Cell. Mol. Neurobiol.* 20, 41–56. doi: 10.1023/A:1006943926765

Falcao, A. M., Marques, F., Novais, A., Sousa, N., Palha, J. A., and Sousa, J. C. (2012). The path from the choroid plexus to the subventricular zone: go with the flow! *Front. Cell. Neurosci.* 6:34. doi: 10.3389/fncel.2012.00034

Fuentealba, L. C., Obernier, K., and Alvarez-Buylla, A. (2012). Adult neural stem cells bridge their niche. *Cell Stem Cell* 10, 698–708. doi: 10.1016/j.stem.2012.05.012

Goldman, S. A., and Chen, Z. (2011). Perivascular instruction of cell genesis and fate in the adult brain. *Nat. Neurosci.* 14, 1382–1389. doi: 10.1038/nn.2963

Graciarena, M., Roca, V., Mathieu, P., Depino, A. M., and Pitossi, F. J. (2013). Differential vulnerability of adult neurogenesis by adult and prenatal inflammation: role of TGF-beta1. *Brain Behav. Immun.* 34, 17–28. doi: 10.1016/j.bbi.2013.05.007

Hatakeyama, J., Wakamatsu, Y., Nagafuchi, A., Kageyama, R., Shigemoto, R., and Shimamura, K. (2014). Cadherin-based adhesions in the apical endfoot are required for active Notch signaling to control neurogenesis in vertebrates. *Development* 141, 1671–1682. doi: 10.1242/dev.102988

Hellstrom, M., Phng, L. K., Hofmann, J. J., Wallgard, E., Coultas, L., Lindblom, P., et al. (2007). Dll4 signalling through Notch1 regulates formation of tip cells during angiogenesis. *Nature* 445, 776–780. doi: 10.1038/nature05571

James, J. M., Gewolb, C., and Bautch, V. L. (2009). Neurovascular development uses VEGF-A signaling to regulate blood vessel ingression into the neural tube. *Development* 136, 833–841. doi: 10.1242/dev.028845

Javaherian, A., and Kriegstein, A. (2009). A stem cell niche for intermediate progenitor cells of the embryonic cortex. *Cereb. Cortex* 19 Suppl. 1, i70–i77. doi: 10.1093/cercor/bhp029

Johansson, P. A. (2014). The choroid plexuses and their impact on developmental neurogenesis. *Front. Neurosci.* 8:340. doi: 10.3389/fnins.2014.00340

Johansson, P. A., Cappello, S., and Gotz, M. (2010). Stem cells niches during development–lessons from the cerebral cortex. *Curr. Opin. Neurobiol.* 20, 400–407. doi: 10.1016/j.conb.2010.04.003

Johansson, P. A., Irmler, M., Acampora, D., Beckers, J., Simeone, A., and Gotz, M. (2013). The transcription factor Otx2 regulates choroid plexus development and function. *Development* 140, 1055–1066. doi: 10.1242/dev.090860

Junghans, D., Hack, I., Frotscher, M., Taylor, V., and Kemler, R. (2005). Beta-catenin-mediated cell-adhesion is vital for embryonic forebrain development. *Dev. Dyn.* 233, 528–539. doi: 10.1002/dvdy.20365

Kokovay, E., Goderie, S., Wang, Y., Lotz, S., Lin, G., Sun, Y., et al. (2010). Adult SVZ lineage cells home to and leave the vascular niche via differential responses to SDF1/CXCR4 signaling. *Cell Stem Cell* 7, 163–173. doi: 10.1016/j.stem.2010.05.019

Kokovay, E., Wang, Y., Kusek, G., Wurster, R., Lederman, P., Lowry, N., et al. (2012). VCAM1 is essential to maintain the structure of the SVZ niche and acts as an environmental sensor to regulate SVZ lineage progression. *Cell Stem Cell* 11, 220–230. doi: 10.1016/j.stem.2012.06.016

Komada, M., Saitsu, H., Kinboshi, M., Miura, T., Shiota, K., and Ishibashi, M. (2008). Hedgehog signaling is involved in development of the neocortex. *Development* 135, 2717–2727. doi: 10.1242/dev.015891

Lehtinen, M. K., Zappaterra, M. W., Chen, X., Yang, Y. J., Hill, A. D., Lun, M., et al. (2011). The cerebrospinal fluid provides a proliferative niche for neural progenitor cells. *Neuron* 69, 893–905. doi: 10.1016/j.neuron.2011.01.023

Leventhal, C., Rafii, S., Rafii, D., Shahar, A., and Goldman, S. A. (1999). Endothelial trophic support of neuronal production and recruitment from the adult mammalian subependyma. *Mol. Cell. Neurosci.* 13, 450–464. doi: 10.1006/mcne.1999.0762

Li, L., Candelario, K. M., Thomas, K., Wang, R., Wright, K., Messier, A., et al. (2014). Hypoxia inducible factor-1α (HIF-1α) is required for neural stem cell maintenance and vascular stability in the adult mouse SVZ. *J. Neurosci.* 34, 16713–16719. doi: 10.1523/JNEUROSCI.4590-13.2014

Liebner, S., Corada, M., Bangsow, T., Babbage, J., Taddei, A., Czupalla, C. J., et al. (2008). Wnt/beta-catenin signaling controls development of the blood-brain barrier. *J. Cell Biol.* 183, 409–417. doi: 10.1083/jcb.200806024

Marques, F., Sousa, J. C., Correia-Neves, M., Oliveira, P., Sousa, N., and Palha, J. A. (2007). The choroid plexus response to peripheral inflammatory stimulus. *Neuroscience* 144, 424–430. doi: 10.1016/j.neuroscience.2006.09.029

McCarty, J. H., Monahan-Earley, R. A., Brown, L. F., Keller, M., Gerhardt, H., Rubin, K., et al. (2002). Defective associations between blood vessels and brain parenchyma lead to cerebral hemorrhage in mice lacking alphav integrins. *Mol. Cell. Biol.* 22, 7667–7677. doi: 10.1128/MCB.22.21.7667-7677.2002

Mirzadeh, Z., Merkle, F. T., Soriano-Navarro, M., Garcia-Verdugo, J. M., and Alvarez-Buylla, A. (2008). Neural stem cells confer unique pinwheel architecture to the ventricular surface in neurogenic regions of the adult brain. *Cell Stem Cell* 3, 265–278. doi: 10.1016/j.stem.2008.07.004

Mollgard, K., Balslev, Y., Lauritzen, B., and Saunders, N. R. (1987). Cell junctions and membrane specializations in the ventricular zone (germinal matrix) of the developing sheep brain: a CSF-brain barrier. *J. Neurocytol.* 16, 433–444. doi: 10.1007/BF01668498

Moreno-Lopez, B., Romero-Grimaldi, C., Noval, J. A., Murillo-Carretero, M., Matarredona, E. R., and Estrada, C. (2004). Nitric oxide is a physiological inhibitor of neurogenesis in the adult mouse subventricular zone and olfactory bulb. *J. Neurosci.* 24, 85–95. doi: 10.1523/JNEUROSCI.1574-03.2004

Nakagomi, N., Nakagomi, T., Kubo, S., Nakano-Doi, A., Saino, O., Takata, M., et al. (2009). Endothelial cells support survival, proliferation, and neuronal differentiation of transplanted adult ischemia-induced neural stem/progenitor cells after cerebral infarction. *Stem Cells* 27, 2185–2195. doi: 10.1002/stem.161

Nakagomi, T., Molnar, Z., Nakano-Doi, A., Taguchi, A., Saino, O., Kubo, S., et al. (2011). Ischemia-induced neural stem/progenitor cells in the pia mater following cortical infarction. *Stem Cells Dev.* 20, 2037–2051. doi: 10.1089/scd.2011.0279

Nie, K., Molnar, Z., and Szele, F. G. (2010). Proliferation but not migration is associated with blood vessels during development of the rostral migratory stream. *Dev. Neurosci.* 32, 163–172. doi: 10.1159/000301135

Ohira, K., Furuta, T., Hioki, H., Nakamura, K. C., Kuramoto, E., Tanaka, Y., et al. (2010). Ischemia-induced neurogenesis of neocortical layer 1 progenitor cells. *Nat. Neurosci.* 13, 173–179. doi: 10.1038/nn.2473

Ottone, C., Krusche, B., Whitby, A., Clements, M., Quadrato, G., Pitulescu, M. E., et al. (2014). Direct cell-cell contact with the vascular niche maintains quiescent neural stem cells. *Nat. Cell Biol.* 16, 1045–1056. doi: 10.1038/ncb3045

Palmer, T. D., Willhoite, A. R., and Gage, F. H. (2000). Vascular niche for adult hippocampal neurogenesis. *J. Comp. Neurol.* 425, 479–494. doi: 10.1002/1096-9861(20001002)425:43.0.CO;2-3

Pluchino, S., Muzio, L., Imitola, J., Deleidi, M., Alfaro-Cervello, C., Salani, G., et al. (2008). Persistent inflammation alters the function of the endogenous brain stem cell compartment. *Brain* 131(Pt 10), 2564–2578. doi: 10.1093/brain/awn198

Ramirez-Castillejo, C., Sanchez-Sanchez, F., Andreu-Agullo, C., Ferron, S. R., Aroca-Aguilar, J. D., Sanchez, P., et al. (2006). Pigment epithelium-derived factor is a niche signal for neural stem cell renewal. *Nat. Neurosci.* 9, 331–339. doi: 10.1038/nn1657

Ruhrberg, C., and Bautch, V. L. (2013). Neurovascular development and links to disease. *Cell. Mol. Life Sci.* 70, 1675–1684. doi: 10.1007/s00018-013-1277-5

Shen, Q., Goderie, S. K., Jin, L., Karanth, N., Sun, Y., Abramova, N., et al. (2004). Endothelial cells stimulate self-renewal and expand neurogenesis of neural stem cells. *Science* 304, 1338–1340. doi: 10.1126/science.1095505

Shen, Q., Wang, Y., Kokovay, E., Lin, G., Chuang, S.-M., Goderie, S. K., et al. (2008). Adult SVZ Stem cells lie in a vascular niche: a quantitative analysis of niche cell-cell interactions. *Cell Stem Cell* 3, 289–300. doi: 10.1016/j.stem.2008.07.026

Sockanathan, S., and Gaiano, N. (2009). Preview. Meninges play a RAdical role in embryonic neural stem cell regulation. *Cell Stem Cell* 5, 455–456. doi: 10.1016/j.stem.2009.10.010

Stenman, J. M., Rajagopal, J., Carroll, T. J., Ishibashi, M., McMahon, J., and McMahon, A. P. (2008). Canonical Wnt signaling regulates organ-specific assembly and differentiation of CNS vasculature. *Science* 322, 1247–1250. doi: 10.1126/science.1164594

Stolp, H. B. (2013). Neuropoietic cytokines in normal brain development and neurodevelopmental disorders. *Mol. Cell. Neurosci.* 53, 63–68. doi: 10.1016/j.mcn.2012.08.009

Stolp, H. B., Turnquist, C., Dziegielewska, K. M., Saunders, N. R., Anthony, D. C., and Molnar, Z. (2011). Reduced ventricular proliferation in the foetal cortex following maternal inflammation in the mouse. *Brain* 134, 3236–3248. doi: 10.1093/brain/awr237

Stolp, H., Neuhaus, A., Sundramoorthi, R., and Molnar, Z. (2012). The long and the short of it: gene and environment interactions during early cortical development and consequences for long-term neurological disease. *Front. Psychiatry* 3:50. doi: 10.3389/fpsyt.2012.00050

Stubbs, D., DeProto, J., Nie, K., Englund, C., Mahmud, I., Hevner, R., et al. (2009). Neurovascular congruence during cerebral cortical development. *Cereb. Cortex* 19 Suppl. 1, i32–i41. doi: 10.1093/cercor/bhp040

Tavazoie, M., Van der Veken, L., Silva-Vargas, V., Louissaint, M., Colonna, L., Zaidi, B., et al. (2008). A specialized vascular niche for adult neural stem cells. *Cell Stem Cell* 3, 279–288. doi: 10.1016/j.stem.2008.07.025

Tepavcevic, V., Lazarini, F., Alfaro-Cervello, C., Kerninon, C., Yoshikawa, K., Garcia-Verdugo, J. M., et al. (2011). Inflammation-induced subventricular zone dysfunction leads to olfactory deficits in a targeted mouse model of multiple sclerosis. *J. Clin. Invest.* 121, 4722–4734. doi: 10.1172/JCI59145

Tomita, S., Ueno, M., Sakamoto, M., Kitahama, Y., Ueki, M., Maekawa, N., et al. (2003). Defective brain development in mice lacking the Hif-1alpha gene in neural cells. *Mol. Cell. Biol.* 23, 6739–6749. doi: 10.1128/MCB.23.19.6739-6749.2003

Vasudevan, A., Long, J. E., Crandall, J. E., Rubenstein, J. L., and Bhide, P. G. (2008). Compartment-specific transcription factors orchestrate angiogenesis gradients in the embryonic brain. *Nat. Neurosci.* 11, 429–439. doi: 10.1038/nn2074

Villeda, S. A., Luo, J., Mosher, K. I., Zou, B., Britschgi, M., Bieri, G., et al. (2011). The ageing systemic milieu negatively regulates neurogenesis and cognitive function. *Nature* 477, 90–94. doi: 10.1038/nature10357

Virgintino, D., Errede, M., Rizzi, M., Girolamo, F., Strippoli, M., Walchli, T., et al. (2013). The CXCL12/CXCR4/CXCR7 ligand-receptor system regulates neuro-glio-vascular interactions and vessel growth during human brain development. *J. Inherit. Metab. Dis.* 36, 455–466. doi: 10.1007/s10545-012-9574-y

4

The rights and wrongs of blood-brain barrier permeability studies: a walk through 100 years of history

Norman R. Saunders[1]*, Jean-Jacques Dreifuss[2], Katarzyna M. Dziegielewska[1], Pia A. Johansson[3], Mark D. Habgood[1], Kjeld Møllgård[4] and Hans-Christian Bauer[5,6]

[1] *Department of Pharmacology and Therapeutics, University of Melbourne, Parkville, VIC, Australia*
[2] *Department of Neuroscience, University of Geneva, Geneva, Switzerland*
[3] *Institute for Stem Cell Research, Helmholtz Center Munich, Munich, Germany*
[4] *Department of Cellular and Molecular Medicine, University of Copenhagen, Copenhagen, Denmark*
[5] *Institute of Tendon and Bone Regeneration, Paracelsus Medical University, Salzburg, Austria*
[6] *Spinal Cord Injury and Tissue Regeneration Center, Paracelsus Medical University, Salzburg, Austria*

Correspondence:
Norman R. Saunders, Department of Pharmacology and Therapeutics, University of Melbourne, Grattan Street, Parkville, VIC 3010, Australia
e-mail: n.saunders@unimelb.edu.au

Careful examination of relevant literature shows that many of the most cherished concepts of the blood-brain barrier are incorrect. These include an almost mythological belief in its immaturity that is unfortunately often equated with absence or at least leakiness in the embryo and fetus. The original concept of a blood-brain barrier is often attributed to Ehrlich; however, he did not accept that permeability of cerebral vessels was different from other organs. Goldmann is often credited with the first experiments showing dye (trypan blue) exclusion from the brain when injected systemically, but not when injected directly into it. Rarely cited are earlier experiments of Bouffard and of Franke who showed methylene blue and trypan red stained all tissues except the brain. The term "blood-brain barrier" "Blut-Hirnschranke" is often attributed to Lewandowsky, but it does not appear in his papers. The first person to use this term seems to be Stern in the early 1920s. Studies in embryos by Stern and colleagues, Weed and Wislocki showed results similar to those in adult animals. These were well-conducted experiments made a century ago, thus the persistence of a belief in barrier immaturity is puzzling. As discussed in this review, evidence for this belief, is of poor experimental quality, often misinterpreted and often not properly cited. The functional state of blood-brain barrier mechanisms in the fetus is an important biological phenomenon with implications for normal brain development. It is also important for clinicians to have proper evidence on which to advise pregnant women who may need to take medications for serious medical conditions. Beliefs in immaturity of the blood-brain barrier have held the field back for decades. Their history illustrates the importance of taking account of all the evidence and assessing its quality, rather than selecting papers that supports a preconceived notion or intuitive belief. This review attempts to right the wrongs. Based on careful translation of original papers, some published a century ago, as well as providing discussion of studies claiming to show barrier immaturity, we hope that readers will have evidence on which to base their own conclusions.

Keywords: blood-brain barrier, blood-cerebrospinal fluid barrier, embryo, fetus, newborn, permeability, tight junctions, transporters

INTRODUCTION

The very first studies of barrier properties in embryos clearly demonstrated the intactness of the interfaces between the blood, brain and cerebrospinal fluid[1]. Thus Wislocki (1920) injected a guinea pig embryo with trypan blue (**Figure 1A**), the same dye, which was first used by Goldmann (1909; 1913 see below). Wislocki (1920) observed that in the embryo, as in adult animals, the dye stained almost all of the tissues of the body, with the notable exception of much of the brain.

Even earlier than this Weed (1917a,b) injected an approximately isotonic solution of potassium ferrocyanide, a small molecule about the same size as sucrose, into the neural tube of E19 and older pig embryos. Weed's results showed that in an E19 pig embryo the potassium ferrocyanide (demonstrated by the Prussian blue reaction) remained entirely within the fluid filling the neural tube (**Figure 1B**). This suggests that even this early in development, shortly after neural tube closure, the

Abbreviations: CNS, central nervous system; CSF, cerebrospinal fluid; HRP, horseradish peroxidase.

[1]Where possible we have worked from original references. Where these were not in English we have given citations of key points in the original language, together with a translation (indicated by italics). Readers will be able to decide for themselves if the translations are accurate and if our deductions from the citations are appropriate.

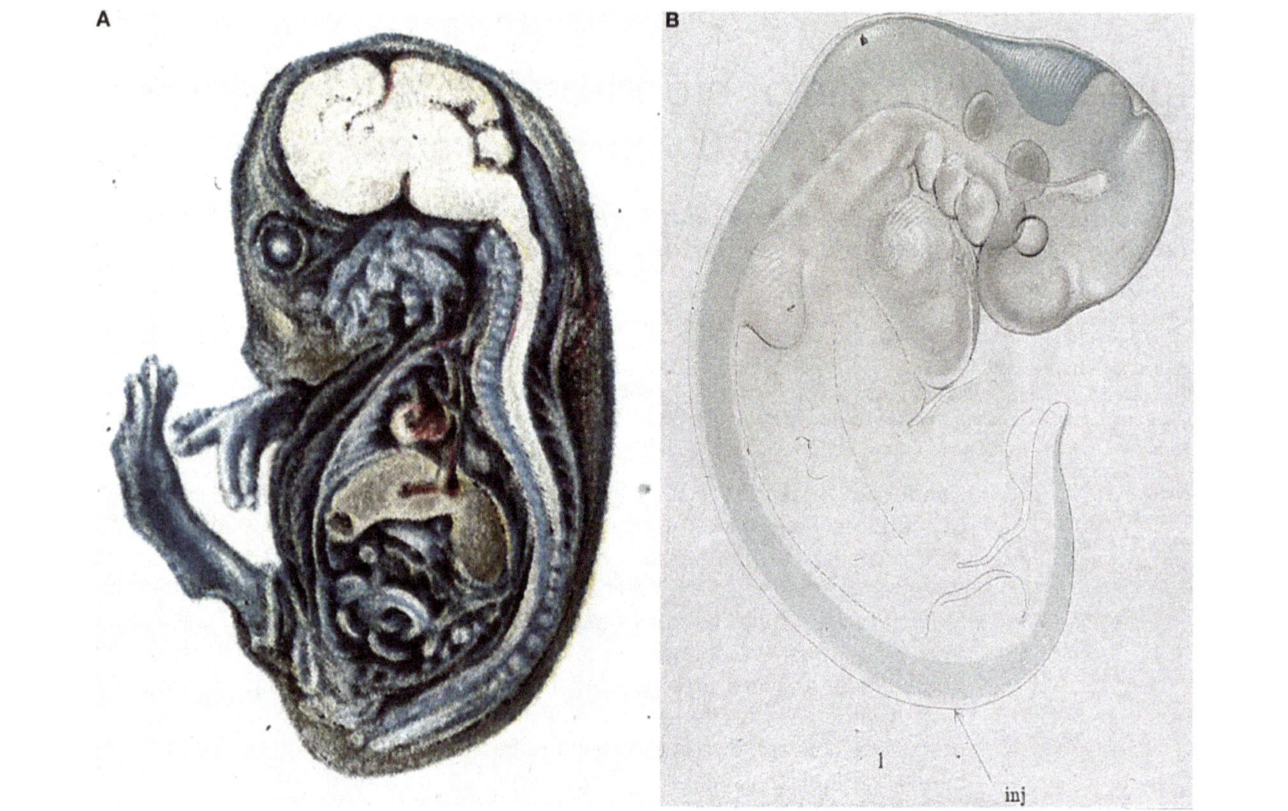

FIGURE 1 | Early demonstration of blood-brain barrier phenomenon in developing brain. (A) Mid gestation guinea pig embryo injected with trypan blue (Wislocki, 1920). Note lack of staining of brain and spinal cord as previously described in adult animals injected with trypan blue (Goldmann, 1909), methylene blue (Bouffard, 1906) and trypan red (Franke, 1905). **(B)** Very early pig embryo (9 mm, E19) injected with isotonic sodium ferrocyanide into spinal canal (arrow) treated with acid (Prussian blue reaction). Note that blue reaction product is confined to CSF, with a small amount of diffusion into brain stem and mid brain tissue, but no staining of somatic tissue. This indicates that the CNS is already a closed compartment separate from the rest of the embryo. From Weed (1917b).

central nervous system (CNS) is separate from the rest of the embryo.

Similar results were obtained in chick embryos by Cohen and Davies (1938). The experiments of Wislocki, Weed and Cohen and Davies are the developmental equivalent of what are sometimes described as Goldmann's 1st and 2nd experiments, in which he reported iv injection (1909) and intrathecal injection (1913) of trypan blue in adult animals of various species. The evidence from the experiments of Weed, Wislocki, Chen and Davies in developing animals for the existence of a barrier between the blood and brain and blood and CSF was as convincing as Goldmann's experiments in adult animals. Yet at some point a belief, which has persisted for nearly 100 years, arose that in embryos, fetuses and even in the newborn and older, the blood-brain barrier is absent, leaky or immature (e.g., Statz and Felgenhauer, 1983; Adinolfi, 1985; Davies and Rudd, 1994; Rodier, 1994, 1995, 2004; Ahmed et al., 1996; ATSDR, 1999, 2007, 2014; Järup, 2003; Costa et al., 2004; Watson et al., 2006; Mhanna et al., 2008; Baldrick, 2010; Ehman, 2010; Srinivasan et al., 2012). These and other authors appear to equate immaturity with "leakiness." The developing brain in all respects is by definition yet to reach a mature adult state and therefore can rightly be described as immature. But this does not tell us whether its brain barriers are "leaky." The real question is their functional status, which seems to us to be more a matter of the relation between barrier functions (which are much more than the presence or absence of passive permeability) that are present at any particular age and stage of brain development. We wondered why such a dogma continues to be accepted in view of overwhelming experimental evidence to the contrary gathered over many decades, for as pointed out by Dobbing (1961): "There has never been a shred of satisfactory evidence in favor of this proposition."

The general explanation seems to be a philosophical rather than an experimentally based one. There seems to have been an underlying assumption, often not clearly enunciated, that because the embryonic and newborn brains are developing, adult barrier mechanisms would necessarily be immature or absent. This was most explicitly stated in "The brain and its environment" by the English physiologist Barcroft (1938): "There is no reason why the brain of the embryo should require an environment of very great chemical constancy. It will of course require a certain minimum of the various materials necessary for growth, but otherwise on first principles we might suppose that the good things of life may exist in and may vary in fetal blood to an extent much greater than in the maternal." However, this is a teleological argument, implying need/requirement or in this case, lack of need/requirement. One could as well argue that a complex organ like the brain would need (require) a specialized environment in which to develop rather than the general "soup" of the embryo as a whole. However, neither argument has any intellectual merit as they are based on opinion rather than experimental evidence. More recently, and in the face of much evidence to the contrary since Barcroft's time, Zheng (2002) has put forward a similar teleological argument: "During early development, the rapid growth of the cerebral cortex perhaps necessities a "leaky" structure of the BBB to accommodate the high demand of blood-borne nutrients for brain growth." However, as we discuss below, the greater entry of some amino acids into the developing brain is a reflection of much higher expression of their transporters in brain endothelial and choroid plexus epithelial cells. This higher expression, which indicates a developmental specialization, is likely to be a reflection of the importance of amino acids for developing brain rather than a manifestation of a non-specific leak.

CONCEPT OF THE BLOOD-BRAIN BARRIER

Before dealing with experimental evidence of brain barriers during development we need to consider the concept of the adult blood-brain barrier itself. This is often attributed to Ehrlich on the basis of his experiments with dyes (e.g., Gröntoft, 1954; Bakay, 1956; Dempsey and Wislocki, 1955; Lee, 1971; Davson et al., 1987; Risau and Seulberger, 1990; Risau and Wolburg, 1990; Hawkins and Davis, 2005; Nag, 2011). However, as pointed out by Bradbury (1995); Ehrlich (1885, 1906) himself never subscribed to the view that the lack of staining of the brain by parenterally administered dyes could be ascribed to some special property of the cerebral endothelial cells. This idea was proposed by Biedl and Kraus (1898); Roux and Borrel (1898), and Lewandowsky (1900) based on comparison of intrathecal and parenteral injections of materials with neurotoxic effects, such as bile salts, after injection by the former route. This was specifically rejected by Ehrlich: "I am unable to accept that the vascular endothelium, as such, exercises different functions in different organs, so that, for example a liver capillary is permeable for certain substances that will not pass through other capillaries" (Ehrlich, 1906). This seems a rather curious conclusion given the description of some of his earlier dye studies (Ehrlich, 1885). In his extensive MD thesis ("Habilitationsschrift") Ehrlich was primarily using dyes as a means of determining the oxygen usage in different organs by their color change (low oxygen or reduction resulting in a colorless state of the dye and on oxygenation resulted in the reverse). He used mainly Alizarin Blue-S (a compound of Alizarin blue and sodium bisulfite) and Indophenol white (which became blue when exposed to oxygen), injected usually subcutaneously into animals of various species. Both of these dyes stained the brain blue, exclusively in gray matter. Under conditions of reduced oxygen (as post mortem) the dyes became colorless. Ehrlich also used dyes treated with acids or heavy metals to give larger particle sizes-alizarin-sodium sulfite-alum and Coerulin-S. These did not stain the brain following subcutaneous injection. To explain this Ehrlich proposed, that "the brain was the most "finely porous" of the organs" he studied. Ehrlich does not say if these "pores" were in blood vessel walls or some other interface between blood and brain tissue. Later Ehrlich (1906) reported on a much larger number of dyes and concluded that acid dyes (with the exception of alizirin) did not stain the gray matter of the brain whereas many basic dyes did. He suggested that dye experiments could be explained by lack of affinity of brain tissue for the dyes rather than to a special property of brain blood vessels. So perhaps Ehrlich could best be described as the reluctant discoverer of the blood-brain barrier phenomenon, but not as the originator of the term "blood-brain barrier."

Many authors, including Spatz (1934), Broman (1941), Davson (1967), Davson et al. (1987), Hawkins and Davis (2005), Engelhardt (2003, 2006), Ribatti et al. (2006), Saunders et al. (2012) have attributed the term "Blut-Hirnschranke" (blood-brain barrier) to Lewandowsky's (1900) publication.

Lewandowsky (1900) used strychnine and sodium ferrocyanide, in much higher doses than the potassium ferrocyanide used by Weed (1917b), who stated that in his experiments it was not toxic. Lewandowsky demonstrated in a variety of animal species that the toxins were effective in much lower doses when injected into the brain than parenterally. He also attributed the lesser penetration of strychnine and sodium ferrocyanide into the brain following subcutaneous injection compared to subarachnoid injection to a difference in the properties of the cerebral vessels compared to other tissues: "...die Hypothese dass die Cappillarwand den Uebertritt bestimmter Stoffe, wie des Natriumferrocyanats verhindert, oder mit anderen Worten, dass seine Affinitat der Capillarzellen des Centralnervensystems nothwendig ist um bestimmte Stoffe an die Nervenzellen hindurchgelangen zu lassen.": *the hypothesis that the capillary wall blocks the transfer of certain molecules like sodium ferrocyanide or in other words, that an affinity of capillary cells of the CNS is necessary in order to allow the transfer of certain molecules to nerve cells.* A close reading of Lewandowsky's original paper reveals that the term "Blut-Hirnschranke" was not actually used, although as indicated by the above quotation, Lewandowsky clearly proposed that cerebral capillaries have specific restrictive properties with respect to some compounds.

The first use of the term "barrier" appears to be by Stern and Gautier (1918a,b), the latter paper is entitled "La barrière qui s'oppose au passage dans le liquide céphalo-rachidien de substances circulant dans le sang présente des différences notables suivant les espèces animales": *The barrier which opposes the movement into the CSF of substances in the blood shows notable differences in different animal species* (Stern and Gautier, 1918b). Stern and colleagues subsequently performed detailed studies of penetration of a wide range of molecules from blood into cerebrospinal fluid (Stern and Gautier, 1921) into brain (Stern and Gautier, 1922) and within the subarachnoid and ventricular CSF (Stern and Gautier, 1923) of adult animals. It was Stern who first described the importance of the interstitial fluid environment of the brain for its normal function, very much in the tradition of Claude Bernard's *milieu interne* (1865).

Malamud et al. (1928), Franceschini (1929) and Joó (1987) appear to be among only a few authors to have acknowledged that Stern was probably the first to coin the term blood-brain barrier ("barrière hémato-encéphalique," Stern and Gautier, 1921). Stern and Gautier were careful to point out that this term did not prejudge either the anatomical nature or functional mechanisms involved. The term "blood-brain barrier" has withstood the test of time, notwithstanding that to people outside the field it is misleading in that it implies an absolute impediment to entry into the brain and does not make it explicitly clear that exchange mechanism are involved—exactly as supposed by Stern when she proposed the term. However, Stern's important contributions to the field of blood-brain barrier biology have either been largely ignored or belittled (see below).

In addition to Lewandowsky's 1900 experiments, Biedl and Kraus (1898) injected bile and bile acids either systemically or directly into the brain. Only in the case of the latter did they see any toxic effects. They ascribed the ineffectiveness of systemically injected bile salts to "the relative impermeability of the capillary walls," although they did not use the term "barrier" to describe this effect. Roux and Borrel (1898) reported on the comparison of subcutaneous and subdural injections of tetanus toxin with the finding that much less toxin is required to provoke central manifestations of tetanus, but only in rabbits; other species were unaffected. Their explanation for the difference was "sans doute, à ce que beaucoup du poison introduit n'arrive pas aux cellules nerveuses et est detruit quelque part dans l'organisme.": without doubt little of the toxin reaches nervous tissue and is destroyed elsewhere in the organism. However, they did not comment on the mechanism that prevented toxin from reaching the brain.

Amongst the most cited papers for the concept of the blood-brain barrier are those of Goldmann (1909, 1913). He compared distribution of the dye trypan blue following parenteral or intrathecal injection. These are sometimes referred to as Goldmann's first and second experiments (Davson, 1976; Bradbury, 1979). Goldmann found that parenterally injected dye did not stain the brain (Goldmann, 1909), whereas it did when injected into the subarachnoid space, (Goldmann, 1913) as illustrated in **Figure 2**. Goldmann is usually given the credit for being the first to use a dye to demonstrate that some dyes administered parenterally do not enter the brain. Goldmann himself acknowledges earlier dye studies of Bouffard (1906) but incorrectly states that Bouffard used trypan blue. Bouffard makes an unreferenced mention of even earlier studies with trypan red and Congo red and describes his own studies with methylene blue. Bouffard (1906) injected this dye by various routes (subcutaneous, intravenous, intramuscular or intracardiac) into mice, guinea pigs and rabbits in single or multiple doses of increasing size. He reported unequivocally that there was no staining of the nervous tissue: "SYSTEME NERVEUX.—Aucune trace de couleur, ni dans les cellules nerveuses, ni dans les éléments

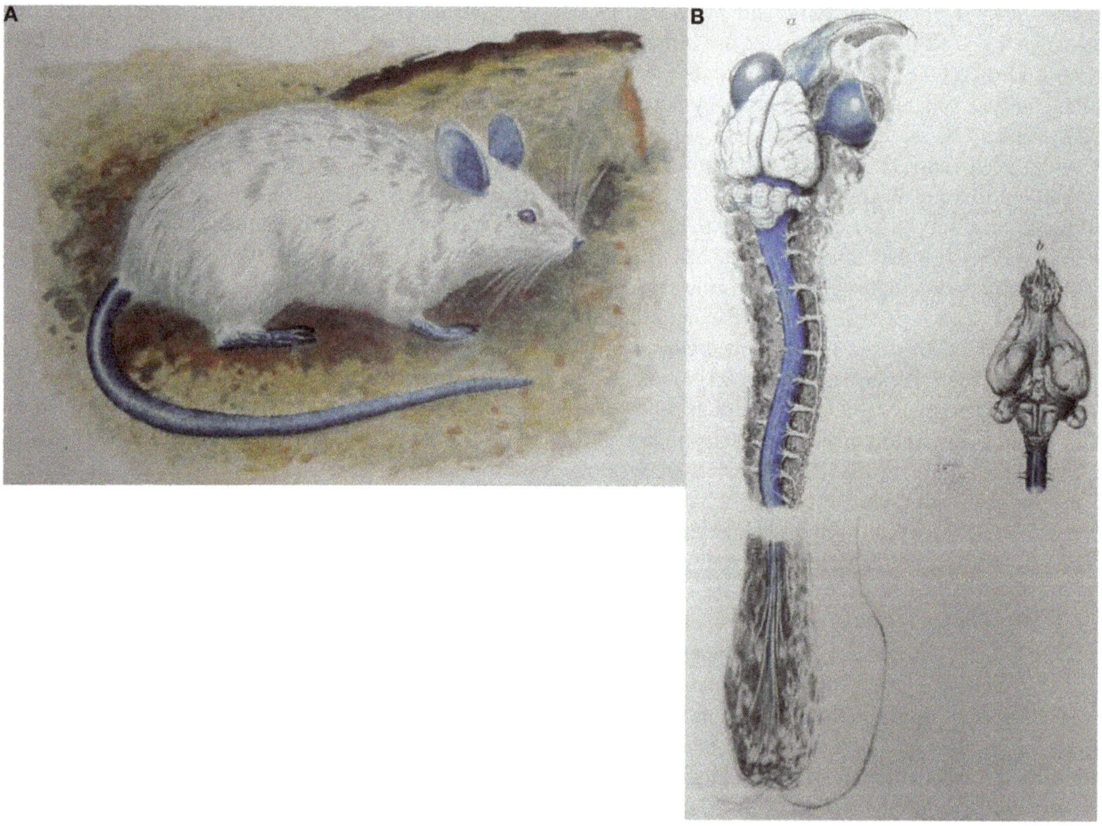

FIGURE 2 | Goldmann's trypan blue injection experiments. (A) Adult rat following systemic injection of trypan blue solution (Goldmann's "1st experiment"). From Goldmann (1909). **(B)** Brain and spinal cord of adult rat following lumbar subarachnoid injection of 0.5 ml, 0.5% trypan blue (Goldmann's "2nd experiment"). From Goldmann (1913).

névrogliques." Bouffard did not report any toxic effects of methylene blue and did not seem to suggest any mechanism to explain the lack of staining of the nervous system. Bouffard (1906) mentioned, but did not reference, an even earlier study by a student of Ehrlich's, Franke, who used trypan red. According to Bouffard, Franke also showed that the dye did not enter the brain although it did enter most other tissues and organs. This citation appears to have been taken from Franke's (1905) thesis, in which Franke stated "Das Trypanrot gehört zu den polytropen Farbstoffen im Sinne EHRLICHS; es wird entsprechend den Beobachtungen, die bei anderen saueren Farbstoffen gemacht worden sind, von allen Organen mit Ausnahme des Nervensystems, aufgenommen": *Trypan red belongs to the polytropic dyes according to Ehrlich; it is taken up,- as observed with other acidic dyes, by all organs except the nervous system.* None of these authors seems to have offered any explanation of the lack of staining of the brain by the different dyes; indeed Goldmann (1913) appears to have been surprised by this observation: "Es ist mir rätselhaft dass grosse Farbstoffmengen, welche bei der intravenösen Applikation in den Gehirngefässen zirkulieren, selbst die feinste Kapillarwand nicht zu durchdringen vermögen": *I fail to understand why high concentrations of dye circulating in the blood vessels after intravenous injection are unable to penetrate even the walls of the finest capillaries* (Goldmann, 1913, p. 45).

Goldmann (1913) did however, remark on the strong staining of the choroid plexus with trypan blue and suggested this represented the site at which dyes were prevented from entering the brain. Goldmann (1909, 1913) reported toxic effects with injected trypan blue and commented that the toxic effects that occurred following subarachnoid injections of the dye were made with amounts of trypan blue that were much less than when injected intravenously, particularly in rabbits. Because the choroid plexus stained very strongly with the dye, Goldmann suggested that it was primarily the choroid plexus that provided a protective mechanism for the brain and that this was the route by which some substances entered the brain. This subsequently led to the use of the term "Weg über den Liquor," although not by Goldmann or by von Monakow to whom it is sometimes attributed.

But Goldmann clearly thought that the choroid plexuses had a protective role in preventing entry of toxic materials into the brain: "Der Plexus vermag andererseits die Zerebrospinalflüssigkeit und damit die Nervensubstanz vor dem Eindringen von Substanzen zu schützen, die sich bei der direkten Einfuhr in den Subarachnoidealraum als ein schweres Gift für die Ganglienzellen erweisen." (Goldmann, 1913, p. 54): *On the other hand the choroid plexus is capable to protect the liquor and therefore also the nervous substance against the influx of substances which when directly transferred into the subarachnoid space are a strong toxin for the ganglionic cells.* He then summarizes his view of the choroid plexus as a protective regulatory mechanism: "Wir kommen somit zu dem Schluß, dass der Plexus ein wichtiger Schutz-und Regulationsmechanismus für das zentrale Nervensystem darstellt, und dass differenten Substanzen Tür und Tor für ihren Eintritt in das zentrale Nervensystem geöffnet werden, wenn die physiologische Eintrittspforte, der Plexus chorioideus, umgangen wird und solche differente Stoffe durch die Lumbalpunktion in eine direkte Berührung mit den Nervenelementen gebracht warden." (Goldmann, 1913, p. 55): *Thus we conclude that the plexus is an important protective-and regulatory mechanism for the CNS and that various substances will freely enter the CNS if the physiological gatekeeper, the choroid plexus, is circumvented by a lumbar puncture, those substances will come into direct contact with the nervous elements.* However it should be noted that Goldmann makes no mention of any protective function of cerebral blood vessels.

ROUTE OF ENTRY FROM BLOOD INTO BRAIN

Stemming from the studies of Goldmann (1909, 1913) described above and supported by von Monakow (1921) there came the suggestion that the choroid plexuses, rather than the cerebral blood vessels, were the CNS protective mechanism and the primary route of entry of nutritive substances into the brain (described by the term "Weg über den Liquor" by later authors). However, this proposed nutritive function of the choroid plexus seems to have been current earlier than this (see Meek, 1907). Stern in particular initially supported this idea in her interpretation of extensive studies of entry of a wide range of molecules from blood into CSF (Stern and Gautier, 1921) and brain (Stern and Gautier, 1922) in which she emphasized the importance of the choroid plexuses in this role. Davson (1956, 1976) considered this an untenable hypothesis and dismissed the idea as "intellectually inadequate" as it did not take account of substantial vascular circulation of the brain parenchyma. This view was shared by Friedemann (1942): "It is utterly unlikely that in an organ of the vital importance of the brain the capillaries should lack their chief uses, namely, mediation of the exchange between blood and tissue and adaptation of blood supply to functional needs" (Friedemann, 1942, p. 126). The idea was also dismissed by several other German authors (e.g., Friedemann and Elkeles, 1931, 1934; Walter, 1934). However, this dismissal is not justified, as these authors have ignored or miss-cited Stern and Rapoport's short papers (e.g., Stern and Rapoport, 1928a,b) from which it is clear that they believed in the existence of two routes of entry from blood into brain: one directly across the blood vessels (endothelial blood-brain barrier) and the other via the choroid plexuses (Goldmann and Stern's blood-brain barrier, now referred to as the epithelial blood-cerebrospinal fluid-barrier). For example, Stern and Rapoport (1928a) reported that in animals subjected to carbon monoxide poisoning, dyes entered brain tissue directly across the cerebral blood vessels, but only sodium ferrocyanide could be detected in the CSF, which was interpreted as suggesting two different routes of entry into the brain, one (for trypan blue or similar colloids) at the vascular endothelial cells of brain capillaries, the other (for sodium ferrocyanide) via the plexuses.

In Geneva Lina Stern, who was a physiologist and biochemist, did not have anybody in her laboratory to perform a thorough post-mortem histology of the brain of the experimental animals. In Moscow she found a competent neuropathologist/histologist Yakov Rapoport, who could localize which cells in the brain had been colored by the injected trypan blue or had been revealed by the Prussian blue reaction. His contribution was therefore of great importance. Unfortunately their cooperation came to an end in the early 1930's. It seems likely that the two disagreed on the respective roles of the blood-CSF and blood-brain barriers.

In contradistinction to her previous short papers with Rapoport, on the "two barriers model," Stern in a short paper (1934) focused her attention on the blood-CSF barrier (which she calls the *barrière hémato-encéphalique*). Stern admits that the use of dyes or of other yes-or-no biological markers to assess the permeability of the barrière hémato-encéphalique (blood-CSF barrier) is open to criticism. "En effet il n'est guère possible de tirer des conclusions sur le comportement du liquide en partant simplement de la pénétration ou de la non-pénétration d'une substance donnée présente [dans le plasma sanguin].": *Actually the composition of the liquid cannot be directly deduced from the passage or non-passage of a substance present in blood plasma.*

According to Stern (1934), the barrier has dual roles of protection and metabolic regulation of the brain. She also introduces the notions of barrier *selectivity* and barrier *resistance*. Thus in this 1934 paper, which was one of the last published in French, Stern makes a very clear statement about the importance of the blood-brain barrier in not only providing protection for the brain but also an appropriate physico-chemical environment for normal brain function: "Partant de l'idée que le liquide céphalo-rachidien represénte le milieu nutritif immédiat des éléments nerveux cérébro-spinaux et que la constance relative de la composition chimique et de l'état physico-chimique de ce milieu est une condition *sine qua non* du fonctionnment normal des centers nerveux, nous avons attributé un rôle de premier plan à l'activité de cet appareil régulateur que représente la barrière hémato-encéphalique.": *Starting with the idea that the CSF represents the immediate nutritive medium for the cells of the brain and spinal cord and that the relative constancy of the chemical composition and physico-chemical state of this medium is the* sine qua non *for normal function of the CNS we have attributed a primary role for this regulatory activity to the blood-brain barrier.* The concept of the blood-brain barrier providing mechanisms that control the internal environment of the brain is a major physiological concept that was decades ahead of its time and really only began to be properly accepted and investigated with the advent of radioactive tracers in the 2nd half of the 20th Century as outlined below.

Stern (1934) does not mention the relative importance of the cerebral vessels (blood-brain barrier) and choroid plexuses (blood-CSF barrier) in these dual functions of protection and regulation of the internal environment of the brain. This remains a technical difficulty to this day. It does seem highly unsatisfactory that later authors did not take account of Stern's direct studies on permeability of the cerebral blood vessels under both normal and pathological conditions. Another extremely important point made by Stern (1934) was her insistence on the necessity of appreciating that the barrier does not have uniform properties with respect to the wide range of molecules that she studied in earlier works: "...le fonctionnement de la barrière ne présente pas un caractère uniforme vis à vis de toutes les substances examinées...": *the function of the barrier is not uniform with respect to all substances studied.* This is an extremely important point, which is often still not realized to this day.

In contrast to the adult brain, in the developing brain it is now clear that the choroid plexuses are indeed the main portal of entry into the brain (Johansson et al., 2008). As will be recounted below, after returning from Geneva to Moscow in 1925 (Dreifuss and Sigrist, 2009) Stern made important contributions to the study of brain barriers in developing animals of a number of species in a series of short papers published in the period 1927–1929. If more notice had been taken of Stern's papers, the longstanding belief in the absence of the blood-brain barrier in the fetus and newborn might have been short-lived.

EARLY DYE STUDIES IN IMMATURE ANIMALS

The important paper of Wislocki (1920), discussed above and illustrated in **Figure 1A**, was rarely cited in most of the literature of the 20th Century, perhaps because it did not fit with the prevailing belief in immaturity of the blood-brain barrier. Even King (1939), who published with Wislocki, does not mention the seminal 1920 paper preferring instead to cite Behnsen (1927) as evidence of barrier immaturity; the deficiencies of the latter study are discussed next. These are perhaps the most cited in support of immaturity or leakiness of the blood-brain barrier (Behnsen, 1926, 1927) particularly his 1927 paper (e.g., Spatz, 1934; King, 1939; Friedemann, 1942; Davson, 1967). In the 1926 paper Behnsen refers to sealing ("Abdichtung") of the barrier in the postnatal animals, and writes in the summary on page 1146 that the blood brain barrier is considerably more leaky (original: "erheblich durchlässiger") than in adult mice as staining with trypan blue appears in young animals more intense generally and also in different places of the CNS compared to the staining pattern of adults. However, in some slightly handicapped adult mice Behnsen also found additional areas in the brain which were stained, that he called those weak spots (orig. "schwache Stellen"), besides those where apparently no barrier exists (orig. "offene Stellen") and puts this in contrast to Goldmann's view that the central nervous is entirely sealed from dye (Goldmann, 1909, 1913). He also suggested: *The fact that the blood-brain barrier in the young is more leaky may also relate to immaturity of tissues and cells and a different level of cellular maturity.* (orig.: "Im Speicherverhalten der nervösen Zellen zeigen sich Unterschiede, die ...auf einen verschiedenen Reifezustand der Zellen zu beziehen sind," Behnsen, 1926. p. 1146). It may be that Behnsen's finding of dye in some parts of the brain was due to the use of an excessive amount of dye (three injections of 1% trypan blue).

Behnsen's paper of 1927 is longer and more detailed and the results and interpretations differ in some respects to the 1926 paper. He speaks more cautiously about an increasing sealing of the barrier during postnatal development and points out that even in adult mice staining can be found in the brain due to local penetration of dye. He commented: "*The sites of dye penetration in the adult animals correspond to the maximal storage in young mice. They are located 1. In the region of Retzius'ependymal wedge in the medulla oblongata; 2. At the attachment sites of the choroid plexus; 3. In the infundibular recess*" (Translation of orig.: "Die Farbstoffdurchtrittstellen der erwachsenen Tiere entsprechen den Speicherungsmaxima der jungen Mäuse...").

Behnsen (1927) himself does not appear to state unequivocally that the barrier is immature in the newborn and his experiments have a number of curious features. As was the case for many barrier studies in the early part of the 20th Century, they involved multiple injections of trypan blue into postnatal (2–3 week old) and adult mice. He reported that areas of the brain that stain for trypan blue at postnatal ages were more extensive than in the adult, but they are located at the same sites, which Behnsen calls "Grenzflächen" i.e., interfaces/membranes between brain and bloodstream or even more generally used by Behnsen: membranes involved in barrier functions are of the same structure in young and adult animals, they only differ gradually in their function. "Die Übereinstimmung der Speicherstellen der erwachsenen Tiere mit denen der jungen macht es sehr wahrscheinlich, daß die Grenzflächen im erwachsenen Zustand, nur graduell verschieden, dieselben örtlichen Bauunterschiede aufweisen, wie sie das Speicherbild für junge Tiere offenbarte." (Behnsen, 1927, p. 570): *The identical storage sites (of dye) in adult animals and in young ones makes it highly likely that the interfaces ("Grenzflächen") in the adult condition differ only gradually, but are otherwise of the same structure as revealed by the dye storage of young animals.*

This is illustrated in two figures reproduced here in **Figure 3**. The distribution of trypan blue is illustrated in sagittal sections of mouse brain from the two ages. However, it is the same line drawing of an adult brain that is used for both ages. This gives the misleading impression that the distribution of the dye in the postnatal brain was wider than it probably was in the actual microscopical slides. This is because the neonatal brain is less well developed particularly with respect to the neocortex. **It is also notable that there is no staining indicated in the postnatal neocortex as this is the region with the least well developed vasculature in the postnatal period compared to the rest of the brain; were the blood-brain barrier to dye to be immature, this is precisely where dye staining would be expected to be apparent.** Bakay (1956) commented that although Behnsen's conclusions are frequently misquoted "they do not reveal a generalized increase in permeability of the barrier."

Behnsen's experiments were repeated in careful detail by Moos and Møllgård (1993). They studied the distribution of trypan blue and Evans blue, a dye that superseded trypan blue from about mid-20th century for blood-brain barrier studies. Moos and Møllgård (1993) used a range of concentrations of the dyes some of which exceeded the binding capacity of plasma albumin to which these dyes bind. Binding of dyes to plasma albumin appears to have been overlooked by the blood-brain barrier field until the observations of Tschirgi (1950), although Ehrlich himself commented that the lack of some of his small molecular weight dyes in urine, was probably accounted for by binding to plasma albumin (Ehrlich, 1885). Also, Stern and colleagues (e.g., Stern et al., 1929) made a distinction in guinea pig embryos and neonatal animals of various species between the blood-brain barrier permeability of low molecular weight sodium ferrocyanide and the lack of penetration of trypan blue, which they described as a colloid. Whether this description reflects knowledge of protein binding or aggregation of the dye in blood is not clear. However, the difference between entry of small lipid insoluble molecules (sodium ferrocyanide in early qualitative experiments and sucrose and inulin in later quantitative experiments) and the lack of entry of trypan blue turned out to be a fundamental distinction in properties of blood-brain and blood-CSF barriers, as will be described below.

Stern et al. (1924) studied the entry of sodium ferrocyanide from blood into CSF in various species at different stages of development. They reported that in the guinea pig the barrier to this molecule was already as in the adult, but in species born at a less mature stage of development (rats, mice, cats) sodium ferrocyanide could be detected in the CSF. Stern and Peyrot (1927) extended the earlier study of Stern et al. (1924) examining entry sodium ferrocyanide into the CSF. In guinea pig fetuses this marker did enter the CSF, but as reported earlier not in the newborn of this species. They confirmed the entry of sodium ferrocyanide in the newborns of rats, mice and cats and in addition rabbits.

Stern and Rapoport (1928a) studied the injection of dyes (trypan blue and Congo red) in neonates of various species. They distinguished clearly between a barrier at the level of the vascular endothelium and the choroid plexus epithelium in dye studies where cellular staining following dye injections, but unlike other authors they thought this was a post mortem phenomenon. In a following year using the same dyes Stern et al. (1929) made the important point that it was necessary to limit the amount dye injected. They stressed that in experiments in adults and developing animals using similar amounts of dye, no dye entered the CSF. But if the amounts were increased substantially (30–40 times than used normally) then staining of the CSF occurred.

Another dye study that is sometimes cited as evidence of barrier immaturity in neonates (e.g., Ribatti et al., 2006) is that of Penta (1932). Penta injected multiple doses of trypan blue or trypan red into postnatal rabbits and cats. Penta seems to have considered that the results of Behnsen and Stern were similar, although as described above Stern et al. (1929) found no entry of trypan blue in the brains of developing animals providing not too much dye was injected. Penta summarized his results as showing that the nervous system of neonates is colored more intensely than that of adults and staining occurred in the regions where the mesenchyme penetrates into the neuraxis. As in many of the adult studies using trypan blue and against the advice of Stern (Stern et al., 1929) Penta mainly used multiple large doses of trypan blue and many of the animals died from the toxic effects of the dye; therefore staining of the brain was hardly surprising. However, Penta did describe one experiment in which much less dye was used in which no staining of the brain (apart from the choroid plexus) occurred, thus confirming Stern's results, without Penta apparently realizing it.

There seems little doubt that at least part of the problem with many early dye studies, both in developing animals and adults, was that the large amounts and multiple injections used led to toxic effects. This might be indicative of a greater fragility of brain barriers in immature animals but should not be interpreted as evidence of an immature or absent blood brain barrier.

The binding of dyes to albumin in plasma was investigated systematically by Moos and Møllgård (1993). They showed that dye only entered the brains of neonatal (one day old) mice and rats if the albumin binding capacity was exceeded, except in regions of the brain known to be devoid of a blood-brain barrier. For concentrations of dye (trypan blue, 1–2%; Evans blue, 0.5–1.0%) that were shown not to exceed the binding capacity of albumin in plasma, neither dye penetrated into the brain by exudation

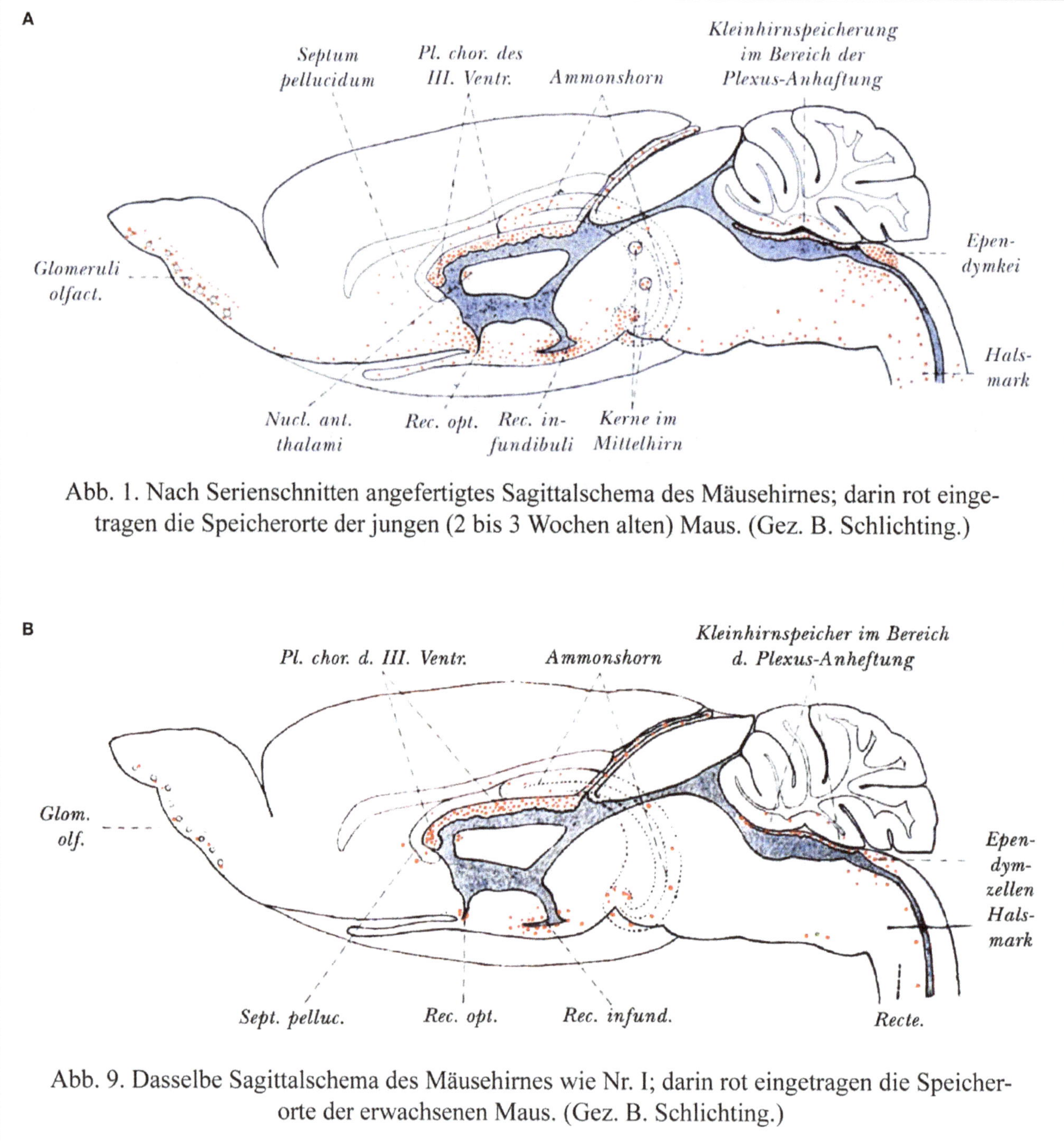

FIGURE 3 | Behnsen's much cited trypan blue experiments. (A) Brain from postnatal mouse injected systemically 3 times with trypan blue at P4–P14. **(B)** Adult mouse brain following systemic injection of trypan blue. Note that as described by Behnsen the dye staining in the postnatal brain is in the same regions as in the adult brain, but more extensive. This is probably a visual artifact due to the use of an outline of an adult mouse brain for both ages. In postnatal mouse brain (P14) the cerebral cortex and cerebellum are less developed than illustrated here. Note also that in the postnatal brain there does not appear to be any dye staining of the neocortex-the region of the developing brain with the least mature blood vessels. From Behnsen (1927).

across cerebral vessel walls in either P10 or adult mice, although there was some staining of choroid plexus epithelial and cerebral endothelial cells. At higher concentrations of the dyes (trypan blue, 2–4%; Evans blue, 2%) at which there was a substantial level of free dye, 60% of neonates and 20% of adults died, with higher proportions at the higher concentrations of dye. Those animals that survived showed various signs of neurotoxicity. Toxic effects of trypan blue had been reported earlier (e.g., Behnsen, 1927; Penta, 1932) but the significance of this in interpretation of barrier studies with dyes seems to have been overlooked by all but

Stern who urged caution in the amount of dye to be injected into neonatal animals (Stern et al., 1929).

LATER STUDIES OF DYES, ALBUMIN AND OTHER MARKERS IN IMMATURE ANIMALS

The use of dyes to study blood-brain barrier permeability in immature animals began to die out in the second half of the 20th Century. This is in contrast to the adult blood-brain barrier field, which continues to place a heavy reliance on dyes, particularly Evans blue, for assessing blood-brain barrier integrity. All of the studies published after 1950 agreed in showing that dyes (usually trypan blue) did not enter the developing brain no matter what age was investigated. The most important of these studies is probably that of Gröntoft (1954) who did experiments in both human fetuses (recent abortions) and newborns. Gröntoft emphasized that the condition of the fetuses was very important in determining whether or not the dye entered the brain. In a series of carefully conducted experiments he showed clearly that when trypan blue was injected as soon as possible after separation of the placenta in human fetuses of a wide range of gestational age, the dye did not stain the brain as a whole, but only those areas (choroid plexus and circumventricular organs) that are outside the blood-brain barrier (**Figure 4**); this was the case even in a very immature embryo of 5 cm in length (approximately 10 weeks post conception). However, when the dye was injected at progressively longer intervals after placental separation of the fetuses (10–30 min depending upon the gestational age) then the whole of the brain stained. Gröntoft carried out similar well-controlled experiments in rabbit fetuses with the same findings.

Grazer and Clemente (1957) injected by various routes solutions of trypan blue into rat embryos from E10.5 to birth. They found no evidence of dye penetration into the brain. Millen and Hess (1958) injected i.p. two doses, 24 h apart, of either trypan blue or sodium ferrocyanide, into neonatal (P0–P8) and adult rats and the animals were examined after 30 min. No staining of the brain for either marker was identified in the neonatal animals apart from the restricted regions (outside the blood-brain barrier) that also stained in the adult. Similar results were reported by Olsson et al. (1968) who injected fluorescently labeled bovine albumin intravascularly in rat embryos as early as E15, compared with neonates and adults.

In the second half of the 20th Century there was a switch from using dyes to using horseradish peroxidase (HRP) as a test of barrier integrity in the developing brain. HRP has a number of problems that are not always well recognized by those that use it. In the context of development the main problem is that, as

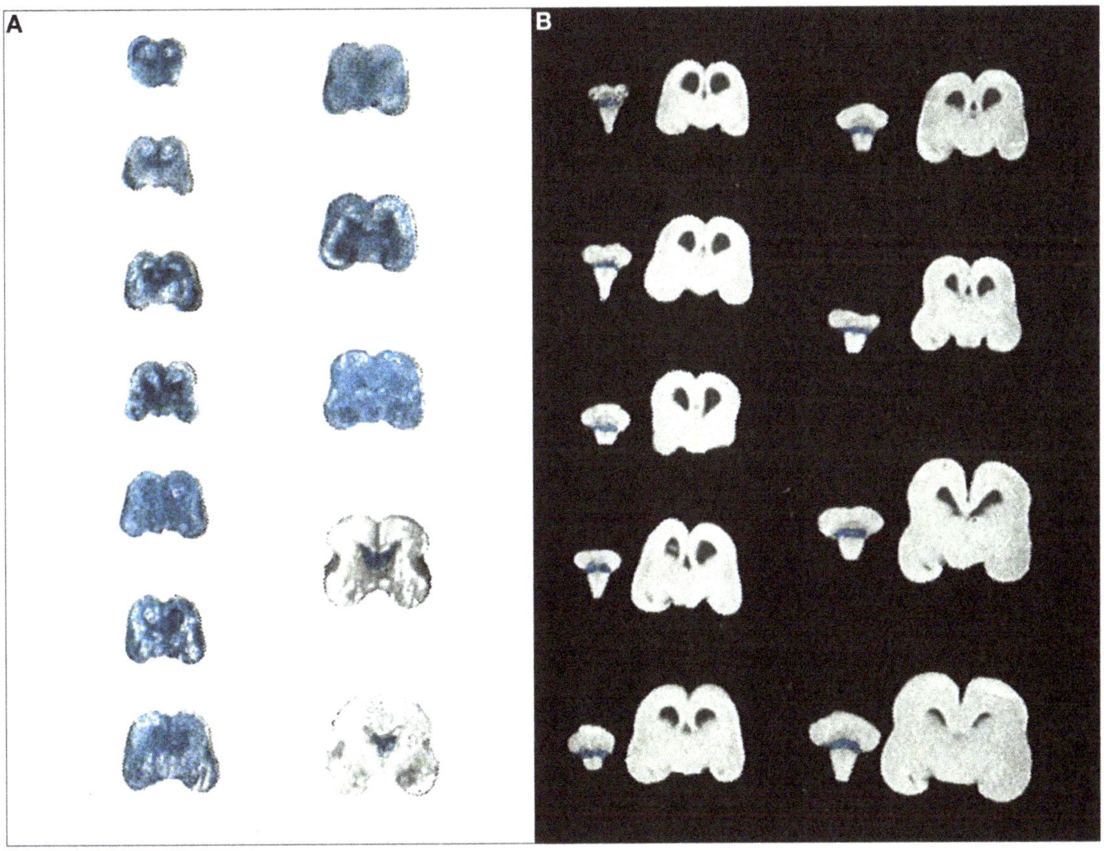

FIGURE 4 | Gröntoft's dye experiments with postmortem aborted human fetuses. (A) Human fetuses (14 cm-18 weeks to 30 cm-31 weeks gestation) injected with trypan blue solution 30 min after caesarian section delivery. **(B)** Human fetuses (14 cm-18 weeks to 30 cm-31 weeks gestation) injected with trypan blue solution 10 min after caesarian section delivery. Note that for the shorter period of anoxia none of the brains stained with trypan blue indicating intact blood-brain barrier to trypan blue even in immature human fetuses. Reproduced with permission from Gröntoft (1954), © Wiley.

with the dyes in earlier experiments, too large a volume or concentration of HRP was injected, thus damaging fragile cerebral blood vessels and giving the appearance of a "leaky" blood-brain barrier (see **Table 1**). Several other authors reported the entry of HRP into brains of very immature embryos, for example chick embryos (Delorme et al., 1970; Delorme, 1972; Bertossi et al., 1992). However, insufficient detail of exactly what was injected makes it difficult to evaluate the results of these studies. The finding that HRP entered the brain at different embryonic ages in the same species or at different stages of brain development in different species suggests that the findings from these studies are likely to have been artefactual. There have been a few reports of

Table 1 | Injection experiments used as test of blood-brain barrier integrity in fetal and neonatal animals.

Authors	Species	Age◇ (days)	Body weight (g)[a]	Injection vol[b] (% total blood vol)	Increase in plasma protein concentration[c]	"Leaky" barrier claimed•	Injected material[d]
Grazer and Clemente, 1957	Rat	E10.5	<0.06	Not stated	–	No	Trypan blue i.p./i.v.[b]
Olsson et al., 1968	Rat	E15	0.14	<5%	–	No	Fluorescein-albumin, Umb.A.
Delorme et al., 1970	Chick	E4.5	0.1	Not stated	3%	Reaction product in neuropil ECS until E10	HRP i.v.
Wakai and Hirokawa, 1978, 1981	Chick	E8	0.5	10%	500%	Yes	HRP i.v.
Dziegielewska et al., 1979, 1980	Sheep	E60	60	7.5%	20%	No	Human plasma protein i.v.
Lossinsky et al., 1986	Mouse	Newborn	1.4	35%	2%	Yes, "massive leakage"	HRP i.v.
Roncali et al., 1986	Chick	E6	0.34	>150%	50%	"Unimpeded extravasation"	HRP intracardiac[e]
Risau et al., 1986	Mouse	E13	0.08	250%	1% increase	"Fully permeable"	HRP intracardiac[e]
Vorbrodt et al., 1986	Mouse	Newborn	1.4	100%	200–300%	Yes**	HRP i.v.
Stewart and Hayakawa, 1987	Mouse	E15	0.26	Not stated	100%*	Yes	HRP i.p.[f]
Dziegielewska et al., 1988	Tammar wallaby	Newborn	0.50	10–20%	25–50%	No	HRP/HSA i.v.
Hulsebosch and Fabian, 1989	Rat	Newborn	5.0	50%*	>400%*	IgG penetration into neuraxis	IgG i.p.[b]
Dermietzel et al., 1992	Rat	E14.5	0.14	100–150%	>100%	Yes	HRP or 40 kDa dextran intracardiac[d]
Ribatti et al., 1993	Chick	E6	0.36[a]	>150%	50%	"Massive diffusion"	HRP or Evans blue, intracardiac
Xu and Ling, 1994	Rat	Newborn	5.0	10%	65%	Yes	Ferritin solution i.v.
Knott et al., 1997	Opossum	P3	0.20	8%*	0.5%*	No	Human albumin i.p.

[a] *Body weights and circulating blood and plasma volumes for chick embryos from Romanoff (1967) and Davis and Garrison (1968). Body weights of fetal rats from unpublished data. Body weights of opossum from Saunders et al. (1989) and unpublished. Weight of youngest animal given.*

[b] *The authors' injection volume when stated has been compared to estimates of circulating blood volume (10% of body weight and allowing a factor of 2 for placental blood volume in the case of fetuses and for extra-embryonic blood volume in chick embryos, although it is doubtful if under the conditions of some of these experiments, much mixing with fetal placental blood would have occurred.*

[c] *The actual circulating blood volume in sheep fetuses has been measured (Dziegielewska et al., 1991). The effect of the amount of injected protein on the plasma protein concentration is also estimated when sufficient information is available. Plasma protein concentrations from Birge et al. (1974, chick embryo) and Dziegielewska et al. (1981, rat fetus).*

[d] *Information is not usually available about the speed of injection nor about the likely distribution volume (e.g., in experiments involving intracardiac injection.*

[e] *In which the normal circulation may not have continued or i.p. injection.*

[f] *In which it is not clear what proportion of the volume and protein will have entered the circulation).*

◇ *Youngest age studied. E is embryonic age from day of conception.*

* *Depending on proportion entering circulation. **But "not detected at E19."*

• *Not all authors of experiments in which marker entered brain tissue from blood vessels describe this as a "leak" or due to immaturity.*

transendothelial passage of markers such as HRP in developing brain (e.g., in tubulovesicular structures, Lossinsky et al., 1986) which may explain the entry of the marker into immature brain in some experiments, as lack of pinocytotic vesicles is a characteristic of adult cerebral endothelial cells.

ENTRY OF SMALL MOLECULAR COMPOUNDS INTO THE BRAIN AND CSF OF IMMATURE ANIMALS

Lina Stern and her colleagues published a preliminary report of studies in a range of species of developing animals (Stern et al., 1924). This was followed by a series of brief papers in the period 1927–1929 on the permeability of the "barrière hémato-encéphalique" to sodium ferrocyanide and several other low molecular weight compounds in fetal guinea pigs and newborns of several species (Stern and Peyrot, 1927; Stern and Rapoport, 1928a,b; Stern et al., 1929). Following injection into fetuses via the uterine horn of pregnant guinea pigs early in gestation, sodium ferrocyanide could be demonstrated by the Prussian blue reaction in the CSF and CNS tissue. However, when sodium ferrocyanide was injected into term embryo or newborn guinea pigs its presence could not be detected in either CSF or CNS tissue. In contrast, when sodium ferrocyanide was injected into the newborns of rabbits, rats, mice, dogs, and cats it could be demonstrated in CSF and nervous system tissue and for several days into the neonatal period. Stern and Peyrot (1927) correlated the cessation of sodium ferrocyanide entry into CSF and nervous tissue with the time of eye opening and suggested that this was the time when the blood-brain barrier ("barrière hémato-encéphalique") to certain substances reached a "normal value," presumably meaning that it reached the adult condition. They concluded that in species born at less mature stages of development (which they suggested probably included human newborns) the "activity" of the barrier was insufficient to protect the CNS against many substances circulating or introduced into the blood.

These qualitative observational results with a small molecule (sodium ferrocyanide 304 Da) foreshadowed quantitative experiments with radiolabelled small molecules such as mannitol (182 Da), sucrose (342 Da), and inulin (5200 Da) in newborns of rats (Ferguson and Woodbury, 1969; Woodbury et al., 1974; Johanson, 1989; Habgood et al., 1993) and fetal sheep (Evans et al., 1974; Dziegielewska et al., 1979), which showed higher CSF/plasma and brain/plasma ratios for the these molecules in immature animals. Although initially interpreted as indicating greater permeability of the blood-brain and blood CSF barriers, it became apparent from measurements of CSF secretion in embryos (Evans et al., 1974; Fossan et al., 1985) and newborns (Bass and Lundborg, 1973; Johanson and Woodbury, 1974) and increase in volume of CSF in rat embryos (Johansson et al., 2006, 2008) that the explanation is more likely to be that the much lower turnover (sink effect) of CSF in the developing brain allowed a greater accumulation of marker in CSF and brain (Bass and Lundborg, 1973; Johansson et al., 2008). However, it took the development of the use of small molecular weight markers that could be both quantified and visualized at the electron microscopic, EM level to show that the route of penetration from blood to CSF of these small markers was via an *intracellular* route in a subpopulation of epithelial cells in the choroid plexuses (Ek et al., 2001, 2003, 2006). These cells appear to be responsible for the transfer of inert dextrans and several plasma proteins from blood into CSF both in the developing and adult brain (Dziegielewska et al., 1991; Liddelow et al., 2009, 2011a). The absolute number of cells involved in this transfer actually increases with age as the choroid plexuses develop, but the CSF/plasma ratios for dextrans and proteins fall, because of the increased turnover of CSF and a larger space into which these markers are diluted (Johansson et al., 2006, 2008).

KERNICTERUS IN THE NEWBORN

One of the persistent beliefs about the blood-brain barrier in the immature organism is that the toxic effects of unconjugated bilirubin that accumulate in the blood of newborn infants suffering from erythroblastosis, generally due to Rhesus blood group incompatibility, are due to "immaturity" of the blood-brain barrier in the newborn. This is a suggestion generally attributed to Spatz (1934) e.g., Broman (1941); Davson (1967), and Lee (1971). Others stated that this was the case but without attribution (e.g., Ganong, 1993; Cotran et al., 1994). Bakay (1956) expressed the view that "the phenomenon of kernicterus appeared to offer irrefutable proof of this theory [that the blood-brain barrier in the newborn is immature]." In his later review Bakay is more circumspect and suggests that the causation of kernicterus has many components of which an immature blood-brain barrier might be one (Bakay, 1968).

Most of Spatz's lengthy paper is taken up with describing and repeating some of Behnsen's (1927) experiments with trypan blue. But he does have a short section on icterus (jaundice) in the adult, with an illustration showing that yellow pigment of bilirubin was confined to dura. He compared this (without illustration) to brain damage (kernicterus) that only occurs in the newborn with the deposition of bilirubin in the brain, characteristically in the basal ganglia and brain stem (**Figure 5**). He does not seem to distinguish between conjugated bilirubin, which accumulates in the circulation of adults sometimes to very high levels, and unconjugated bilirubin that accumulates in newborns because the activity of the conjugating liver enzyme, glucuronyl transferase, is very low at birth and normally increases during the first days of life. These two forms of bilirubin had been identified earlier (van den Bergh and Müller, 1916). What was not known in the 1930s was that unconjugated bilirubin binds tightly to plasma albumin and a key factor (but not the only one) in the occurrence of kernicterus is when the binding capacity of albumin for unconjugated bilirubin is exceeded; this form of bilirubin which is highly lipid soluble (in contrast to conjugated bilirubin) enters the brain without restraint.

It is noteworthy that clinicians, who have had to deal with the problem of kernicterus in the newborn for many years, rarely seem to have invoked the state of maturity of the blood-brain barrier in the neonate as a major factor in the occurrence of kernicterus (e.g., Iskander et al., 2014), although it has occasionally been mentioned (e.g., Zuelzer and Mudgett, 1950; Spiegel-Adolf et al., 1954; Ernster et al., 1957); rather they developed clinical treatments aimed at reducing the level of unconjugated bilirubin in infants who were at risk: exchange transfusion (Allen et al., 1950; Gerrard, 1952) barbiturate induction of glucuronyl

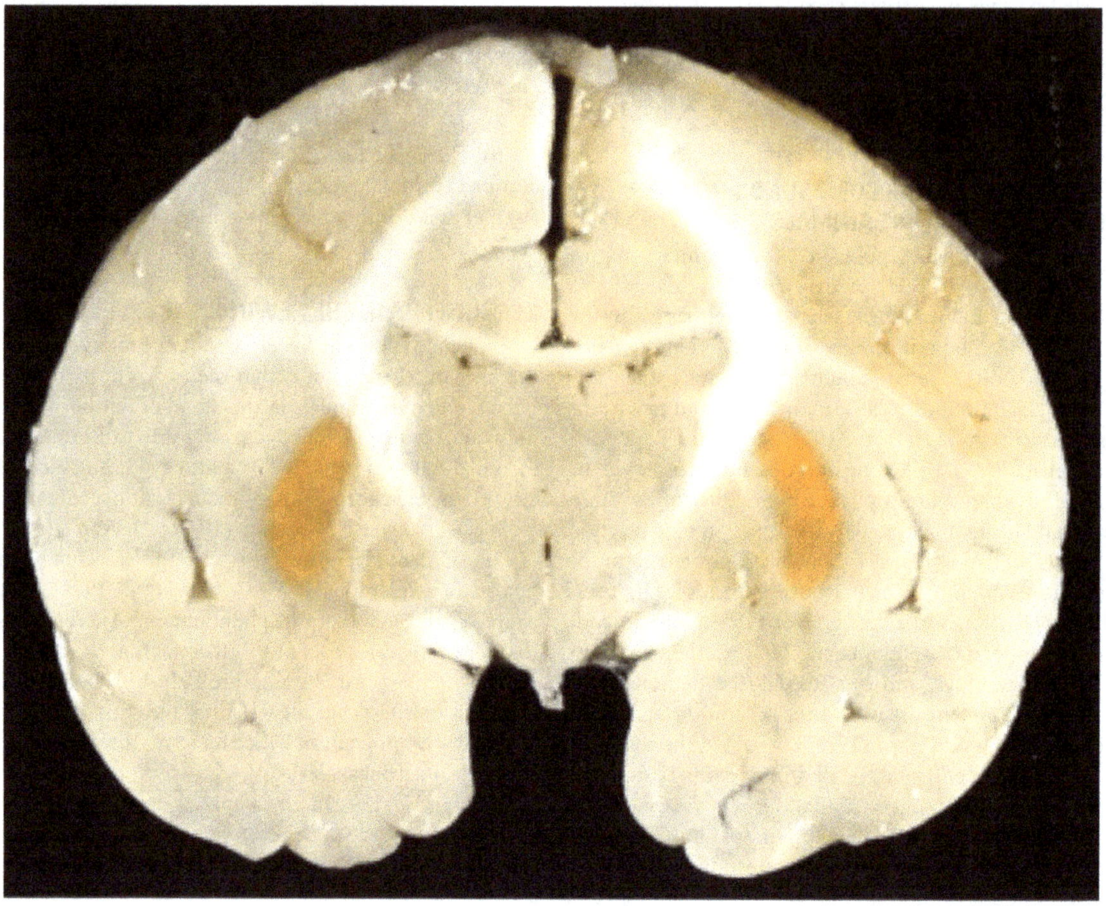

FIGURE 5 | Kernicterus in brain of neonatal monkey with jaundice. Note staining of putamen (one of the basal ganglia), which does not occur in adult brain as jaundice in adults, is generally due to high levels of conjugated bilirubin to which the blood brain barrier is impermeable. From Windle (1969).

transferase and phototherapy (Lucey, 1971) as well as prevention by immunization of Rh-ve women against the D blood group antigen (Clarke, 1989). But the linking of blood-brain barrier immaturity to kernicterus has persisted amongst other groups of scientists and clinicians for decades after Spatz (1934). A good example is a physiologist, (Ganong, 1993) who stated that: "Bile pigments do not enter the brain in the adult but in the fetus and newborn infant the blood-brain barrier is not developed." Following correspondence with one author (NRS) in later editions Ganong (1999) modified this to state that "the bilirubin penetrates the brain of infants with erythroblastosis at least in part because the blood-brain barrier is more permeable in infancy"; he was not willing to take account of the effect of binding of unconjugated bilirubin to plasma albumin. Similar wording has been retained by the new authors of Ganong's Review of Medical Physiology (Barrett et al., 2012) following his unfortunate demise. Some aspects of bilirubin neural toxicity are discussed by Palmela et al. (submitted).

Some pathologists have also considered that kernicterus is due to immaturity of the blood-brain barrier (Cotran et al., 1994). A detailed consideration of kernicterus is beyond the scope of this review. But comprehensive papers are available both on the pathogenesis and treatment particularly by Wennberg and his colleagues (e.g., Wennberg, 2000; Ahlfors and Wennberg, 2004; Wennberg et al., 2006) and in Volpe (2008). However, it is becoming increasingly clear that the mechanisms involved in whether or not kernicterus occurs in newborns are much more complex than the absolute level of unconjugated bilirubin and the binding capacity of albumin in plasma. These complexities have been reviewed by Ghersi-Egea et al. (2009) and include the finding that bilirubin is a substrate for several ABC efflux transporters, which would thus be expected to contribute to limiting the entry of bilirubin into the brain.

EXPERIMENTS WITH RADIOISOTOPICALLY LABELED MOLECULES IN DEVELOPING ANIMALS

The introduction of radiolabelled markers was a major advance in experimental approaches to understanding blood-brain barrier mechanisms. The use of inert markers of permeability such as sucrose and inulin has been mentioned above. In this section we shall deal briefly with experiments involving the use of P^{32} and amino acids labeled with ^{3}H or ^{14}C. Compared to inert markers there are potential problems with metabolically active radiolabelled molecules such as amino acids. Thus it needs to be shown that the radioactive tag is still attached to the molecule and that the measured radioactivity is due to transfer into the brain separate from its metabolic incorporation, for example into proteins.

^{32}PHOSPHORUS

Bakay (1953, 1956) studied the uptake of ^{32}P into brain and other organs following parenteral injection into pregnant (3rd–4th week), newborn, up to 7 weeks postnatal rabbits and in the adult. Animals were killed 24 h after injection and various organs dissected out. In some cases radioautographs of the heads or brains of fetuses were prepared. The results showed a much higher uptake of ^{32}P in the younger the animals. In fetuses and newborns the brain/blood ratio was >1, compared to about 0.3 in the adult, which Bakay (1953) interpreted as indicating that the vascular permeability in the fetal brain is increased. He discusses whether the increased permeability reflects a leaky, incompletely formed blood-brain barrier or increased metabolism and faster turnover in the developing nervous system. He concluded that neither explanation was satisfactory. Bakay (1953) observed that in the radioautographs of fetal brain the distribution of ^{32}P was almost uniform whereas in the brain of the mother it was concentrated in the choroid plexuses and the lining of the ventricles. Rather puzzlingly he took this as evidence that there is a blood-brain barrier to ^{32}P in the fetus but that its permeability is greater than in the adult.

AMINO ACID TRANSPORT

In early experiments with radiolabelled amino acids there was a similar finding of a much greater entry of some (but not all) into the developing than adult brain of several species (Himwich et al., 1957; Roberts et al., 1959; Purpura and Carmichael, 1960; Lajtha and Toth, 1961; Seta et al., 1972; Baños et al., 1978) but as with ^{32}P it was not possible to distinguish between cerebral endothelial cell transport and metabolic incorporation into brain tissue in accounting for the greater uptake in developing brain. Some authors interpreted such results as indicating "lesser effectiveness" of the blood-brain barrier for amino acids in young animals (e.g., Kuttner et al., 1961; Lee, 1971). The problem of determining cerebral transport of amino acids across the blood-brain barrier without the complication of metabolic contamination of brain samples was solved by Oldendorf (1971) who developed a short pass technique in which exposure of amino acid or other metabolically active molecules to the brain from the cerebrovascular circulating blood was limited to one circulation time, thus being too quick for significant metabolic incorporation to occur. The technique was adapted for newborn and postnatal animals by Oldendorf's students (Braun et al., 1980; Cornford et al., 1982; Pardridge and Mietus, 1982) and by Lefauconnier and Trouvé (1983), Al-Sarraf (2002), and Al-Sarraf et al. (1997). These experiments showed that many amino acids and other metabolically active compounds were transported into developing brain at much higher rates than in the adult; this was interpreted as reflecting the greater metabolic demand of the developing brain rather than immaturity of the blood-brain barrier. However, some authors have continued to suggest that greater uptake may reflect barrier immaturity (e.g., Watson et al., 2006).

Thus it has been clear for sometime that transport mechanisms at the brain barrier interfaces determine the composition of the internal environment of developing brain and supply essential nutrients and other molecules important for growth and differentiation of the brain. What has been lacking until recently is information on the presence and expression of specific transporters in the brain barrier interfaces. This is now available from expression studies of isolated cerebral endothelial cells from neonatal mice (Daneman et al., 2010a) and from choroid plexuses of fetal mice and rats compared to the adult (Liddelow et al., 2012, submitted). Many of these so called Slc transporters are expressed at higher levels in the developing brain compared to the adult, thus accounting for the earlier observations of higher entry of specific amino acids into the developing brain. There are differences in the expression patterns of these Slc transporters in the cerebral endothelial cells and in the choroid plexus epithelial cells and many more are expressed at higher levels in the fetal choroid plexus (see reviews by Saunders et al., 2013 and Liddelow et al., submitted). This reflects the greater importance of the choroid plexuses for transport into the brain compared to the vasculature at very early stages of brain development. The plexuses develop much earlier than the blood supply (Johansson et al., 2008). The findings also help to explain a number of important observations on developmentally different effects of amino acids on brain function. For example it was reported many years ago that glutamate is toxic to the brain if administered in the neonatal period (Olney and Ho, 1970) which some attributed to "immaturity" of the blood-brain barrier (Viña et al., 1997). However, it can now be seen that the barrier contribution to toxicity is much more likely to be due to greater transport of glutamate by e.g., Slc1a4 (see Saunders et al., 2012).

THE PARACELLULAR PATHWAY AND TIGHT JUNCTIONS IN BARRIER INTERFACES IN THE DEVELOPING BRAIN

The concept of the paracellular pathway is an important tenet of epithelial biology that was extended to cerebral endothelial interfaces. It arose from some ingenious experiments of Frömter and Diamond (1972). These authors measured transepithelial resistance in a variety of epithelia *in vitro* by passing a microelectrode over the external surface of the epithelium. They observed that when the electrode tip was over the region of the border between adjacent cells there was a marked drop in resistance across the epithelium. Frömter and Diamond proposed that this indicated a low resistance pathway across the epithelium for water and ion flow. They subsequently extended this concept to include the paracellular pathway as the route by which small lipid insoluble molecules such as sucrose crossed epithelia (Diamond, 1974). The physical basis for the paracellular pathway is the junctional complex between adjacent cells and in particular the tight junction component of the complex (Brightman and Reese, 1969). However, there are some important limitations to this interpretation of the sites of low resistance across epithelia. Firstly the dimensions of the tip of the microelectrodes used by Frömter and Diamond was about 5 μM compared to the intercellular space at the level of tight junctions, which is measured in nanometers, if not zero where adjacent cell membranes are fused. Thus an alternative explanation for the low resistance pathway is that there is an intracellular pathway close to the border of the cell membrane between adjacent cells.

Diamond (1974) seems to have acknowledged this possibility as he suggested that in some epithelia the low resistance pathway might be due to "leaky" cells, although he thought this would be exceptional. Secondly, water and ions cannot yet be visualized with sufficient resolution for their route across epithelia to be defined. Until recently this was also the case for low molecular weight compounds such as sucrose and inulin; however, this problem has been solved by the use of biotin labeled small molecular sized compounds that can be visualized at both the light and electron microscopical level. At least in the case of choroid plexus epithelial and cerebral endothelial cells in the South American opossum, *Monodelphis domestica*, the intercellular junctions are impermeable to a compound biotin ethylenediamine that is smaller than sucrose (Ek et al., 2001, 2003, 2006). In addition it was found that biotin labeled markers transfer across a subpopulation of plexus epithelial cells and not between them (Ek et al., 2001, 2003, 2006; Liddelow et al., 2009). These studies require independent replication, preferably in several different species, but they indicate that the earliest vessels growing into the brain are structurally well enough developed for their tight junctions to be impermeable to even very small molecules. These results also suggest that the presence of a low resistance pathway across epithelial cells, rather than the paracellular route, as envisaged by Diamond (1974) as an exceptional situation may indeed exist.

Over many years the results of ultrastructural studies of tight junctions in the cerebral vasculature and choroid plexuses of the developing brain have been conflicting. Two of the earliest ultrastructural studies of the developing mammalian brain barriers were those of Donahue and Pappas, (1961, rat cerebral capillaries) and Tennyson and Pappas (1964, rabbit choroid plexus). Most of their descriptions dealt with subcellular structures, but they do comment on and illustrate what in those days were called terminal bars that were present in the earliest embryos examined (E14). These appear to correspond to structures associated with what were subsequently described as tight junctions (Brightman and Reese, 1969). Particularly considering that the 1960s were early days for electron microscopy of developing brain tissue (which in those days was regarded as very difficult to fix adequately) the micrographs of Donahue and Pappas and Tennyson and Pappas are of high quality and show clearly well formed intercellular tight junctions. Tennyson (1975) published a more comprehensive paper on choroid plexus development in human and rabbit fetuses. It includes illustrations of what she now refers to as "tight junctions" in the earliest rabbit fetuses studied (E15).

Subsequent to the early paper of Tennyson and Pappas (1964) there have been numerous transmission electron microscope studies of tight junctions in the developing brain, mainly in chick embryos (Delorme et al., 1970; Delorme, 1972; Roy et al., 1974) rodents (Stewart and Hayakawa, 1994) fetal sheep (Møllgård and Saunders, 1975, 1977; Møllgård et al., 1976, 1979) but also some in human fetuses (Møllgård and Saunders, 1975, 1986; Virgintino et al., 2004). Most, but not all, seem to agree that the typical appearance of closely apposed cell membranes of adjacent cerebral endothelial cells appears very early in brain development, although some authors (e.g., Stewart and Wiley, 1981) nonetheless conclude that the blood-brain barrier at these early stages is more permeable than in the adult. This was based on citing papers showing greater entry of both metabolically active and inert molecules into the developing brain and a high concentration of protein in CSF (cf. Sections 6, 8, and 11).

Some authors also used HRP in an attempt to delineate the age at which there was a change from blood-brain barrier permeability to one of impermeability. However, insofar as the methodological information is available it seems likely that in many experiments excessive volumes or concentrations of HRP solution or other markers were injected, thus mechanically disrupting the fragile blood vessels (e.g., Wakai and Hirokawa, 1978, 1981; Risau et al., 1986; Stewart and Hayakawa, 1987; Bertossi et al., 1988; Ribatti et al., 1993; and see **Table 1**). Also HRP has toxic effects and may give rise to anomalous permeability results, even in adult animals (e.g., Mazariegos et al., 1984). Nevertheless Tauc et al. (1984) were able to show that tight junctions in the choroid plexuses of rat embryos at least as early as E14 were impermeable to HRP. These observations were supported by freeze fracture studies showing a similarly early development of tight junction structure.

Møllgård et al. (1976) carried out a quantitative study of freeze fracture tight junction complexity in fetal sheep embryonic choroid plexus. This showed that there were only minor changes in junctional complexity over a large period of development in contrast to reports in the same species of large developmental changes in apparent permeability from blood to CSF for small molecular markers (Evans et al., 1974; Dziegielewska et al., 1979). It should be noted that the large change in apparent permeability was probably mainly due to an increase in CSF secretion rate (see above), but this does not diminish the significance of the finding that the freeze fracture appearance of choroid plexus tight junctions appeared very early in development.

Dermietzel et al. (1977) published a detailed freeze fracture study of the development of intercellular junctions of the chick embryo choroid plexus from E5, the day on which it begins to differentiate. A junctional network of strands was apparent by E6 and by E9 intercellular zonula occludens were more or less complete.

Attempts to correlate expression of individual tight junction genes with some supposed age when cerebral blood vessels stop being leaky, seem doomed to failure unless experiments are conducted under adequate physiological conditions. The findings that different tight junction genes are expressed at different ages and that the junctions become molecularly more complex with age seem more likely to reflect changes in the mechanical properties of tight junctions in the face of increasing hydrostatic pressure (systemic blood pressure) during embryonic and fetal development (Evans et al., 1974; Dziegielewska et al., 1979). The question of whether or not there is a stage of early vascularization of the brain when the blood vessels are leaky is a functional one that can only be answered by permeability experiments conducted under reasonably physiological conditions. In spite of several attempts (e.g., Risau et al., 1986; Mizee et al., 2013; Ben-Zvi et al., 2014, see also Bauer et al., 2014) there is no convincingly demonstrated link between the expression of one particular gene and the supposed sealing of blood vessels entering the CNS tissue, apart from Nitta et al. (2003) who showed increased permeability to small molecules (<800 Da) in claudin 5-deficient mice; this was attributed to tight junction permeability although not confirmed at the ultrastructural level.

IONIC GRADIENTS BETWEEN CSF AND PLASMA IN THE DEVELOPING BRAIN

Some of the most convincing evidence that some critical brain barrier properties develop very early in the embryo comes from studies of ion gradients between CSF and plasma. In the adult the ionic composition of CSF is characteristically different from that of plasma and is also appreciably more stable. This reflects the importance of a homeostatically constant environment that is a prerequisite for normal brain function (Davson, 1967; Davson and Segal, 1996). The gradients are set up by ion pumps in the epithelial cells of the choroid plexuses (Damkier et al., 2013). Similar pumps in the cerebral vascular endothelial cells may also contribute via the extracellular fluid of the brain (Davson and Segal, 1996). An essential structural component of this homeostatic mechanism is the presence of tight junctions between the adjacent cells of the choroid plexus epithelium and cerebrovascular endothelium. Thus in development, if even a single ion gradient is present, it indicates the presence of both a cellular ion pump and functional integrity of the tight junctions, as without the latter a gradient simply cannot be established. In the 1970s–80s there were several studies in a variety of species showing the presence of ion gradients between CSF and plasma (Flexner, 1938; Bito and Myers, 1970; Bradbury et al., 1972; Amtorp and Sørensen, 1974; Sedlácek, 1975; Mitchell et al., 1982; Nattie et al., 1984). More recently gene expression studies have shown that key ion channel and transporter genes are expressed very early embryonic life in the choroid plexuses (Liddelow et al., 2012, 2013).

CONCENTRATION AND ORIGIN OF PROTEINS IN CSF IN DEVELOPING BRAIN

One of the pieces of evidence sometimes put forward in favor of immaturity or leakiness of the blood-brain barrier in the developing brain is that the CSF in fetal and newborn animals contains a much higher concentration of protein than in the adult (Adinolfi et al., 1976; Adinolfi and Haddad, 1977; Ramey and Birge, 1979; Adinolfi, 1985; Fishman, 1992). Strictly speaking the composition of CSF is much more determined by movements of molecules across the choroid plexuses rather than entry via the blood vessels and brain interstitial fluid, although clinicians frequently (but erroneously) interpret CSF changes as reflecting changes in permeability of the blood-brain barrier. Since the middle of the last century it has been known that the concentration of protein in human newborn CSF (e.g., Spiegel-Adolf et al., 1954; Nasralla et al., 1958) is higher than in the adult (Davson and Segal, 1996) and even more so if the infants are prematurely born (e.g., Otila, 1948; Bauer et al., 1965). Results from these and other studies are summarized in **Table 2**. The mean values reported for healthy term babies were in the range 63–115 mg/100 ml. For pre-term infant the mean values in different series were generally higher (up to nearly 190 mg/100 ml). Little information about human fetal CSF is known but Adinolfi published important studies on CSF and plasma proteins obtained from aborted human fetuses (Adinolfi et al., 1976; Adinolfi and Haddad, 1977; Adinolfi, 1985). These studies showed that the concentration of total protein and of individual proteins such as a-fetoprotein, transferrin and IgG were much higher than reported for live-born infants; the highest

Table 2 | Total protein concentration (mg/100 ml) in CSF of full term and pre-term infants estimated during the first few days of life.

Authors	Mean (mg/100 ml)	S.E.M	Range	*n*	Condition
FULL TERM					
Spiegel-Adolf et al., 1954	103	9.9	–	14	Normal
Widell, 1958	80.9	6.2	–	11	Healthy
Nasralla et al., 1958	115	5.8	46–194	34	Normal
Naidoo, 1968	63	1.6	32–240	135	Healthy
Piliero and Lending, 1959	70	6.0	25–90	35	Normal
Watson, 1964	77	5.3	26–180	51	Cerebral anoxia
Heine et al., 1981[a]	73.0	17.6	53–95	10	No cereb meningitis
Ahmed et al., 1996	80.8	30.8*	–	17	Prev. healthy
Chadwick et al., 2011	106	–	94–115***	54	No meningitis
Srinivasan et al., 2012	78^	137**	60–100	130	Normal
PRE TERM					
Otila, 1948[b]	100	5.5	50–138	19	Healthy
Nasralla et al., 1958[c]	167	6.4	81–259	49	Normal
Gyllenswärd and Malmström, 1962[d]	176	26	57–292	9	Healthy
Bauer et al., 1965[e]	187	28	30–1600	70	Various
Bartolozzi et al., 1967[f]	62	4.3	12–144	59	Normal
Cole et al., 1974[g]	120	10	–	9	Normal
Sarff et al., 1976	90	–	20–170		No meningitis
Statz and Felgenhauer, 1983[h]	139	77*	68–240	10	No pathology
Mhanna et al., 2008[i]	180^	–	124–270	10	Suspect sepsis
Srinivasan et al., 2012[j]	104^	203**	79–131	148	Normal

[a]0–4 weeks. No data on birth weights or gestational age.
[b]Birth weights 920-2150 g, Table 19, p. 91.
[c]Birth weights ≤ 4.5 lbs, Table 2, p. 1404.
[d]Birth weights ≤ 2000 g, Table 5, p. 60.
[e]Birth weights 800–2620 g, Figure 1, p. 1018.
[f]Birth weights ≤ 2500 g, Figure 2, p. 299.
[g]Birth weights 1080–1710 g, Table 1, p. 724.
[h]27–32 weeks, Table 3, p. 158.
[i]27 weeks, values less at younger and older ages.
[j]28–35 weeks, Tables II, p730 and III, p731.
**S.D. **95th percentile. ***CIs. ^Median.*

individual total protein value reported was 730 mg/100 ml at 24 weeks gestation (Adinolfi et al., 1976) although it needs to be born in mind that the CSF samples were obtained from aborted fetuses of uncertain physiological state.

Similar results, however, have been obtained for numerous animal species where it was possible to obtain CSF and plasma samples from a wide range of stages of fetal and neonatal development collected under good physiological conditions. The results from animal studies have been reviewed by Saunders (1977, 1992) and by Dziegielewska and Saunders (1988). One of the earliest studies was by Klosovskii (1963) in cat embryos in which CSF protein concentration was up to 22 times that in the adult. Klosovskii correctly interpreted this as having some nutritive function in the developing brain rather than ascribing it to barrier immaturity. The concentration of total protein and of individual proteins in fetal CSF is much higher than in the newborn and adult, but if samples were obtained early enough in development the level was lower than a peak that occurred in all species probably coinciding with the period of maximum neurogenesis. Although Adinolfi (1985) and others interpreted the high CSF concentration of protein in CSF in the developing brain as evidence of a leaky blood-brain and/or blood-CSF barrier there is now substantial evidence that it is a consequence of specific transport of proteins from blood to CSF via a subpopulation of choroid plexus epithelial cells (Dziegielewska et al., 1980, 1991; Habgood et al., 1992; Knott et al., 1997; Johansson et al., 2006, 2008; Liddelow et al., 2009, 2011a,b). In addition it should be noted that the concentration of protein in any space is a function of its amounts and volume in which they distribute. As has been shown by Johansson et al. (2008) the *amount* of protein in the adult CSF is actually greater in the fetus due to a combination of expanding of the ventricular system and increased CSF flow.

INDUCTION OF TIGHT JUNCTIONS IN BRAIN BARRIER INTERFACES

Another widespread misconception is that astrocytes are essential for the induction of tight junctions in cerebral blood vessels in the developing brain. In adult brain end feet of astrocytes encircle cerebral capillaries (Caley and Maxwell, 1970; Xu and Ling, 1994). They are thought to make significant contributions to blood-brain barrier functions (Abbott et al., 2006). The belief that astrocytes may be involved in tight junction formation in the developing brain seems to stem largely from *in vitro* experiments. In culture the presence of either astrocytes or conditioned medium from cultured astrocytes produced cells with more complex tight junctions (Tao-Cheng et al., 1987) and was essential for the preparation of cerebral endothelial monolayers with high transendothelial resistance (Dehouck et al., 1990; Rubin et al., 1991). Janzer and Raff (1987) are frequently cited as supporting the notion that astrocytes are essential for tight junction formation *in vivo*. However, Holash et al. (1993) showed their results were an artifact (see Saunders et al., 2012, for further discussion). It seems to have been overlooked that there are no astrocytes present in the developing brain when it is first vascularized (Caley and Maxwell, 1970; Daneman et al., 2010a). As first shown by Stewart and Wiley (1981) using chick-quail chimeras, tight junction formation in cerebral vessels is induced by some factor in the neural tissue of the developing brain. The vessels are tight to proteins and small molecules from as early as vessels first grow into the neural tissue (Bauer et al., 1993, 1995; Ek et al., 2006). It is not yet clear what the induction factor(s) is/are. However it seems that the pericytes make an important contribution to tight junction formation (Daneman et al., 2010b). The main period of differentiation of astrocytes and their association with capillaries occur in rodents in the first 3 weeks of postnatal life (Caley and Maxwell, 1970). It may be that astrocytes contribute to tight junction-induction during this period of intense vascularization, and subsequent maintenance of tight junctions, but they are not involved in earlier stages of vascularization of the brain.

WHY IS IT IMPORTANT TO UNDERSTAND FUNCTIONING OF BARRIER MECHANISMS IN THE DEVELOPING BRAIN?

It seems unsatisfactory that this belief in the "immaturity" or leakiness of the blood-brain barrier has persisted into the 21st Century in spite of much evidence to the contrary as reviewed above. There are two quite different reasons why it is important to understand the functional status of barrier mechanisms in the developing brain. The first is that they are likely to be important for different features of brain development at different stages in its development. This is suggested for example, by changes in gene expression for different efflux and influx mechanisms in both the cerebral vasculature and choroid plexuses during brain development (Virgintino et al., 2000, 2007; Daneman et al., 2010a; Liddelow et al., 2012; Kratzer et al., 2013).

The other reason is that it is clinically important. At present because of a lack of information on the extent to which drugs enter the developing brain of the embryo following administration to the mother, the general advice given by doctors to pregnant women is to avoid taking drugs. However, this is not very helpful advice in the case of patients with severe medical conditions requiring continued treatment such as epilepsy (Forsberg and Wide, 2011) depression and anxiety (El Marroun et al., 2014; Ornoy and Koren, 2014) psychosis (Galbally et al., 2014) cancer (van Hasselt et al., 2014), or severe hypertension (Brown and Garovic, 2014).

In the US it has been estimated that between 30 and 35% of women have taken psychoactive drugs during pregnancy (Goldberg and Nissim, 1994). In a study of nearly 100,000 pregnancies, Andrade et al. (2004) found that 64% of pregnant women received a drug prescription. In a four nation study in Europe (De Vigan et al., 1999) an average of 36% of women interviewed used at least one drug during the first trimester of pregnancy. There was substantial national variation (22.5% in Glasgow and 50 and 40% in two centers in France). Because drugs are not systematically investigated for possible deleterious effects on the developing brain the clinical management of pregnant women may be a difficult decision between what is best for the mother and limiting potential damage to the developing fetal brain. This lack of knowledge not only makes it difficult for doctors to make rational decisions about when to and when not to medicate, but commonly results in non-compliance to prescribed medication, terminating medication or self-medication, as well as alternative natural remedies being used by mothers (Wood et al., 2014). The only information available to clinicians at present consists of collections of reports of adverse effects or lack of such effects in compendia such as Yaffe's index (Briggs et al., 2008) or national data organizations such as the US Food and Drug Administration (FDA) or the Australian Drug Evaluation Committee in pregnancy, which classify drugs into categories A/B/C/D/X, where A are drugs shown to be safe for the human fetus and X known to induce birth defects (see Teratology Society Public Affairs Committee, 1994). The majority of drugs fall into categories B and C, drugs for which there are not enough data in humans to know whether they are safe for the fetus. The consequences of the currently inadequate state of knowledge about the safety of medications administered during pregnancy have been highlighted by Kennedy (2011). This classification has been under sustained criticism from the Teratology Society in the US (Teratology Society Public Affairs Committee, 1994, 2007) primarily on the grounds that the lack of knowledge about drugs used in pregnancy generates difficulties in making clinical decisions and causing considerable anxiety in patients. This classification is now being abandoned in the US, in favor of a new pregnancy and lactation-labeling rule designed to improve risk versus benefit assessment of drugs used in pregnant and nursing mothers (Ramoz and Patel-Shori, 2014).

Drug use during pregnancy is likely to increase in the future due to higher average ages of mothers, increasing the likelihood of pregnancy complications as well as a higher incidence of premature births with significant medical interventions as a consequence. There is also a growing apprehension that environmental toxins may affect the developing brain. One review listed over 200 industrial compounds known to be neurotoxic in humans and experimental studies have shown over 1000 substances (Grandjean and Landrigan, 2006); this list probably only represents a very small fraction of all chemicals that are neurotoxic. It is particularly inappropriate that public bodies such as the Agency for Toxic Substances and Disease registry (ATSDR) at the Centre for Disease Control in the US should perpetuate statements about immaturity of the blood-brain barrier based on out of date information and mythology. This has been discussed in detail by Ek et al. (2012) but this discussion appears to have had no impact on current reports published by the ATSDR. A more hopeful sign is that the CDC has recently convened meetings to discuss developing a more systematic approach to safer medication use in pregnancy (Broussard et al., 2014).

Recent gene expression studies in developing animal brains (Daneman et al., 2010a; Liddelow et al., 2012, submitted; Kratzer et al., 2013) suggest that many of the protective efflux mechanism that prevent entry of drugs and toxins into the adult brain are present and in some cases more highly expressed in blood vessels and choroid plexuses of the developing brain. However, expression does not necessarily equate with functional effectiveness, so there is an urgent need for systematic drug studies in pregnant and newborn animals and people, in order to define clearly the potential hazards or lack of hazards, when drugs are administered to pregnant women.

SUMMARY

In conclusion, it seems that many of the most strongly held beliefs about the early history of the blood-brain barrier are incorrect. The blood-brain barrier was not described first by Ehrlich (1885); indeed he did not believe that there were any differences in permeability of cerebral blood vessels compared to the rest of the body. Lewandowsky (1900) did not coin the term blood-brain barrier ("Blut-Hirnschranke"). The first person to use this term seems to have been Stern (Stern and Gautier, 1921). Goldmann (1909) was not the first person to demonstrate that some dyes (in his experiments trypan blue) do not enter the brain following parenteral injection. This appears to have been first reported by Franke (1905) who used trypan red. Behnsen (1927) although frequently cited as providing evidence for immaturity of the blood-brain barrier did not do so. Other claims of barrier immaturity or leakiness in developing animals in dye injection experiments can be explained by use of excessive volumes or concentrations of material injected into fragile animals. Early induction of tight junctions in cerebral vessels does not involve astrocytes. At least in the choroid plexus the route of transfer from blood to CSF is intracellular and not via the paracellular pathway.

The importance of discarding the notion of blood-brain barrier immaturity or leakiness in the developing brain lies in the fact that this belief has impeded research into these mechanisms in brain development and their possible relevance for normal and abnormal brain development, as well as the need for systematic studies of therapeutic agents used to treat pregnant women. Therapeutic advice to such patients should be based on evidence, not fear of the unknown.

AUTHOR CONTRIBUTIONS

All of the listed authors contributed to the conception, design, research, drafting and final approval of the work. They each agree to be accountable for all aspects of the work.

REFERENCES

Abbott, N. J., Rönnbäck, L., and Hansson, E. (2006). Astrocyte-endothelial interactions at the blood-brain barrier. *Nat. Rev. Neurosci.* 7, 41–53. doi: 10.1038/nrn1824

Adinolfi, M. (1985). The development of the human blood-brain barrier. *Dev. Med. Child. Neurol.* 27, 532–537. doi: 10.1111/j.1469-8749.1985.tb04581.x

Adinolfi, M., Beck, S. E., Haddad, S. A., and Seller, M. J. (1976). Permeability of the blood-cerebrospinal fluid barrier to plasma proteins during foetal and perinatal life. *Nature* 259, 140–141. doi: 10.1038/259140a0

Adinolfi, M., and Haddad, S. A. (1977). Levels of plasma proteins in human and rat fetal CSF and the development of the blood-CSF barrier. *Neuropädiatrie* 8, 345–353. doi: 10.1055/s-0028-1091530

Ahlfors, C. E., and Wennberg, R. P. (2004). Bilirubin-albumin binding and neonatal jaundice. *Semin. Perinatol.* 28, 334–339. doi: 10.1053/j.semperi.2004.09.002

Ahmed, A., Hickey, S. M., Ehrett, S., Trujillo, M., Brito, F., Goto, C., et al. (1996). Cerebrospinal fluid values in the term neonate. *Pediatr. Infect. Dis. J.* 15, 298–303. doi: 10.1097/00006454-199604000-00004

Allen, F. H. Jr., Diamond, L. K., and Vaughan, V. C. (1950). Erythroblastosis fetalis. VI. Prevention of kernicterus. *Am. J. Dis. Child.* 80, 779–791.

Al-Sarraf, H. (2002). Transport of 14C-gamma-aminobutyric acid into brain, cerebrospinal fluid and choroid plexus in neonatal and adult rats. *Brain Res. Dev. Brain Res.* 139, 121–129. doi: 10.1016/S0165-3806(02)00537-0

Al-Sarraf, H., Preston, J. E., and Segal, M. B. (1997). Changes in the kinetics of the acidic amino acid brain and CSF uptake during development in the rat. *Dev. Brain Res.* 102, 127–134. doi: 10.1016/S0165-3806(97)00089-8

Amtorp, O., and Sørensen, S. C. (1974). The ontogenetic development of concentration differences for protein and ions between plasma and cerebrospinal fluid in rabbits and rats. *J. Physiol.* 243, 387–400.

Andrade, S. E., Gurwitz, J. H., Davis, R. L., Chan, K. A., Finkelstein, J. A., Fortman, K., et al. (2004). Prescription drug use in pregnancy. *Am. J. Obstet. Gynecol.* 191, 398–407. doi: 10.1016/j.ajog.2004.04.025

ATSDR. (2014). *Agency for Toxic Substances and Disease Registry Home Page.* Available online at: http://www.atsdr.cdc.gov (retrieved August 29 2014).

ATSDR. Tp46. (1999). Available online at: http://www.atsdr.cdc.gov/ToxProfiles/tp46.pdf (retrieved August 29 2014).

ATSDR. Tp13. (2007). Available online at: http://www.atsdr.cdc.gov/ToxProfiles/tp13.pdf (retrieved August 29 2014).

Bakay, L. (1953). Studies on blood-brain barrier with radioactive phosphorus. III. Embryonic development of the barrier. *Arch. Neurol. Psychiatry* 70, 30–39. doi: 10.1001/archneurpsyc.1953.02320310036002

Bakay, L. (1956). "Development of the blood-brain barrier," in *The Blood-Brain Barrier, with Special Regard to the use of Radioactive Isotopes*, ed L. Bakay (Springfield, IL: Thomas), 77–149.

Bakay, L. (1968). Changes in barrier effect in pathological states. *Prog. Brain Res.* 29, 315–339. doi: 10.1016/S0079-6123(08)64165-5

Baldrick, P. (2010). Juvenile animal testing in drug development – Is it useful? *Regul. Toxicol. Pharmacol.* 57, 291–299. doi: 10.1016/j.yrtph.2010.03.009

Baños, G., Daniel, P. M., and Pratt, O. E. (1978). The effect of age upon the entry of some amino acids into the brain, and their incorporation into cerebral protein. *Dev. Med. Child. Neurol.* 20, 335–346.

Barcroft, J. (1938). *The Brain and its Environment 1. The Activity of the Brain in Mid-Foetal Life.* New Haven, CT: Yale University Press.

Barrett, K. E., Barman, S. M., Boitano, S., and Brooks, H. L. (2012). *Ganong's Review of Medical Physiology. 24th Edn.* New York, NY: McGraw Hill Lange.

Bartolozzi, G., Ciampolini, M., Franchini, F., and Marianelli, L. (1967). Studio delle protein liquorate nel prematuro. I Richerche lettroforetiche. *Riv. Clin. Pediatr.* 80, 296–309.

Bass, N. H., and Lundborg, P. (1973). Postnatal development of bulk flow in the cerebrospinal fluid system of the albino rat: clearance of carboxyl-(14C)inulin after intrathecal infusion. *Brain Res.* 52, 323–332. doi: 10.1016/0006-8993(73)90668-9

Bauer, C. H., New, M. I., and Miller, J. (1965). Cerebrospinal fluid protein values of premature infants. *J. Pediatr.* 66, 1017–1022. doi: 10.1016/S0022-3476(65)80086-5

Bauer, H., Sonnleitner, U., Lametschwandtner, A., Steiner, M., Adam, H., and Bauer, H. C. (1995). Ontogenic expression of the erythroid-type glucose transporter (Glut 1) in the telencephalon of the mouse: correlation to the tightening of the blood-brain barrier. *Brain Res. Dev. Brain Res.* 86, 317–325. doi: 10.1016/0165-3806(95)00044-E

Bauer, H. C., Bauer, H., Lametschwandtner, A., Amberger, A., Ruiz, P., and Steiner, M. (1993). Neovascularization and the appearance of morphological characteristics of the blood–brain barrier in the embryonic mouse central nervous system. *Brain Res. Dev. Brain Res.* 75, 269–278. doi: 10.1016/0165-3806(93)90031-5

Bauer, H.-C., Kritzbai, I. A., Bauer, H., and Traweger, A. (2014). "You Shall Not Pass" – Tight junctions of the Blood Brain Barrier. *Front. Neurosci.* 8:392. doi: 10.3389/fnins.2014.00392

Behnsen, G. (1926). Farbstoffversuche mit Trypanblau an der Schranke zwischen Blut und Zentralnervensystem der wachsenden Maus. *Münch. Med. Wochenschrift* 73, 1143–1147.

Behnsen, G. (1927). Über die Farbstoffspeicherung im Zentralnervensystem der weissen Maus in verschiedenen Alterszuständen. *Z. Zellforsch. Mikrosk. Anat.* 4, 515–572. doi: 10.1007/BF00637105

Ben-Zvi, A., Lacoste, B., Kur, E., Andreone, B. J., and Mayshar, Y., Yan, H., et al. (2014). Mfsd2a is critical for the formation and function of the blood–brain barrier. *Nature* 509, 573–590. doi: 10.1038/nature13324

Bernard, C. (1865). *Introduction a l'étude de la Médecine Expérimentale.* Paris: Balliere.

Bertossi, M., Mancini, L., Favia, A., Nico, B., Ribatti, D., Virgintino, D., et al. (1992). Permeability-related structures in developing and mature microvessels of the chicken optic tectum. *Biol. Struct. Morphog.* 4, 144–152.

Bertossi, M., Ribatti, D., Nico, B., Mancini, L., Lozupone, E., and Roncali. L. (1988). The barrier systems in the choroidal plexuses of the chick embryo studied by means of horseradish peroxidase. *J. Submicrosc. Cytol. Pathol.* 20, 385–395.

Biedl, A., and Kraus, R. (1898). Über eine bisher unbekannte toxische Wirkung der Gallensäuren auf das Centralnervensystem. *Centralblatt. Inn. Med.* 19, 1185–1200.

Birge, W. J., Rose, A. D., Haywood, J. R., and Doolin, P. F. (1974). Development of the blood-cerebrospinal fluid barrier to proteins and differentiation of cerebrospinal fluid in the chick embryo. *Dev. Biol.* 41, 245–254. doi: 10.1016/0012-1606(74)90303-0

Bito, L. Z., and Myers, R. E. (1970). The ontogenesis of haematoencephalic cation transport in the rhesus monkey. *J. Physiol. (Lond.)* 208, 153–170.

Bouffard, G. (1906). Injection des couleurs de benzidine aux animaux normaux. *Ann. d. l'Inst. Pasteur. Paris* 20, 539–548.

Bradbury, M. W. B. (1979). *The Concept of a Blood-Brain Barrier.* Chichester: Wiley.

Bradbury, M. W. B. (1995). "Developing views of the blood-brain barrier," in *New Concepts of a Blood-Brain Barrier*, eds J. Greenwood, D. J. Begley, and M. B. Segal (New York, NY: Plenum), 1–9.

Bradbury, M. W. B., Crowder, J., Desai, S., Reynolds, J. M., Reynolds, M., and Saunders, N. R. (1972). Electrolytes and water in the brain and cerebrospinal fluid of the foetal sheep and guinea pig. *J. Physiol. (Lond.)* 227, 591–610.

Braun, L. D., Cornford, E. M., and Oldendorf, W. H. (1980). Newborn rabbit blood–brain barrier is selectively permeable and differs substantially from the adult. *J. Neurochem.* 34, 147–152. doi: 10.1111/j.1471-4159.1980.tb04633.x

Briggs, G. G., Freeman, R. K., and Yaffe, S. J. (2008). *Drugs in Pregnancy and Lactation.* Philadelphia, PA: Walters Kluwer.

Brightman, M. W., and Reese, T. S. (1969). Junctions between intimately apposed cell membranes in the vertebrate brain. *J. Cell. Biol.* 40, 48–77. doi: 10.1083/jcb.40.3.648

Broman, T. (1941). The possibilities of the passage of substances from the blood to the central nervous system (Is there a blood-brain-barrier and a blood-cerebrospinal fluid barrier?). *Acta Psychol. Scand.* 16, 1–25. doi: 10.1111/j.1600-0447.1941.tb07398.x

Broussard, C. S., Frey, M. T., Hernandez-Diaz, S., Greene, M. F., Chambers, C. D., Sahin, L., et al. (2014). Developing a systematic approach to safer medication use during pregnancy: summary of a centers for disease control and prevention-convened meeting. *Am. J. Obstet. Gynecol.* 211, 208–214. doi: 10.1016/j.ajog.2014.05.040

Brown, C. M., and Garovic, V. D. (2014). Drug treatment of hypertension in pregnancy. *Drugs* 74, 283–229 doi: 10.1007/s40265-014-0187-7

Caley, D. W., and Maxwell, D. S. (1970). Development of the blood vessels and extracellular spaces during postnatal maturation of rat cerebral cortex. *J. Comp. Neurol.* 138, 31–47. doi: 10.1002/cne.901380104

Chadwick, S. L., Wilson, J. W., Levin, J. E., and Martin, J. M. (2011). Cerebrospinal fluid characteristics in infants who present to the Emergency Department with fever. *Pediatr. Infect. Dis. J.* 30, e63–e67. doi: 10.1097/INF.0b013e31820ad2ba

Clarke, C. A. (1989). Preventing rhesus babies: the Liverpool research and follow up. *Arch. Dis. Child.* 64, 1734–1749. doi: 10.1136/adc.64.12.1734

Cohen, H., and Davies, S. (1938). The Morphology and permeability of the roof of the fourth ventricle in some mammalian embryos. *J. Anat.* 72, 430–455.

Cole, V. A., Durbin, G., Olaffson, A., Reynolds, E. O. R., Rivers, R., and Smith, J. (1974). Pathogenesis of intraventricular haemorrhage in newborn infants. *Arch. Dis. Child.* 49, 722–728. doi: 10.1136/adc.49.9.722

Cornford, E. M., Braun, L. D., and Oldendorf, W. H. (1982). Developmental modulations of blood-brain barrier permeability as an indicator of changing nutritional requirements in the brain. *Pediatr. Res.* 16, 324–328. doi: 10.1203/00006450-198204000-00017

Costa, L. G., Aschner, M., Vitalone, A., Syversen, T., and Soldin, O. P. (2004). Developmental neuropathology of environmental agents. *Ann. Rev. Pharmacol. Toxicol.* 44, 87–110. doi: 10.1146/annurev.pharmtox.44.101802.121424

Cotran, R. S., Kumar, V., Robbins, S. L., and Schoen, F. J. (1994). *Robbins Pathologic Basis of Disease, 5th Edn.* Philadelphia, PA: W. B. Saunders.

Dale, H. (1954). Paul Ehrlich. *Br. Med. J.* 1, 659–663. doi: 10.1136/bmj.1.4863.659

Damkier, H. H., Brown, P. D., and Praetorius, J. (2013). Cerebrospinal fluid secretion by the choroid plexus. *Physiol. Rev.* 93, 1847–1892. doi: 10.1152/physrev.00004.2013

Daneman, R., Zhou, L., Agalliu, D., Cahoy, J. D., Kaushal, A., and Barres, B. A. (2010a). The mouse blood-brain barrier transcriptome: a new resource for understanding the development and function of brain endothelial cells. *PLoS ONE* 5:e13741. doi: 10.1371/journal.pone.0013741

Daneman, R., Zhou, L., Kebede, A. A., and Barres, B. A. (2010b). Pericytes are required for blood-brain barrier integrity during embryogenesis. *Nature* 468, 562–566. doi: 10.1038/nature09513

Davies, P. A., and Rudd, P. T. (1994). *Neonatal Meningitis.* Cambridge: MacKeith Press.

Davis, J. E., and Garrison, N. E. (1968). Mean weights of chick embryos correlated with the stages of Hamburger and Hamilton. *J. Morph.* 124, 79–82. doi: 10.1002/jmor.1051240105

Davson, H. (1956). *Physiology of the Ocular and Cerebrospinal Fluids.* London: Churchill.

Davson, H. (1967). *Physiology of the Cerebrospinal Fluid.* London: Churchill.

Davson, H. (1976). Review lecture: the blood-brain barrier. *J. Physiol. (Lond.)* 255, 1–28.

Davson, H., Welch, K., and Segal, M. B. (1987). *Physiology and Pathophysiology of the Cerebrospinal Fluid.* Edinburgh: Churchill Livingstone.

Davson, H., and Segal, M. B. (1996). *Physiology of the CSF and Blood-Brain Barriers.* Boca Raton, FL: CRC Press.

Dehouck, M.-P., Meìresse, S., Delorme, P., Fruchart, J.-C., and Cecchelli, R. (1990). An easier, reproducible, and mass-production method to study the blood–brain barrier *in vitro*. *J. Neurochem.* 54, 1798–1801. doi: 10.1111/j.1471-4159.1990.tb01236.x

Delorme, P. (1972). Differenciation ultrastructurale des jonctions intercellulaires de l'endothelium des capillaires télencéphaliques chez l'embryon de poulet. *Z. Zellforsch. Mikrosk. Anat.* 133, 571–582. doi: 10.1007/BF00307137

Delorme, P., Gayet, J., and Grignon, G. (1970). Ultrastructural study on transcapillary exchanges in the developing telencephalon of the chicken. *Brain Res.* 22, 269–283. doi: 10.1016/0006-8993(70)90471-3

Dempsey, E. W., and Wislocki, G. B. (1955). An electron microscopic study of the blood-brain barrier in the rat, employing silver nitrate as a vital stain. *J. Biophys. Biochem. Cytol.* 1, 245–256. doi: 10.1083/jcb.1.3.245

Dermietzel, R., Krause, D., Kremer, M., Wang, C., and Stevenson, B. (1992). Pattern of glucose transporter (Glut 1) expression in embryonic brains is related to maturation of blood-brain barrier tightness. *Dev. Dyn.* 193, 152–163. doi: 10.1002/aja.1001930207

Dermietzel, R., Meller, K., Tetzlaff, W., and Waelsch, M. (1977). *In vivo* and *in vitro* formation of the junctional complex in choroid epithelium. A freeze-etching study. *Cell Tissue Res.* 181, 427–441. doi: 10.1007/BF00221766

De Vigan, C., De Walle, H. E. K., Cordier, S., Goujard, J., Knill-Jines, R., Aymé, S., et al. (1999). Therapeutic drug use during pregnancy: a comparison in four European countries. *J. Clin. Epidemiol.* 52, 977–982. doi: 10.1016/S0895-4356(99)00091-8

Diamond, J. M. (1974). Tight and leaky junctions of epithelia: a perspective on kisses in the dark. *Fed. Proc.* 33, 2220–2224.

Dobbing, J. (1961). The blood-brain barrier. *Physiol. Rev.* 41, 130–188.

Donahue, S., and Pappas, G. D. (1961). The fine structure of capillaries in the cerebral cortex of the rat at various stages of development. *Am. J. Anat.* 108, 331–347. doi: 10.1002/aja.1001080307

Dreifuss, J.-J., and Sigrist, N. T. (2009). Lina Stern, l'académicienne genevoise persécutée en URSS. *Rev. Med. Suisse* 5, 593–597. Available online at: http://rms.medhyg.ch/article.php?ID_ARTICLE=RMS_194_0593

Dziegielewska, K. M., Evans, C. A., Lai, P. C., Lorscheider, F. L., Malinowska, D. H., Møllgård, K., et al. (1981). Proteins in cerebrospinal fluid and plasma of fetal rats during development. *Dev. Biol.* 83, 193–200. doi: 10.1016/S0012-1606(81)80024-3

Dziegielewska, K. M., Evans, C. A. N., Malinowska, D. H., Møllgård, K., Reynolds, M. L., and Saunders, N. R. (1980). Blood-cerebrospinal fluid transfer of plasma proteins during fetal development in the sheep. *J. Physiol. (Lond.)* 300, 457–465.

Dziegielewska, K. M., Evans, C. A. N., Malinowska, D. H., Møllgård, K., Reynolds, J. M., Reynolds, M. L., et al. (1979). Studies of the development of brain barrier systems to lipid insoluble molecules in fetal sheep. *J. Physiol. (Lond.)* 292, 207–231.

Dziegielewska, K. M., Habgood, M. D., Møllgård, K., Stagaard, M., and Saunders, N. R. (1991). Species-specific transfer of plasma albumin from blood into different cerebrospinal fluid compartments in the fetal sheep. *J. Physiol. (Lond.)* 439, 215–237.

Dziegielewska, K. M., Hinds, L. A., Møllgård, K., Reynolds, M. L., and Saunders, N. R. (1988). Blood-brain, blood-cerebrospinal fluid and cerebrospinal fluid-brain barriers in a marsupial (*Macropus eugenii*) during development. *J. Physiol. (Lond)* 403, 367–388.

Dziegielewska, K. M., and Saunders, N. R. (1988). "The development of the blood-brain barrier: proteins in fetal and neonatal CSF, their nature and origins," in *Handbook of Human Growth and Developmental Biology. Vol 1. Neural, Sensory, Motor and Integrative Development*, eds E. Meisami and P. S. Timiras (Boca Raton, FL: CRC Press), 169–191.

Ehman, K. (2010)."Development of the mammalian nervous system," in *Reproductive Toxicolgy, 3rd Edn.*, eds R. W. Kapp and R. W. Tyl (New York, NY: Informa), 51–67.

Ehrlich, P. (1885). *Das Sauerstoffbedürfnis des Organismus. Eine Farbenanalytische Studie.* Berlin: Hirschwald.

Ehrlich, P. (1906). "The relations existing between chemical constitution, distribution and pharmacological action," in *Collected Studies on Immunity New York: John Wiley & Sons, translated by C Bolduana from Ch XXXIV of Gesammelte Arbeiten zur Immunitätsforschung*, ed P. Ehrlich (Berlin: Hirschwald), 1904.

Ek, C. J., Dziegielewska, K. M., Habgood, M. D., and Saunders, N. R. (2012). Barriers in the developing brain and neurotoxicology. *Neurotoxicology* 33, 586–604. doi: 10.1016/j.neuro.2011.12.009

Ek, C. J., Habgood, M. D., Dziegielewska, K. M., and Saunders, N. R. (2003). Structural characteristics and barrier properties of the choroid plexuses in developing brain of the opossum (*Monodelphis domestica*). *J. Comp. Neurol.* 460, 451–464. doi: 10.1002/cne.10661

Ek, C. J., Habgood, M. D., Dziegielewska, K. M., and Saunders, N. R. (2006). Functional effectiveness of the blood-brain barrier to small water-soluble molecules in developing and adult opossum (*Monodelphis domestica*). *J. Comp. Neurol.* 496, 13–26. doi: 10.1002/cne.20885

Ek, J., Habgood, M. D., Dziegielewska, K. M., and Saunders, N. R. (2001). Permeability of the blood-brain and blood-CSF barriers to small molecular weight lipid insoluble markers during postnatal development in the opossum, *Monodelphis domestica. J. Physiol. (Lond.)* 536, 841–853. doi: 10.1111/j.1469-7793.2001.00841.x

El Marroun, H., White, T., Verhuist, F. C., and Tiemeier, H. (2014). Maternal use of antidepressant or anxiolytic medication during pregnancy and childhood neurodevelopmental outcomes: a systematic review. *Eur. Child. Adolesc. Psychiatry* 23, 973–992. doi: 10.1007/s00787-014-0558-3

Engelhardt, B. (2003). Development of the blood-brain barrier. *Cell Tissue Res.* 314, 119–129. doi: 10.1007/s00441-003-0751-z

Engelhardt, B. (2006). "Development of the blood-brain interface," in *Blood-Brain Barriers*, Vol. 1, eds R. Dermietzel, D. C. Spray, and M. Nedergaard (Weinheim: Wiley-VCH), 11–39.

Ernster, L., Herlin, L., and Zetterstrom, R. (1957). Experimental studies on the pathogenesis of kernicterus. *Pediatrics* 20, 647–652.

Evans, C. A. N., Reynolds, J. M., Reynolds, M. L., Saunders, N. R., and Segal, M. B. (1974). The development of a blood-brain barrier mechanism in foetal sheep. *J. Physiol. (Lond.)* 238, 371–386.

Ferguson, R. K., and Woodbury, D. M. (1969). Penetration of 14C-inulin and 14C-sucrose into brain, cerebrospinal fluid, and skeletal muscle of developing rats. *Exp. Brain Res.* 7, 181–194. doi: 10.1007/BF00239028

Fishman, R. A. (1992). *Cerebrospinal Fluid in Diseases of the Nervous System, 2nd Edn.* Philadelphia, FL: WB *Saunders*.

Flexner, L. B. (1938). Changes in the chemistry and nature of the cerebrospinal fluid during fetal life in the pig. *Am. J. Physiol.* 124, 131–135.

Forsberg, L., and Wide, K. (2011). Long-term consequences after exposure to antiepileptic drugs in utero.*Ther. Adv. Drug Saf.* 2, 227–234. doi: 10.1177/2042098611419003

Fossan, G., Cavanagh, M. E., Evans, C. A. N., Malinowska, D. H., Møllgård, K., Reynolds, M. L., et al. (1985). CSF-brain permeability in the immature sheep fetus: a CSF-brain barrier. *Dev. Brain Res.* 18, 113–124. doi: 10.1016/0165-3806(85)90255-X

Franceschini, P. (1929). Sulla presenza di elementi connettivali nel sistema nervoso centrale e sopra alcune particlarità di struttura dele meningi molli die plessi coroidei. A proposito della cosi detta barriera "emato-encefalica". *Sperimentale* 83, 419–445.

Franke, E. (1905). *Therapeutische Versuche bei Trypanosomenerkrankung.* Dissertation, Giessen.

Frömter, E., and Diamond, J. (1972). Route of passive ion permeation in epithelia. *Nat. New Biol.* 235, 9–13. doi: 10.1038/newbio235009a0

Friedemann, U. (1942). Blood-brain barrier. *Physiol. Rev.* 22, 125–145.

Friedemann, U., and Elkeles, A. (1931). Über die Permeabilität der Blut-Hirnschranke für Bakteriengifte. I. Mitteilung. 1. Experimentelle Untersuchungen über die Diphtherie-Vergiftung. *Z. Exp. Med.* 74, 293–319.

Friedemann, U., and Elkeles, A. (1934). The blood-brain barrier in infectious diseases: its permeability to toxins in relation to their electrical charges. *Lancet* 7, 719–724. doi: 10.1016/S0140-6736(00)92558-3

Galbally, M., Snellen, M., and Power, J. (2014). Antipsychotic drugs in pregnancy: a review of their maternal and fetal effects. *Ther. Adv. Drug Saf.* 5, 100–107. doi: 10.1177/2042098614522682

Ganong, W. B. (1993). *Review of Medical Physiology. 16th Edn.* East Norwalk, CT: Appleton & Lange.

Ganong, W. B. (1999). *Review of Medical Physiology. 19th Edn.* Stamford, CT: Appleton & Lange.

Gerrard, J. (1952). Kernicterus. *Brain* 75, 526–570. doi: 10.1093/brain/75.4.526

Ghersi-Egea, J.-F., Gazzin, S., and Strazielle, N. (2009). Blood-brain interfaces and bilirubin-induced neurological diseases. *Curr. Pharm. Des.* 15, 2893–2907. doi: 10.2174/138161209789058147

Goldberg, H. L., and Nissim, R. (1994). Psychotropic drugs in pregnancy and lactation. *Int. J. Psychiatr. Med.* 24, 129–147. doi: 10.2190/2BF1-0718-WE7F-A9F7

Goldmann, E. E. (1909). Die äussere und innere Sekretion des gesunden und kranken Organismus im Lichte der 'vitalen Färbung.' *Beiträg Klinische Chirurgie* 64, 192–265.

Goldmann, E. E. (1913). Vitalfärbung am Zentralnervensyatem. Beitrag zur Physio-Pathologie des plexus chorioideus und der Hirnhäute. *Abh preuss, Akad Wiss Phys-Math Kl* 1, 1–60.

Grandjean, P., and Landrigan, P. J. (2006). Developmental neurotoxicity of industrial chemicals. *Lancet* 368, 2167–2178. doi: 10.1016/S0140-6736(06)69665-7

Grazer, F. M., and Clemente, C. D. (1957). Developing blood-brain barrier to trypan blue. *Proc. Soc. Exp. Biol. Med.* 94, 758–760. doi: 10.3181/00379727-94-23077

Gröntoft, O. (1954). Intracranial haemorrhage and blood-brain barrier problems in the newborn. *Acta Pathol. Microbiol. Scand. Suppl.* 100, 1–109.

Gyllenswärd, Å., and Malmström, S. (1962). The cerebrospinal fluid of newborn infants. *Acta Paediatr.* 135, 54–62. doi: 10.1111/j.1651-2227.1962.tb08658.x

Habgood, M. D., Knott, G. W., Dziegielewska, K. M., and Saunders, N. R. (1993). The nature of the blood-CSF barrier permeability decrease during postnatal brain development in the rat. *J. Physiol. (Lond.)* 468, 73–83.

Habgood, M. D., Sedgwick, J. E. C., Dziegielewska, K. M., and Saunders, N. R. (1992). A developmentally regulated blood-cerebrospinal fluid transfer mechanism for albumin in immature rats. *J. Physiol. (Lond.)* 456, 181–192.

Hawkins, B. T., and Davis, T. P. (2005). The Blood-brain barrier/neurovascular unit in health and disease. *Pharmacol. Rev.* 57, 173–185. doi: 10.1124/pr.57.2.4

Heine, W., Hobusch, D., and Drescher, U. (1981). Eiweissgehalt des Liquors und Blut-Liquor-relation der Glucose und Electrolyte im Säuglings-und Kindersalter. Helv. *Paediatr. Acta* 36, 217–227.

Himwich, W. A., Petersen, J. C., and Allen, M. L. (1957). Hematoencephalic exchange as a function of age. *Neurology* 7, 705–710. doi: 10.1212/WNL.7.10.705

Holash, J. A., Noden, D. M., and Stewart, P. A. (1993). Re-evaluating the role of astrocytes in blood-brain barrier induction. *Dev. Dyn.* 197, 14–25. doi: 10.1002/aja.1001970103

Hulsebosch, C. E., and Fabian, R. H. (1989). Penetration of IgGs into the neuraxis of the neonatal rat. *Neurosci. Lett.* 98, 13–18. doi: 10.1016/0304-3940(89)90365-0

Hüntelmann, A. C. (2010). Legend of science. External constructions by the extended family - the biography of Paul Ehrlich. *Interdisciplines* 2, 13–36. doi: 10.2390/indi-v1-i2-17

Iskander, I., Gamaleldin, R., El Houchi, S., El Shenawy, A., Seoud, I., El Gharbawi, N., et al. (2014). Serum bilirubin and bilirubin/albumin ratio as predictors of bilirubin encephalopathy. *Pediatrics* 134, e1330–e1339. doi: 10.1542/peds.2013-1764

Janzer, R. C., and Raff, M. C. (1987). Astrocytes induce blood-brain barrier properties in endothelial cells. *Nature* 325, 253–257. doi: 10.1038/325253a0

Järup, L. (2003). Hazards of heavy metal contamination. *Br. Med. Bull.* 68, 167–182. doi: 10.1093/bmb/ldg032

Johanson, C. E. (1989). "Ontogeny and Phylogeny of the blood-brain barrier," in *Implications of the Blood Brain Barrier and its Manipulation, Vol. 1. Basic aspects*, ed E. A. Neuwelt (New York, NY: Plenum), 157–198.

Johanson, C. E., and Woodbury, D. M. (1974). "Changes in CSF flow and extracellular space in the developing rat," in *Drugs and the Developing Brain*, eds A. Vernadakis and N. Weiner (New York, NY: Plenum), 281–287.

Johansson, P. A., Dziegielewska, K. M., Ek, C. J., Habgood, M. D., Liddelow, S. A., Potter, A. M., et al. (2006). Blood–CSF barrier function in the rat embryo. *Eur. J. Neurosci.* 24, 65–76. doi: 10.1111/j.1460-9568.2006.04904.x

Johansson, P. A., Dziegielewska, K. M., Liddelow, S. A., and Saunders, N. R. (2008). The blood-CSF barrier explained: when development is not immaturity. *Bioessays* 30, 237–248. doi: 10.1002/bies.20718

Joó, F. (1987). Current aspects of the development of the blood-brain barrier. *Int. J. Dev. Neurosci.* 5, 369–372. doi: 10.1016/0736-5748(87)90013-X

Kennedy, D. S. (2011). A to X: the problem of categorisation of drugs in pregnancy—an Australian perspective. *Med. J. Aust.* 195, 572–574. doi: 10.5694/mja11.11119

King, L. S. (1939). The hematoencephalic barrier. *Arch. Neurol. Psychiatr.* 41, 51–72. doi: 10.1001/archneurpsyc.1939.02270130061003

Knott, G. W., Dziegielewska, K. M., Habgood, M. D., Li, Z. S., and Saunders, N. R. (1997). Albumin transfer across the choroid plexus of South American opossum (*Monodelphis domestica*). *J. Physiol.(Lond.)* 499, 179–194.

Klosovskii, B. N. (1963). *The Development of the Brain and its Disturbance by Harmful Factors Translated by Haigh, B.* Oxford: Pergamon.

Kratzer, I., Liddelow, S. A., Saunders, N. R., Dziegielewska, K. M., Strazielle, N., and Ghersi-Egea, J. F. (2013). Developmental changes in the transcriptome of the rat choroid plexus in relation to neuroprotection. *Fluid Barriers CNS* 10:25. doi: 10.1186/2045-8118-10-25

Kuttner, R., Sims, J. A., and Gordon, M. W. (1961). The uptake of a metabolically inert amino acid by brain and other organs. *J. Neurochem.* 6, 311–317. doi: 10.1111/j.1471-4159.1961.tb13481.x

Lajtha, A., and Toth, J. (1961). The brain barrier system-II. Uptake and transport of amino acids by the brain. *J. Neurochem.* 8, 216–225. doi: 10.1111/j.1471-4159.1961.tb13545.x

Lee, J. C. (1971). Evolution of the concept of the blood-brain barrier concept. *Prog. Neuropathol.* 1, 84–145.

Lefauconnier, J.-M., and Trouvé, R. (1983). Developmental changes in the pattern of amino acid transport at the blood-brain barrier in rats. *Brain Res.* 283, 175–182. doi: 10.1016/0165-3806(83)90095-0

Lewandowsky, M. (1900). Zur Lehre von der Cerebrospinalflüssgkeit. *Z. Clin. Med.* 40, 480–494.

Liddelow, S., Dziegielewska, K. M., Ek, C. J., Johansson, P. A., Potter, A., and Saunders, N. R. (2009). Cellular transfer of macromolecules across the developing choroid plexus of *Monodelphis domestica*. *Eur. J. Neurosci.* 29, 253–266. doi: 10.1111/j.1460-9568.2008.06571.x

Liddelow, S., Dziegielewska, K. M., Noor, N., Potter, A. M., and Saunders, N. R. (2011a). Modification of choroid plexus protein transfer from blood to cerebrospinal fluid in response to altered plasma protein composition during development. *Eur. J. Neurosci.* 33, 391–400. doi: 10.1111/j.1460-9568.2010.07509.x

Liddelow, S. A., Dziegielewska, K. M., Ek, C. J., Habgood, M. D., Bauer, H., Bauer, H.-C., et al. (2013). Mechanisms that determine the internal environment of the developing brain: a transcriptomic, functional and ultrastructural approach. *PLoS ONE* 8:e65629. doi: 10.1371/journal.pone.0065629

Liddelow, S. A., Dziegielewska, K. M., Møllgård, K., Phoenix, T. N., Temple, S., VandeBerg, J. L., et al. (2011b). Sparc/osteonectin, an endogenous mechanism for targeting albumin to the blood-CSF interface during brain development. *Eur. J. Neurosci.* 34, 1062–1073. doi: 10.1111/j.1460-9568.2011.07821.x

Liddelow, S. A., Temple, S., Møllgård, K., Gehwold, R., Wagner, A., Bauer, H., et al. (2012). Molecular characterisation of transport mechanisms at the developing mouse blood-CSF interface: a transcriptome approach. *PLoS ONE* 7:e33554. doi: 10.1371./journal.pone.0033554

Lossinsky, A. S., Vorbrodt, A. W., and Wisniewski, H. M. (1986). Characterization of endothelial cell transport in the developing mouse blood-brain barrier. *Dev. Neurosci.* 8, 61–75. doi: 10.1159/000112242

Lucey, J. F. (1971). Changing concepts regarding exchange transfusions and neonatal jaundice. *Clin. Obstet. Gynecol.* 14, 586–593. doi: 10.1097/00003081-197106000-00020

Malamud, W., Fuchs, D. M., and Malamud, N. (1928). Barrier between the blood and the cerebrospinal fluid. 1. Changes in permeability in mental disease. *Arch. Neurol. Psychiatry* 20, 780–798. doi: 10.1001/archneurpsyc.1928.02210160121010

Mazariegos, M. R., Tice, L. W., and Hand, A. R. (1984). Alteration of tight junctional permeability in the rat parotid gland after isoproterenol stimulation. *J. Cell Biol.* 98, 1865–1877. doi: 10.1083/jcb.98.5.1865

Meek, W. J. (1907). A study of the choroid plexus. *J. Comp. Neurol.* 17, 286–306.

Mhanna, M. J., Alesseh, H., Gori, A., and Aziz, H. F. (2008). Cerebrospinal fluid values in very low birth weight infants with suspected sepsis at different ages. *Pediatr. Crit. Care Med.* 9, 294–298. doi: 10.1097/01.PCC.0b013e31816c6e12

Millen, J. W., and Hess, A. (1958). The blood-brain barrier: an experimental study with vital dyes. *Brain* 81, 248–257. doi: 10.1093/brain/81.2.248

Mitchell, W., Kim, C. S., O'Tuama, L. A., Pritchard, J. B., and Pick, J. R. (1982). Choroid plexus, brain and kidney Na+,K+-ATPase: comparative activities in fetal, newborn and young adult rabbits. *Neurosci. Lett.* 31, 37–40. doi: 10.1016/0304-3940(82)90050-7

Mizee, M. R., Wooldrik, D., Lakeman, K. A., van het Hof, B., Drexhage, J. A., Geerts, D., et al. (2013). Retinoic acid induces blood-brain barrier development. *J. Neurosci.* 33, 1660–1671. doi: 10.1523/JNEUROSCI.1338-12.2013

Møllgård, K., Lauritzen, B., and Saunders, N. R. (1979). Double replica technique applied to choroid plexus from early foetal sheep: completeness and complexity of tight junctions. *J. Neurocytol.* 8, 139–149. doi: 10.1007/BF01175557

Møllgård, K., Malinowska, D. H., and Saunders, N. R. (1976). Lack of correlation between tight junction morphology and permeability properties in developing choroid plexus. *Nature* 264, 293–294. doi: 10.1038/264293a0

Møllgård, K., and Saunders, N. R. (1975). Complex tight junctions of epithelial and of endothelial cells in early foetal brain. *J. Neurocytol.* 4, 453–468. doi: 10.1007/BF01261375

Møllgård, K., and Saunders, N. R. (1986).The development of the human blood-brain and blood-CSF barriers. *Neuropathol. Appl. Neurobiol.* 12, 337–358. doi: 10.1111/j.1365-2990.1986.tb00146.x

Møllgård, K., and Saunders, N. R. (1977). A possible transepithelial pathway via endoplasmic reticulum in foetal sheep choroid plexus. *Proc. R. Soc. Lond. B Biol. Sci.* 199, 321–326. doi: 10.1098/rspb.1977.0142

Moos, T., and Møllgård, K. (1993). Cerebrovascular permeability to azo dyes and plasma proteins in rodents of different ages. *Neuropathol. Appl. Neurobiol.* 19, 120–127. doi: 10.1111/j.1365-2990.1993.tb00416.x

Nag, S. (2011). Morphology and properties of brain endothelial cells, Ch 1 in the blood-brain and other neural barriers: reviews and protocols. *Methods Mol. Biol.* 686, 3–35. doi: 10.1007/978-1-60761-938-3_1

Naidoo, B. T. (1968). The cerebrospinal fluid in the healthy newborn infant. *S. Afr. Med. J.* 42, 933–935.

Nasralla, M., Gawronska, E., and Hsia, D. Y.-Y. (1958). Studies on the relation between serum and spinal fluid bilirubin during early infancy. *J. Clin. Invest.* 37, 1403–1412. doi: 10.1172/JCI103730

Nattie, E. E., Edwards, W. H., and Marin-Padilla, M. (1984). Newborn puppy cerebral acid-base regulation in experimental asphyxia and recovery. *J. Appl. Physiol.* 56, 1178–1186.

Nitta, T., Hata, M., Gotoh, S., Seo, Y., Sasaki, H., Hashimoto, N., et al. (2003). Size-selective loosening of the blood-brain barrier in claudin-5-deficient mice. *J. Cell Biol.* 161, 653–660. doi: 10.1083/jcb.200302070

Oldendorf, W. M. (1971). Brain uptake of radiolabeled amino acids, amines, and hexoses after arterial injection. *Am. J. Physiol.* 221, 1629–1639.

Olney, J. W., and Ho, O. L. (1970). Brain damage in infant mice following oral intake of glutamate, aspartate or cysteine. *Nature* 227, 609–611. doi: 10.1038/227609b0

Olsson, Y., Klatzo, I., Sourander, P., and Steinwall, O. (1968). Blood-brain barrier to albumin in embryonic new born and adult rats. *Acta Neuropathol.* 16, 117–124. doi: 10.1007/BF00691305

Ornoy, A., and Koren, G. (2014). Selective serotonin reuptake inhibitors in human pregnancy: on the way to resolving the controversy. *Semin. Fetal Neonatal Med.* 19, 188–194. doi: 10.1016/j.siny.2013.11.007

Otila, E. (1948). Studies on the cerebrospinal fluid in premature infants. *Acta Paediatr.* 35(Suppl. 8), 9–100.

Pardridge, W. M., and Mietus, L. J. (1982). Kinetics of neutral amino acid transport through the blood-brain barrier of the newborn rabbit. *J. Neurochem.* 38, 955–962. doi: 10.1111/j.1471-4159.1982.tb05335.x

Penta, P. (1932). Sulla colorazione vitale del sistema nervosa negli centrale animali neonati. *Riv. Neurol.* 5, 62–80.

Piliero, S. J., and Lending, M. (1959). Protein studies in normal newborn infants. Paper electrophoresis of cerebrospinal fluid and serum. *Am. J. Dis. Child.* 97, 785–789. doi: 10.1001/archpedi.1959.02070010787004

Purpura, D. P., and Carmichael, M. W. (1960). Characteristics of blood-brain barrier to gamma-aminobutyric acid in neonatal cat. *Science* 131, 410–412. doi: 10.1126/science.131.3398.410

Ramey, B. A., and Birge, W. H. (1979). Development of cerebrospinal fluid and the blood-cerebrospinal fluid barrier in rabbits. *Dev. Biol.* 68, 292–298. doi: 10.1016/0012-1606(79)90261-6

Ramoz, L. L., and Patel-Shori, N. M. (2014). Recent changes in pregnancy and lactation labeling: retirement of risk categories. *Pharmacotherapy* 34, 389–395. doi: 10.1002/phar.1385

Ribatti, D., Nico, B., and Bertossi, M. (1993). The development of the blood-brain barrier in the chick. Studies with Evans blue and horseradish peroxidase. *Ann. Anat.* 175, 85–88. doi: 10.1016/S0940-9602(11)80247-5

Ribatti, D., Nico, B., Crivellato, E., and Artico, M. (2006). Development of the blood-brain barrier: a historical point of view. *Anat. Rec. B New Anat.* 289B, 3–8. doi: 10.1002/ar.b.20087

Risau, W., Hallmann, R., and Albrecht, U. (1986). Differentiation-dependent expression of proteins in brain endothelium during development of the blood–brain barrier. *Dev. Biol.* 117, 537–545. doi: 10.1016/0012-1606(86)90321-0

Risau, W., and Seulberger, H. (1990). "Angiogenesis and differentiation of blood-brain barrier endothelium. Ch 1," in *Pathophysiology of the Blood-Brain Barrier*, Vol. 14, eds B. B. Johansson, C. H. Owman, and H. Widner (Amsterdam: Elsevier), 3–9.

Risau, W., and Wolburg, H. (1990). Development of the blood–brain barrier. *Trends Neurosci.* 13, 174–178. doi: 10.1016/0166-2236(90)90043-A

Roberts, R. B., Flexner, J. B., and Flexner, L. B. (1959). Biochemical and physiological differentiation during morphogenesis. XXIII. Further observations relating to the synthesis of amino acids and proteins by the cerebral cortex and liver of the mouse. *J. Neurochem.* 4, 78–90. doi: 10.1111/j.1471-4159.1959.tb13176.x

Rodier, P. M. (1994). Vulnerable periods and processes during central nervous system development. *Environ. Health Perspect.* 102, 121–124. doi: 10.1289/ehp.94102121

Rodier, P. M. (1995). Developing brain as a target of toxicity. *Environ. Health Perspect.* 103, 73–76. doi: 10.1289/ehp.95103s673

Rodier, P. M. (2004). Environmental causes of central nervous system maldevelopment. *Pediatrics* 113, 1076–1083. Available online at: http://pediatrics.aappublications.org/content/113/Supplement_3/1076.full.html

Romanoff, A. L. (1967). *Biochemistry of the Avian Embryo*. New York, NY: Wiley.

Roncali, L., Nico, B., Ribatti, D., Bertossi, M., and Mancini, L. (1986). Microscopical and ultrastructural investigations on the development of the blood-brain barrier in the chick embryo optic tectum. *Acta Neuropathol.* 70, 193–201. doi: 10.1007/BF00686072

Roux, E., and Borrel, A. (1898). Tétanos cérébral et immunité contre le tétanus. *Ann. Institut Pasteur* 12, 225–239.

Roy, S., Hirano, A., Kochen, J. A., and Zimmerman, H. M. (1974). The fine structure of cerebral blood vessels in chick embryo. *Acta Neuropath.* 30, 277–285. doi: 10.1007/BF00697010

Rubin, L. L., Hall, D. E., Porter, S., Barbu, K., Cannon, C., Horner, H. C., et al. (1991). A cell culture model of the blood-brain barrier. *J. Cell Biol.* 115, 1725–1735. doi: 10.1083/jcb.115.6.1725

Sarff, L. D., Platt, L. H., and McCracken, G. H. Jr. (1976). Cerebrospinal fluid evaluation in neonates: comparison of high-risk infants with and without meningitis. *J. Pediatr.* 88, 473–477. doi: 10.1016/S0022-3476(76)80271-5

Saunders, N. R. (1977). Ontogeny of the blood-brain barrier. *Exp. Eye Res.* 25(Suppl.), 523–550. doi: 10.1016/S0014-4835(77)80046-8

Saunders, N. R. (1992). "Ontogenetic development of brain barrier mechanisms," in *Physiology and Pharmacology of the Blood Brain-barrier. Vol. 103. Handbook of Experimental Pharmacology*, ed M. W. B. Bradbury (Berlin: Springer-Verlag), 327–369.

Saunders, N. R., Adam, E., Reader, M., and Møllgård, K. (1989). *Monodelphis domestica* (grey short-tailed opossum): an accessible model for studies of early neocortical development. *Anat. Embryol.* 180, 227–236. doi: 10.1007/BF00315881

Saunders, N. R., Daneman, R., Dziegielewska, K. M., and Liddelow, S. A. (2013). Transporters of the blood-brain and blood-CSF interfaces in development and in the adult. *Mol. Aspects Med.* 34, 742–752. doi: 10.1016/j.mam.2012.11.006

Saunders, N. R., Liddelow, S. A., and Dziegielewska, K. M. (2012). Barrier mechanisms in the developing brain. *Front. Neuropharmacol.* 3:46. doi: 10.3389/fphar.2012.00046

Sedlácek, J. (1975). Some basic chemical components of the cerebrospinal fluid in developing chick embryos. *Physiol. Bohemoslov.* 24, 305–313.

Seta, K., Sershen, H., and Lajtha, A. (1972). Cerebral amino acid uptake *in vivo* in newborn mice. *Brain Res.* 47, 415–425. doi: 10.1016/0006-8993(72)90649-X

Spatz, H. (1934). Die Bedeutung der vitalen Färbung für die Lehre vom Stoffaustausch zwischen dem Zentralnervensystem and dem iibrigen Körper. *Arch. F. Psychiatr.* 101, 267–358. doi: 10.1007/BF01789978

Spiegel-Adolf, M., Baird, H. W. 3rd., Szekely, E. G., and Wycis, H. T. (1954). Cerebrospinal fluid studies in infant children with cerebral palsy and other neurologic disorders. *Pediatrics* 14, 215–221.

Srinivasan, L., Shah, S. S., Padula, M. A., Abbasi, S., McGowan, K. L., and Harris, M. C. (2012). Cerebrospinal fluid reference ranges in term and preterm infants in the neonatal intensive care unit. *J. Pediatr.* 161, 729–734. doi: 10.1016/j.jpeds.2012.03.051

Statz, A., and Felgenhauer, K. (1983). Development of the blood-CSF barrier. *Dev. Med. Child Neurol.* 25, 152–161. doi: 10.1111/j.1469-8749.1983.tb13738.x

Stern, L. (1934). A propos de la méthod d'investigation du fonctionnement de la barrière hémato-encéphalique. *C. R. Soc. Biol.* 115, 1059–1061.

Stern, L., Battelli, F., and Peyrot, R. (1924). Fonctionnement de la barrière hémato-encéphalique (H.-E.) chez les divers animaux au cours de leur développement. *Schw. Med. Wschr.* 5, 313.

Stern, L., and Gautier, R. (1918a). Passage simultané des substances dans le liquide céphalo-rachidien et dans les centres nerveux. *R. C. R. d. Ia Soc. de Phys. et d'hist. natur. de Genève* 35, 58–60.

Stern, L., and Gautier, R. (1918b). Le passage dans le liquide céphalo-rachidien de substances introduites dans la circulation et leur action sur le système nerveux central chez les différentes espèces animales. *R. C. R. d. Ia Soc. de Phys. et d'hist. natur. de Genève* 35, 91–94.

Stern, L., and Gautier, R. (1921). Recherches sur le liquide céphalo-rachidien. 1. Les rapports entre le liquide céphalo-rachidien et la circulation sanguine. *Arch. Int. Physiol.* 17, 138–192. doi: 10.3109/13813452109146211

Stern, L., and Gautier, R. (1922). Recherches sur le liquide céphalo-rachidien. II. Les rapports entre le liquide céphalo-rachidien et les éléments nerveux de l'axe cérébro-spinal. *Arch. Int. Physiol.* 17, 391–448. doi: 10.3109/13813452209146219

Stern, L., and Gautier, R. (1923). Recherches sur le liquide céphalo-rachidien. II. Rapports entre le liquide céphalo-rachidien et des espaces ventriculaires et cellui des espaces sous-arachnodiens. *Arch. Int. Physiol.* 20, 403–436. doi: 10.3109/13813452309145975

Stern, L., and Peyrot, R. (1927). Le fonctionnment de la barrière hémato-encéphalique aux divers stades de développement chez les diverses especes animals. *C. R. Soc. Biol.* 96, 1124–1126.

Stern, L., and Rapoport, J. L. (1928a). Les rapports entre l'augmentation de la perméabilité de la barrière hémato-encéphalique et les altérations de son substratum morphologique. *C. R. Soc. Biol.* 98, 1515–1517.

Stern, L., and Rapoport, J. L. (1928b). Les échanges entre le liquide céphalorachidien et les éléments nerveux cérébro-spinaux. *C. R. Soc. Biol.* 98, 1518–1519.

Stern, L., Rapoport, J. L., and Lokschina, E.-S. (1929). Le fonctionnement de la barrière hémato-encéphalique chez les nouveau nés. *C. R. Soc. Biol.* 100, 231–223.

Stewart, P. A., and Hayakawa, E. M. (1987). Interendothelial junctional changes underlie the developmental "tightening" of the blood brain barrier. *Brain Res.* 429, 271–281. doi: 10.1016/0165-3806(87)90107-6

Stewart, P. A., and Hayakawa, K. (1994). Early ultrastructural changes in blood-brain barrier vessels of the rat embryo. *Brain Res. Dev. Brain Res.* 78, 25–34. doi: 10.1016/0165-3806(94)90005-1

Stewart, P. A., and Wiley, M. J. (1981). Developing nervous tissue induces formation of blood-brain barrier characteristics in invading endothelial cells: a study using quail-chick transplantation chimeras. *Dev. Biol.* 84, 183–192. doi: 10.1016/0012-1606(81)90382-1

Tao-Cheng, J. H., Nagy, Z., and Brightman, M. W. (1987). Tight junctions of brain endothelium *in vitro* are enhanced by astroglia. *J. Neurosci.* 7, 3293–3299.

Tauc, M., Vignon, X., and Bouchaud, C. (1984). Evidence for the effectiveness of the blood–CSF barrier in the fetal rat choroid plexus. A freeze-fracture and peroxidase diffusion study. *Tissue Cell* 16, 65–74. doi: 10.1016/0040-8166(84)90019-3

Tennyson, V. (1975). "Ultrastructural characteristics of the telencephalic and myelencephalic choroid plexus in fetus of man and rabbit, and a comparison with the adult choroid plexus in rabbit," in *The Choroid Plexus in Health and Disease*, eds M. G. Netsky and S. Shuangshati (Bristol: John Wright & Sons), 36–71.

Tennyson, V. M., and Pappas, G. D. (1964). Fine structure of the developing telencephalic and myelencephalic choroid plexus in the rabbit. *J. Comp. Neurol.* 123, 379–412. doi: 10.1002/cne.901230307

Teratology Society Public Affairs Committee. (1994). FDA Classification of drugs for teratogenic risk. *Teratology* 49, 446–447. doi: 10.1002/tera.1420490603

Teratology Society Public Affairs Committee. (2007). Teratology public affairs committee position paper: pregnancy labeling for prescription drugs: ten years later. *Birth Defects Res. A Clin. Mol. Teratol.* 79, 627–630. doi: 10.1002/bdra.20389

Tschirgi, R. D. (1950). Protein complexes and the impermeability of the blood-brain barrier to dyes. *Am. J. Physiol.* 163, 756.

van den Bergh, H. A. A., and Müller, P. (1916). Über eine direkte und indirekte Diazoreaktion auf Bilirubin. *Biochem. Zeitschrift* 77, 90–103.

van Hasselt, J. G., van Calsteren, K., Heyns, L., Han, S., Mhallem Gziri, M., Schellens, J. H., et al. (2014). Optimizing anti-cancer drug treatment in pregnant cancer patients: pharmacokinetic analysis of gestation-induced changes for doxorubicin, epirubicin, docetaxel and paclitaxel. *Ann. Oncol.* 25, 2059–2065. doi: 10.1093/annonc/mdu140

Vein, A. A. (2008). Science and fate: Lina Stern (1878-1968), a neurophysiologist and biochemist. *J. Hist. Neurosci.* 17, 195–206. doi: 10.1080/09647040601138478

Viña, J. R., DeJoseph, M. R., Hawkins, P. A., and Hawkins, R. A. (1997). Penetration of glutamate into brain of 7-day-old rats. *Metab. Brain Dis.* 12, 219–227. doi: 10.1007/BF02674614

Virgintino, D., Errede, M., Girolamo, F., Capobianco, C., Robertson, D., Vimercati, A., et al. (2007). Fetal blood-brain barrier P-glycoprotein contributes to brain protection during human development. *J. Neuropathol. Exp. Neurol.* 67, 50–61. doi: 10.1097/nen.0b013e31815f65d9

Virgintino, D., Errede, M., Robertson, D., Capobianco, C., Girolamo, F., Vimercati, A., et al. (2004). Immunolocalization of tight junction proteins in the adult and developing human brain. *Histochem. Cell Biol.* 122, 51–59. doi: 10.1007/s00418-004-0665-1

Virgintino, D., Robertson, D., Benagiano, V., Errede, M., Bertossi, M., Ambrosi, G., et al. (2000). Immunogold cytochemistry of the blood-brain barrier glucose transporter GLUT1 and endogenous albumin in the developing human brain. *Brain Res. Dev. Brain Res.* 123, 95–101. doi: 10.1016/S0165-3806(00)00086-9

Volpe, J. J. (2008). "Bilirubin and brain injury," in *Neurology of the Newborn, 5th Edn.*, ed J. J. Volpe (Philadelphia, PA: W. B. Saunders), 619–651.

von Monakow, C. (1921). Der Kreislauf des Liquor cerebro-spinalis. *Schweiz Arch. Neurol. Psychiatry* 8, 233–234.

Vorbrodt, A. W., Lossinsky, A. S., and Wisniewski, H. M. (1986). Localization of alkaline phosphatase activity in endothelia of developing and mature mouse blood-brain barrier. *Dev. Neurosci.* 8, 1–13. doi: 10.1159/000112236

Wakai, S., and Hirokawa, N. (1978). Development of the blood-brain barrier to horseradish peroxidase in the chick embryo. *Cell Tissue Res.* 195, 195–203. doi: 10.1007/BF00236719

Wakai, S., and Hirokawa, N. (1981). Development of blood-cerebrospinal fluid barrier to horseradish peroxidase in the avian choroidal epithelium. *Cell Tissue Res.* 214, 271–278. doi: 10.1007/BF00249211

Walter, K. (1934). Die allgemeinen Grundlagen des Stoffaustausches zwischen dem Zentralnervensystem und dem übrigen Körper. *Archiv für Psychiatrie* 10, 195–230. doi: 10.1007/BF01789976

Watson, D. (1964). Modern methods for determining cerebrospinal fluid protein. *Clin. Chem.* 10, 412–416.

Watson, R. E., Desesso, J. M., Hurtt, M. E., and Cappon, G. D. (2006). Postnatal growth and morphological Development of the brain: a species comparison. *Birth Defects Res. B. Dev. Reprod. Toxicol.* 77, 471–484. doi: 10.1002/bdrb.20090

Weed, L. H. (1917a). An anatomical consideration of the cerebro-spinal fluid. *Anat. Res.* 12, 461–496. doi: 10.1002/ar.1090120405

Weed, L. H. (1917b). The development of the cerebrospinal fluid spaces in pig and in man. *Contrib. Embryol. Carnegie Inst.* 5, 3–116.

Wennberg, R. P. (2000). The blood-brain barrier and bilirubin encephalopathy. *Cell. Mol. Neurobiol.* 20, 97–109. doi: 10.1023/A:1006900111744

Wennberg, R. P., Ahlfors, C. E., Bhutani, V. K., Johnson, L. H., and Shapiro, S. M. (2006). Toward understanding kernicterus: a challenge to improve the management of jaundiced newborns. *Pediatrics* 117, 474–485. doi: 10.1542/peds.2005-0395

Widell, S. (1958). On the cerebrospinal fluid in normal children and in patients with acute abacterial meningoencephalitis. *Acta Paediatr.* 47(Suppl.), 115. doi: 10.1111/j.1651-2227.1958.tb07687.x

Wiesendanger, M. (2010). Constantin von Monakow (1853-1930) and Lina Stern (1878-1968). *Schweiz Arch. Neurol. Psychiatry* 161, 140–144.

Windle, W. F. (1969). Brain Damage by asphyxia at birth. *Sci. Am.* 221, 76–84. doi: 10.1038/scientificamerican1069-76

Wislocki, G. B. (1920). Experimental studies on fetal absorption. I. The vitality stained fetus. *Contrib. Embryol. Carnegie Inst.* 11, 45–60.

Wood, K. E., Sinclair, L. L., Rysgaard, C. D., Strathman, F. G., McMillin, G. A., and Krasowski, M. D. (2014). Retrospective analysis of the diagnostic yield of newborn drug testing. *BMC Pregnancy Childbirth* 14:250. doi: 10.1186/1471-2393-14-250

Woodbury, D. M., Johanson, C., and Brønsted, M. (1974). "Maturation of the blood-brain and blood-cerebrospinal fluid barriers and transport systems," in *Narcotics and the Hypothalamus*, eds E. Zimmerman and R. George (New York, NY: Raven Press), 225–247.

Xu, J., and Ling, E.-A. (1994). Studies of the ultrastructure and permeability of the blood-brain barrier in the developing corpus callosum in postnatal rat brain using electron dense tracers. *J. Anat.* 184, 227–237.

Zheng, W. (2002). "Blood-brain barrier and blood-CSF barrier in metal-induced neurotoxicities," in *Handbook of Neurotoxicology*, Vol. 1, ed E. J. Massaro (Totowa, NJ: Humana Press), 161–193.

Zuelzer, W. W., and Mudgett, R. T. (1950). KERNICTERUS: etiologic study based on an analysis of 55 cases. *Pediatrics* 6, 453–474.

5

Choroid plexus in developmental and evolutionary perspective

Brent Roy Bill[1†] and Vladimir Korzh[2,3]*

[1] *Semel Institute for Neuroscience and Human Behavior, University of California Los Angeles, Los Angeles, CA, USA*
[2] *Agency for Science, Technology and Research of Singapore, Institute of Molecular and Cell Biology, Singapore, Singapore*
[3] *National University of Singapore, Department of Biological Sciences, Singapore, Singapore*

Correspondence:
Vladimir Korzh, Institute of Molecular and Cell Biology, A-STAR (Agency for Science, Technology and Research), 61 Biopolis Dr., Proteos, Singapore 138673, Singapore
e-mail: vlad@imcb.a-star.edu.sg

†Present address:
Brent Roy Bill, Department of Biology, The University of Texas at Tyler, Tyler, TX, USA

The blood-cerebrospinal fluid boundary is present at the level of epithelial cells of the choroid plexus. As one of the sources of the cerebrospinal fluid (CSF), the choroid plexus (CP) plays an important role during brain development and function. Its formation has been studied largely in mammalian species. Lately, progress in other model animals, in particular the zebrafish, has brought a deeper understanding of CP formation, due in part to the ability to observe CP development *in vivo*. At the same time, advances in comparative genomics began providing information, which opens a possibility to understand further the molecular mechanisms involved in evolution of the CP and the blood-cerebrospinal fluid boundary formation. Hence this review focuses on analysis of the CP from developmental and evolutionary perspectives.

Keywords: brain-CSF, transgenics, epithelium, vasculature, stroma, glia

WHAT IS THE CHOROID PLEXUS?

The choroid plexus (CP) is a set of ependymal-derived structures that regulate the composition of cerebrospinal fluid (CSF). Historically, the term "CP" (from Latin: chorion–delicate, plexus–knot) was defined by the vasculature; however, it now refers to multiple layers and cell types that form this organ (Strong, 1956; Netsky et al., 1975; Johanson, 2003; Redzic et al., 2005; Bill et al., 2008; Garcia-Lecea et al., 2008). The CP structure is conserved in vertebrate species, and consists of: a fenestrated vasculature core, an interstitial stromal layer, and a single layer of polarized cuboidal epithelia. Endothelial-derived and epithelial-derived basement membranes flank the stroma providing for a unique method of semipermeable filtration (Johanson et al., 2011). In most vertebrates there are four CP's: CPIII, CPIV, and two lateral CPs, inset within each ventricle. Due to differences in cortical development, teleosts have only two CPs, the diencephalic and myelencephalic CP (dCP and mCP) homologous with the midline CPs (CPIII and IV, respectively). For simplicity, we will primarily focus on comparisons between mCP and CPIV development.

Despite vital roles in development, physiology, and protection of the brain, the CP has remained outside of a sphere of interest for many mainstream neuroscientists. There are numerous reasons why this is the case including: reductionist approaches that refine work to a targeted neural tissue, a misconception that the CSF is only for metabolic support and waste removal, and a limited view of the pathologies that affect the CP. A renaissance in CP research has occurred over the past few years placing the CP as a critical modulator of the central nervous system elucidating roles during sleep, appetite, neural transmitter availability, and development of the brain (Zappaterra and Lehtinen, 2012). It has been implicated in over 30 multi-systemic disorders (Emerich et al., 2005; Lavezzi et al., 2013). Furthermore, it has presented itself as a potential target for pharmaceutical and cell-based treatments for Amblyopia, Stroke, Parkinson's disease, Huntington's disease, and Alzheimer's disease (Borlongan et al., 2004a,b; Emerich et al., 2006; Luo et al., 2013; Spatazza et al., 2013; Bolos et al., 2014). This clearly illustrates the need for a better understanding of the development and function of this vital organ.

A strong case can be made that the CP should be considered one of the circumventricular organs (Weindl and Joynt, 1973; Tsuneki, 1986; Ganong, 2000; Joly et al., 2007), as they have many similarities; for example, location at a periphery of the brain in close proximity to the ventricles, high levels of vascularization, functional roles in endocrine signaling, the production of proteins for secretion into the CSF, and the presence of fenestrated vessels (Molnar and Stolp; Richardson, this volume). However, the barrier function performed by the epithelia tight junctions of the CP has generated discussion as to its inclusion amongst circumventricular organs (Jeong et al., 2008; Umans and Taylor, 2012). Hence attempts to analyze the evolutionary and developmental origins of CP and some circumventricular organs such as subcommissural organ might shed light on this topic.

Comparative genomics early on demonstrated its importance for analysis of expression of imprinted genes in the developing CP (Overall et al., 1997), and genes critical for its development (Johansson et al., 2013). Recently, the detailed characterization of CP development in teleosts (Bill et al., 2008; Garcia-Lecea et al., 2008) and the significant progress in genome sequencing of model animals, including several fish (see, for example, Howe et al., 2013; Venkatesh et al., 2014) opened new horizons for advancement of comparative genomics of the CP on a much broader scale.

DEVELOPMENT OF CP IN MAMMALS

In all vertebrates, the CPs develop in a posterior to anterior order with the CP of the IVth ventricle developing prior to more anterior CPs (Netsky et al., 1975; Knott et al., 1997; Garcia-Lecea et al., 2008). This is unlike many other developmental processes that progress from anterior to posterior, including, but not limited to, somitogenesis and neurodifferentiation (Korzh et al., 1993; Kimmel et al., 1995). It is tempting to link this sequence of events with other preceding neurodevelopmental events such as, closure of the neural tube in amphibians and mammals, which is a bidirectional process progressing both anteriorly and posteriorly from the hindbrain (Copp et al., 2003; Korzh, 2014).

The hindbrain roof plate epithelium has been considered to serve two major roles: the dorsal organizing center (Liem et al., 1997; Lee and Jessell, 1999; Lee et al., 2000; Millonig et al., 2000; Broom et al., 2012), and the source of the intermediate epithelium that transforms into cerebrospinal fluid-producing epithelium of the CPIV (Wilting and Christ, 1989; Thomas and Dziadek, 1993). As a dorsal organizing center, the hindbrain roof plate epithelium influences dorsal neuroectoderm, by secreting signaling molecules, such as BMPs and WNTs, to direct transcription in domains along the dorsal-ventral axis, specifically within the rhombic lip (Chizhikov and Millen, 2004; Currle et al., 2005). Reciprocal Notch signaling maintains the boundary between the hindbrain roof plate epithelium and the rhombic lip (Broom et al., 2012). Given that the cells of the CP epithelium and vascular are drawn to this location, it is tempting to hypothesize that the hindbrain roof plate epithelium secretes factors that recruit these cell types.

It is thought that in mammals the hindbrain roof plate epithelium is primarily derived from the dorsal most neural ectoderm of the lateral rhombic lips, and these cells differ at the molecular level along the anterior-posterior and dorsal-ventral axes (Awatramani et al., 2003; Chizhikov et al., 2006; Hunter and Dymecki, 2007). The hindbrain roof plate epithelium consists of three distinct fields (**Figure 1**). The two primary fields are the medial and lateral fields, and they are distinct in developmental timing and mitotic activity. The lateral field expresses several molecular markers that further separate it into the lateral-anterior

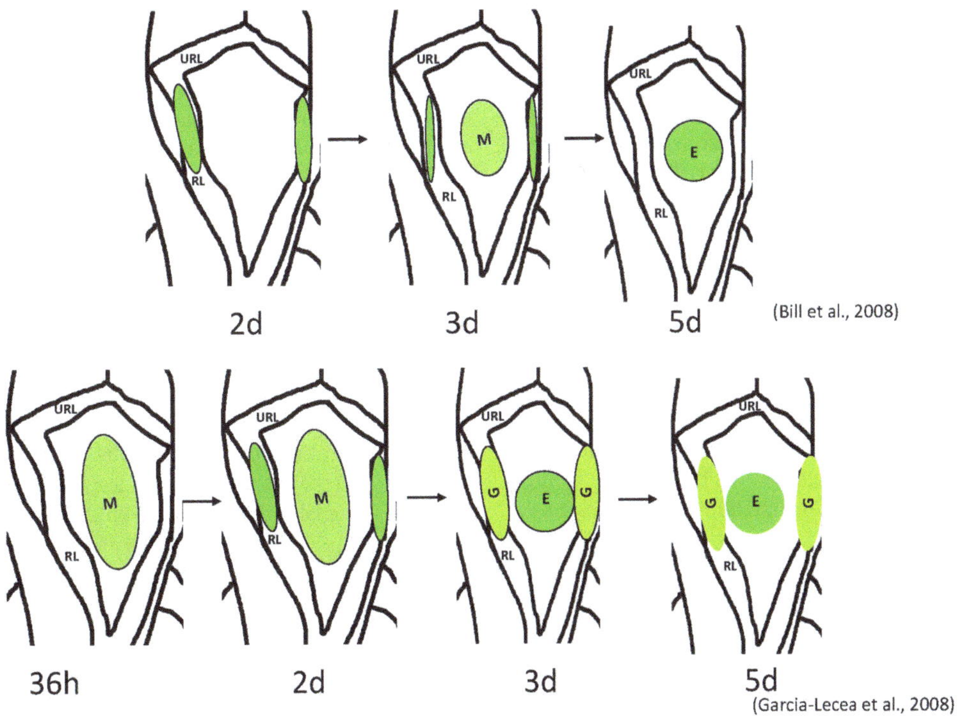

FIGURE 1 | Schemata of formation of the choroid plexus of IV ventricle in zebrafish as revealed by analysis of different transgenics. Above– mn16Et, below – Gateways. The cytosolic GFP, first detected the lateral clusters, could be detected in the prospective epithelial cells of mn16Et at 3 dpf, i.e., after these coalesced toward the midline. This mimics events of the CP morphogenesis as hypothesized in mammals. In contrast, in the Gateway transgenics, the GFP is rather prominent in the midline cluster prior to its coalescence, i.e. during a stage of *tela choroidea*. Abbreviations: E, epidermal cells of the prospective choroid plexus of IV ventricle; G, glial cells of the prospective choroid plexus of IV ventricle; M, midline cluster; RL, rhombic lips; URL, upper rhombic lips.

and lateral-posterior fields (Hunter and Dymecki, 2007). It appears that the lateral fields are the primary contributor of cells to CPIV, which initially develops as an invagination of the hindbrain roof plate epithelium (Awatramani et al., 2003). CPIV will subsequently receive migratory cells directly from the rhombic lip (Hunter and Dymecki, 2007). The fate-mapping studies of these fields lead to a number of questions. What is the fate of the midline field of hindbrain roof plate epithelium, and what are its contributions to CPIV development? Are the midline and lateral fields the sole source of cells present in the CPIV differentiated epithelium? Does the hindbrain roof plate epithelium also contribute to the CPIV vasculature or stroma? Is there a roof plate at the hindbrain (myelencephalon) level adjacent to the CPIV (mCP)? What genes are involved in specification of the different cell lineages in the CPIV? Are there cell adhesion molecules present on the cellular surface of developing CPIV cells that restrict cell type mixing, or do they segregate by developmental turnover as previously determined for the lateral CP (Liddelow et al., 2010)?

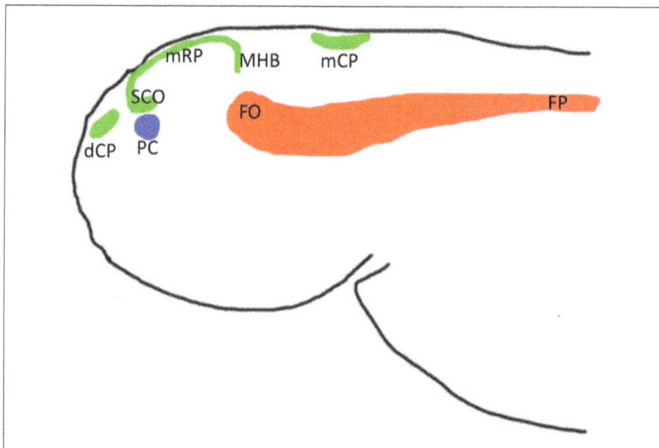

FIGURE 2 | Schemata of location of anterior midline structures of the neural tube in zebrafish based on analysis of several enhancer-trap transgenics. Abbreviations: dCP, choroid plexus of diencephalon; mCP, choroid plexus of myelencephalon; FO, flexural organ; FP, floor plate; mRP, metencephalon (midbrain) roof plate; PC, posterior commissure; SCO, subcommissural organ; MHB, midbrain hindbrain boundary.

CAN FISH PROVIDE INFORMATION RELEVANT TO CP DEVELOPMENT IN MAMMALS?

Given that all vertebrates, including fish have brain ventricles (Lowery and Sive, 2005), it is reasonable to expect that the molecular mechanisms underlying their formation were conserved during evolution, at least to some extent. For example, the Engrailed family of evolutionarily conserved transcriptional repressors plays an important role during formation of the midbrain-hindbrain boundary and adjacent tissues, the posterior midbrain and cerebellum. Engrailed loss-of-function mutations result in a reduction and/or loss of these structures, whereas gain-of-function mutations in Engrailed family members expressed at the dorsal midline cause misspecification of roof plate cells thus perturbing axonal navigation and interfering with the development of structures deriving from the dorsal neuroepithelium, such as the CP, epiphysis and subcommissural organ in fish, birds and rodents (Araki and Nakamura, 1999; Ristoratore et al., 1999; Louvi and Wassef, 2000). This suggests that the developmental program of the CP and some circumventricular organs is evolutionarily conserved opening a possibility to study these processes in the abundantly available and transparent embryos of fish (**Figure 2**). Indeed, the first *in vivo* studies of several enhancer-trap transgenic lines of zebrafish expressing cytosolic GFP (**Table 1**) brought about significant progress in understanding the development of CP.

THE FATE OF THE MIDLINE FIELD AND SPECIFICATION OF CP LINEAGES

As mentioned above, cell fate studies of CPIV in mice demonstrated a role of cells of the rhombic lips (lateral fields) in this process; however, the role of the hindbrain roof plate epithelium, in the absence of suitable markers, is not well-understood (Awatramani et al., 2003; Landsberg et al., 2005; Hunter and Dymecki, 2007). Interestingly, in zebrafish, a very similar developmental scenario can be proposed based upon observations of formation of the mCP. In the zebrafish transgenic line, mn16Et GFP expression is initially confined to the rhombic lips (lateral clusters), then spreads toward the midline. In time, only the midline cluster remains fluorescent (Bill et al., 2008). This could be interpreted in a manner similar to that in mice, i.e., that the lateral clusters of the rhombic lips are the only structures giving rise to the *tela choroidea*, the primordium of the CP.

Fortunately, zebrafish are amenable to large-scale genetic manipulation, thus additional *in vivo* markers for *tela choroidea* and CP were generated within our large-scale screen for enhancer-trap lines in zebrafish (Parinov et al., 2004; Kondrychyn et al., 2009). This provided the opportunity to study CP formation in real time. In particular, the transgenic line Gateways (sqet33e20Et) revealed formation of the dCP and mCP, each from several distinct cell groups, which is similar to that during formation of CPs in mice (Currle et al., 2005; Garcia-Lecea et al., 2008). The following phases of mCP formation were defined: (i) the *tela choroidea* forms from the neuroepithelial cells of the IVth ventricle roof, simultaneously the vasculature grows toward the final mCP location; (ii) some cells of the rhombic lips join the *tela choroidea* by migrating from the upper and lateral rhombic lips, reminiscent of the migration observed in mice and mn16Et zebrafish; (iii) the *tela choroidea* coalesces forming the button-like structure (medial cluster or mCP epithelial cells) in the roof of the IVth ventricle; (iv) the capillary encircles the structure and invades its interior; (v) as the *tela choroidea* coalesces, the remaining cells of the lateral clusters develop an astroglial phenotype, and (vi) these cells later converge with the medial cluster due to a reduction of the ventricle and ventricular roof. Therefore, this analysis revealed contribution into the mCP from at least four different cell lineages—the primary medial cluster derived from a roof of IVth ventricle, the secondary cells of medial cluster derived from lateral rhombic lips, the endothelial cells of the invading vasculature, and astroglial cells of the rhombic lips. Based on morphological criteria, the former two lineages contribute to the epithelial and stromal components of the CP, and the latter two correspond to endothelial and astroglial components. To support

Table 1 | Zebrafish transgenic lines that label the choroid plexus.

Transgenic line	Tissue	Genes linked	References
sqet33Et	CP, dorsal interneurons, NCC, meninx	*zic3-zic6*	Kondrychyn et al., 2011; Winata et al., 2013
sqet3310Et	CP (epithelium), roof and floor plates, pigment and olfactory		Kondrychyn et al., 2011
sqet33e20Et (Gateways)	CP (medial and lateral clusters, tela choroidea, epithelium and glia), roof plate, NCC, CVOs, lens, pronephros, olfactory	*csrnp1b, sulf1, slc05A1*	Jiao et al., 2011; Kondrychyn et al., 2011
sqKR19Et	Expression pattern identical to that in SqET33-E20—CP (medial and lateral clusters, tela choroidea, epithelium and glia), roof plate, NCC, CVOs, lens, pronephros, olfactory	*sema3gb*	Teh et al., 2010
sqet33-mi84Et	CP (vasculature), general vasculature	*pard3*	Kondrychyn et al., 2011
sqgw18aEt	CP, roof plate, ear, eyes	Not mapped	Kondrychyn et al., 2011
sqgw19cEt	CP, roof plate, ventral neurons of spinal cord	Not mapped	Kondrychyn et al., 2011
sqgw42aEt	CP (epithelium), roof plate, ventral neurons	*csrnp1b, sulf1, slc05A1*	Garcia-Lecea et al., 2008
sqgw84bEt	CP, roof plate, pronephros, neurons	*slc22A13*	Kondrychyn et al., 2011
mn16Et	Lateral and medial clusters, tela choroidea, epithelium.	Not mapped	Bill et al., 2008

and develop this idea further more experimental evidence will be required. Nevertheless, based on unpublished results of other zebrafish transgenics, it is clear that these highlight events somewhat different from those seen in mn16Et and Gateways. It is critical that these transgenic and other developmental markers of CP be characterized, as they will further delineate unique contributions of different cell populations into the CP.

ANTERIOR ROOF PLATE: DISAPPEARING ACT OR MODIFYING MORPHOGENESIS?

The study of formation of the midline signaling structures in zebrafish transgenics revealed similar organization of the roof and floor plates along the spinal cord. During late neurulation, when the primitive lumen is reduced into a central canal, the roof plate is extended significantly along the dorsal-ventral axis, whereas floor plate is extended a little (Kondrychyn et al., 2013; Korzh, 2014). This organization reverses anteriorly, where starting from the myelencephalon level the floor plate progressively extends along the dorsal-ventral axis and the roof plate either is converted into other dorsal midline structures such as CP, or is significantly reduced as it happens at the level of mesencephalon (Korzh, 2007, 2014). Several observations support this interpretation. First, none of several roof plate transgenics analyzed so far express a fluorescent marker in the roof plate only; other expression domains represent the neural crest derivatives, interneurons, CP (see **Table 1**), i.e., structures derived from common progenitors (Papan and Campos-Ortega, 1999; Garcia-Lecea et al., 2008).

This raises an intriguing question: does the roof plate disappear partially and/or convert into other structures (CP or circumventricular organs)? Is this unique to bony fish? As mentioned above, there are several studies documenting the roof plate at the myelencephalon level in terrestrial vertebrates (Liem et al., 1997; Lee and Jessell, 1999; Lee et al., 2000; Millonig et al., 2000). Hence, the dorsal neural tube of bony fish may be evolutionary ancient and reminiscent of a common ancestor of vertebrates. And yet a presence of the most of circumventricular organs in zebrafish and terrestrial vertebrates (except those at the telencephalon level) makes this doubtful. One should not forget that current theories of formation of CP in bony fish and mammals still differ somewhat (Awatramani et al., 2003; Landsberg et al., 2005; Hunter and Dymecki, 2007; Korzh, 2007, 2014; Garcia-Lecea et al., 2008). Perhaps, the roof plate development in terrestrial vertebrates could be studied *in vivo*, at some point, or with help from comparative genomics, and results of such studies will contribute toward solving this interesting evolutionary puzzle.

Since the CP occupies a position at the dorsal midline, it is reasonable to predict that it forms by early neural progenitors found in this place. The roof plate occupies the dorsal midline of spinal cord. This poses a question, does the roof plate occupy the dorsal midline of the fourth (myelencephalic) ventricle, or do these cells somewhat differ? Dorsal neuroepithelium of the spinal cord prior to conversion into the roof plate undergoes topological transformation without cell migration. As a result the cells polarized initially along the medial-lateral axis become polarized along dorsal-ventral axis and elongate (Kondrychyn et al., 2013). In contrast, cells of midline dorsal neuroepithelium at the myelencephalic level fail to undergo such transformation. Instead, they coalesce into a cluster representing the epithelial lineage of CP. In parallel, the lateral clusters develop as glial cells morphologically reminiscent of the roof plate, but their presence is limited by an extent of 2–3 rhombomeres proximal to the medial cluster. These will fuse later on with the medial cluster as the glial lineage of the same CP (Garcia-Lecea et al., 2008). Each of these clusters represents approximately one half of the myelencephalic roof plate progenitors. Hence one may speculate that a ventricle separates the roof plate progenitors into two lateral clusters, and that the ventricle formation drives morphogenetic transformation of the dorsal midline progenitors into CP.

Hence at least for now there is no reason to believe that at the level of brain ventricles the roof plate is maintained. This consideration is supported by analysis of the roof plate formation in other brain regions, for example, the mesencephalon. At this level one more cavity reminiscent of a ventricle forms early on in parallel with the myelencephalon (hindbrain, IVth) and diencephalon (IIIrd) *bona fide* ventricles. This transient cavity known as the opthocoele develops an equivalent of the Sylvius aqueduct connecting two ventricles. At this level the roof plate cells are not as elongated as those at the spinal cord level, but they do have morphological similarity to the spinal cord roof plate. So, it seems we may formulate a simple hypothesis: "The roof plate is present at the dorsal midline of the neural tube only in absence of ventricles. In presence of ventricles it is converted into other derivatives, such as CP, etc."

Does the roof plate contribute into any other midline derivatives? One of these is the subcommissural organ. It has been suggested that the subcommissural organ is derived from the neuroepithelial cells that line the lumen of the dorsal-caudal aspect of the diencephalon (Huh et al., 2009). In view of the fact that the subcommissural organ expresses several transgenes as the roof plate and/or CP, we suggest that this organ, located posterior and ventral to the epiphysis and, immediately below the posterior commissure, develops as the modified extension of the mesencephalic roof plate (Korzh, 2014).

GENES OF THE DORSAL MIDLINE

At the molecular level, there are at least two differences that have been identified in development of the CP in mammals and teleosts. First, *Otx2* null mice fail to develop all four CP; however, in teleosts, *otx2* expression appears limited to the diencephalon (Li et al., 1994; Johansson et al., 2013) thus potentially restricting its effects on the dCP. Despite several morpholinos designed for knockdown of Otx2 and available zebrafish mutants, the CPs in Otx2-deficient animals have not been investigated further. Second, transthyretinin (*TTR*), a common marker of the CP in amniotes, is not expressed in the CP of amphibians and teleost fish (Power et al., 2000). Given that in these species high levels of *ttr* are produced by the liver, future studies will be required to determine whether liver-derived *ttr* can functionally substitute for CP-derived *ttr*.

There are many more similarities in expression of molecular markers in the CP. Clusterin is the cytoprotective secreted chaperone protein linked to protection of cells from oxidative stress, and its deficiency has been implicated in Alzheimer's, metabolic and cardiovascular diseases (Trougakos, 2013; Park et al., 2014). Despite being vertebrate-specific, when expressed in *Drosophila,* Clusterin increases resistance to heat-shock, wet starvation, oxidative stress and increases the lifespan of flies (Lee et al., 2012). During mouse development its expression is enriched in the CP and ependyma (Charnay et al., 2008), and in zebrafish, it is expressed in developing mCP (Jiao et al., 2011). Clusterin may represent the earliest CSF protein secreted by the CP that suppresses proteotoxic stress. Clusterin expression is regulated by Notch signaling (Jiao et al., 2011). The developmental roles of both Notch and Shh signaling are conserved between fish and mammals, and Notch is known to regulate CP development (Hunter and Dymecki, 2007; Bill et al., 2008; Garcia-Lecea et al., 2008; Nielsen and Dymecki, 2010).

There are also several areas that will require more research to determine the similarities and differences in developmental activity of evolutionary conserved genes. The CPIII fails to develop in the Gli3-deficient mouse embryos (Grove et al., 1998). In zebrafish Gli3 is broadly expressed in the dorsal neural tube (Tyurina et al., 2005); however functional studies of CP in the Gli3-deficient zebrafish have not been performed. Amongst genes expressed in the CP of both mice and zebrafish, there are several Msx genes (Nishikawa et al., 1994; Landsberg et al., 2005; Thisse and Thisse, 2005); however, systematic comparisons will need to be performed and their specific roles in CP development established. Lastly, Gdf7 marks the primordium of the CP epithelium in mice, and has been utilized by many studies to drive expression within the CPIV (Currle et al., 2005); however, *gdf7* expression and function have not been analyzed in zebrafish in sufficient detail. These studies will be critical to determine the level of evolutionary conservation of developmental mechanisms of the CP and fill in a gap in this knowledge using molecular tools already available.

Translation of teleost findings to the mammalian systems could also be highly informative. The transposon-mediated enhancer-trap study identified several cell populations that contribute to the formation of the CP, and the insertion sites mapped identified the mCP-associated genes. In particular, the Gateway (sqet33e20Et) transgene has been mapped into a region containing *csrnp1a* (*axud1*), *sulf1*, and *slc5a1* (Garcia-Lecea et al., 2008). Transposon insertions of two other transgenic lines with expression in the CP (sqgw42aEt and sqgw45cEt) were mapped into the same genomic area supporting a role for one of these genes in the CP development or function. *csrnp1*, whose expression is controlled by Shh and PDGF, was proposed to be involved in regulating cell migration. It is essential for the development of neural-crest-derived cephalic structures (Schmahl et al., 2007; Feijoo et al., 2009). *slc5a1* (*sglt1*) has been studied for its role in glucose re-absorption in kidney and intestine (Gorboulev et al., 2012). Given that the functionally related glucose transporter 1 (GLUT1) is expressed in the CP of mammals, as well as that of bony and cartilaginous fish, this would make *slc5a1,* which encodes the sodium/glucose cotransporter rather interesting to investigate further despite the fact that its expression pattern might preclude a localized function (Farrell and Pardridge, 1991; Farrell et al., 1992; Planas et al., 2000; Jensen et al., 2010; Balmaceda-Aguilera et al., 2012). *sulf1* is expressed in the developing CP of mice (Ohto et al., 2002; Kalus et al., 2009; Ratzka et al., 2010), where its deficiency causes only minor defects or no defects in development of the CP probably due to functional redundancy with other Sulf genes (Holst et al., 2007; Kalus et al., 2009). Its orthologue in zebrafish is also expressed in the CP along with two other related genes—*sulf2* and *sulf2a* (Gorsi et al., 2010). Since *sulf1* has been linked to formation of the BBB, it is probably the best candidate gene, which expression is mimicked in the Gateways. Coincidentantly, the posttranslational modification of components of the extracellular matrix by sulfation plays an important role in regulation of cellular signaling (FGF, Hh, and Wnt) and mutations affecting components of sulfation machinery and its substrates are known to cause a variety of developmental defects linked to deficient cell signaling (Luders et al., 2003).

Lastly, several of the genes, specifically those that mediate the tight junctions between the CP epithelial cells are conserved across multiple phyla. These are not specific to the CP alone, but are a consistent feature between blood-CSF barrier, which is mediated at the level of epithelial cells of the CP (Dziegielewska et al., 2001); and BBB, which in all vertebrates is mediated at the level of endothelial cells of brain microvessels except sharks and rays, where it is at the level of astrocytes (Abbott et al., 2006; Bundgaard and Abbott, 2008). In the blood-CSF barrier the tight junction (or *zonula occludens*, ZO) is located in apical regions between adjacent epithelial cells, and filters the blood-to-CSF passage of hydrophilic molecules and ions (Johanson, 2003). Tight junctions are dynamic multimolecular complexes of membrane-associated proteins active in intracellular signaling, which include ZO proteins and claudins and a number of other proteins (Luissint et al., 2012). In the zebrafish there are three maternally-expressed genes encoding ZO proteins, so the ZO proteins are available from the very beginning of development (Kiener et al., 2007). Claudin 5a is also expressed in the brain during a period prior to and during CP formation (Zhang et al., 2010). Although a systematic analysis of genes expressed in the CP epithelia in evolutionary perspective is still in its infancy, there is a progress in this area. Hence, we will know to which extent the CP epithelium is conserved in evolution rather soon.

DEVELOPMENT OF THE CP VASCULATURE

The vasculature of the human CPIV is supplied by branches that originate primarily from the posterior inferior cerebellar artery, and to a lesser extent the anterior inferior cerebellar artery (mostly in the anterior CP portion closest to the foramen of Lushka). In rare cases, branches of the superior cerebellar, the basilar artery, or other arteries extend branches to supply the CP (Sharifi et al., 2005). Once inside the CP the vessels become highly branched and interconnected providing a vast network. The vessels are unique from other brain regions in that they lack the endothelial barrier protein and astrocytic processes in the basement membrane (Bouchaud et al., 1989; Rosenstein et al., 1992), and contain 60–80 nm transcellular pores or fenestrations, allowing for the exit of substrates into the stroma (Strazielle and Ghersi-Egea, 2000; Stan et al., 2012). The fenestrations are covered by diaphragms that have tufts of heparan sulfate proteoglycans extending into the lumen suggesting a role in selective permeability (Stan et al., 2012). The dilation of these vessels is mediated by pericytes, innervating nerves, and interepithelial pressure sensors (Mortazavi et al., 2014), and has a direct effect on the composition of the CSF; therefore, they are highly regulated in response to CSF conditions independent of the physiological blood pressure (Scala et al., 2011). A specialized basement membrane, critical for serum filtering, is secreted by the vasculature very similar to that secreted by the fenestrated vasculature of the kidney (Johanson et al., 2011).

DEVELOPMENT OF THE MAMMALIAN CP VASCULATURE

In human, the posterior inferior cerebellar artery and anterior inferior cerebellar artery begin sprouting at 44 and 40 days, respectively, and the posterior inferior cerebellar artery terminates in the CP at 52 days. Its arrival is concurrent with that of the first epithelial cells suggesting that signaling from the roof plate is critical for angiogenesis (Macchi et al., 2005). Development of the posterior inferior cerebellar artery is highly variable, with a variety of origins and paths consistent with a model in which hypoxia induces angiogenic factors, for example VEGF, and consequently angiogenic sprouting induced (Macchi et al., 2005; Yang et al., 2010). Angiogenic sprouting has been described in detail for the CP vasculature in other organisms as well. Strong described the process in 14-day rabbit embryos observing a reorganization of vessels occurring, with the pontobulbar artery running into the area that develops as the *tela choroidea* (Strong, 1956). Over the next few days the vasculature continues to develop, and anastomose being drawn into each progressive epithelial invagination (Strong, 1956). A second more rapid angiogenic process, called splitting angiogenesis or intussusceptive angiogenesis, is involved in the enumeration of vessels within the invaginations. This process was inferred from the identification of pillar structures bisecting larger vessels of the CP by electron microscopy (Scala et al., 2011). This developmental process has been primarily described in other tissues; however, it could be extrapolated to the CP vasculature. Intussusceptive angiogenesis describes three separate processes for vascular enumeration: microvascular growth, arborization, and remodeling (Makanya et al., 2009).

The zebrafish is one of the premiere animal models for studying vascular development due to its ability to develop without a functioning circulatory system or blood (Stainier, 2001), and large number of transgenics that label the vasculature (Lawson and Weinstein, 2002; Jin et al., 2005, 2007; Rehn et al., 2011; Trinh le et al., 2011; Zhou et al., 2011; Sacilotto et al., 2013). Unfortunately, the vasculature structure of the adult mCP has not been characterized as it has been in mammals. This is primarily due to an emphasis within the zebrafish community on early developmental processes, thus mCP characterization has been limited to the first 6 days post fertilization (dpf). Angiogenic sprouting occurs from the middle cerebral vessel at 48 hpf creating the dorsal longitudinal vein. The dorsal longitudinal vein extends along the dorsal midline turning at ~50 hpf to fuse with either left or right posterior cerebral vein (Bill et al., 2008; Lenard et al., 2013). The tip cells of the dorsal longitudinal vein and posterior cerebral vein initiate this junction, subsequently rearranging, and splitting to produce a multicellular lumen (Lenard et al., 2013). Consistent with events in the mammalian CPIV, the angiogenic sprout arrival occurs simultaneous to the migration of the epithelial field suggesting that the roof plate organizer is required to attract both sets of cells to their final localization. A secondary branch forms off of the main dorsal longitudinal vein branch and then fuses with the opposing posterior cerebral vein, and a third branch forms to connect the left and right posterior cerebral veins. We named this connecting vessel the trans-choroid plexus branch as it crosses near the posterior margin of mCP (Bill et al., 2008). Further branching between the dorsal longitudinal vein, posterior cerebral vein, and trans-choroid plexus branch are observed by 5 dpf internal to the mCP region defined by transgenic lines that label the mCP epithelia. The resulting structure is highly fragile and prone to hemorrhage (Bill, 2008) much like the mammalian CP (Scott and Bergevin, 2005). Given this fragility, it is not surprising, that the CP vasculature is constantly being repaired utilizing bone marrow-derived endothelial progenitors (Zhang et al., 2002). Unfortunately, processes such as invagination of the mCP, intussusceptive angiogenesis, and the integration of bone marrow-derived endothelial progenitors have not been studied in zebrafish. One striking difference is that the zebrafish appears to have a relatively invariant growth profile, while the vascular growth in humans is much more variable. There are two potential reasons for its invariant nature in the zebrafish. The first is that the corresponding period of zebrafish developmental program is much more rapid than that in human (2 h vs. 8 days). The increased developmental window could allow for competing attractive and repulsive angiogenic factors time to alter the trajectory of the main vessel. A second hypothesis could be related to the levels of oxygen that are driving vascular development. We know that the zebrafish are able to survive for up to 7 dpf without a functioning circulatory system, due to the permeability of the embryo to oxygen; therefore, hypoxic conditions within the developing brain would be much more common during human development. This would lead to involvement of competing angiogenic factors as other brain regions would attempt to obtain oxygen, and thus development would take a much more tortuous path.

At the molecular level sprouting angiogenesis, intussusceptive angiogenesis, and development of fenestrations are controlled by interactions between the VEGF, NOTCH, and SHH signaling pathways (Kamba et al., 2006; Nielsen and Dymecki, 2010; Yang et al., 2010; Dimova et al., 2013). The CP epithelial cells continuously secrete VEGF at high levels even in adults suggesting multiple roles for VEGF in vascular development (Esser et al., 1998), while the endothelial cells express the VEGF receptors. While these processes have been investigated extensively in the tail of the zebrafish, work on the cranial vasculature has lagged behind, and very little is known about the genes required for the dorsal longitudinal vein attraction to the mCP, branching, and production of the fenestrated vessels. Part of the problem is a general role of some of these pathways (Notch and Shh) in morphogenesis of the CP (Garcia-Lecea et al., 2008). In the future, extension of the developmental and molecular studies of the mCP vasculature will be required to determine the extent of conservation.

DEVELOPMENT OF THE CP STROMA

The stroma lies between the vascular basement membrane and the epithelial basement membrane. It contains a wide variety of cells including: fibroblasts, telocytes, stem cells, dendritic cells, leukocytes, macrophages, kolmer cells (a specialized monocyte, also called epiplexus cells), and in some cases T-cells (Strazielle and Ghersi-Egea, 2000; Nataf et al., 2006; Popescu et al., 2012). The stroma is hypothesized to function as a stem cell niche with the nestin-positive fibroblasts and telocytes supporting myeloid progenitors and neural stem cells, respectively (Nataf et al., 2006; Popescu et al., 2012).

The stroma develops from invagination of the mesenchyme that lies dorsal to the hindbrain roof plate epithelium, and progressively transitions to being composed of high levels of connective tissues with low density of mesenchymal cells (Shuangshoti and Netsky, 1966). Little is known about the development of this region; however, there are indications that the stromal composition may be highly dynamic and change during development, and in response to immunologic insult. For example, it is hypothesized that the fibroblast niche provides different developmental signals during development than during adulthood based on the progeny of the myeloid progenitors; embryonic-derived progenitors produce dendritic cells, while adult-derived progenitors produce macrophages (Nataf et al., 2006). Another difference is that kolmer cells are only present in the adult CP (Strazielle and Ghersi-Egea, 2000). Given the immunologic complexity of the stroma, much of the cell diversity is driven by immunologic insult, or CNS injury (Mitchell et al., 2009; Wojcik et al., 2011; Hasegawa-Ishii et al., 2013; Shechter et al., 2013; Szmydynger-Chodobska et al., 2013). Previous analysis in zebrafish failed to demonstrate presence of unlabelled cells in the mCP of transgenics suggesting that all cell lineages except vasculature derive from GFP-positive cells (Garcia-Lecea et al., 2008). This raises a criticism regarding contribution of mesenchymal cells into the mCP of this species; however, as mentioned all analyses on zebrafish have focused on early development opening the possibility that the mesenchymal-derived cells enter at later developmental time points. New *in vitro* systems and transgenics in combination with high-resolution bioimaging may lead to a much better definition of this portion of the mCP.

CONCLUSIONS

The CP has been a popular organ system to investigate in a variety of vertebrates including fish, lizards, amphibians, birds, and mammals; however, the number of systematic studies that look at a single feature of the CP across the phyla have been very few, and primarily restricted to the CP epithelia. Given the CP's importance in a variety of physiologic brain functions and pathologies, we suggest a need for these types of studies, as they provide valuable insights into understanding CP development and function. In this review, we have tried to highlight how several studies in the zebrafish have expanded our knowledge of CP development in general, and shed light on several aspects that remain not fully understood, including developmental fate of the medial group of hindbrain roof cells. Based on comparisons of fish and mice, we observe that the CP derives from cells that share their origin with the roof plate and neural crest, and its development is driven by the evolutionary conserved molecular determinants. Indeed, this is a renaissance in CP research, and there are many questions that are yet to be answered. For example, what are the tropic factors that are secreted from the dorsal organizing center to attract the vasculature and epithelia cells to their final location? What are the molecular differences that exist within the CP, as cells can be derived from either the roof plate or neural crest? What is the molecular identity of the stem cell niche? And lastly, to what extent are features of the CP conserved? Given an abundance of modern developmental tools (transgenics and cell transplantation), and genomic technologies (single cell transcriptome and genome engineering), we are poised to answer these questions, and feel that they can be answered soon.

ACKNOWLEDGMENTS

Authors are indebted to the collective input of colleagues from the Steve Ekker, Lisa Schimenti and Vladimir Korzh laboratories, where most of experimental data in support of our ideas have been generated and personnel of the Fish Facilities of the University of Minnesota and the Institute of Molecular and Cell Biology, Singapore for care and maintenance of fish.

REFERENCES

Abbott, N. J., Ronnback, L., and Hansson, E. (2006). Astrocyte-endothelial interactions at the blood-brain barrier. *Nat. Rev. Neurosci.* 7, 41–53. doi: 10.1038/nrn1824

Araki, I., and Nakamura, H. (1999). Engrailed defines the position of dorsal di-mesencephalic boundary by repressing diencephalic fate. *Development* 126, 5127–5135.

Awatramani, R., Soriano, P., Rodriguez, C., Mai, J. J., and Dymecki, S. M. (2003). Cryptic boundaries in roof plate and choroid plexus identified by intersectional gene activation. *Nat. Genet.* 35, 70–75. doi: 10.1038/ng1228

Balmaceda-Aguilera, C., Cortes-Campos, C., Cifuentes, M., Peruzzo, B., Mack, L., Tapia, J. C., et al. (2012). Glucose transporter 1 and monocarboxylate transporters 1, 2, and 4 localization within the glial cells of shark blood-brain-barriers. *PLoS ONE* 7:e32409. doi: 10.1371/journal.pone.0032409

Bill, B. R. (2008). *Utilization of Forward and Reverse Genetic Approaches to Inform Ocular and Choroid Plexus Development. Molecular, Cellular, Developmental Biology, and Genetics.* Minneapolis, MN: University of Minnesota.

Bill, B. R., Balciunas, D., McCarra, J. A., Young, E. D., Xiong, T., Spahn, A. M., et al. (2008). Development and Notch signaling requirements of the zebrafish choroid plexus. *PLoS ONE* 3:e3114. doi: 10.1371/journal.pone.0003114

Bolos, M., Antequera, D., Aldudo, J., Kristen, H., Bullido, M. J., and Carro, E. (2014). Choroid plexus implants rescue Alzheimer's disease-like pathologies by modulating amyloid-beta degradation. *Cell. Mol. Life Sci.* 71, 2947–2955. doi: 10.1007/s00018-013-1529-4

Borlongan, C. V., Skinner, S. J., Geaney, M., Vasconcellos, A. V., Elliott, R. B., and Emerich, D. F. (2004a). Intracerebral transplantation of porcine choroid plexus provides structural and functional neuroprotection in a rodent model of stroke. *Stroke* 35, 2206–2210. doi: 10.1161/01.STR.0000138954.25825.0b

Borlongan, C. V., Skinner, S. J., Geaney, M., Vasconcellos, A. V., Elliott, R. B., and Emerich, D. F. (2004b). Neuroprotection by encapsulated choroid plexus in a rodent model of Huntington's disease. *Neuroreport* 15, 2521–2525. doi: 10.1097/00001756-200411150-00018

Bouchaud, C., Le Bert, M., and Dupouey, P. (1989). Are close contacts between astrocytes and endothelial cells a prerequisite condition of a blood-brain barrier? The rat subfornical organ as an example. *Biol. Cell* 67, 159–165.

Broom, E. R., Gilthorpe, J. D., Butts, T., Campo-Paysaa, F., and Wingate, R. J. (2012). The roof plate boundary is a bi-directional organiser of dorsal neural tube and choroid plexus development. *Development* 139, 4261–4270. doi: 10.1242/dev.082255

Bundgaard, M., and Abbott, N. J. (2008). All vertebrates started out with a glial blood-brain barrier 4-500 million years ago. *Glia* 56, 699–708. doi: 10.1002/glia.20642

Charnay, Y., Imhof, A., Vallet, P. G., Hakkoum, D., Lathuiliere, A., Poku, N., et al. (2008). Giannakopoulos, Clusterin expression during fetal and postnatal CNS development in mouse. *Neuroscience* 155, 714–724. doi: 10.1016/j.neuroscience.2008.06.022

Chizhikov, V. V., and Millen, K. J. (2004). Mechanisms of roof plate formation in the vertebrate CNS. *Nat. Rev. Neurosci.* 5, 808–812. doi: 10.1038/nrn1520

Chizhikov, V. V., Lindgren, A. G., Currle, D. S., Rose, M. F., Monuki, E. S., and Millen, K. J. (2006). The roof plate regulates cerebellar cell-type specification and proliferation. *Development* 133, 2793–2804. doi: 10.1242/dev.02441

Copp, A. J., Greene, N. D., and Murdoch, J. N. (2003). The genetic basis of mammalian neurulation. *Nat. Rev. Genet.* 4, 784–793. doi: 10.1038/nrg1181

Currle, D. S., Cheng, X., Hsu, C. M., and Monuki, E. S. (2005). Direct and indirect roles of CNS dorsal midline cells in choroid plexus epithelia formation. *Development* 132, 3549–3559. doi: 10.1242/dev.01915

Dimova, I., Hlushchuk, R., Makanya, A., Styp-Rekowska, B., Ceausu, A., Flueckiger, S., et al. (2013). Inhibition of Notch signaling induces extensive intussusceptive neo-angiogenesis by recruitment of mononuclear cells. *Angiogenesis* 16, 921–937. doi: 10.1007/s10456-013-9366-5

Dziegielewska, K. M., Ek, J., Habgood, M. D., and Saunders, N. R. (2001). Development of the choroid plexus. *Microsc Res. Tech.* 52, 5–20. doi: 10.1002/1097-0029(20010101)52:1<5::AID-JEMT3>3.0.CO;2-J

Emerich, D. F., Skinner, S. J., Borlongan, C. V., Vasconcellos, A. V., and Thanos, C. G. (2005). The choroid plexus in the rise, fall and repair of the brain. *Bioessays* 27, 262–274. doi: 10.1002/bies.20193

Emerich, D. F., Thanos, C. G., Goddard, M., Skinner, S. J., Geany, M. S., Bell, W. J., et al. (2006). Extensive neuroprotection by choroid plexus transplants in excitotoxin lesioned monkeys. *Neurobiol. Dis.* 23, 471–480. doi: 10.1016/j.nbd.2006.04.014

Esser, S., Wolburg, K., Wolburg, H., Breier, G., Kurzchalia, T., and Risau, W. (1998). Vascular endothelial growth factor induces endothelial fenestrations *in vitro*. *J. Cell Biol.* 140, 947–959. doi: 10.1083/jcb.140.4.947

Farrell, C. L., and Pardridge, W. M. (1991). Blood-brain barrier glucose transporter is asymmetrically distributed on brain capillary endothelial lumenal and ablumenal membranes: an electron microscopic immunogold study. *Proc. Natl. Acad. Sci. U.S.A.* 88, 5779–5783. doi: 10.1073/pnas.88.13.5779

Farrell, C. L., Yang, J., and Pardridge, W. M. (1992). GLUT-1 glucose transporter is present within apical and basolateral membranes of brain epithelial interfaces and in microvascular endothelia with and without tight junctions. *J. Histochem. Cytochem.* 40, 193–199. doi: 10.1177/40.2.1552163

Feijoo, C. G., Sarrazin, A. F., Allende, M. L., and Glavic, A. (2009). Cysteine-serine-rich nuclear protein 1, Axud1/Csrnp1, is essential for cephalic neural progenitor proliferation and survival in zebrafish. *Dev. Dyn.* 238, 2034–2043. doi: 10.1002/dvdy.22006

Ganong, W. F. (2000). Circumventricular organs: definition and role in the regulation of endocrine and autonomic function. *Clin. Exp. Pharmacol. Physiol.* 27, 422–427. doi: 10.1046/j.1440-1681.2000.03259.x

Garcia-Lecea, M., Kondrychyn, I., Fong, S. H., Ye, Z. R., and Korzh, V. (2008). *In vivo* analysis of choroid plexus morphogenesis in zebrafish. *PLoS ONE* 3:e3090. doi: 10.1371/journal.pone.0003090

Gorboulev, V., Schurmann, A., Vallon, V., Kipp, H., Jaschke, A., Klessen, D., et al. (2012). Na(+)-D-glucose cotransporter SGLT1 is pivotal for intestinal glucose absorption and glucose-dependent incretin secretion. *Diabetes* 61, 187–196. doi: 10.2337/db11-1029

Gorsi, B., Whelan, S., and Stringer, S. E. (2010). Dynamic expression patterns of 6-O endosulfatases during zebrafish development suggest a subfunctionalisation event for sulf2. *Dev. Dyn.* 239, 3312–3323. doi: 10.1002/dvdy.22456

Grove, E. A., Tole, S., Limon, J., Yip, L., and Ragsdale, C. W. (1998). The hem of the embryonic cerebral cortex is defined by the expression of multiple Wnt genes and is compromised in Gli3-deficient mice. *Development* 125, 2315–2325.

Hasegawa-Ishii, S., Shimada, A., Inaba, M., Li, M., Shi, M., Kawamura, N., et al. (2013). Selective localization of bone marrow-derived ramified cells in the brain adjacent to the attachments of choroid plexus. *Brain Behav. Immun.* 29, 82–97. doi: 10.1016/j.bbi.2012.12.010

Holst, C. R., Bou-Reslan, H., Gore, B. B., Wong, K., Grant, D., Chalasani, S., et al. (2007). Secreted sulfatases Sulf1 and Sulf2 have overlapping yet essential roles in mouse neonatal survival. *PLoS ONE* 2:e575. doi: 10.1371/journal.pone.0000575

Howe, K., Clark, M. D., Torroja, C. F., Torrance, J., Berthelot, C., Muffato, M., et al. (2013). The zebrafish reference genome sequence and its relationship to the human genome. *Nature* 496, 498–503. doi: 10.1038/nature12111

Huh, M. S., Todd, M. A., and Picketts, D. J. (2009). SCO-ping out the mechanisms underlying the etiology of hydrocephalus. *Physiology* 24, 117–126. doi: 10.1152/physiol.00039.2008

Hunter, N. L., and Dymecki, S. M. (2007). Molecularly and temporally separable lineages form the hindbrain roof plate and contribute differentially to the choroid plexus. *Development* 134, 3449–3460. doi: 10.1242/dev.003095

Jensen, P. J., Gunter, L. B., and Carayannopoulos, M. O. (2010). Akt2 modulates glucose availability and downstream apoptotic pathways during development. *J. Biol. Chem.* 285, 17673–17680. doi: 10.1074/jbc.M109.079343

Jeong, J. Y., Kwon, H. B., Ahn, J. C., Kang, D., Kwon, S. H., Park, J. A., et al. (2008). Functional and developmental analysis of the blood-brain barrier in zebrafish. *Brain Res. Bull.* 75, 619–628. doi: 10.1016/j.brainresbull.2007.10.043

Jiao, S., Dai, W., Lu, L., Liu, Y., Zhou, J., Li, Y., et al. (2011). The conserved clusterin gene is expressed in the developing choroid plexus under the regulation of notch but not IGF signaling in zebrafish. *Endocrinology* 152, 1860–1871. doi: 10.1210/en.2010-1183

Jin, S. W., Beis, D., Mitchell, T., Chen, J. N., and Stainier, D. Y. (2005). Cellular and molecular analyses of vascular tube and lumen formation in zebrafish. *Development* 132, 5199–5209. doi: 10.1242/dev.02087

Jin, S. W., Herzog, W., Santoro, M. M., Mitchell, T. S., Frantsve, J., Jungblut, B., et al. (2007). A transgene-assisted genetic screen identifies essential regulators of vascular development in vertebrate embryos. *Dev. Biol.* 307, 29–42. doi: 10.1016/j.ydbio.2007.03.526

Johanson, C. (2003). "The choroid plexus—CSF nexus," in *Neuroscience in Medicine,* ed P. M. Conn (Totowa, NJ: Humana Press), 165–195.

Johanson, C. E., Stopa, E. G., and McMillan, P. N. (2011). The blood-cerebrospinal fluid barrier: structure and functional significance. *Methods Mol. Biol.* 686, 101–131. doi: 10.1007/978-1-60761-938-3_4

Johansson, P. A., Irmler, M., Acampora, D., Beckers, J., Simeone, A., and Gotz, M. (2013). The transcription factor Otx2 regulates choroid plexus development and function. *Development* 140, 1055–1066. doi: 10.1242/dev.090860

Joly, J. S., Osorio, J., Alunni, A., Auger, H., Kano, S., and Retaux, S. (2007). Windows of the brain: towards a developmental biology of circumventricular and other neurohemal organs. *Semin. Cell Dev. Biol.* 18, 512–524. doi: 10.1016/j.semcdb.2007.06.001

Kalus, I., Salmen, B., Viebahn, C., von Figura, K., Schmitz, D., D'Hooge, R., et al. (2009). Differential involvement of the extracellular 6-O-endosulfatases Sulf1 and Sulf2 in brain development and neuronal and behavioural plasticity. *J. Cell. Mol. Med.* 13, 4505–4521. doi: 10.1111/j.1582-4934.2008.00558.x

Kamba, T., Tam, B. Y., Hashizume, H., Haskell, A., Sennino, B., Mancuso, M. R., et al. (2006). VEGF-dependent plasticity of fenestrated capillaries in the normal adult microvasculature. *Am. J. Physiol. Heart Circ. Physiol.* 290, H560–H576. doi: 10.1152/ajpheart.00133.2005

Kiener, T. K., Sleptsova-Friedrich, I., and Hunziker, W. (2007). Identification, tissue distribution and developmental expression of tjp1/zo-1, tjp2/zo-2 and tjp3/zo-3 in the zebrafish, *Danio rerio. Gene Expr. Patterns* 7, 767–776. doi: 10.1016/j.modgep.2007.05.006

Kimmel, C. B., Ballard, W. W., Kimmel, S. R., Ullmann, B., and Schilling, T. F. (1995). Stages of embryonic development of the zebrafish. *Dev. Dyn.* 203, 253–310. doi: 10.1002/aja.1002030302

Knott, G. W., Dziegielewska, K. M., Habgood, M. D., Li, Z. S., and Saunders, N. R. (1997). Albumin transfer across the choroid plexus of South American opossum (*Monodelphis domestica*). *J. Physiol.* 499(Pt 1), 179–194.

Kondrychyn, I., Garcia-Lecea, M., Emelyanov, A., Parinov, S., and Korzh, V. (2009). Genome-wide analysis of Tol2 transposon reintegration in zebrafish. *BMC Genomics* 10:418. doi: 10.1186/1471-2164-10-418

Kondrychyn, I., Teh, C., Garcia-Lecea, M., Guan, Y., Kang, A., and Korzh, V. (2011). Zebrafish Enhancer TRAP transgenic line database ZETRAP 2.0. *Zebrafish* 8, 181–182. doi: 10.1089/zeb.2011.0718

Kondrychyn, I., Teh, C., Sin, M., and Korzh, V. (2013). Stretching morphogenesis of the roof plate and formation of the central canal. *PLoS ONE* 8:e56219. doi: 10.1371/journal.pone.0056219

Korzh, V. (2007). Transposons as tools for enhancer trap screens in vertebrates. *Genome Biol.* 8(Suppl. 1):S8. doi: 10.1186/gb-2007-8-s1-s8

Korzh, V. (2014). Stretching cell morphogenesis during late neurulation and mild neural tube defects. *Dev. Growth Differ.* 56, 425–433. doi: 10.1111/dgd.12143

Korzh, V., Edlund, T., and Thor, S. (1993). Zebrafish primary neurons initiate expression of the LIM homeodomain protein Isl-1 at the end of gastrulation. *Development* 118, 417–425.

Landsberg, R. L., Awatramani, R. B., Hunter, N. L., Farago, A. F., DiPietrantonio, H. J., Rodriguez, C. I., et al. (2005). Hindbrain rhombic lip is comprised of discrete progenitor cell populations allocated by Pax6. *Neuron* 48, 933–947. doi: 10.1016/j.neuron.2005.11.031

Lavezzi, A. M., Matturri, L., Del Corno, G., and Johanson, C. E. (2013). Vulnerability of fourth ventricle choroid plexus in sudden unexplained fetal and infant death syndromes related to smoking mothers. *Int. J. Dev. Neurosci.* 31, 319–327. doi: 10.1016/j.ijdevneu.2013.04.006

Lawson, N. D., and Weinstein, B. M. (2002). *In vivo* imaging of embryonic vascular development using transgenic zebrafish. *Dev. Biol.* 248, 307–318. doi: 10.1006/dbio.2002.0711

Lee, K. J., and Jessell, T. M. (1999). The specification of dorsal cell fates in the vertebrate central nervous system. *Annu. Rev. Neurosci.* 22, 261–294. doi: 10.1146/annurev.neuro.22.1.261

Lee, K. J., Dietrich, P., and Jessell, T. M. (2000). Genetic ablation reveals that the roof plate is essential for dorsal interneuron specification. *Nature* 403, 734–740. doi: 10.1038/35001507

Lee, Y. N., Shim, Y. J., Kang, B. H., Park, J. J., and Min, B. H. (2012). Over-expression of human clusterin increases stress resistance and extends lifespan in Drosophila melanogaster. *Biochem. Biophys. Res. Commun.* 420, 851–856. doi: 10.1016/j.bbrc.2012.03.087

Lenard, A., Ellertsdottir, E., Herwig, L., Krudewig, A., Sauteur, L., Belting, H. G., et al. (2013). *In vivo* analysis reveals a highly stereotypic morphogenetic pathway of vascular anastomosis. *Dev. Cell* 25, 492–506. doi: 10.1016/j.devcel.2013.05.010

Li, Y., Allende, M. L., Finkelstein, R., and Weinberg, E. S. (1994). Expression of two zebrafish orthodenticle-related genes in the embryonic brain. *Mech. Dev.* 48, 229–244. doi: 10.1016/0925-4773(94)90062-0

Liddelow, S. A., Dziegielewska, K. M., Vandeberg, J. L., and Saunders, N. R. (2010). Development of the lateral ventricular choroid plexus in a marsupial, *Monodelphis domestica. Cerebrospinal Fluid Res.* 7:16. doi: 10.1186/1743-8454-7-16

Liem, K. F. Jr., Tremml, G., and Jessell, T. M. (1997). A role for the roof plate and its resident TGFbeta-related proteins in neuronal patterning in the dorsal spinal cord. *Cell* 91, 127–138. doi: 10.1016/S0092-8674(01)80015-5

Louvi, A., and Wassef, M. (2000). Ectopic engrailed 1 expression in the dorsal midline causes cell death, abnormal differentiation of circumventricular organs and errors in axonal pathfinding. *Development* 127, 4061–4071.

Lowery, L. A., and Sive, H. (2005). Initial formation of zebrafish brain ventricles occurs independently of circulation and requires the nagie oko and snakehead/atp1a1a.1 gene products. *Development* 132, 2057–2067. doi: 10.1242/dev.01791

Luders, F., Segawa, H., Stein, D., Selva, E. M., Perrimon, N., Turco, S. J., et al. (2003). Slalom encodes an adenosine 3′-phosphate 5′-phosphosulfate transporter essential for development in Drosophila. *EMBO J.* 22, 3635–3644. doi: 10.1093/emboj/cdg345

Luissint, A. C., Artus, C., Glacial, F., Ganeshamoorthy, K., and Couraud, P. O. (2012). Tight junctions at the blood brain barrier: physiological architecture and disease-associated dysregulation. *Fluids Barriers CNS* 9:23. doi: 10.1186/2045-8118-9-23

Luo, X. M., Lin, H., Wang, W., Geaney, M. S., Law, L., Wynyard, S., et al. (2013). Recovery of neurological functions in non-human primate model of Parkinson's disease by transplantation of encapsulated neonatal porcine choroid plexus cells. *J. Parkinsons Dis.* 3, 275–291. doi: 10.3233/JPD-130214

Macchi, V., Porzionato, A., Guidolin, D., Parenti, A., and De Caro, R. (2005). Morphogenesis of the posterior inferior cerebellar artery with three-dimensional reconstruction of the late embryonic vertebrobasilar system. *Surg. Radiol. Anat.* 27, 56–60. doi: 10.1007/s00276-004-0303-6

Makanya, A. N., Hlushchuk, R., and Djonov, V. G. (2009). Intussusceptive angiogenesis and its role in vascular morphogenesis, patterning, and remodeling. *Angiogenesis* 12, 113–123. doi: 10.1007/s10456-009-9129-5

Millonig, J. H., Millen, K. J., and Hatten, M. E. (2000). The mouse Dreher gene Lmx1a controls formation of the roof plate in the vertebrate CNS. *Nature* 403, 764–769. doi: 10.1038/35001573

Mitchell, K., Yang, H. Y., Berk, J. D., Tran, J. H., and Iadarola, M. J. (2009). Monocyte chemoattractant protein-1 in the choroid plexus: a potential link between vascular pro-inflammatory mediators and the CNS during peripheral tissue inflammation. *Neuroscience* 158, 885–895. doi: 10.1016/j.neuroscience.2008.10.047

Mortazavi, M. M., Griessenauer, C. J., Adeeb, N., Deep, A., Bavarsad Shahripour, R., Loukas, M., et al. (2014). The choroid plexus: a comprehensive review of its history, anatomy, function, histology, embryology, and surgical considerations. *Childs Nerv. Syst.* 30, 205–214. doi: 10.1007/s00381-013-2326-y

Nataf, S., Strazielle, N., Hatterer, E., Mouchiroud, G., Belin, M. F., and Ghersi-Egea, J. F. (2006). Rat choroid plexuses contain myeloid progenitors capable of differentiation toward macrophage or dendritic cell phenotypes. *Glia* 54, 160–171. doi: 10.1002/glia.20373

Netsky, M. G., Shuangshoti, S., Tennyson, V. M., Brightman, M. W., Becker, N. H., Sutton, C. H., et al. (1975). *The Choroid Plexus in Health and Disease.* Charlottesville, VA: University Press of Virginia.

Nielsen, C. M., and Dymecki, S. M. (2010). Sonic hedgehog is required for vascular outgrowth in the hindbrain choroid plexus. *Dev. Biol.* 340, 430–437. doi: 10.1016/j.ydbio.2010.01.032

Nishikawa, K., Nakanishi, T., Aoki, C., Hattori, T., Takahashi, K., and Taniguchi, S. (1994). Differential expression of homeobox-containing genes Msx-1 and Msx-2 and homeoprotein Msx-2 expression during chick craniofacial development. *Biochem. Mol. Biol. Int.* 32, 763–771.

Ohto, T., Uchida, H., Yamazaki, H., Keino-Masu, K., Matsui, A., and Masu, M. (2002). Identification of a novel nonlysosomal sulphatase expressed in the floor plate, choroid plexus and cartilage. *Genes Cells* 7, 173–185. doi: 10.1046/j.1356-9597.2001.00502.x

Overall, M., Bakker, M., Spencer, J., Parker, N., Smith, P., and Dziadek, M. (1997). Genomic imprinting in the rat: linkage of Igf2 and H19 genes and opposite parental allele-specific expression during embryogenesis. *Genomics* 45, 416–420. doi: 10.1006/geno.1997.4933

Papan, C., and Campos-Ortega, J. A. (1999). Region-specific cell clones in the developing spinal cord of the zebrafish. *Dev. Genes Evol.* 209, 135–144. doi: 10.1007/s004270050237

Parinov, S., Kondrichin, I., Korzh, V., and Emelyanov, A. (2004). Tol2 transposon-mediated enhancer trap to identify developmentally regulated zebrafish genes *in vivo*. *Dev. Dyn.* 231, 449–459. doi: 10.1002/dvdy.20157

Park, S., Mathis, K. W., and Lee, I. K. (2014). The physiological roles of apolipoprotein J/clusterin in metabolic and cardiovascular diseases. *Rev. Endocr. Metab. Disord.* 15, 45–53. doi: 10.1007/s11154-013-9275-3

Planas, J. V., Capilla, E., and Gutierrez, J. (2000). Molecular identification of a glucose transporter from fish muscle. *FEBS Lett.* 481, 266–270. doi: 10.1016/S0014-5793(00)02020-2

Popescu, B. O., Gherghiceanu, M., Kostin, S., Ceafalan, L., and Popescu, L. M. (2012). Telocytes in meninges and choroid plexus. *Neurosci. Lett.* 516, 265–269. doi: 10.1016/j.neulet.2012.04.006

Power, D. M., Elias, N. P., Richardson, S. J., Mendes, J., Soares, C. M., and Santos, C. R. (2000). Evolution of the thyroid hormone-binding protein, transthyretin. *Gen. Comp. Endocrinol.* 119, 241–255. doi: 10.1006/gcen.2000.7520

Ratzka, A., Mundlos, S., and Vortkamp, A. (2010). Expression patterns of sulfatase genes in the developing mouse embryo. *Dev. Dyn.* 239, 1779–1788. doi: 10.1002/dvdy.22294

Redzic, Z. B., Preston, J. E., Duncan, J. A., Chodobski, A., and Szmydynger-Chodobska, J. (2005). The choroid plexus-cerebrospinal fluid system: from development to aging. *Curr. Top. Dev. Biol.* 71, 1–52. doi: 10.1016/S0070-2153(05)71001-2

Rehn, K., Wong, K. S., Balciunas, D., and Sumanas, S. (2011). Zebrafish enhancer trap line recapitulates embryonic aquaporin 1a expression pattern in vascular endothelial cells. *Int. J. Dev. Biol.* 55, 613–618. doi: 10.1387/ijdb.103249kp

Ristoratore, F., Carl, M., Deschet, K., Richard-Parpaillon, L., Boujard, D., Wittbrodt, J., et al. (1999). The midbrain-hindbrain boundary genetic cascade is activated ectopically in the diencephalon in response to the widespread expression of one of its components, the medaka gene Ol-eng2. *Development* 126, 3769–3779.

Rosenstein, J. M., Krum, J. M., Sternberger, L. A., Pulley, M. T., and Sternberger, N. H. (1992). Immunocytochemical expression of the endothelial barrier antigen (EBA) during brain angiogenesis. *Brain Res. Dev. Brain Res.* 66, 47–54. doi: 10.1016/0165-3806(92)90138-M

Sacilotto, N., Monteiro, R., Fritzsche, M., Becker, P. W., Sanchez-Del-Campo, L., Liu, K., et al. (2013). Analysis of Dll4 regulation reveals a combinatorial role for Sox and Notch in arterial development. *Proc. Natl. Acad. Sci. U.S. A.* 110, 11893–11898. doi: 10.1073/pnas.1300805110

Scala, G., Corona, M., Langella, E., and Maruccio, L. (2011). Microvasculature of the buffalo (*Bubalus bubalis*) choroid plexuses: structural, histochemical, and immunocytochemical study. *Microsc. Res. Tech.* 74, 67–75. doi: 10.1002/jemt.20875

Schmahl, J., Raymond, C. S., and Soriano, P. (2007). PDGF signaling specificity is mediated through multiple immediate early genes. *Nat. Genet.* 39, 52–60. doi: 10.1038/ng1922

Scott, D. E., and Bergevin, M. (2005). Fine structural correlates of the choroid plexus of the lateral cerebral ventricle of the human fetal brain. *Anat. Rec.* 282, 8–12. doi: 10.1002/ar.a.20104

Sharifi, M., Ciolkowski, M., Krajewski, P., and Ciszek, B. (2005). The choroid plexus of the fourth ventricle and its arteries. *Folia Morphol.* 64, 194–198.

Shechter, R., Miller, O., Yovel, G., Rosenzweig, N., London, A., Ruckh, J., et al. (2013). Recruitment of beneficial M2 macrophages to injured spinal cord is orchestrated by remote brain choroid plexus. *Immunity* 38, 555–569. doi: 10.1016/j.immuni.2013.02.012

Shuangshoti, S., and Netsky, M. G. (1966). Histogenesis of choroid plexus in man. *Am. J. Anat.* 118, 283–316. doi: 10.1002/aja.1001180114

Spatazza, J., Lee, H. H., Di Nardo, A. A., Tibaldi, L., Joliot, A., Hensch, T. K., et al. (2013). Choroid-plexus-derived Otx2 homeoprotein constrains adult cortical plasticity. *Cell Rep.* 3, 1815–1823. doi: 10.1016/j.celrep.2013.05.014

Stainier, D. Y. (2001). Zebrafish genetics and vertebrate heart formation. *Nat. Rev. Genet.* 2, 39–48. doi: 10.1038/35047564

Stan, R. V., Tse, D., Deharvengt, S. J., Smits, N. C., Xu, Y., Luciano, M. R., et al. (2012). The diaphragms of fenestrated endothelia: gatekeepers of vascular permeability and blood composition. *Dev. Cell* 23, 1203–1218. doi: 10.1016/j.devcel.2012.11.003

Strazielle, N., and Ghersi-Egea, J. F. (2000). Choroid plexus in the central nervous system: biology and physiopathology. *J. Neuropathol. Exp. Neurol.* 59, 561–574.

Strong, L. H. (1956). Early development of the ependyma and vascular pattern of the fourth ventricular choroid plexus in the rabbit. *Am. J. Anat.* 99 249–290. doi: 10.1002/aja.1000990204

Szmydynger-Chodobska, J., Gandy, J. R., Varone, A., Shan, R., and Chodobski, A. (2013). Synergistic interactions between cytokines and AVP at the blood-CSF barrier result in increased chemokine production and augmented influx of leukocytes after brain injury. *PLoS ONE* 8:e79328. doi: 10.1371/journal.pone.0079328

Teh, C., Chudakov, D. M., Poon, K. L., Mamedov, I. Z., Sek, J. Y., Shidlovsky, K., et al. (2010). Optogenetic *in vivo* cell manipulation in KillerRed-expressing zebrafish transgenics. *BMC Dev. Biol.* 10:110. doi: 10.1186/1471-213X-10-110

Thisse, B., and Thisse, C. (2005). Functions and regulations of fibroblast growth factor signaling during embryonic development. *Dev. Biol.* 287, 390–402. doi: 10.1016/j.ydbio.2005.09.011

Thomas, T., and Dziadek, M. (1993). Capacity to form choroid plexus-like cells *in vitro* is restricted to specific regions of the mouse neural ectoderm. *Development* 117, 253–262.

Trinh le, A., Hochgreb, T., Graham, M., Wu, D., Ruf-Zamojski, F., Jayasena, C. S., et al. (2011). A versatile gene trap to visualize and interrogate the function of the vertebrate proteome. *Genes Dev.* 25, 2306–2320. doi: 10.1101/gad.174037.111

Trougakos, I. P. (2013). The molecular chaperone apolipoprotein J/clusterin as a sensor of oxidative stress: implications in therapeutic approaches - a mini-review. *Gerontology* 59, 514–523. doi: 10.1159/000351207

Tsuneki, K. (1986). A survey of occurrence of about seventeen circumventricular organs in brains of various vertebrates with special reference to lower groups. *J. Hirnforsch.* 27, 441–470.

Tyurina, O. V., Guner, B., Popova, E., Feng, J., Schier, A. F., Kohtz, J. D., et al. (2005). Zebrafish Gli3 functions as both an activator and a repressor in Hedgehog signaling. *Dev. Biol.* 277, 537–556. doi: 10.1016/j.ydbio.2004.10.003

Umans, R. A., and Taylor, M. R. (2012). Zebrafish as a model to study drug transporters at the blood-brain barrier. *Clin. Pharmacol. Ther.* 92, 567–570. doi: 10.1038/clpt.2012.168

Venkatesh, B., Lee, A. P., Ravi, V., Maurya, A. K., Lian, M. M., Swann, J. B., et al. (2014). Elephant shark genome provides unique insights into gnathostome evolution. *Nature* 505, 174–179. doi: 10.1038/nature12826

Weindl, A., and Joynt, R. J. (1973). Barrier properties of the subcommissural organ. *Arch. Neurol.* 29, 16–22. doi: 10.1001/archneur.1973.00490250034004

Wilting, J., and Christ, B. (1989). An experimental and ultrastructural study on the development of the avian choroid plexus. *Cell Tissue Res.* 255, 487–494. doi: 10.1007/BF00218783

Winata, C. L., Kondrychyn, I., Kumar, V., Srinivasan, K. G., Orlov, Y., Ravishankar, A., et al. (2013). Genome wide analysis reveals Zic3 interaction with distal regulatory elements of stage specific developmental genes in zebrafish. *PLoS Genet.* 9:e1003852. doi: 10.1371/journal.pgen.1003852

Wojcik, E., Carrithers, L. M., and Carrithers, M. D. (2011). Characterization of epithelial V-like antigen in human choroid plexus epithelial cells: potential role in CNS immune surveillance. *Neurosci. Lett.* 495, 115–120. doi: 10.1016/j.neulet.2011.03.051

Yang, J., Dombrowski, S. M., Deshpande, A., Krajcir, N., and Luciano, M. G. (2010). VEGF/VEGFR-2 changes in frontal cortex, choroid plexus, and

CSF after chronic obstructive hydrocephalus. *J. Neurol. Sci.* 296, 39–46. doi: 10.1016/j.jns.2010.06.012

Zappaterra, M. W., and Lehtinen, M. K. (2012). The cerebrospinal fluid: regulator of neurogenesis, behavior, and beyond. *Cell. Mol. Life Sci.* 69, 2863–2878. doi: 10.1007/s00018-012-0957-x

Zhang, J., Piontek, J., Wolburg, H., Piehl, C., Liss, M., Otten, C., et al. (2010). Establishment of a neuroepithelial barrier by Claudin5a is essential for zebrafish brain ventricular lumen expansion. *Proc. Natl. Acad. Sci. U.S.A.* 107, 1425–1430. doi: 10.1073/pnas.0911996107

Zhang, Z. G., Zhang, L., Jiang, Q., and Chopp, M. (2002). Bone marrow-derived endothelial progenitor cells participate in cerebral neovascularization after focal cerebral ischemia in the adult mouse. *Circ. Res.* 90, 284–288. doi: 10.1161/hh0302.104460

Zhou, T., Wang, L., Zhu, K. Y., Dong, M., Xu, P. F., Chen, Y., et al. (2011). Dominant-negative C/ebpalpha and polycomb group protein Bmi1 extend short-lived hematopoietic stem/progenitor cell life span and induce lethal dyserythropoiesis. *Blood* 118, 3842–3852. doi: 10.1182/blood-2010-12-327908

6

The Drosophila blood-brain barrier: development and function of a glial endothelium

Stefanie Limmer, Astrid Weiler, Anne Volkenhoff, Felix Babatz and Christian Klämbt*

Institut für Neuro- und Verhaltensbiologie, Universität Münster, Münster, Germany

***Correspondence:**
Christian Klämbt, Institut für Neuro- und Verhaltensbiologie, Universität Münster, Badestr. 9, 48140 Münster, Germany
e-mail: klaembt@uni-muenster.de

The efficacy of neuronal function requires a well-balanced extracellular ion homeostasis and a steady supply with nutrients and metabolites. Therefore, all organisms equipped with a complex nervous system developed a so-called blood-brain barrier, protecting it from an uncontrolled entry of solutes, metabolites or pathogens. In higher vertebrates, this diffusion barrier is established by polarized endothelial cells that form extensive tight junctions, whereas in lower vertebrates and invertebrates the blood-brain barrier is exclusively formed by glial cells. Here, we review the development and function of the glial blood-brain barrier of *Drosophila melanogaster*. In the Drosophila nervous system, at least seven morphologically distinct glial cell classes can be distinguished. Two of these glial classes form the blood-brain barrier. Perineurial glial cells participate in nutrient uptake and establish a first diffusion barrier. The subperineurial glial (SPG) cells form septate junctions, which block paracellular diffusion and thus seal the nervous system from the hemolymph. We summarize the molecular basis of septate junction formation and address the different transport systems expressed by the blood-brain barrier forming glial cells.

Keywords: Drosophila, glia, blood-brain barrier, septate junction formation, transmembrane transporter, astrocyte-neuron lactate shuttle hypothesis

INTRODUCTION

In all animals, an efficient separation of metabolic and ionic balance between nervous system and circulation is necessary. This in consequence led to the evolution of the so-called blood-brain barrier (Abbott et al., 2006). Vertebrates are characterized by a highly vascularized nervous system, while the insect nervous system floats in the hemolymph, which circulates through the body by the action of a primitive heart (**Figures 1A–C**). In the mammalian nervous system, the blood-brain barrier is established by an interplay of polarized endothelial cells and pericytes that leads to the formation of endothelial tight junctions (Armulik et al., 2010, 2011; Daneman et al., 2010b). These tight junctions prevent uncontrolled paracellular leakage of solutes into the brain. In more primitive vertebrates such as in elasmobranch fish (sharks, skates, and rays), but also in some bony fish (sturgeon), the blood-brain barrier is formed by perivascular astrocytes. These glial cells form interdigitating lamellae but do not establish tight junctions (Bundgaard and Abbott, 2008). A morphologically similar blood-brain barrier is found in insects. Here, only the outer surface of the nervous system, which is formed exclusively by glial cells, contacts the hemolymph. Although this glial barrier appears to be related to the evolutionary ancestral form of the blood-brain barrier, Drosophila has only recently emerged as a genetic model to study blood-brain barrier biology (Carlson et al., 2000; Abbott et al., 2006). Here, we summarize what is currently known on the organization and the physiological properties of the Drosophila blood-brain barrier.

Why is Drosophila a good system to study blood-brain barrier properties? One of the advantages is that the nervous system is small and almost all cells are known. In addition, geneticists established rich resource and tool kits, which allow the easy manipulation of individual cells at any time of development (Dietzl et al., 2007; Venken et al., 2011; Jenett et al., 2012; Li et al., 2014). The basis of neuronal transmission is identical in flies and man and, moreover, even complex behavioral aspects appear to be controlled by similar mechanisms (Davis, 2011; Anholt and Mackay, 2012). Thus, based on the overwhelming wealth of data documenting the evolutionary conservation of central biological processes, one can expect that work on the Drosophila blood-brain barrier, which correctly should be termed hemolymph-brain barrier, might provide further insights into the general biology of this essential boundary.

THE NERVOUS SYSTEM OF DROSOPHILA

Drosophila is a holometabolic insect. Following 1 day of embryogenesis, three larval stages spread over the next 4 days. During the subsequent pupal stage, which covers another 5 days, metamorphosis takes place and the imago, the adult fly, emerges. Accordingly, the nervous system of Drosophila develops in two phases.

The larval nervous system originates from stem cells called neuroblasts that delaminate in five waves shortly after gastrulation into the interior of the embryo (Campos-Ortega and Hartenstein, 1997). Analysis of the nervous system is simplified by the fact that the thoracic and abdominal segments are mostly alike and

---

Abbreviations: ABC, ATP binding cassette; ATP, Adenosine triphosphate; FACS, fluorescence-activated cell sorting; GCM, Glial Cells Missing; GFP, green flourescent protein; GPCR, G protein-coupled receptor; IPC, Insulin-Producing Cell; RNA, Ribonucleic acid; SPG, subperineurial glia; TCA cycle, tricarboxylic acid cycle; UDP, Uridine diphosphate.

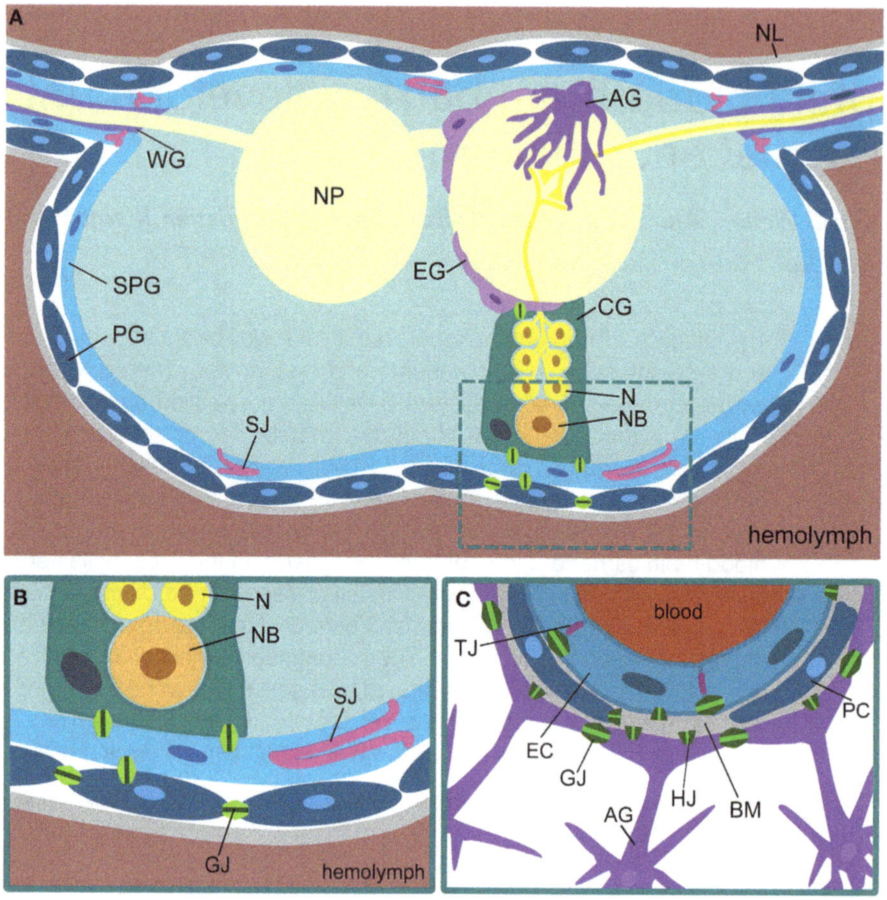

FIGURE 1 | Comparison of Drosophila and mammalian blood-brain barriers. (A) Schematic view of a cross-section of a Drosophila ventral nerve cord. The nervous system is covered by a sheath of extracellular matrix, called neural lamella (NL). The outermost glial layer consists of perineurial glial cells (PG). The subperineurial glia (SPG) forms pleated septate junctions (SJ) and blocks paracellular transport. Neurons (N) project into the neuropil (NP). Neuronal cell bodies and neuroblasts (NB) are surrounded by cortex glia (CG). The neuropil is covered by ensheathing glia (EG). Astrocytes (AG) invade the neuropil. In the peripheral nerves, wrapping glia (WG) ensheath axons. **(B)** In Drosophila, the blood-brain barrier is built by perineurial and subperineurial glia. The latter form septate junctions (SJ) to prevent paracellular diffusion. The different glial cells are connected via gap junctions (GJ). **(C)** The mammalian blood-brain barrier is built by endothelial cells (EC) that form tight junctions (TJ) to prevent paracellular diffusion. The endothelium is in close contact with pericytes (PC). Both are surrounded by the basal membrane (BM). Gap junctions (GJ) can be found between the endothelial cells and between the astrocytes (AG). Gap junction hemichannels (HJ) can be found in all the cell types.

thus, a large part of the nervous system called ventral nerve cord represents an array of repeated and almost identical neuromeric units. Currently, the identity and the lineage of all neuroblasts are known and by the end of embryogenesis about 650 neurons and 65 glial cells are found in each neuromer of the ventral nerve cord (Broadus et al., 1995; Landgraf et al., 1997; Schmid et al., 1999; Wheeler et al., 2006; Beckervordersandforth et al., 2008; Rickert et al., 2011). The brain lobes of the Drosophila larvae originate from somewhat less well-defined head neuroblasts (Urbach and Technau, 2003). The neuronal circuits established by the many neurons in the larval brain are currently being deciphered by analyzing serial TEM sections of a larval brain (Cardona et al., 2010). Thus, it can be anticipated that within the next years the complete anatomical building plan of the larval nervous system is known.

The adult nervous system, including the elaborate compound eyes, develops during early pupal stages. Neuroblast proliferation is reactivated at the end of the larval stage to generate a large number of neurons, particularly in the two brain lobes. When fully developed, the fly central nervous system harbors about 30,000 neurons (Lovick et al., 2013). Upon GFP labeling of neurons or glial cells and subsequent FACS sorting we counted about 25,000 neuronal and 10,000 glial cells per adult brain (Limmer et al., unpublished).

DROSOPHILA GLIAL CELLS

As in primitive vertebrates, the Drosophila blood-brain barrier is formed by glial cells (Stork et al., 2008). The fly nervous system harbors seven morphologically and molecularly distinct glial subtypes, namely midline glia, perineurial glia, subperineurial glia (SPG), cortex glia, ensheathing glia, astrocytes, and wrapping glia (**Figures 1A,B**) (Ito et al., 1995; Pereanu et al., 2005; Silies et al., 2007; Awasaki et al., 2008; Stork et al., 2008, 2012, 2014; Hartenstein, 2011). The entire nervous system is covered by a layer of perineurial glial cells. These cells participate in blood-brain barrier function although their exact contribution is currently unknown. The subjacent glial cell layer is represented by the SPG cells. These flat and interdigitating cells form elaborate septate junctions, which prevent paracellular diffusion (Bainton et al., 2005; Stork et al., 2008; Mayer et al., 2009). The cortex glial cells engulf neuronal stem cells and their progeny and most likely exert some nutritional functions. The ensheathing glial cells form a sheath around the neuropil area, which lacks cell bodies and harbors only axons and dendrites. Astrocytes invade the neuropil to modulate synaptic transmission as it is known from their vertebrate homologs (Awasaki et al., 2008; Stork et al., 2014). The wrapping glia is mostly found in the peripheral nervous system where these cells engulf individual axons (Pereanu et al., 2005; Awasaki et al., 2008; Franzdóttir et al., 2009).

All glial subtypes are generated in the Drosophila embryo and emerge from stem cells programmed by the expression of the gene *glial cells missing* (*gcm*) (Hosoya et al., 1995; Jones et al., 1995; Vincent et al., 1996). The presence of the Gcm transcription factor specifies glial identity except for the midline glia, which requires the activity of the master regulator gene *single minded* (Crews et al., 1988). Gcm subsequently activates a cascade of transcription factors. The transcription factor Pointed promotes glial differentiation and the Zn-finger protein Tramtrack inhibits neuronal differentiation in glial cells (Klaes et al., 1994; Giesen et al., 1997). Together with other transcriptional regulators such as Prospero, Distal-less and Deadringer, these factors most likely are involved in specifying the glial subtype identity (Shandala et al., 2003; Thomas and van Meyel, 2007; Schmidt et al., 2011). The relevant transcriptional regulators that specify blood-brain barrier identity are currently unknown.

THE DROSOPHILA BLOOD-BRAIN BARRIER

The establishment of the Drosophila blood-brain barrier occurs at the end of embryogenesis and requires the SPG cells. Only 16 of these cells are formed in every neuromere and four additional SPG cells are generated along every segmental nerve (Beckervordersandforth et al., 2008; von Hilchen et al., 2013). During larval stages, when the animal grows in size by a factor of 100, and likewise during metamorphosis, no additional SPG cells are formed but the blood-brain barrier remains intact (Awasaki et al., 2008; Stork et al., 2008; Unhavaithaya and Orr-Weaver, 2012). Thus, the few SPG cells generated during embryonic stages must grow enormously in size during development, and at the same time they have to maintain their elaborate junctional contacts that prevent paracellular diffusion (see below).

Once the SPG cells are born at about mid-embryogenesis, they form numerous filopodia-like processes and eventually spread to touch their neighbors at the end of embryogenesis (Schwabe et al., 2005). The SPG cells now establish a contiguous, very flat, endothelial-like sheet that covers the entire nervous system and the cell contact zones interdigitate extensively. Interestingly, in cuttlefish as well as in sturgeon, the glial blood-brain barrier also involves highly overlapping glial lamellae (Lane and Abbott, 1992; Bundgaard and Abbott, 2008). In Drosophila, glial cells of the blood-brain barrier in addition form extensive septate junctions that further restrict the paracellular diffusion between different glial cells (Carlson et al., 2000; Schwabe et al., 2005; Stork et al., 2008). The first experimental confirmation of the physiological relevance of septate junctions for blood-brain barrier integrity was provided by the genetic analysis of the septate junction component NeurexinIV. In the absence of this protein, which is homologous to the Caspr protein found in septate-like junctions in vertebrate paranodes, the blood-brain barrier is permissive to even large molecules like dextran and in consequence, the high potassium content of the hemolymph can spread into the nervous system where it blocks any neuronal activity (Baumgartner et al., 1996).

The SPG cells are very large: a single SPG can cover the size of one half of the eye imaginal disc thus covering an area equivalent to about 10,000 epithelial cells (Silies et al., 2007). In order to achieve this enormous cell growth, the SPG cells undergo polyploidization (Unhavaithaya and Orr-Weaver, 2012). All SPG cells form a polarized endothelium that in most areas does not even reach a thickness of 1 μm. The thin nature of these barrier-forming cells has hindered detailed electron microscopic studies for a long time. Only the ability to label individual cells with GFP using subperineurial specific Gal4 driver strains such as *gliotactin-Gal4* or *moodyGal4* has allowed the description of the intricate morphology of these cells (Schwabe et al., 2005; Silies et al., 2007; Stork et al., 2008; Hatan et al., 2011; Unhavaithaya and Orr-Weaver, 2012). Currently, only few molecular markers for the blood-brain barrier are available. The multidrug resistance protein Mdr65 was shown to reside in the apical domain of the SPG cell, whereas the GPCR Moody is found at the basal portion of the cell (DeSalvo et al., 2011).

FORMATION OF SEPTATE JUNCTIONS

The most characteristic feature of the SPG is the formation of extensive septate junctions. This type of cell-cell junction has been particularly well studied in ectodermal cells, such as tracheal cells (Tepass and Hartenstein, 1994). Septate junctions are a complex crystalline array of comb-like structures built by a bewildering number of different proteins that connect individual cells, as revealed by freeze-fracture studies (**Figure 2**) (Lane and Swales, 1979; Lane, 1991). The cell-cell distance in these junctions is about 20 nm and thus a bit larger than in tight junctions that seal the brain endothelial cells in mammals (Farquhar and Palade, 1963, 1965). Many membrane-associated proteins are known to be involved in septate junction formation (**Table 1**). The core group of septate junction proteins contains the cation pump ATPalpha, the claudin family members Megatrachea and Sinous, the Ig-domain protein Neuroglian, the potassium pump subunit Nervana2, the Caspr homolog NeurexinIV and the two cytoplasmic proteins Coracle and Varicose (Oshima and Fehon, 2011, see also references in **Table 1**). These proteins recruit a large number of additional membrane proteins that together build the septate junctions (**Table 1**). Loss of most of these proteins results in the disruption of septate junctions.

Septate junction structure becomes even more elaborate at tricellular junctions. Here, septate junction strands of three cells meet and appear to be linked to a central core in the extracellular space between three neighboring cells (**Figure 2**). The tricellular junctions are among the first junctional complexes

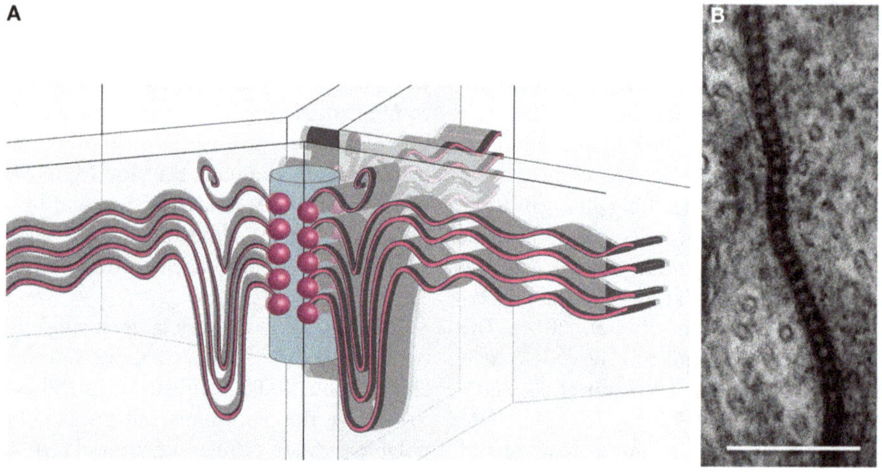

FIGURE 2 | Organization of tricellular junctions. (A) Schematic view of septate junctions at tricellular contacts according to the tricellular plug model (Graf et al., 1982; Noirot-Timothée et al., 1982; Schulte et al., 2003). Septate junctions (red sinuous lines) span the membranes of two adjacent cells. At a central core (blue cylinder), emanating from transmembrane proteins (red balls), the septate junctions extend. **(B)** Transmission electron microscopic image of pleated septate junctions between two SPG cells.

to differentiate and are characterized by several specific proteins such as Gliotactin or Macroglobin (Auld et al., 1995; Genova and Fehon, 2003; Schulte et al., 2003; Padash-Barmchi et al., 2010; Bätz et al., 2014; Furuse et al., 2014; Oda et al., 2014). Possibly septate junction formation initiates from these positions to match the stretch growth of the SPG cells during larval development (**Figure 2**). The extent of septate junction formation is in part controlled by the G protein-coupled receptor Moody (Bainton et al., 2005; Schwabe et al., 2005). The Moody protein is continuously required for septate junction formation and a temporal lack of *moody* function, evoked by conditional RNA interference, results in a transient opening of the blood-brain barrier (Bainton et al., 2005). It is important to note that Moody, like possibly other developmentally required proteins, may affect both, development and the physiology of the blood-brain barrier. Indeed some effects of Moody on barrier function, such as increased cocaine sensitivity, can be seen under experimental conditions (Bainton et al., 2005). However, in the normal life of a fly no serious defects are observed when *moody* function is lacking. It was noted by Schwabe et al. (2005) that *moody* mutations are lethal, but it was also mentioned that few homozygous females and hemizygous males survive to adulthood. Interestingly, homozygous *moody* flies can be easily kept as a living stock, suggesting that blood-brain barrier physiology can be efficiently regulated by additional pathways.

How Moody signaling regulates septate junction dynamics remains unclear. *moody* null mutants show normal septate junction morphology but a somewhat reduced junctional length (Schwabe et al., 2005). In addition, Moody was shown to affect the formation of actin-rich structures along the lateral borders of the SPG cells, which also contributes to the effects on blood-brain barrier integrity (Hatan et al., 2011).

In conclusion, SPG cells are intimately interconnected by septate junctions. They set up a tight seal around the nervous system, such that metabolite import into the brain, and the exit of waste products and xenobiotics out of the nervous system can be tightly controlled.

TRANSPORT OF METABOLITES ACROSS THE BLOOD-BRAIN BARRIER

A classical function of the blood-brain barrier is to control transport of ions and metabolites. Once the septate junctions are formed between individual SPG cells, paracellular diffusion is blocked. This, in consequence, calls for efficient and highly active transport mechanisms that shuttle all required metabolites into the brain. The relevant transporters are mostly defined by bioinformatic criteria and their expression has been globally addressed by tissue specific transcriptomics and is summarized in FlyAtlas (Chintapalli et al., 2013).

Metabolite transport across the SPG cell layer not only requires an efficient uptake mechanism into the SPG cells, but also an efficient secretion of metabolites into the nervous system. This aspect may not be confined to the blood-brain barrier, since glial cells in general and in particular SPG cells establish extensive gap junctions, which is similarly observed in endothelial cells (**Figure 1**) (Lane and Swales, 1979; Lane, 1991; Holcroft et al., 2013; Gaete et al., 2014). Thus, once metabolites have entered the blood-brain barrier forming cells, they might be easily distributed throughout the whole nervous system via these intercellular connections. Gap junctions are a hallmark of invertebrate glia and most glial cells express several Drosophila innexins, which constitute the functional connexin homologs of invertebrates (Holcroft et al., 2013). The direct coupling of glial cells by gap junctions is also reflected by glial Ca^{2+} waves, which can be seen in the blood-brain barrier, the cortex and the astrocyte glial population (Melom and Littleton, 2013; Spéder and Brand, 2014; Stork et al., 2014).

In addition to the transport of metabolites into the brain, waste products and xenobiotics need to be shuttled out of the brain. In vertebrates, chemoprotection is mediated by ATP-binding

Table 1 | Septate junction proteins.

Gene	Vertebrate homolog	Structural domains	Function	References
ATPα	NA^+/K^+ ATPase α-subunit		Ion pump ATPase	Genova and Fehon, 2003
nervana 2	NA^+/K^+ ATPase β-subunit		Ion pump ATPase	Genova and Fehon, 2003
boudin		Ly-6, GPI	Secreted, non-autonomous	Hijazi et al., 2009
coiled		Ly-6, GPI	Homophilic adhesion, symmetrical expression of adjacent cells necessary	Nilton et al., 2010; Syed et al., 2011
crimpled		Ly-6, GPI		Nilton et al., 2010
crooked		Ly-6, GPI		Nilton et al., 2010
retroactive		Ly-6	Chitin cable formation	Moussian et al., 2006
Contactin	Contactin	Ig, FnIII, GPI	Cell-adhesion	Faivre-Sarrailh et al., 2004
Fasciclin III		Ig	Cell-adhesion	Narasimha et al., 2008
Lachesin		Ig, GPI	Cell-adhesion	Llimargas et al., 2004
Neuroglian	Neurofascin 155	Ig, FnIII	Cell-adhesion	Genova and Fehon, 2003
Neurexin IV	Caspr/Paranodin	Laminin G and EGF domains	Cell-adhesion	Baumgartner et al., 1996
coracle	Protein 4.1	FERM	Linker protein	Fehon et al., 1994
kune-kune	Claudin	PDZ-domain	Cell-adhesion	Nelson et al., 2010
megatrachea	Claudin	PDZ-domain	Cell-adhesion	Jaspers et al., 2012
sinuous	Claudin	PDZ-domain	Cell-adhesion	Wu and Beitel, 2004
discs large	hDLG/Sap97	MAGUK, SH3, PDZ, guanylate kinase domain	Linker protein	Woods et al., 1996
scribble	hscrib1	PDZ-Domain, LRR	Linker protein	Bilder and Perrimon, 2000
Gliotactin	Neuroligin3	Noncatalytic cholinesterase like molecule	Cell-adhesion	Auld et al., 1995
Macroglobulin complement-related	α2M	Thioester protein (TEP) family		Bätz et al., 2014; Hall et al., 2014
Melanotransferrin	MTF	Iron binding, GPI	Iron-binding, endocytosis	Tiklová et al., 2010
varicose	Pals2	MAGUK	Linker protein	Wu et al., 2007
wunen		Lipid phosphat phosphatase		Ile et al., 2012
yurt				Laprise et al., 2009

The known Drosophila septate junction proteins are listed. Structural domains and the predicted molecular functions are indicated. Ly-6, lymphocyte antigen-6; GPI, glycosyl phosphatidylinositol; Ig, immunoglobuline; FnIII, fibronectin type III; EGF, epidermal growth factor; MAGUK, membrane-associated guanylate kinases; SH3, SRC homology 3; LRR, leucine-rich repeat.

cassette (ABC) transporters such as the Multidrug-resistance protein 1 (Mdr1). Quite similar, *mdr65* performs related functions in the Drosophila nervous system (Mayer et al., 2009). In line with this, Mdr65 levels are elevated upon exposure to insecticides (Dermauw and Van Leeuwen, 2014). Mdr65 belongs to a large class of transporters with 56 members in Drosophila of which several are expressed in the nervous system (Dermauw and Van Leeuwen, 2014). Their function, however, is largely unknown and will not be further discussed here.

Neural cells need to take up specific lipids from the hemolymph, which feeds into specific anabolic pathways (Palm et al., 2012) or is directly used as energy source during ß-oxidation (Palanker et al., 2009). In the following we will focus on metabolite import across the blood-brain barrier and review the main classes of the relevant transport systems. Due to space constrains, however, we will neglect lipid metabolism. We anticipate that the wealth of tools available in Drosophila will promote a deeper understanding of the physiological roles of this important barrier.

WATER HOMEOSTASIS

Mechanisms for controlling influx and efflux of water are essential for osmotic control of fluids in the nervous system. Water can enter the nervous system through aquaporins, small membrane-spanning proteins that form channels to facilitate water flow along the osmotic gradient. 14 aquaporins are known in humans and in particular aquaporin-4 (AQP4) has been linked to blood-brain barrier function. AQP4 localizes to astrocyte endfeet at the CSF-CNS and blood-CNS barriers and is crucially required for the regulation of water homeostasis and the definition of the extracellular space in the CNS (Nagelhus and Ottersen, 2013; Papadopoulos and Verkman, 2013).

The Drosophila genome harbors eight aquaporin-encoding genes (FlyBase, CV: water transmembrane transporter activity, **Table 2**). The DRIP protein has the highest sequence similarity to vertebrate AQP4 but shows no prominent CNS expression (Chintapalli et al., 2013). *big brain* (*bib*) was initially identified as a neurogenic gene and encodes a protein related to aquaporins (Rao et al., 1990). Although Bib has water transport properties, this function is still controversial (Tatsumi et al., 2009). The Drosophila aquaporin most prominently expressed in the CNS is CG7777 (Chintapalli et al., 2013), but currently no functional analysis has been performed.

ION HOMEOSTASIS

The hemolymph is an ion rich fluid (**Table 3**). In particular the high potassium concentration, which is characteristic for the invertebrate hemolymph, would be problematic for normal neuronal function. In the mammalian blood, potassium levels are only around 1–5 mM and thus almost a factor of 10 lower compared to the Drosophila hemolymph. The blood-brain barrier prevents any uncontrolled influx of ions into the nervous system. In consequence, the potassium concentration in the Drosophila brain fluid is about 5 mM or less (Armstrong et al., 2012).

The Drosophila genome harbors a large number of proteins linked to potassium influx or export (Chintapalli et al., 2013). However, only in few cases, their relevance for regulated ion transport across the blood-brain barrier has been demonstrated. One example is the Fray kinase and its target Ncc69, the homolog of the human SLC12 $Na^+/K^+/Cl^-$ cotransporter (Leiserson et al., 2000, 2011). Ncc69 is expressed in SPG cells and *Ncc69* mutant larvae develop a peripheral neuropathy with fluid accumulations between glia and axons (Leiserson et al., 2011). The effect of Ncc69 on CNS physiology is not reported. Several other ion transport proteins of the SLC12 family are also expressed in the Drosophila brain (Sun et al., 2010) but their possible glial functions are unexplored.

In a genetic screen for temperature-sensitive conditional seizure mutants the glial-specific Na^+/Ca^{2+}, K^+ exchanger Zydeco was identified. Zydeco is mostly expressed by the cortex glia and not by the blood-brain barrier glia (Guan et al., 2005; Melom and Littleton, 2013). In addition to channels, active ion pumps such as the Na^+/K^+ ATPase are involved in regulating ion homeostasis in the brain. The two Drosophila nervana genes (*nrv1* and *nrv2*) encode beta subunits of the Na^+/K^+ ATPase. Nrv2 and the ATPase alpha are expressed in the SPG, where they are localized to septate junctions. Hypomorphic mutants for the ATPase alpha subunit show a bang and ouabain sensitivity (Schubiger et al., 1994). Septate junction formation, however, does not depend on ATPase function (Genova and Fehon, 2003; Paul et al., 2007).

UPTAKE OF AMINO ACIDS INTO THE NERVOUS SYSTEM

Amino acids are not only required for protein synthesis, but particular amino acids or their direct derivatives are also used as neurotransmitters. Cells are able to generate most amino acids from intermediates of the citric acid cycle. However, some amino acids cannot be produced and thus their uptake and transport is essential. In Drosophila, 10 proteinogenic L-amino acids are essential: tryptophan, phenylalanine, leucine, histidine, valine, isoleucine, lysine, methionine, arginine, and threonine (Boudko, 2012). Therefore, specific transport systems for these amino acids must be expressed by the SPG cells.

In vertebrates, nine distinct amino acid transport systems have been reported to be present at the brain capillary endothelium (Smith, 2000): the X-system is a high affinity, sodium-independent transport system for anionic amino acids, the L-system transports large neutral amino acids, the A-and ASC-systems transport small neutral amino acids, the Y^+-system is a sodium-independent cationic amino acid transport system, the B^{o+}-system represents a high affinity transport system and transports both neutral and basic amino acids and the ß-system is a low capacity, sodium-dependent transporter for taurine and ß-alanine. The N-system mediates the sodium-dependent transport of L-glutamine, L-histidine and L-asparagine and the T-system transports thyroid hormones.

Two well-known X-system transporters are EAAT1 and EAAT2, which in mammals are expressed by astrocytes (Rothstein et al., 1994). In Drosophila, both proteins have been described, but are expressed in glial cells other than the blood-brain barrier cells (Soustelle et al., 2002; Freeman et al., 2003; Stacey et al., 2010). In total, 51 Drosophila genes are annotated to have an "organic acid transmembrane transporter activity" or as "amino acid transporter" (**Table 4**). For a few of these proteins

Table 2 | Drosophila Aquaporins.

Gene	CG number	Human homolog	CNS expression			References
			FlyAtlas	BDGP	Literature	
drip	*CG9023*	AQP1, AQP4	–	–	No	Kaufmann et al., 2005
big brain	*CG4722*	AQP4	Yes	Yes	Yes	Rao et al., 1990
aquaporin	*CG12251*	AQP12	No	No	–	
CG7777	*CG7777*	AQP1	Yes	No	Yes	Kaufmann et al., 2005
CG17664	*CG17664*	MIWC, AQP4	No	–	No	Kaufmann et al., 2005
CG17662	*CG17662*	MIWC, AQP4	No	–	–	
CG4019	*CG4019*	MIWC, AQP4	Low	No	No	Kaufmann et al., 2005
CG5398	*CG5398*	AQP2	No	–	No	Kaufmann et al., 2005

All predicted Drosophila aquaporins (FlyBase, CV: water transmembrane transporter activity) are listed. Information about the CNS expression of each gene were obtained from FlyAtlas, the Berkely Drosophila Genome Project (BDGP), and the literature shown. AQP, aquaporin; MIWC, mercurial-insensitive water channel.

Table 3 | Ion concentration in the hemolymph.

$[Na^+]$ [mM]	$[K^+]$ [mM]	$[Cl^-]$ [mM]	$[Mg^{2+}]$ [mM]	$[Ca^{2+}]$ [mM]	Remark/method	References
THIRD INSTAR LARVAL						
52 ± 1	36 ± 1	30 ± 1	–	–	Photometry and chemical methods	Croghan and Lockwood, 1960
56.5	40.2	42.2	41.6	15.9	Physical and chemical methods	Begg and Cruickshank, 1962
~45	~23	–	–	–	Ion-selective microelectrodes	Naikkhwah and O'Donnell, 2011
ADULT						
70 – 110	26				Ion-selective microelectrodes	Naikkhwah and O'Donnell, 2011
123.7 ± 9.2	28.4 ± 2.4				Ion-selective microelectrodes	MacMillan and Hughson, 2014

Drosophila third instar larval and adult hemolymph concentrations of selected ions are listed. The method of concentration determination is indicated.

expression in CNS glial cells has been noted (Soustelle et al., 2002; Besson et al., 2005; Augustin et al., 2007; Grosjean et al., 2008; Featherstone, 2011). In some cases, expression in the blood-brain barrier was found (e.g., CG15088, Thimgan et al., 2006) but functional analysis is lacking so far.

ENERGY SUPPLY OF THE BRAIN

The energy expenditure for normal neuronal function is enormous. The human brain requires about 20% of the total resting oxygen consumption of the entire body although it comprises only about 2% of the body mass. Likewise in flies, just the photoreceptor cells in the retina consume about 10% of the total ATP production (Laughlin et al., 1998). Therefore, an efficient transport of energy-rich nutrients such as sugars needs to be established at the blood-brain barrier.

THE ASTROCYTE-NEURON LACTATE SHUTTLE HYPOTHESIS

The intense metabolic interactions between glial cells and neurons led to the astrocyte-neuron lactate shuttle (ANLS) hypothesis (Pellerin and Magistretti, 1994, 2012; Allaman et al., 2011). In the mammalian brain, the main energy source is glucose, which is shuttled into the nervous system via the Glut1 transporter. Glut1 is asymmetrically expressed in endothelial cells and is also found in astrocytes surrounding the endothelium (Leybaert, 2005). Glucose that is taken up by astrocytes is then metabolized through glycolysis to lactate or pyruvate. These small C_3 metabolites are then released into the extracellular space to be utilized by neurons, which is supported by experimental and as well as theoretical considerations (Rouach et al., 2008; Jolivet et al., 2009; Harris et al., 2012). Enhanced neuronal activity might be linked to an increase in Glut1 expression, which would account for increased energy supply (Leybaert, 2005). This energetic coupling may be of more general relevance, since also the survival of myelinated axons depends on metabolic support by the corresponding glial cells (Fünfschilling et al., 2012; Lee et al., 2012). In invertebrates, a similar compartmentalization of energy metabolism is likely to be established as well. In the honeybee retina, glucose is exclusively taken up by glial cells and alanine, which is generated from pyruvate through transamination, seems to be shuttled to neurons to fuel the TCA cycle (Tsacopoulos et al., 1994).

TREHALOSE TRANSPORTERS IN THE DROSOPHILA BLOOD-BRAIN BARRIER

Several different sugars are present in the Drosophila hemolymph (**Table 5**). The main carbohydrate found in the insect hemolymph is trehalose, a non-reducing disaccharide with two D-glucose units linked by an α, α-1,1-glycosidic bond. Smaller amounts of glucose and fructose are also found, but their respective concentrations appear to vary depending on the metabolic state of the animal (Blatt and Roces, 2001). Upon feeding, carbohydrates are taken up by the intestinal epithelium and glucose is secreted into the hemolymph. The glucose is then shuttled to the fat body, where trehalose is synthesized from glucose-6-phosphate and UDP-glucose by the enzyme Trehalose phosphate synthase,

Table 4 | Drosophila amino acid transporters.

Gene	CG	Human homolog	CNS expression			Function	References
			FlyAtlas	BDGP	Literature		
	CG13248	SLC7	Yes	Yes	Yes	Cationic AA transporter; putative arginine transporter	Romero-Calderón and Krantz, 2006; Park et al., 2011
	CG5535	SLC7	Yes		No	Cationic AA transporter	Romero-Calderón and Krantz, 2006
	CG12531	SLC7	Yes			Cationic AA transporter	Romero-Calderón and Krantz, 2006
	CG7255	SLC7	No		No	Cationic AA transporter	Romero-Calderón and Krantz, 2006
slimfast	CG11128	SLC7	No			Cationic AA transporter	
Jhl-21	*CG12317*	SLC7	Yes			L-AA transporter; lysine and other neutral AA transport light chain of heterodimeric transporter	Freeman et al., 2003; Reynolds et al., 2009
pathetic	*CG3424*	SLC36	Yes	Yes	Yes	AA transporter; alanine, glycine transporter	Goberdhan et al., 2005
minidiscs	*CG3297*	SLC7	Yes	Yes		AA transporter	Reynolds et al., 2009
Nutrient Amino Acid transporter 1	*CG3252*	SLC6	No		No/yes	K^+/AA symporter; L-/D-amino acid transporter Neutral AA transporter	Thimgan et al., 2006; Miller et al., 2008; Romero-Calderón et al., 2008
	CG17119	CTNS	Yes			AA transporter; lysosomal L-cysteine transporter	Romero-Calderón and Krantz, 2006
	CG1139	SLC36	No	No		AA transporter; cysteine, alanine, glycine transport	Goberdhan et al., 2005; Romero-Calderón and Krantz, 2006
	CG1607	SLC7	Yes			AA transporter	Romero-Calderón and Krantz, 2006
	CG13384	SlC36	Yes			AA transporter	Romero-Calderón and Krantz, 2006
	CG13743	SLC38	Yes			AA transporter	Romero-Calderón and Krantz, 2006
	CG7708	SLC5	Yes	Yes		AA transporter; Proline/Na^+ symporter; Choline transporter	Romero-Calderón and Krantz, 2006
	CG7888	SLC36	Yes			AA transporter	Romero-Calderón and Krantz, 2006
	CG9413	SLC7	Yes			AA transporter	Romero-Calderón and Krantz, 2006
List	*CG15088*	SLC6	Yes		Yes	K^+/AA symporter; neuro-transmitter/Na^+ symporter	Romero-Calderón and Krantz, 2006; Thimgan et al., 2006; Kasuya et al., 2009
	CG30394	SLC38	Yes			AA transporter	Romero-Calderón and Krantz, 2006

(Continued)

Table 4 | Continued

Gene	CG	Human homolog	CNS expression			Function	References
			FlyAtlas	BDGP	Literature		
tadr	*CG9264*	SLC7	Yes			AA transporter	
	CG4991	SLC36	Yes			AA transporter	Romero-Calderón and Krantz, 2006
	CG1628	SLC25	Yes			AA transporter; L-ornithine transporter	Romero-Calderón and Krantz, 2006
	CG8785	SLC36	No			AA transporter	Romero-Calderón and Krantz, 2006
	CG12943	SLC36	No			AA transporter	Romero-Calderón and Krantz, 2006
	CG13646	no	No			AA transporter	Romero-Calderón and Krantz, 2006
	CG32079	SLC36	No		No	AA transporter	Romero-Calderón and Krantz, 2006
	CG32081	SLC36	No			AA transporter	
hoepel1	*CG12787*	OCA2	Yes			L-tyrosine transporter	
hoepel2	*CG15624*	OCA2	Yes			L-tyrosine transporter	
kazachoc	*CG5594*	SLC12	Yes	Yes	Yes	K^+/Cl^- symporter; AA transporter	Hekmat-Scafe et al., 2006; Sun et al., 2010 Filippov et al., 2003
	CG31547	SLC12	Yes		Yes	AA transporter; $Na^+/K^+/Cl^-$ symporter	Filippov et al., 2003; Romero-Calderón and Krantz, 2006; Sun et al., 2010
Ncc69	*CG4357*	SLC12	Yes		No/yes	$Na^+/K^+/Cl^-$ cotransporter; AA transporter	Filippov et al., 2003; Romero-Calderón and Krantz, 2006; Sun et al., 2010; Leiserson et al., 2011
	CG12773	SLC12	Yes		No/yes	AA transporter; $Na^+/K^+/Cl^-$ symporter	Filippov et al., 2003; Romero-Calderón and Krantz, 2006; Sun et al., 2010
	CG1698	SLC6	No		No	K^+/Cl^- symporter	Romero-Calderón and Krantz, 2006; Thimgan et al., 2006
karmoisin	*CG12286*	SLC16	Yes			Monocarboxylic acid transporter	
Silnoon	*CG8271*	SLC16	Yes			Secondary active monocarboxylate transporter; Butyrate, lactate transport	Jang et al., 2008
outsiders	*CG8062*	SLC16	No			Monocarboxylic acid transporter	
Dietary and metabolic glutamate transporter	*CG5304*	SLC17	Yes		No	High affinity inorganic phosphate/Na^+ symporter; Glutamate transporter; Na^+-independent glutamate transporter	Laridon et al., 2008; Shim et al., 2011

(Continued)

Table 4 | Continued

Gene	CG	Human homolog	CNS expression			Function	References
			FlyAtlas	BDGP	Literature		
Eaat 1	*CG3747*	SLC1	Yes		Yes	Glutamate/Na^+ symporter; L-aspartate transporter; Na^+/Dicarboxylate symporter; L-Glutamate transporter	Besson et al., 2000; Freeman et al., 2003; Rival et al., 2004
Eaat 2	*CG3159*	SLC1	Yes		Yes	Glutamate/Na^+ transporter; L-aspartate Taurine transporter; Na^+/Dicarboxylate symporter	Besson et al., 2000, 2005, 2011; Soustelle et al., 2002 Freeman et al., 2003
genderblind	*CG6070*	SLC7	Yes	Yes	Yes	AA transporter Glutamate transporter	Augustin et al., 2007, Grosjean et al., 2008
Ntl	*CG7075*	SLC6	No		No	Neurotransmitter/Na^+ symporter; Glycine transporter	Thimgan et al., 2006; Romero-Calderón et al., 2008
Vesicular GABA transporter	*CG8394*	SLC3	Yes		Yes	GABA/H^+ symporter; AA transporter	Romero-Calderón et al., 2008; Fei et al., 2010
Vesicular glutamate transporter	*CG9887*	SLC17	Yes		Yes	High affinity inorganic phosphate/Na^+ symporter; L-glutamate transporter	Daniels et al., 2004
	CG1732	SLC6	Yes	Yes	Yes	GABA/Na^+ symporter	Romero-Calderón and Krantz, 2006; Thimgan et al., 2006
	CG4476	SLC6	Yes		No	K^+/AA symporter; Neurotransmitter/Na^+ symporter	Romero-Calderón and Krantz, 2006; Thimgan et al., 2006
	CG16700	SLC36	Yes			AA transporter; GABA/H^+ symporter	Romero-Calderón and Krantz, 2006
	CG5549	SLC6	No		Yes	Glycine/Na^+ symporter	Romero-Calderón and Krantz, 2006; Thimgan et al., 2006
	CG8850	SLC6	No		No	K^+/AA symporter; Na^+/AA symporter	Romero-Calderón and Krantz, 2006; Thimgan et al., 2006
	CG13796	No	No			Glycine/Na^+ symporter	Romero-Calderón and Krantz, 2006
	CG15279	SLC5	No		No	Cation/Na^+ symporter	Romero-Calderón and Krantz, 2006; Thimgan et al., 2006

Amino acid transporters annotated in FlyBase as "organic acid transmembrane transporter activity" or as "amino acid transporter" are listed. Information about the CNS expression of each gene was obtained from FlyAtlas, the Berkely Drosophila Genome Project (BDGP), or literature. The predicted function of each protein is indicated. SLC, solute carrier; AA, amino acid; OCA2, oculocutaneous albinism II; GABA, γ-Aminobutyric acid.

which is encoded by an essential gene in Drosophila (Tps1, CG4104, Chen and Haddad, 2004). Among others, trehalose is used for the maintenance of energy metabolism during fasting and non-feeding periods (Friedman, 1978; Arrese and Soulages, 2010; Chen et al., 2010).

These observations suggest that specific sugar transporters exist, which import either trehalose or glucose into the brain. Two dedicated trehalose transporters, Tret1-1 and Tret1-2, have been described in *Drosophila melanogaster* (Kikawada et al., 2007). A comparison with other insect species shows that only one trehalose transporter gene is conserved in insects whereas the second trehalose transporter gene found in *Drosophila melanogaster* (*Tret1-2*) arose from a recent gene duplication event. Tret1-1 but not Tret1-2 is able to transport trehalose when expressed in Xenopus oocytes suggesting that the two trehalose transporters exert non-redundant functions (Kanamori et al., 2010). Trehalose transporters belong to the solute carrier 2 (SLC2) facilitated glucose transporter family with strongest homology to the human SLC2A8 protein. According to microarray data, Tret1-1 is strongly expressed in the brain. Tret1-2 is expressed only at very low levels. Its function is currently unknown (Kanamori et al., 2010). In conclusion, the Trehalose transporter is in a prime

Table 5 | Sugar concentration in the insect hemolymph.

Organism	Trehalose	Glucose	Fructose	Remark	References
A. mori, G. mellonella, T. polyphemus, P. cecropia	2–13 mg/ml	0–2.8 mg/ml	Not tested	Based on chromatography and chemical methods	Wyatt and Kalf, 1957
Several insects	2–50 mg/ml	Generally low amounts, but *Apis mellifica* 6–32 mg/ml, *Phormia regina* 7–12.5 mg/ml	Generally low amounts, but *Apis mellifica* 2–16 mg/ml	Review on hemolymph composition in insects	Jeuniaux, 1971
Apis mellifica	40 mg/ml	10 mg/ml	10 mg/ml	HPLC, trehalose concentration changes depending on metabolic rate	Blatt and Roces, 2001
Drosophila larvae	60 mg/ml	50 mg/ml	Not tested	Commercial kit	Lee and Park, 2004
Drosophila larvae	13.7–17.2 mg/ml	5.4–7.2 mg/ml	Not tested	Commercial kit	Broughton et al., 2008
Drosophila larvae	6 mg/ml	1 mg/ml	Not tested	Commercial kit	Pasco and Léopold, 2012
Drosophila adults	17.2 mg/ml	1.8 mg/ml	Not tested	Commercial kit	Broughton et al., 2008

Trehalose, glucose, and fructose concentrations in the hemolymph of different organisms and developmental stages are listed. Methods for concentration measurements are indicated.

position to control the import of high-energy carbohydrates at the blood-brain barrier.

CARBOHYDRATE TRANSPORTERS IN THE DROSOPHILA BLOOD-BRAIN BARRIER

In total, 78 genes of Drosophila harbor a sugar transporter motif (Interpro domain search; IPR005829, **Table 6**). Most of the encoded proteins, however, probably will not transport sugar across the plasma membrane but, as the SLC35 member Meigo, organize intracellular trafficking of different sugars to ensure glycosylation (Sekine et al., 2013). As an alternative to trehalose, other sugars such as glucose or fructose could be taken up by the nervous system to meet the high neuronal energy demand. In vertebrates, the SLC2 family includes Glut2 and Glut5 transporters, which have been characterized as glucose and fructose transporters (Douard and Ferraris, 2008; Kellett et al., 2008; Mueckler and Thorens, 2013). No clear homolog of Glut2 and Glut5 can be identified in Drosophila, so it remains uncertain whether fructose can be imported into the nervous system. Interestingly, however, a fructose receptor (Gr43a) has been shown to be expressed on several CNS neurons (Miyamoto et al., 2012). Thus, a possible explanation for the apparent lack of Glut2 or Glut5 homologs is that fructose might be either generated in the brain or that the fructose sensing CNS neurons form dendrites that leave the CNS to detect fructose in the hemolymph.

Unlike in the Drosophila hemolymph, glucose is the main energy supply in the mammalian blood. Glucose is transported by Glut1 and Glut3, which are also members of the SLC2 family. For both of these facilitated glucose transporters, glucose, galactose, and mannose transport activities have been found (Uldry and Thorens, 2004). Glut1 functions in the mammalian endothelial blood-brain barrier and in astrocytes, whereas Glut3 is expressed by neurons (Leino et al., 1997). In Drosophila, Glut1 is specifically expressed in the embryonic nervous system and microarray data indicate continued expression in brain tissue (FlyBase). Future work needs to discriminate whether Glut1 is expressed in neurons or glial cells or both. In contrast, Glut3 is only expressed in imaginal discs of late larval stages and in adult testis (FlyBase). Thus, Glut1 might be responsible for glucose uptake into the nervous system. In support of this notion, loss of *glut1* function is lethal (Saito et al., 2002) and expression of *glut1* is able to improve locomotor behavior and survival of flies when mitochondrial activity is reduced in glial cells (Besson et al., 2010).

In addition, members of the SLC5A family (SLC5A1 and SLC5A2) have been shown to mediate sodium-dependent glucose uptake (Featherstone, 2011). One Drosophila SLC5A family member is CG9657, which is also expressed in glial cells (Freeman et al., 2003).

BLOOD-BRAIN BARRIER AND HORMONAL FUNCTION

In addition to the control of metabolism, the blood-brain barrier must also permit the entry and exit of hormones into or out of the nervous system. This is especially true for the Drosophila neuroendocrine system, which consists of neurosecretory cells (NSCs) in the brain. The Drosophila genome encodes eight insulin-like peptides (Dilps), which are the functional homologs

Table 6 | Drosophila sugar transporters.

Gene	CG	Human homolog	CNS expression FlyAtlas	CNS expression BDGP	Function	Reference
	CG10960	SLC2A8 (Glut8)	Yes	Yes	glucose transporter	
Tret1-1	*CG30035*	SLC2A8 (Glut8)	Yes		glucose transporter; trehalose transport	Kikawada et al., 2007; Kanamori et al., 2010
Glut1	*CG1086*	SLC2	Yes	Yes	glucose transporter	
	CG1213	SLC2	Yes		glucose transporter	
sut1	*CG8714*	SLC2	Yes		sugar/H$^+$ symporter; glucose transporter	
Glut3	*CG3853*	SLC2	No		sugar transporter; glucose transporter	
Tret1-2	*CG8234*	SLC2A8 (Glut8)	No		fructose transporter; glucose transporter;	Kanamori et al., 2010
sut2	*CG17975*	SLC2	No		sugar/H$^+$ symporter; glucose transporter	
sut3	*CG17976*	SLC2	No		sugar/H$^+$ symporter; glucose transporter	
sut4	*CG1380*	SLC2	No		sugar/H$^+$ symporter; glucose transporter	
	CG1208	SLC2	Yes		glucose transporter	
	CG7882	SLC2	No		glucose transporter	
	CG8249	SLC2	No		glucose transporter	
	CG4797	SLC2	Yes		glucose transporter	
	CG8837	SLC2	Yes		transporter activity	
	CG15406	SLC2	No		fructose transporter	
	CG4607	SLC2	Yes		substrate-specific transporter	
	CG3285	SLC2	No		transporter activity	
	CG33281	SLC2	No		monosaccaride transporter	
	CG6484	SLC2	No		glucose transporter	
	CG33282	SLC2	No		monosaccaride transporter	
	CG15408	SLC2	No		fructose transporter	
	CG14605	SLC2	No		transmembrane transporter activity	
	CG14606	SLC2	No		hexose transporter	
	CG11976	SLC2	Yes		monosaccaride transporter	
	CG3168	SLC22/SV2	Yes	Yes	transporter activity	Altenhein et al., 2006
	CG6126	SLC22	Yes	Yes	organic cation transporter	
Orct	*CG6331*	SLC22	Yes	Yes	organic cation transporter	
	CG3790	SLC22	Yes		carnitine transporter	
	CG6356	SLC22	Yes		secondary active organic cation transporter	
	CG7084	SLC22	Yes		secondary active organic cation transporter	
	CG7442	SLC22	Yes		secondary active organic cation transporter	
Orct2	*CG13610*	SLC22	Yes	Yes	organic cation transporter	
	CG8654	SLC22	Yes	Yes	secondary active organic cation transporter	
	CG10486	SLC22	No		secondary active organic cation transporter	
	CG16727	SLC22	No		organic cation transporter	
	CG17751	SLC22	No		secondary active organic cation transporter	
	CG17752	SLC22	No		secondary active organic cation transporter	

(Continued)

Table 6 | Continued

Gene	CG	Human homolog	CNS expression		Function	Reference
			FlyAtlas	BDGP		
	CG14855	SLC22	Yes		secondary active organic cation transporter	
	CG14856	SLC22	No		secondary active organic cation transporter	
	CG6006	SLC22	Yes		carnitine transporter	
	CG6231	SLC22	Yes		secondary active organic cation transporter	
	CG7333	SLC22	No		secondary active organic cation transporter	
	CG5592	SLC22	No		secondary active organic cation transporter	
	CG7342	SLC22	No		secondary active organic cation transporter	
	CG42269	SLC22	No		secondary active organic cation transporter	
	CG7458	SLC22	No		secondary active organic cation transporter	
	CG8925	SLC22	No		carnitine transporter	
	CG9317	SLC22	Yes		secondary active organic cation transporter	
Csat	*CG2675*	SLC35	Yes		UDP-galactose transporter; sugar/H^+ symporter	Segawa et al., 2002
Efr	*CG3774*	SLC35	Yes		nucleotide-sugar transporter; GDP-fuctose transporter	
frc	*CG3874*	SLC35	Yes		triose-phosphate transporter; pyrimidine nucleotide-sugar transporter	
meigo	*CG5802*	SLC35	Yes		UDP-N-acetylglucosamine transporter	
sll	*CG7623*	SIC35	Yes		UDP-N-acetylglucosamine transporter; 3′-phosphoadenosine 5′-phosphosulfate transporter	
Papst2	*CG7853*	SLC35	Yes		UDP-N-acetylglucosamine transporter; 3′-phosphoadenosine 5′-phosphosulfate transporter	
Gfr	*CG9620*	SLC35	Yes		GDP-fucose transporter	
	CG33181	SLC41	Yes		cation transporter	
	CG11537	HIAT1	Yes		carbohydrate transporter	
Prp38	*CG30342*	PRPF38	Yes		pre-mRNA-splicing factor	
	CG7009	FTSJ1	Yes		tRNA methyltransferase activity	
slv	*CG8717*	SLC50	Yes		sweet sugar transporter	
rtet	*CG5760*	MFSD	Yes		sugar transporter	
	CG15096	SLC17	Yes		high affinity inorganic phosphate/Na^+ symporter	
	CG30344 (CG8054)	SLC46	Yes		transporter activity	Freeman et al., 2003
	CG6901	SVOP	No		transporter activity	
	CG12783	SV2	No		transporter activity	
	CG30345	SLC46	No		transporter activity	
	CG15553	SLC46	No		transporter activity	

(Continued)

Table 6 | Continued

Gene	CG	Human homolog	CNS expression		Function	Reference
			FlyAtlas	BDGP		
	CG14160	–	No		transporter activity	
	CG17929	–	No		transporter activity	
	CG17930	–	No		transporter activity	
	CG32053	–	No		transporter activity	
	CG32054	–	No		transporter activity	
	CG42825	–	No		transporter activity	
	CG31103	SV2	No		transporter activity	
	CG33233	SV2	No		transporter activity	
	CG4324	SVOPL	No		organic cation transporter	
	CG5078	HIAT1	No		carbohydrate transporter	

Carbohydrate transporters harboring a sugar transporter motif (Interpro domain search, IPR005829) are listed. Information about the CNS expression of each gene was obtained as indicated. The predicted function of each protein is noted. SLC, solute carrier; HIAT, hippocampus abundant transcript 1; PRPF, pre-mRNA processing factor; FTSJ1, FtsJ RNA methyltransferase homolog 1; MFSD10, major facilitator superfamily domain containing 10; SVOP, SV2 related protein homolog; SV2, synaptic vesicle glycoprotein 2; SVOPL, SVOP-like.

of vertebrate insulin and insulin-like growth factors (IGFs) that affect a wide range of processes (Erion and Sehgal, 2013; Shim et al., 2013). Dilp2, 3 and 5 are expressed by 14 insulin-producing cells (IPCs) and released into the hemolymph to regulate growth, metabolism, reproduction, and life span (Nässel et al., 2013). A key trigger of Dilp release from IPCs is food intake. The associated increase in hemolymph sugar and amino acid levels is sensed by the fat body and causes release of the leptin-like peptide Unpaired 2 (Upd2), which acts on IPCs via GABAergic neurons (Rajan and Perrimon, 2012). However, how this fat body-derived signal passes the blood-brain barrier or how it is sensed by the surface glia and then further transmitted into the nervous system is not known.

An additional fat body derived signal coordinates the second wave of neurogenesis at the end of larval stages, which must be matched to the nutritional status of the animal. This still elusive signal triggers expression of Dilp6 in the SPG, which in turn activates the proliferation of larval neuroblasts (Chell and Brand, 2010; Sousa-Nunes et al., 2011). Interestingly, both, the expression and the secretion of Dilp6 from the SPG cells depend on the presence of gap junctions in these cells (Spéder and Brand, 2014).

Moreover, the blood-brain barrier influences the physiology of the animal. It is known that some hemolymph proteins modulate the mating behavior of Drosophila (Lazareva et al., 2007). Interestingly, the sex of the blood-brain barrier matters and male-specific factors of the blood-brain barrier are required for normal male courtship behavior (Hoxha et al., 2013). These aspects of blood-brain barrier function are currently not extensively studied but it appears likely, that in the near future more surprising findings will be made.

CONCLUSIONS

Nervous system function strongly depends on a well-balanced ion and metabolite milieu. To ensure this homeostasis in the brain, the blood-brain barrier fulfills a variety of functions. It seals the brain from circulation and, in consequence, active transport systems are required for all solutes that have to be shuttled into or out of the brain. Therefore, a number of specific transporters must be expressed in the barrier forming cells. In Drosophila, as in primitive vertebrates, the blood-brain barrier is formed by glia. To date, our knowledge about essential transporters expressed in the glia is very limited. However, genomic information and transcriptomic data as already available for the mouse (Daneman et al., 2010a) will soon enable us to identify many relevant genes in Drosophila and the wealth of genetic tools will ease their analysis. One of the future challenges will be to decipher how the metabolic supply through the blood-brain barrier is matched to neuronal activity. In light of the apparently well-conserved blood-brain barrier, functional studies using Drosophila are expected to deepen our understanding of how the blood-brain barrier keeps our nervous system functional.

ACKNOWLEDGMENTS

We are thankful to S. Rumpf and N. Saunders for comments on the manuscript. Work in the lab of Christian Klämbt is supported by the Deutsche Forschungsgemeinschaft (DFG, SFB 1009). Stefanie Limmer is supported by a postdoctoral fellowship of the DFG.

REFERENCES

Abbott, N. J., Rönnbäck, L., and Hansson, E. (2006). Astrocyte-endothelial interactions at the blood-brain barrier. *Nat. Rev. Neurosci.* 7, 41–53. doi: 10.1038/nrn1824

Allaman, I., Bélanger, M., and Magistretti, P. J. (2011). Astrocyte-neuron metabolic relationships: for better and for worse. *Trends Neurosci.* 34, 76–87. doi: 10.1016/j.tins.2010.12.001

Altenhein, B., Becker, A., Busold, C., Beckmann, B., Hoheisel, J. D., and Technau, G. M. (2006). Expression profiling of glial genes during Drosophila embryogenesis. *Dev. Biol.* 296, 545–560. doi: 10.1016/j.ydbio.2006.04.460

Anholt, R. R. H., and Mackay, T. F. C. (2012). Genetics of aggression. *Annu. Rev. Genet.* 46, 145–164. doi: 10.1146/annurev-genet-110711-155514

Armstrong, G. A. B., Rodríguez, E. C., and Meldrum Robertson, R. (2012). Cold hardening modulates K+ homeostasis in the brain of *Drosophila melanogaster* during chill coma. *J. Insect Physiol.* 58, 1511–1516. doi: 10.1016/j.jinsphys.2012.09.006

Armulik, A., Genové, G., and Betsholtz, C. (2011). Pericytes: developmental, physiological, and pathological perspectives, problems, and promises. *Dev. Cell* 21, 193–215. doi: 10.1016/j.devcel.2011.07.001

Armulik, A., Genové, G., Mäe, M., Nisancioglu, M. H., Wallgard, E., Niaudet, C., et al. (2010). Pericytes regulate the blood-brain barrier. *Nature* 468, 557–561. doi: 10.1038/nature09522

Arrese, E. L., and Soulages, J. L. (2010). Insect fat body: energy, metabolism, and regulation. *Annu. Rev. Entomol.* 55, 207–225. doi: 10.1146/annurev-ento-112408-085356

Augustin, H., Grosjean, Y., Chen, K., Sheng, Q., and Featherstone, D. E. (2007). Nonvesicular release of glutamate by glial xCT transporters suppresses glutamate receptor clustering *in vivo*. *J. Neurosci.* 27, 111–123. doi: 10.1523/JNEUROSCI.4770-06.2007

Auld, V. J., Fetter, R. D., Broadie, K., and Goodman, C. S. (1995). Gliotactin, a novel transmembrane protein on peripheral glia, is required to form the blood-nerve barrier in Drosophila. *Cell* 81, 757–767. doi: 10.1016/0092-8674(95)90537-5

Awasaki, T., Lai, S.-L., Ito, K., and Lee, T. (2008). Organization and postembryonic development of glial cells in the adult central brain of Drosophila. *J. Neurosci.* 28, 13742–13753. doi: 10.1523/JNEUROSCI.4844-08.2008

Bainton, R. J., Tsai, L. T.-Y., Schwabe, T., DeSalvo, M., Gaul, U., and Heberlein, U. (2005). moody encodes two GPCRs that regulate cocaine behaviors and blood-brain barrier permeability in Drosophila. *Cell* 123, 145–156. doi: 10.1016/j.cell.2005.07.029

Bätz, T., Förster, D., and Luschnig, S. (2014). The transmembrane protein Macroglobulin complement-related is essential for septate junction formation and epithelial barrier function in Drosophila. *Development* 141, 899–908. doi: 10.1242/dev.102160

Baumgartner, S., Littleton, J. T., Broadie, K., Bhat, M. A., Harbecke, R., Lengyel, J. A., et al. (1996). A Drosophila neurexin is required for septate junction and blood-nerve barrier formation and function. *Cell* 87, 1059–1068. doi: 10.1016/S0092-8674(00)81800-0

Beckervordersandforth, R. M., Rickert, C., Altenhein, B., and Technau, G. M. (2008). Subtypes of glial cells in the Drosophila embryonic ventral nerve cord as related to lineage and gene expression. *Mech. Dev.* 125, 542–557. doi: 10.1016/j.mod.2007.12.004

Begg, M., and Cruickshank, W. J. (1962). A partial analysis of Drosophila larval hæmolymph. *Proc. R Soc. Edinb. B Biol.* 68, 215–236. doi: 10.1017/S0080455X00001053

Besson, M.-T., Dupont, P., Fridell, Y.-W. C., and Liévens, J.-C. (2010). Increased energy metabolism rescues glia-induced pathology in a Drosophila model of Huntington's disease. *Hum. Mol. Genet.* 19, 3372–3382. doi: 10.1093/hmg/ddq249

Besson, M.-T., Ré, D. B., Moulin, M., and Birman, S. (2005). High affinity transport of taurine by the Drosophila aspartate transporter dEAAT2. *J. Biol. Chem.* 280, 6621–6626. doi: 10.1074/jbc.M412440200

Besson, M. T., Sinakevitch, I., Melon, C., Iché-Torres, M., and Birman, S. (2011). Involvement of the Drosophila taurine/aspartate transporter dEAAT2 in selective olfactory and gustatory perceptions. *J. Comp. Neurol.* 519, 2734–2757. doi: 10.1002/cne.22649

Besson, M. T., Soustelle, L., and Birman, S. (2000). Selective high-affinity transport of aspartate by a Drosophila homologue of the excitatory amino-acid transporters. *Curr. Biol.* 10, 207–210. doi: 10.1016/S0960-9822(00)00339-0

Bilder, D., and Perrimon, N. (2000). Localization of apical epithelial determinants by the basolateral PDZ protein Scribble. *Nature* 403, 676–680. doi: 10.1038/35001108

Blatt, J., and Roces, F. (2001). Haemolymph sugar levels in foraging honeybees (*Apis mellifera* carnica): dependence on metabolic rate and *in vivo* measurement of maximal rates of trehalose synthesis. *J. Exp. Biol.* 204, 2709–2716.

Boudko, D. Y. (2012). Molecular basis of essential amino acid transport from studies of insect nutrient amino acid transporters of the SLC6 family (NAT-SLC6). *J. Insect Physiol.* 58, 433–449. doi: 10.1016/j.jinsphys.2011.12.018

Broadus, J., Skeath, J. B., Spana, E. P., Bossing, T., Technau, G., and Doe, C. Q. (1995). New neuroblast markers and the origin of the aCC/pCC neurons in the Drosophila central nervous system. *Mech. Dev.* 53, 393–402. doi: 10.1016/0925-4773(95)00454-8

Broughton, S., Alic, N., Slack, C., Bass, T., Ikeya, T., Vinti, G., et al. (2008). Reduction of DILP2 in Drosophila triages a metabolic phenotype from lifespan revealing redundancy and compensation among DILPs. *PLoS ONE* 3:e3721. doi: 10.1371/journal.pone.0003721

Bundgaard, M., and Abbott, N. J. (2008). All vertebrates started out with a glial blood-brain barrier 4-500 million years ago. *Glia* 56, 699–708. doi: 10.1002/glia.20642

Campos-Ortega, J., and Hartenstein, V. (1997). *The Embryonic Development of Drosophila Melanogaster*. 2nd Edn. Berlin: Springer-Verlag. doi: 10.1007/978-3-662-22489-2

Cardona, A., Saalfeld, S., Preibisch, S., Schmid, B., Cheng, A., Pulokas, J., et al. (2010). An integrated micro- and macroarchitectural analysis of the Drosophila brain by computer-assisted serial section electron microscopy. *PLoS Biol* 8:e1000502. doi: 10.1371/journal.pbio.1000502

Carlson, S. D., Juang, J. L., Hilgers, S. L., and Garment, M. B. (2000). Blood barriers of the insect. *Annu. Rev. Entomol.* 45, 151–174. doi: 10.1146/annurev.ento.45.1.151

Chell, J. M., and Brand, A. H. (2010). Nutrition-responsive glia control exit of neural stem cells from quiescence. *Cell* 143, 1161–1173. doi: 10.1016/j.cell.2010.12.007

Chen, J., Tang, B., Chen, H., Yao, Q., Huang, X., Chen, J., et al. (2010). Different functions of the insect soluble and membrane-bound trehalase genes in chitin biosynthesis revealed by RNA interference. *PLoS ONE* 5:e10133. doi: 10.1371/journal.pone.0010133

Chen, Q., and Haddad, G. G. (2004). Role of trehalose phosphate synthase and trehalose during hypoxia: from flies to mammals. *J. Exp. Biol.* 207, 3125–3129. doi: 10.1242/jeb.01133

Chintapalli, V. R., Wang, J., Herzyk, P., Davies, S. A., and Dow, J. A. (2013). Data-mining the FlyAtlas online resource to identify core functional motifs across transporting epithelia. *BMC Genomics* 14:518. doi: 10.1186/1471-2164-14-518

von Hilchen, C. M., Bustos, Á. E., Giangrande, A., Technau, G. M., and Altenhein, B. (2013). Predetermined embryonic glial cells form the distinct glial sheaths of the Drosophila peripheral nervous system. *Development* 140, 3657–3668. doi: 10.1242/dev.093245

Crews, S. T., Thomas, J. B., and Goodman, C. S. (1988). The Drosophila single-minded gene encodes a nuclear protein with sequence similarity to the per gene product. *Cell* 52, 143–151. doi: 10.1016/0092-8674(88)90538-7

Croghan, P. C., and Lockwood, A. P. M. (1960). The composition of the hemolymph of the larva of *Drosophila melanogaster*. *J. Exp. Biol.* 37, 339–343.

Daneman, R., Zhou, L., Agalliu, D., Cahoy, J. D., Kaushal, A., and Barres, B. A. (2010a). The mouse blood-brain barrier transcriptome: a new resource for understanding the development and function of brain endothelial cells. *PLoS ONE* 5:e13741. doi: 10.1371/journal.pone.0013741

Daneman, R., Zhou, L., Kebede, A. A., and Barres, B. A. (2010b). Pericytes are required for blood-brain barrier integrity during embryogenesis. *Nature* 468, 562–566. doi: 10.1038/nature09513

Daniels, R. W., Collins, C. A., Gelfand, M. V., Dant, J., Brooks, E. S., Krantz, D. E., et al. (2004). Increased expression of the Drosophila vesicular glutamate transporter leads to excess glutamate release and a compensatory decrease in quantal content. *J. Neurosci.* 24, 10466–10474. doi: 10.1523/JNEUROSCI.3001-04.2004

Davis, R. L. (2011). Traces of Drosophila memory. *Neuron* 70, 8–19. doi: 10.1016/j.neuron.2011.03.012

Dermauw, W., and Van Leeuwen, T. (2014). The ABC gene family in arthropods: comparative genomics and role in insecticide transport and resistance. *Insect Biochem. Mol. Biol.* 45, 89–110. doi: 10.1016/j.ibmb.2013.11.001

DeSalvo, M. K., Mayer, N., Mayer, F., and Bainton, R. J. (2011). Physiologic and anatomic characterization of the brain surface glia barrier of Drosophila. *Glia* 59, 1322–1340. doi: 10.1002/glia.21147

Dietzl, G., Chen, D., Schnorrer, F., Su, K.-C., Barinova, Y., Fellner, M., et al. (2007). A genome-wide transgenic RNAi library for conditional gene inactivation in Drosophila. *Nature* 448, 151–156. doi: 10.1038/nature05954

Douard, V., and Ferraris, R. P. (2008). Regulation of the fructose transporter GLUT5 in health and disease. *Am. J. Physiol. Endocrinol. Metab.* 295, E227–E237. doi: 10.1152/ajpendo.90245.2008

Erion, R., and Sehgal, A. (2013). Regulation of insect behavior via the insulin-signaling pathway. *Front. Physiol.* 4:353. doi: 10.3389/fphys.2013.00353

Faivre-Sarrailh, C., Banerjee, S., Li, J., Hortsch, M., Laval, M., and Bhat, M. A. (2004). Drosophila contactin, a homolog of vertebrate contactin, is required for septate junction organization and paracellular barrier function. *Development* 131, 4931–4942. doi: 10.1242/dev.01372

Farquhar, M. G., and Palade, G. E. (1963). Junctional complexes in various epithelia. *J. Cell Biol.* 17, 375–412. doi: 10.1083/jcb.17.2.375

Farquhar, M. G., and Palade, G. E. (1965). Cell junctions in amphibian skin. *J. Cell Biol.* 26, 263–291. doi: 10.1083/jcb.26.1.263

Featherstone, D. E. (2011). Glial solute carrier transporters in Drosophila and mice. *Glia* 59, 1351–1363. doi: 10.1002/glia.21085

Fehon, R. G., Dawson, I. A., and Artavanis-Tsakonas, S. (1994). A Drosophila homologue of membrane-skeleton protein 4.1 is associated with septate junctions and is encoded by the coracle gene. *Development* 120, 545–557.

Fei, H., Chow, D. M., Chen, A., Romero-Calderón, R., Ong, W. S., Ackerson, L. C., et al. (2010). Mutation of the Drosophila vesicular GABA transporter disrupts visual figure detection. *J. Exp. Biol.* 213, 1717–1730. doi: 10.1242/jeb.036053

Filippov, V., Aimanova, K., and Gill, S. S. (2003). Expression of an Aedes aegypti cation-chloride cotransporter and its Drosophila homologues. *Insect Mol. Biol.* 12, 319–331. doi: 10.1046/j.1365-2583.2003.00415.x

Franzdóttir, S. R., Engelen, D., Yuva-Aydemir, Y., Schmidt, I., Aho, A., and Klämbt, C. (2009). Switch in FGF signalling initiates glial differentiation in the Drosophila eye. *Nature* 460, 758–761. doi: 10.1038/nature08167

Freeman, M. R., Delrow, J., Kim, J., Johnson, E., and Doe, C. Q. (2003). Unwrapping glial biology: Gcm target genes regulating glial development, diversification, and function. *Neuron* 38, 567–580. doi: 10.1016/S0896-6273(03)00289-7

Friedman, S. (1978). Trehalose regulation, one aspect of metabolic homeostasis. *Ann. Rev. Entomol* 23, 389–407. doi: 10.1146/annurev.en.23.010178.002133

Fünfschilling, U., Supplie, L. M., Mahad, D., Boretius, S., Saab, A. S., Edgar, J., et al. (2012). Glycolytic oligodendrocytes maintain myelin and long-term axonal integrity. *Nature* 485, 517–521. doi: 10.1038/nature11007

Furuse, M., Izumi, Y., Oda, Y., Higashi, T., and Iwamoto, N. (2014). Molecular organization of tricellular tight junctions. *Tissue Barriers* 2, e28960. doi: 10.4161/tisb.28960

Gaete, P. S., Lillo, M. A., and Figueroa, X. F. (2014). Functional role of connexins and pannexins in the interaction between vascular and nervous system. *J. Cell. Physiol.* 229, 1336–1345. doi: 10.1002/jcp.24563

Genova, J. L., and Fehon, R. G. (2003). Neuroglian, Gliotactin, and the Na^+/K^+ ATPase are essential for septate junction function in Drosophila. *J. Cell Biol.* 161, 979–989. doi: 10.1083/jcb.200212054

Giesen, K., Hummel, T., Stollewerk, A., Harrison, S., Travers, A., and Klämbt, C. (1997). Glial development in the Drosophila CNS requires concomitant activation of glial and repression of neuronal differentiation genes. *Development* 124, 2307–2316.

Goberdhan, D. C. I., Meredith, D., Boyd, C. A. R., and Wilson, C. (2005). PAT-related amino acid transporters regulate growth via a novel mechanism that does not require bulk transport of amino acids. *Development* 132, 2365–2375. doi: 10.1242/dev.01821

Graf, F., Noirot-Timothée, C., and Noirot, C. (1982). The specialization of septate junctions in regions of tricellular junctions. I. Smooth septate junctions (=continuous junctions). *J. Ultrastruct. Res.* 78, 136–151. doi: 10.1016/S0022-5320(82)80019-1

Grosjean, Y., Grillet, M., Augustin, H., Ferveur, J.-F., and Featherstone, D. E. (2008). A glial amino-acid transporter controls synapse strength and courtship in Drosophila. *Nat. Neurosci.* 11, 54–61. doi: 10.1038/nn2019

Guan, Z., Saraswati, S., Adolfsen, B., and Littleton, J. T. (2005). Genome-wide transcriptional changes associated with enhanced activity in the Drosophila nervous system. *Neuron* 48, 91–107. doi: 10.1016/j.neuron.2005.08.036

Hall, S., Bone, C., Oshima, K., Zhang, L., McGraw, M., Lucas, B., et al. (2014). Macroglobulin complement-related encodes a protein required for septate junction organization and paracellular barrier function in Drosophila. *Development* 141, 889–898. doi: 10.1242/dev.102152

Harris, J. J., Jolivet, R., and Attwell, D. (2012). Synaptic energy use and supply. *Neuron* 75, 762–777. doi: 10.1016/j.neuron.2012.08.019

Hartenstein, V. (2011). Morphological diversity and development of glia in Drosophila. *Glia* 59, 1237–1252. doi: 10.1002/glia.21162

Hatan, M., Shinder, V., Israeli, D., Schnorrer, F., and Volk, T. (2011). The Drosophila blood brain barrier is maintained by GPCR-dependent dynamic actin structures. *J. Cell Biol.* 192, 307–319. doi: 10.1083/jcb.201007095

Hekmat-Scafe, D. S., Lundy, M. Y., Ranga, R., and Tanouye, M. A. (2006). Mutations in the K+/Cl- cotransporter gene kazachoc (kcc) increase seizure susceptibility in Drosophila. *J. Neurosci.* 26, 8943–8954. doi: 10.1523/JNEUROSCI.4998-05.2006

Hijazi, A., Masson, W., Augé, B., Waltzer, L., Haenlin, M., and Roch, F. (2009). boudin is required for septate junction organisation in Drosophila and codes for a diffusible protein of the Ly6 superfamily. *Development* 136, 2199–2209. doi: 10.1242/dev.033845

Holcroft, C. E., Jackson, W. D., Lin, W.-H., Bassiri, K., Baines, R. A., and Phelan, P. (2013). Innexins Ogre and Inx2 are required in glial cells for normal postembryonic development of the Drosophila central nervous system. *J. Cell Sci.* 126, 3823–3834. doi: 10.1242/jcs.117994

Hosoya, T., Takizawa, K., Nitta, K., and Hotta, Y. (1995). glial cells missing: a binary switch between neuronal and glial determination in Drosophila. *Cell* 82, 1025–1036. doi: 10.1016/0092-8674(95)90281-3

Hoxha, V., Lama, C., Chang, P. L., Saurabh, S., Patel, N., Olate, N., et al. (2013). Sex-specific signaling in the blood-brain barrier is required for male courtship in Drosophila. *PLoS Genet.* 9:e1003217. doi: 10.1371/journal.pgen.1003217

Ile, K. E., Tripathy, R., Goldfinger, V., and Renault, A. D. (2012). Wunen, a Drosophila lipid phosphate phosphatase, is required for septate junction-mediated barrier function. *Development* 139, 2535–2546. doi: 10.1242/dev.077289

Ito, K., Urban, J., and Technau, G. M. (1995). Distribution, classification, and development ofDrosophila glial cells in the late embryonic and early larval ventral nerve cord. *Roux's Arch. Dev. Biol.* 204, 284–307. doi: 10.1007/BF02179499

Jang, C., Lee, G., and Chung, J. (2008). LKB1 induces apical trafficking of Silnoon, a monocarboxylate transporter, in *Drosophila melanogaster*. *J. Cell Biol.* 183, 11–17. doi: 10.1083/jcb.200807052

Jaspers, M. H. J., Nolde, K., Behr, M., Joo, S.-H., Plessmann, U., Nikolov, M., et al. (2012). The claudin Megatrachea protein complex. *J. Biol. Chem.* 287, 36756–36765. doi: 10.1074/jbc.M112.399410

Jenett, A., Rubin, G. M., Ngo, T.-T. B., Shepherd, D., Murphy, C., Dionne, H., et al. (2012). A GAL4-driver line resource for Drosophila neurobiology. *Cell Rep.* 2, 991–1001. doi: 10.1016/j.celrep.2012.09.011

Jeuniaux, C. (1971). "Hemolymph-Arthropoda," in *Chemical Zoology*, eds M. Florkin and B. T. Scheer (New York; London: Academic Press), 64–118.

Jolivet, R., Magistretti, P. J., and Weber, B. (2009). Deciphering neuron-glia compartmentalization in cortical energy metabolism. *Front. Neuroenergetics* 1:4. doi: 10.3389/neuro.14.004.2009

Jones, B. W., Fetter, R. D., Tear, G., and Goodman, C. S. (1995). glial cells missing: a genetic switch that controls glial versus neuronal fate. *Cell* 82, 1013–1023. doi: 10.1016/0092-8674(95)90280-5

Kanamori, Y., Saito, A., Hagiwara-Komoda, Y., Tanaka, D., Mitsumasu, K., Kikuta, S., et al. (2010). The trehalose transporter 1 gene sequence is conserved in insects and encodes proteins with different kinetic properties involved in trehalose import into peripheral tissues. *Insect Biochem. Mol. Biol.* 40, 30–37. doi: 10.1016/j.ibmb.2009.12.006

Kasuya, J., Kaas, G. A., and Kitamoto, T. (2009). A putative amino acid transporter of the solute carrier 6 family is upregulated by lithium and is required for resistance to lithium toxicity in Drosophila. *Neuroscience* 163, 825–837. doi: 10.1016/j.neuroscience.2009.07.027

Kaufmann, N., Mathai, J. C., Hill, W. G., Dow, J. A. T., Zeidel, M. L., and Brodsky, J. L. (2005). Developmental expression and biophysical characterization of a *Drosophila melanogaster* aquaporin. *Am. J. Physiol. Cell Physiol.* 289, C397–C407. doi: 10.1152/ajpcell.00612.2004

Kellett, G. L., Brot-Laroche, E., Mace, O. J., and Leturque, A. (2008). Sugar absorption in the intestine: the role of GLUT2. *Annu. Rev. Nutr.* 28, 35–54. doi: 10.1146/annurev.nutr.28.061807.155518

Kikawada, T., Saito, A., Kanamori, Y., Nakahara, Y., Iwata, K.-I., Tanaka, D., et al. (2007). Trehalose transporter 1, a facilitated and high-capacity trehalose transporter, allows exogenous trehalose uptake into cells. *Proc. Natl. Acad. Sci. U.S.A.* 104, 11585–11590. doi: 10.1073/pnas.0702538104

Klaes, A., Menne, T., Stollewerk, A., Scholz, H., and Klämbt, C. (1994). The Ets transcription factors encoded by the Drosophila gene pointed direct glial cell differentiation in the embryonic CNS. *Cell* 78, 149–160. doi: 10.1016/0092-8674(94)90581-9

Landgraf, M., Bossing, T., Technau, G. M., and Bate, M. (1997). The origin, location, and projections of the embryonic abdominal motorneurons of Drosophila. *J. Neurosci.* 17, 9642–9655.

Lane, N. J. (1991). Morphology of glial blood-brain barriers. *Ann. N.Y. Acad. Sci.* 633, 348–362. doi: 10.1111/j.1749-6632.1991.tb15626.x

Lane, N. J., and Abbott, N. J. (1992). Freeze-fracture evidence for a novel restricting junction at the blood-brain barrier of the cuttlefish *Sepia officinalis*. *J. Neurocytol.* 21, 295–303. doi: 10.1007/BF01224762

Lane, N. J., and Swales, L. S. (1979). Intercellular junctions and the development of the blood-brain barrier in *Manduca sexta*. *Brain Res.* 168, 227–245. doi: 10.1016/0006-8993(79)90166-5

Laprise, P., Lau, K. M., Harris, K. P., Silva-Gagliardi, N. F., Paul, S. M., Beronja, S., et al. (2009). Yurt, Coracle, Neurexin IV and the Na+,K+-ATPase form a novel group of epithelial polarity proteins. *Nature* 459, 1141–1145. doi: 10.1038/nature08067

Laridon, B., Callaerts, P., and Norga, K. (2008). Embryonic expression patterns of Drosophila ACS family genes related to the human sialin gene. *Gene Expr. Patterns* 8, 275–283. doi: 10.1016/j.gep.2007.12.003

Laughlin, S. B., de Ruyter van Steveninck, R. R., and Anderson, J. C. (1998). The metabolic cost of neural information. *Nat. Neurosci.* 1, 36–41. doi: 10.1038/236

Lazareva, A. A., Roman, G., Mattox, W., Hardin, P. E., and Dauwalder, B. (2007). A role for the adult fat body in Drosophila male courtship behavior. *PLoS Genet.* 3:e16. doi: 10.1371/journal.pgen.0030016

Lee, G., and Park, J. H. (2004). Hemolymph sugar homeostasis and starvation-induced hyperactivity affected by genetic manipulations of the adipokinetic hormone-encoding gene in *Drosophila melanogaster*. *Genetics* 167, 311–323. doi: 10.1534/genetics.167.1.311

Lee, Y., Morrison, B. M., Li, Y., Lengacher, S., Farah, M. H., Hoffman, P. N., et al. (2012). Oligodendroglia metabolically support axons and contribute to neurodegeneration. *Nature* 487, 443–448. doi: 10.1038/nature11314

Leino, R. L., Gerhart, D. Z., van Bueren, A. M., McCall, A. L., and Drewes, L. R. (1997). Ultrastructural localization of GLUT 1 and GLUT 3 glucose transporters in rat brain. *J. Neurosci. Res.* 49, 617–626.

Leiserson, W. M., Forbush, B., and Keshishian, H. (2011). Drosophila glia use a conserved cotransporter mechanism to regulate extracellular volume. *Glia* 59, 320–332. doi: 10.1002/glia.21103

Leiserson, W. M., Harkins, E. W., and Keshishian, H. (2000). Fray, a Drosophila serine/threonine kinase homologous to mammalian PASK, is required for axonal ensheathment. *Neuron* 28, 793–806. doi: 10.1016/S0896-6273(00)00154-9

Leybaert, L. (2005). Neurobarrier coupling in the brain: a partner of neurovascular and neurometabolic coupling? *J. Cereb. Blood Flow Metab.* 25, 2–16. doi: 10.1038/sj.jcbfm.9600001

Li, H.-H., Kroll, J. R., Lennox, S. M., Ogundeyi, O., Jeter, J., Depasquale, G., et al. (2014). A GAL4 driver resource for developmental and behavioral studies on the larval CNS of Drosophila. *Cell Rep.* 8, 897–908. doi: 10.1016/j.celrep.2014.06.065

Llimargas, M., Strigini, M., Katidou, M., Karagogeos, D., and Casanova, J. (2004). Lachesin is a component of a septate junction-based mechanism that controls tube size and epithelial integrity in the Drosophila tracheal system. *Development* 131, 181–190. doi: 10.1242/dev.00917

Lovick, J. K., Ngo, K. T., Omoto, J. J., Wong, D. C., Nguyen, J. D., and Hartenstein, V. (2013). Postembryonic lineages of the Drosophila brain: I. Development of the lineage-associated fiber tracts. *Dev. Biol.* 384, 228–257. doi: 10.1016/j.ydbio.2013.07.008

MacMillan, H. A., and Hughson, B. N. (2014). A high-throughput method of hemolymph extraction from adult Drosophila without anesthesia. *J. Insect Physiol.* 63, 27–31. doi: 10.1016/j.jinsphys.2014.02.005

Mayer, F., Mayer, N., Chinn, L., Pinsonneault, R. L., Kroetz, D., and Bainton, R. J. (2009). Evolutionary conservation of vertebrate blood-brain barrier chemoprotective mechanisms in Drosophila. *J. Neurosci.* 29, 3538–3550. doi: 10.1523/JNEUROSCI.5564-08.2009

Melom, J. E., and Littleton, J. T. (2013). Mutation of a NCKX eliminates glial microdomain calcium oscillations and enhances seizure susceptibility. *J. Neurosci.* 33, 1169–1178. doi: 10.1523/JNEUROSCI.3920-12.2013

Miller, M. M., Popova, L. B., Meleshkevitch, E. A., Tran, P. V., and Boudko, D. Y. (2008). The invertebrate B(0) system transporter, D. melanogaster NAT1, has unique d-amino acid affinity and mediates gut and brain functions. *Insect Biochem. Mol. Biol.* 38, 923–931. doi: 10.1016/j.ibmb.2008.07.005

Miyamoto, T., Slone, J., Song, X., and Amrein, H. (2012). A fructose receptor functions as a nutrient sensor in the Drosophila brain. *Cell* 151, 1113–1125. doi: 10.1016/j.cell.2012.10.024

Moussian, B., Tång, E., Tonning, A., Helms, S., Schwarz, H., Nüsslein-Volhard, C., et al. (2006). Drosophila Knickkopf and Retroactive are needed for epithelial tube growth and cuticle differentiation through their specific requirement for chitin filament organization. *Development* 133, 163–171. doi: 10.1242/dev.02177

Mueckler, M., and Thorens, B. (2013). The SLC2 (GLUT) family of membrane transporters. *Mol. Aspects Med.* 34, 121–138. doi: 10.1016/j.mam.2012.07.001

Nagelhus, E. A., and Ottersen, O. P. (2013). Physiological roles of aquaporin-4 in brain. *Physiol. Rev.* 93, 1543–1562. doi: 10.1152/physrev.00011.2013

Naikkhwah, W., and O'Donnell, M. J. (2011). Salt stress alters fluid and ion transport by Malpighian tubules of *Drosophila melanogaster*: evidence for phenotypic plasticity. *J. Exp. Biol.* 214, 3443–3454. doi: 10.1242/jeb.057828

Narasimha, M., Uv, A., Krejci, A., Brown, N. H., and Bray, S. J. (2008). Grainy head promotes expression of septate junction proteins and influences epithelial morphogenesis. *J. Cell Sci.* 121, 747–752. doi: 10.1242/jcs.019422

Nässel, D. R., Kubrak, O. I., Liu, Y., Luo, J., and Lushchak, O. V. (2013). Factors that regulate insulin producing cells and their output in Drosophila. *Front. Physiol.* 4:252. doi: 10.3389/fphys.2013.00252

Nelson, K. S., Furuse, M., and Beitel, G. J. (2010). The Drosophila Claudin Kune-kune is required for septate junction organization and tracheal tube size control. *Genetics* 185, 831–839. doi: 10.1534/genetics.110.114959

Nilton, A., Oshima, K., Zare, F., Byri, S., Nannmark, U., Nyberg, K. G., et al. (2010). Crooked, coiled and crimpled are three Ly6-like proteins required for proper localization of septate junction components. *Development* 137, 2427–2437. doi: 10.1242/dev.052605

Noirot-Timothée, C., Graf, F., and Noirot, C. (1982). The specialization of septate junctions in regions of tricellular junctions. II. Pleated septate junctions. *J. Ultrastruct. Res.* 78, 152–165. doi: 10.1016/S0022-5320(82)80020-8

Oda, Y., Otani, T., Ikenouchi, J., and Furuse, M. (2014). Tricellulin regulates junctional tension of epithelial cells at tricellular contacts via Cdc42. *J. Cell Sci.* doi: 10.1242/jcs.150607. [Epub ahead of print].

Oshima, K., and Fehon, R. G. (2011). Analysis of protein dynamics within the septate junction reveals a highly stable core protein complex that does not include the basolateral polarity protein Discs large. *J. Cell Sci.* 124, 2861–2871. doi: 10.1242/jcs.087700

Padash-Barmchi, M., Browne, K., Sturgeon, K., Jusiak, B., and Auld, V. J. (2010). Control of Gliotactin localization and levels by tyrosine phosphorylation and endocytosis is necessary for survival of polarized epithelia. *J. Cell Sci.* 123, 4052–4062. doi: 10.1242/jcs.066605

Palanker, L., Tennessen, J. M., Lam, G., and Thummel, C. S. (2009). Drosophila HNF4 regulates lipid mobilization and β-oxidation. *Cell Metab.* 9, 228–239. doi: 10.1016/j.cmet.2009.01.009

Palm, W., Sampaio, J. L., Brankatschk, M., Carvalho, M., Mahmoud, A., Shevchenko, A., et al. (2012). Lipoproteins in *Drosophila melanogaster*–assembly, function, and influence on tissue lipid composition. *PLoS Genet.* 8:e1002828. doi: 10.1371/journal.pgen.1002828

Papadopoulos, M. C., and Verkman, A. S. (2013). Aquaporin water channels in the nervous system. *Nat. Rev. Neurosci.* 14, 265–277. doi: 10.1038/nrn3468

Park, D., HadŽiæ, T., Yin, P., Rusch, J., Abruzzi, K., Rosbash, M., et al. (2011). Molecular organization of Drosophila neuroendocrine cells by dimmed. *Curr. Biol.* 21, 1515–1524. doi: 10.1016/j.cub.2011.08.015

Pasco, M. Y., and Léopold, P. (2012). High sugar-induced insulin resistance in Drosophila relies on the lipocalin Neural Lazarillo. *PLoS ONE* 7:e36583. doi: 10.1371/journal.pone.0036583

Paul, S. M., Palladino, M. J., and Beitel, G. J. (2007). A pump-independent function of the Na,K-ATPase is required for epithelial junction function and tracheal tube-size control. *Development* 134, 147–155. doi: 10.1242/dev.02710

Pellerin, L., and Magistretti, P. J. (1994). Glutamate uptake into astrocytes stimulates aerobic glycolysis: a mechanism coupling neuronal activity to glucose utilization. *Proc. Natl. Acad. Sci. U.S.A.* 91, 10625–10629. doi: 10.1073/pnas.91.22.10625

Pellerin, L., and Magistretti, P. J. (2012). Sweet sixteen for ANLS. *J. Cereb. Blood Flow Metab.* 32, 1152–1166. doi: 10.1038/jcbfm.2011.149

Pereanu, W., Shy, D., and Hartenstein, V. (2005). Morphogenesis and proliferation of the larval brain glia in Drosophila. *Dev. Biol.* 283, 191–203. doi: 10.1016/j.ydbio.2005.04.024

Rajan, A., and Perrimon, N. (2012). Drosophila cytokine unpaired 2 regulates physiological homeostasis by remotely controlling insulin secretion. *Cell* 151, 123–137. doi: 10.1016/j.cell.2012.08.019

Rao, Y., Jan, L. Y., and Jan, Y. N. (1990). Similarity of the product of the Drosophila neurogenic gene big brain to transmembrane channel proteins. *Nature* 345, 163–167. doi: 10.1038/345163a0

Reynolds, B., Roversi, P., Laynes, R., Kazi, S., Boyd, C. A. R., and Goberdhan, D. C. I. (2009). Drosophila expresses a CD98 transporter with an evolutionarily conserved structure and amino acid-transport properties. *Biochem. J.* 420, 363–372. doi: 10.1042/BJ20082198

Rickert, C., Kunz, T., Harris, K.-L., Whitington, P. M., and Technau, G. M. (2011). Morphological characterization of the entire interneuron population reveals principles of neuromere organization in the ventral nerve cord of Drosophila. *J. Neurosci.* 31, 15870–15883. doi: 10.1523/JNEUROSCI.4009-11.2011

Rival, T., Soustelle, L., Strambi, C., Besson, M.-T., Iché, M., and Birman, S. (2004). Decreasing glutamate buffering capacity triggers oxidative stress and neuropil degeneration in the Drosophila brain. *Curr. Biol.* 14, 599–605. doi: 10.1016/j.cub.2004.03.039

Romero-Calderón, R., and Krantz, D. E. (2006). Transport of polyamines in Drosophila S2 cells: kinetics, pharmacology and dependence on the plasma membrane proton gradient. *Biochem. J.* 393, 583. doi: 10.1042/BJ20050981

Romero-Calderón, R., Uhlenbrock, G., Borycz, J., Simon, A. F., Grygoruk, A., Yee, S. K., et al. (2008). A glial variant of the vesicular monoamine transporter is required to store histamine in the drosophila visual system. *PLoS Genet.* 4:e1000245. doi: 10.1371/journal.pgen.1000245

Rothstein, J. D., Martin, L., Levey, A. I., Dykes-Hoberg, M., Jin, L., Wu, D., et al. (1994). Localization of neuronal and glial glutamate transporters. *Neuron* 13, 713–725. doi: 10.1016/0896-6273(94)90038-8

Rouach, N., Koulakoff, A., Abudara, V., Willecke, K., and Giaume, C. (2008). Astroglial metabolic networks sustain hippocampal synaptic transmission. *Science* 322, 1551–1555. doi: 10.1126/science.1164022

Saito, M., Awasaki, T., and Hama, C. (2002). Genetic analyses of essential genes in cytological region 61D1-2 to 61F1-2 of *Drosophila melanogaster*. *Mol. Genet. Genomics* 268, 446–454. doi: 10.1007/s00438-002-0770-6

Schmid, A., Chiba, A., and Doe, C. Q. (1999). Clonal analysis of Drosophila embryonic neuroblasts: neural cell types, axon projections and muscle targets. *Development* 126, 4653–4689.

Schmidt, I., Franzdóttir, S. R., Edenfeld, G., Rodrigues, F., Zierau, A., and Klämbt, C. (2011). Transcriptional regulation of peripheral glial cell differentiation in the embryonic nervous system of Drosophila. *Glia* 59, 1264–1272. doi: 10.1002/glia.21123

Schubiger, M., Feng, Y., Fambrough, D. M., and Palka, J. (1994). A mutation of the Drosophila sodium pump alpha subunit gene results in bang-sensitive paralysis. *Neuron* 12, 373–381. doi: 10.1016/0896-6273(94)90278-X

Schulte, J., Tepass, U., and Auld, V. J. (2003). Gliotactin, a novel marker of tricellular junctions, is necessary for septate junction development in Drosophila. *J. Cell Biol.* 161, 991–1000. doi: 10.1083/jcb.200303192

Schwabe, T., Bainton, R. J., Fetter, R. D., Heberlein, U., and Gaul, U. (2005). GPCR signaling is required for blood-brain barrier formation in drosophila. *Cell* 123, 133–144. doi: 10.1016/j.cell.2005.08.037

Segawa, H., Kawakita, M., and Ishida, N. (2002). Human and Drosophila UDP-galactose transporters transport UDP-N-acetylgalactosamine in addition to UDP-galactose. *Eur. J. Biochem.* 269, 128–138. doi: 10.1046/j.0014-2956.2001.02632.x

Sekine, S. U., Haraguchi, S., Chao, K., Kato, T., Luo, L., Miura, M., et al. (2013). Meigo governs dendrite targeting specificity by modulating Ephrin level and N-glycosylation. *Nat. Neurosci.* 16, 683–691. doi: 10.1038/nn.3389

Shandala, T., Takizawa, K., and Saint, R. (2003). The dead ringer/retained transcriptional regulatory gene is required for positioning of the longitudinal glia in the Drosophila embryonic CNS. *Development* 130, 1505–1513. doi: 10.1242/dev.00377

Shim, J., Gururaja-Rao, S., and Banerjee, U. (2013). Nutritional regulation of stem and progenitor cells in Drosophila. *Development* 140, 4647–4656. doi: 10.1242/dev.079087

Shim, M. S., Kim, J. Y., Lee, K. H., Jung, H. K., Carlson, B. A., Xu, X. M., et al. (2011). l(2)01810 is a novel type of glutamate transporter that is responsible for megamitochondrial formation. *Biochem. J.* 439, 277–286. doi: 10.1042/BJ20110582

Silies, M., Yuva, Y., Engelen, D., Aho, A., Stork, T., and Klämbt, C. (2007). Glial cell migration in the eye disc. *J. Neurosci.* 27, 13130–13139. doi: 10.1523/JNEUROSCI.3583-07.2007

Smith, Q. R. (2000). Transport of glutamate and other amino acids at the blood-brain barrier. *J. Nutr.* 130, 1016S–1022S.

Sousa-Nunes, R., Yee, L. L., and Gould, A. P. (2011). Fat cells reactivate quiescent neuroblasts via TOR and glial insulin relays in Drosophila. *Nature* 471, 508–512. doi: 10.1038/nature09867

Soustelle, L., Besson, M.-T., Rival, T., and Birman, S. (2002). Terminal glial differentiation involves regulated expression of the excitatory amino acid transporters in the Drosophila embryonic CNS. *Dev. Biol.* 248, 294–306. doi: 10.1006/dbio.2002.0742

Spéder, P., and Brand, A. H. (2014). Gap junction proteins in the blood-brain barrier control nutrient-dependent reactivation of drosophila neural stem cells. *Dev. Cell.* 30, 309–321. doi: 10.1016/j.devcel.2014.05.021

Stacey, S. M., Muraro, N. I., Peco, E., Labbé, A., Thomas, G. B., Baines, R. A., et al. (2010). Drosophila glial glutamate transporter Eaat1 is regulated by fringe-mediated notch signaling and is essential for larval locomotion. *J. Neurosci.* 30, 14446–14457. doi: 10.1523/JNEUROSCI.1021-10.2010

Stork, T., Bernardos, R., and Freeman, M. R. (2012). Analysis of glial cell development and function in Drosophila. *Cold Spring Harb. Protoc.* 2012, 1–17. doi: 10.1101/pdb.top067587

Stork, T., Engelen, D., Krudewig, A., Silies, M., Bainton, R. J., and Klämbt, C. (2008). Organization and function of the blood-brain barrier in Drosophila. *J. Neurosci.* 28, 587–597. doi: 10.1523/JNEUROSCI.4367-07.2008

Stork, T., Sheehan, A., Tasdemir-Yilmaz, O. E., and Freeman, M. R. (2014). Neuron-glia interactions through the heartless FGF receptor signaling pathway mediate morphogenesis of Drosophila astrocytes. *Neuron* 83, 388–403. doi: 10.1016/j.neuron.2014.06.026

Sun, Q., Tian, E., Turner, R. J., and Ten Hagen, K. G. (2010). Developmental and functional studies of the SLC12 gene family members from *Drosophila melanogaster*. *Am. J. Physiol. Cell Physiol.* 298, C26–C37. doi: 10.1152/ajpcell.00376.2009

Syed, M. H., Krudewig, A., Engelen, D., Stork, T., and Klämbt, C. (2011). The CD59 family member leaky/coiled is required for the establishment of the blood-brain barrier in Drosophila. *J. Neurosci.* 31, 7876–7885. doi: 10.1523/JNEUROSCI.0766-11.2011

Tatsumi, K., Tsuji, S., Miwa, H., Morisaku, T., Nuriya, M., Orihara, M., et al. (2009). Drosophila big brain does not act as a water channel, but mediates cell adhesion. *FEBS Lett.* 583, 2077–2082. doi: 10.1016/j.febslet.2009.05.035

Tepass, U., and Hartenstein, V. (1994). The development of cellular junctions in the Drosophila embryo. *Dev. Biol.* 161, 563–596. doi: 10.1006/dbio.1994.1054

Thimgan, M. S., Berg, J. S., and Stuart, A. E. (2006). Comparative sequence analysis and tissue localization of members of the SLC6 family of transporters in adult *Drosophila melanogaster*. *J. Exp. Biol.* 209, 3383–3404. doi: 10.1242/jeb.02328

Thomas, G. B., and van Meyel, D. J. (2007). The glycosyltransferase Fringe promotes delta-notch signaling between neurons and glia, and is required for subtype-specific glial gene expression. *Development* 134, 591–600. doi: 10.1242/dev.02754

Tiklová, K., Senti, K.-A., Wang, S., Gräslund, A., and Samakovlis, C. (2010). Epithelial septate junction assembly relies on melanotransferrin iron binding and endocytosis in Drosophila. *Nat. Cell Biol.* 12, 1071–1077. doi: 10.1038/ncb2111

Tsacopoulos, M., Veuthey, A. L., Saravelos, S. G., Perrottet, P., and Tsoupras, G. (1994). Glial cells transform glucose to alanine, which fuels the neurons in the honeybee retina. *J. Neurosci.* 14, 1339–1351.

Uldry, M., and Thorens, B. (2004). The SLC2 family of facilitated hexose and polyol transporters. *Pflugers Arch.* 447, 480–489. doi: 10.1007/s00424-003-1085-0

Unhavaithaya, Y., and Orr-Weaver, T. L. (2012). Polyploidization of glia in neural development links tissue growth to blood-brain barrier integrity. *Genes Dev.* 26, 31–36. doi: 10.1101/gad.177436.111

Urbach, R., and Technau, G. M. (2003). Molecular markers for identified neuroblasts in the developing brain of Drosophila. *Development* 130, 3621–3637. doi: 10.1242/dev.00533

Venken, K. J. T., Simpson, J. H., and Bellen, H. J. (2011). Genetic manipulation of genes and cells in the nervous system of the fruit fly. *Neuron* 72, 202–230. doi: 10.1016/j.neuron.2011.09.021

Vincent, S., Vonesch, J. L., and Giangrande, A. (1996). Glide directs glial fate commitment and cell fate switch between neurones and glia. *Development* 122, 131–139.

Wheeler, S. R., Kearney, J. B., Guardiola, A. R., and Crews, S. T. (2006). Single-cell mapping of neural and glial gene expression in the developing Drosophila CNS midline cells. *Dev. Biol.* 294, 509–524. doi: 10.1016/j.ydbio.2006.03.016

Woods, D. F., Hough, C., Peel, D., Callaini, G., and Bryant, P. J. (1996). Dlg protein is required for junction structure, cell polarity, and proliferation control in Drosophila epithelia. *J. Cell Biol.* 134, 1469–1482. doi: 10.1083/jcb.134.6.1469

Wu, V. M., and Beitel, G. J. (2004). A junctional problem of apical proportions: epithelial tube-size control by septate junctions in the Drosophila tracheal system. *Curr. Opin. Cell Biol.* 16, 493–499. doi: 10.1016/j.ceb.2004.07.008

Wu, V. M., Yu, M. H., Paik, R., Banerjee, S., Liang, Z., Paul, S. M., et al. (2007). Drosophila Varicose, a member of a new subgroup of basolateral MAGUKs, is required for septate junctions and tracheal morphogenesis. *Development* 134, 999–1009. doi: 10.1242/dev.02785

Wyatt, G. R., and Kalf, G. F. (1957). The chemistry of insect hemolymph II. Trehalose and other carbohydrates. *J. Gen. Physiol.* 40, 833–847. doi: 10.1085/jgp.40.6.833

7

The inner CSF–brain barrier: developmentally controlled access to the brain via intercellular junctions

Sophie Whish[1], Katarzyna M. Dziegielewska[1], Kjeld Møllgård[2], Natassya M. Noor[1], Shane A. Liddelow[1,3], Mark D. Habgood[1], Samantha J. Richardson[4] and Norman R. Saunders[1]*

[1] *Department of Pharmacology and Therapeutics, University of Melbourne, Parkville, VIC, Australia*
[2] *Department of Cellular and Molecular Medicine, Institute of Cellular and Molecular Medicine, University of Copenhagen, Copenhagen, Denmark*
[3] *Department of Neurobiology, Stanford University, Palo Alto, CA, USA*
[4] *School of Medical Sciences, RMIT University, Bundoora, VIC, Australia*

***Correspondence:**
Norman R. Saunders, Department of Pharmacology and Therapeutics, University of Melbourne, Grattan Street, Parkville, VIC 3010, Australia
e-mail: n.saunders@unimelb.edu.au

In the adult the interface between the cerebrospinal fluid and the brain is lined by the ependymal cells, which are joined by gap junctions. These intercellular connections do not provide a diffusional restrain between the two compartments. However, during development this interface, initially consisting of neuroepithelial cells and later radial glial cells, is characterized by "strap" junctions, which limit the exchange of different sized molecules between cerebrospinal fluid and the brain parenchyma. Here we provide a systematic study of permeability properties of this inner cerebrospinal fluid-brain barrier during mouse development from embryonic day, E17 until adult. Results show that at fetal stages exchange across this barrier is restricted to the smallest molecules (286Da) and the diffusional restraint is progressively removed as the brain develops. By postnatal day P20, molecules the size of plasma proteins (70 kDa) diffuse freely. Transcriptomic analysis of junctional proteins present in the cerebrospinal fluid-brain interface showed expression of adherens junctional proteins, actins, cadherins and catenins changing in a development manner consistent with the observed changes in the permeability studies. Gap junction proteins were only identified in the adult as was claudin-11. Immunohistochemistry was used to localize at the cellular level some of the adherens junctional proteins of genes identified from transcriptomic analysis. N-cadherin, β- and α-catenin immunoreactivity was detected outlining the inner CSF-brain interface from E16; most of these markers were not present in the adult ependyma. Claudin-5 was present in the apical-most part of radial glial cells and in endothelial cells in embryos, but only in endothelial cells including plexus endothelial cells in adults. Claudin-11 was only immunopositive in the adult, consistent with results obtained from transcriptomic analysis. These results provide information about physiological, molecular and morphological-related permeability changes occurring at the inner cerebrospinal fluid-brain barrier during brain development.

Keywords: cerebrospinal fluid, brain development, barriers, permeability, ventricular zone

INTRODUCTION

The exchange of molecules between the brain and the periphery is restricted by specific cellular and biochemical mechanisms present at several interfaces between these two compartments: the blood–brain barrier proper, the blood–cerebrospinal fluid (CSF) barrier, the blood-arachnoid barrier and the (inner) CSF–brain barrier only present during brain development (Møllgård et al., 1987; Saunders et al., 2012). The morphological basis of blood–brain and blood–CSF barriers is the presence of tight junctions between cerebral vascular endothelial cells and choroid plexus epithelial cells respectively. These junctions restrict free diffusion between the blood, the brain parenchyma and the CSF (for reviews see Saunders et al., 1999, 2000, 2012; Dziegielewska and Saunders, 2002; Ek et al., 2012; Engelhardt and Liebner, 2014). Much less is known about the development of CSF–brain interface. Junctions between cells lining the ventricular system of the developing brain were first described on the basis of conventional electron microscopy as modified tight or intermediate junctions, or as desmosomes (Tennyson and Pappas, 1962; Duckett, 1968; Levitt et al., 1981). Subsequent studies characterized these junctions in fetal sheep using thin-section and freeze-fracture electron microscopy and established that they had a very different structural arrangement compared with tight junctions. Unlike tight junctions, which appear to join cells in a "belt-like fashion" at their luminal lateral cell membranes, these novel junctions, named "strap junctions," appeared to encircle cells from their ventricular surface (Møllgård et al., 1987) and were shown to

Abbreviations: CSF, cerebrospinal fluid; RNA-Seq, RNA sequencing; BDA, biotinylated dextran amine; BED; biotin ethylenediamine; kDa, kilodalton.

hinder the free diffusion of solutes from the CSF into the fetal brain (Fossan et al., 1985). In contrast to tight junctions of blood–brain and blood–CSF barriers, which are present from the earliest stages of brain development and remain throughout adulthood (Møllgård and Saunders, 1986; Mishra and Teale, 2012; Saunders et al., 2012), strap junctions are only present during development, with minimal gap junctions between some neuroepithelial cells; in the mature brain only gap junctions are present (Brightman and Reese, 1969; Møllgård and Saunders, 1986; Møllgård et al., 1987; Iliff et al., 2012). Additional evidence for the presence of a developmentally regulated CSF–brain barrier came from a study examining the cellular distribution of native and foreign albumins injected into fetal and neonatal lateral ventricles of rats (Cavanagh and Warren, 1985). This study showed that both types of albumin were distributed in some (but not all) cells lining the ventricles suggesting specialized uptake rather than paracellular unrestricted diffusion (Cavanagh and Warren, 1985).

The fetal-specific interface that separates CSF from the brain's internal milieu is thought to control the transfer and diffusion of solutes into the brain and play an important role in restricting access of protein, present in high concentration in fetal CSF (Dziegielewska et al., 1980, 1981, 1986, 1989; Adinolfi, 1985; Dziegielewska and Saunders, 1988), across the ventricular zone, which initially consists of neuroepithelial cells that subsequently differentiate to radial glial cells prior to neurogenesis. This, combined with an increase in colloidal osmotic pressure due to the high protein concentration responsible for the expansion of the ventricles and outward growth of the brain (Desmond and Jacobson, 1977), are fundamental mechanisms controlling normal brain development (Saunders, 1992; Johansson et al., 2008; Saunders et al., 2012). The presence of this diffusion restraint during brain development has been suggested to be important for normal cortical development (Stolp et al., 2011b) and its disturbance is thought to contribute to several neurodevelopmental pathologies such as autism (Stolp, 2013; Stolp et al., 2013).

The present study is the first comprehensive investigation into the permeability properties of the inner CSF-brain interface during development, using lipid insoluble molecular markers with a range of sizes from 286 to 70,000 Da. We report that permeability of this barrier in mouse brain gradually changes from highly restrictive at fetal ages to an unrestricted diffusion in the adult. Molecular characterization, using RNA sequencing performed at a fetal and adult age, identified several known junctional proteins that are expressed at the CSF-brain barrier in a developmentally regulated manner. In addition to the transcriptomic analysis we also demonstrated that the change in the permeability characteristics coincided with changes in the cellular distribution of several junctional proteins such as cadherins, catenins and claudin-5. We propose that these junctional proteins are involved in the formation of strap junctions and in regulation of the changing diffusional properties of this barrier.

MATERIALS AND METHODS

ANIMAL EXPERIMENTATION

Ethics statement

All experimental protocols were approved by the Animal Ethics Committee, University of Melbourne (Application ID 1112115.2).

Animal experiments

Time-mated pregnant Swiss Pro mice were obtained from the Animal Resource Centre Pty. Ltd. (ARC, Perth, Australia). Animals were housed in the Biomedical Sciences Animal Facility (University of Melbourne) in sterile micro-isolator cages at 20°C on a 12 h light/dark cycle with food and water *ad libitum*.

Ages of mice used for permeability studies and for estimates of total protein concentration in plasma and CSF were: embryonic day (E) 17, E19 and postnatal day (P) 0, P10, P20 and adult (20–25 g). For transcriptome analysis, RNA-Seq, ventricular/ependymal layer was dissected out from fetal brains at E17/18, and adult (see below). For morphological studies paraffin embedded sections from fetal stages, E15/16, E17-19 and postnatal stages, P15, P20 and adult mice brains were used. These were obtained from previous studies (Liddelow et al., 2012).

Anesthesia

In experiments involving fetal animals, pregnant mice (E17–E19) were anesthetized by an intraperitoneal (i.p.) injection of urethane (30% in distilled water, Veterinary Companies of Australia (VCA), Australia). Two doses of 0.2 ml were given 20 min apart. Animals were monitored during this process and pain reflexes were observed. When the pain reflexes were no longer evident, mice were placed supine on a heated pad (33°C) and the uterine horns were exposed. Each fetus was removed consecutively from the uterine horn. After all fetuses were removed, the mother was killed by transection of the heart.

Postnatal pups of both sexes (P0, P10, and P20) and adult female mice were individually anesthetized using inhaled Isoflurane (VCA). Once deep anesthesia was obtained the animals were placed under the dissecting microscope, and several experimental procedures were conducted as described below.

Total protein concentration

Blood and CSF were collected from 3 to 4 pups at each age and from 3 to 4 adults. Blood was collected from the heart of terminally anesthetized animals using either a heparinized 1 ml syringe with a 26-gauge needle (adults) or a heparinized pulled glass micro-capillary (fetuses and postnatal pups) and centrifuged to separate plasma. CSF was collected from the *cisterna magna* via gentle suction using a fine glass micro-capillary and PVC tubing to obtain paired samples. CSF samples were inspected under a microscope for blood contamination (Habgood et al., 1993). For fetal animals CSF samples were pooled from several littermates to obtain a large enough volume. Plasma and CSF samples were stored at −20°C until use.

Total protein concentrations in plasma and CSF samples were estimated using the Bradford method (Bradford, 1976) and Protein Standard (Binding Sites, UK). All dilutions of the standards in the range of 1–10 ug/100 ul (in triplicate) and samples (in duplicate) were made in sterile saline. Plasma samples were diluted 1000x while CSF ranged from 100x to 10x depending on the age (Dziegielewska et al., 1979). The volume of both the standards and the samples was always 100 μl as described in the original method (Bradford, 1976). The concentration of the total protein in each sample was measured from constructed concentration curves and expressed in mg 100 ml^{-1} a standard unit in the field (Dziegielewska et al., 1979, 1989).

CSF-brain barrier permeability experiments

Rhodamine–conjugated biotinylated dextran amines, BDAs, of molecular masses 3000 Da (3 kDa), 10000 Da (10 kDa) and 70000Da (70 kDa) and a 286 Da biotin ethylenediamine hydrobromide (BED) obtained from Molecular Probes (USA) were used in these experiments. Three to four individual mice from at least two separate litters were obtained for each experiment. All probes were diluted in sterile saline (25 $mgml^{-1}$) and were injected into the right ventricle of anesthetized animals via a glass microcapillary and gentle pressure (see **Figure 1**). Injected volumes are listed in **Table 1**. Following injection the markers were allowed to distribute for a further 2–3 min (fetal), 5 min (postnatal ages to P20) or 10 min (adults) so that each dextran would flow into the contralateral ventricle. Brains of animals injected with fluorescence BDAs were dissected out from the skull and fixed by immersion in 4% paraformaldehyde (PFA) for 24 h at 4°C. Brains from pups injected with BED were fixed in Bouin's fixative for 24 h and processed for paraffin embedding (see below).

Fluorescence microscopy

At the end of permeability experiments and following fixation, brains were embedded in high gel strength 4% Agar (Sigma Aldrich) and sectioned in the coronal plane at 80 μm using a vibrating microtome (Leica). All sections containing the lateral ventricles were collected for analysis. Each section was mounted on a glass slide using fluorescence mounting medium (DAKO). Slides were kept at 4°C and covered with foil to restrict light exposure. All sections were viewed with an Olympus BX50 fluorescent light microscope with a filter specific for rhodamine. Digitized photographs were taken using an Olympus DP70 camera that was attached to the microscope and processed in Adobe Photoshop CC® (Adobe® Systems Incorporated, USA). The brightness and color balance functions were used to obtain images with a background close to black to enhance contrast and to standardize obtained images.

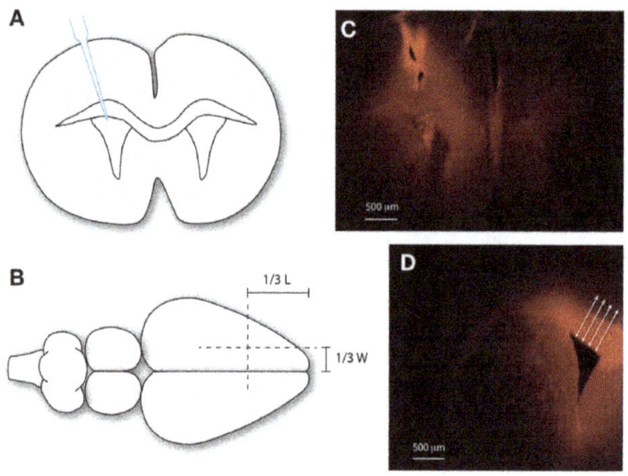

FIGURE 1 | Injection of biotin dextran amines into the ventricular system of mice. Schematic diagrams **(A,B)** and images **(C,D)** illustrating the methods used to inject dextrans into the lateral ventricles of mouse brain. **(A)** Micropipette injection of dextran into lateral ventricle. **(B)** Illustrates surface landmarks for injection site. **(C)** Distribution of dextran following injection. **(D)** Method used to measure diffusion distance of dextrans (red) using ImageJ64. Mean of 10 measurements, spanning the ventricular zone at right angles to ventricular surface (arrows). Scale bars 500 μm in **(C,D)**. L, length; W, width.

Table 1 | Volumes and times of injected probes at different ages.

Age	Volume	Time
E17, P0	1 μl	2, 3 min
P5, P10	5 μl	5 min
P20, Adult	10 μl	5, 10 min

Immunohistochemistry

Paraffin-embedded coronal sections from mice from fetal ages E15-16, E17-19 and postnatal ages P15, P20 and adult were obtained from previous studies (Liddelow et al., 2012). Prior to immunohistochemical processing sections were deparaffinized and rehydrated in xylene followed by a series of graded alcohols, treated with a 0.5% solution of hydrogen peroxide in methanol for 15 min to quench endogenous peroxidase, and then rinsed in TRIS buffered saline (TBS, 5 mM Tris-HCl, 146 mM NaCl, pH 7.6). Non-specific binding was removed by incubation for 30 min with blocking buffer (ChemMate antibody diluent S2022, DakoCytomation, Glostrup, Denmark) at room temperature. The sections were incubated overnight at 4°C with rabbit polyclonal or mouse monoclonal antibodies against claudin-5, claudin-11, α-catenin, β-catenin and N-cadherin (details in **Table 2**). Following primary antibody incubation the sections were washed with TBS and incubated for 30 min with the REAL EnVision™ Detection System, Peroxidase/DAB+, Rabbit/Mouse, (K5007) from DakoCytomation. The sections were counterstained with Mayer's hematoxylin and dehydrated in graded alcohols followed by xylene and coverslipped with DPX mounting medium. Control sections were incubated with mouse IgG1, IgG2a or non-specific unrelated rabbit antibodies, as well as subjected to omission of primary or secondary antibodies. These were always blank.

Sections were viewed with an Olympus bright field microscope and photographs taken with only brightness manipulated to obtain comparable images. Three to four sections from a minimum of three brains at each age were developed with each antibody.

Detection of BED

Brains from BED injected fetal mice were paraffin-embedded as described previously (Liddelow et al., 2011) and 5 μm serial coronal sections cut through the cortex encompassing

Table 2 | Antibodies used for immunohistochemistry.

Antigen	Manufacturer	Code no.	Species	Dilution
Cadherin N	Abcam	ab12221	Rabbit	1:500
Catenin a E	Santa cruz	sc-7894	Rabbit	1:100
Catenin ß	Zymed	13-8400	Mouse	1:100
Claudin 5	Abcam	ab15108	Rabbit	1:150
Claudin 11	Abcam	ab53041	Rabbit	1:1500

the lateral ventricles. Five sections spanning the whole lateral ventricular system were processed for histological staining using the ABC detection method (Vector laboratories) and 3, 3′–diaminobenzidine (DAB) chromagen substrate developer (DAKO) following manufactures' instructions. De-waxing, rehydration, dehydration and mounting of sections with DPX were performed as described above. Sections from brains not injected with BED served as controls and these were always blank.

RNA sequencing analysis

The lateral aspect of the ventricular zone of E17/18 and adult mouse brains was carefully dissected (**Figure 1**). Tissue from five brains, collected from three different litters, was pooled randomly to obtain three equal samples at each age and was processed for RNA sequencing.

RNA extraction

Total RNA was extracted from pools of E17/18 lateral ventricular zone and adult lateral ependymal zone ($n = 3$ for both ages) using the RNeasy Mini Kit, Qiashredder columns and gDNA removal columns (Qiagen, Valencia, CA, USA) according to standard supplier protocol. Total RNA samples were quantified using a NanoDrop ND-1000 UV-VIS spectrophotometer (Thermo Scientific, Wilmington, DE, USA).

Illumina next generation RNA sequencing

As previously described for an RNA-Seq study of developing choroid plexus (Liddelow et al., 2013) sequencing was performed at the Australian Genome Research Facility (Melbourne, VIC, Australia). A cDNA library was prepared from 10 μg of total RNA using the mRNA-Seq Sample Preparation Kit (Illumina, San Diego, CA, USA) according to standard manufacturer protocol. Quality of the library was verified using a DNA 1000 chip using the Agilent 2100 Bioanalyzer (Agilent) and quantified by fluorimetry. Only samples with an RNA Integrity Number close to 10.0 were kept for further sequencing experiments. The library was subjected to 100 bp single end read cycles of sequencing on an Illumina HiSeq 2000 sequencer as per manufacturer protocol. Cluster generation was performed on a c-Bot (Illumina) with a single read cluster generation kit.

RNA sequencing data analysis

Short reads were trimmed to remove ambiguous bases from the start and segments with low quality scores from the end, as indicated by the ascii character "B" in Illumina 1.5 phred score encoding. Trimmed reads were mapped with Bowtie version 0.12.7 (Langmead et al., 2009) to the Ensembl (Hubbard et al., 2009) rat genome, release 61. Reads that did not map uniquely were discarded. The number of reads mapped to nuclear genes was determined with HTSeq (Anders et al., 2015) version 0.4.7p4, using the default "union" counting option. Differential expression between the adult and embryonic samples was detected using an exact test in the Bioconductor (Gentleman et al., 2004) edgeR package, version 2.4.0 (Robinson et al., 2010), with common dispersion used to estimate variance between samples. Genes considered significantly differentially expressed were those with a p-value of less than 0.05 after Benjamini-Hochberg false discovery rate correction. A combination of gene ontology annotation and manual curation was used to select genes encoding proteins that form part of a cell junction. Gene ontology descriptions for rat were downloaded from Biomart (Hubbard et al., 2009), and genes with "junction" mentioned in their gene ontology description were selected. Junction genes of interest were then extracted from this list. Similar searches were carried for other functional categories as described in the Results/Discussion below. For initial analysis genes with >100 sequence reads and age-related fold changes (FC) >2.0 ($\log_2$FC > 1.0) were collated and are summarized in **Tables 1–4**. For more specific analysis of some particular function categories a lower cut-off of 10 sequence reads was used. Complete sequencing data have been deposited in the Gene

Table 3 | RNASeq expression of junction-associated genes in embryonic day 17 (E17) and adult ependymal cells.

(A) E17 expression		(B) Adult expression	
Gene ID	**FPKM (AVE)**	**Gene ID**	**FPKM (AVE)**
Actb	805.8	*Cldn11*	304.7
Ctnnb1	114.6	*Actb*	115.8
Actr1a	39.1	*Gja1*	35.8
Cdh2	23.4	*Pkp4*	31.2
Actr2	14.2	*Ctnnb1*	29.0
Actl6b	7.7	*Actr1a*	10.3
Ctnna2	4.6	*Actr1b*	6.8
Actr3	4.3	*Actr2*	6.0
Pcdhgc3	3.8	*Gjc3*	5.5
Ctnnd2	3.8	*Jam3*	3.5
Actr10	2.7	*Ctnna1*	2.6
Actr1b	2.1	*Actn4*	2.2
Actg1	2.0	*Ctnnd2*	2.0
Ctnnbip1	1.6	*Cdh2*	1.9
Ctnna1	1.4	*Gjb1*	1.9
Actn4	1.3	*Ctnna2*	1.3
Ctnnbl1	1.3	*Actr10*	1.2
Cdh13	1.2	*Actr3b*	1.1
Cldn5	1.0	*Pcdhgc3*	1.1
Cdh11	0.8	*Actr3b*	1.1
Cdh4	0.7	*Actl6b*	0.9
Actr3b	0.7	*Pcdh10*	0.8
Pkp4	0.6	*Tjp1*	0.7
Pcdh10	0.5	*Cdh13*	0.5
Gja1	0.3	*Jam2*	0.4
Pcdh17	0.3	*Cldn5*	0.3
Tjp1	0.2	*Ctnnbip1*	0.3
Jam2	0.2	*Cdh11*	0.2
Jam3	0.2	*Ctnnbl1*	0.2
Cldn11	0.0	*Pcdh17*	0.2
Gjb1	0.0	*Actg1*	0.2
Gjc3	0.0	*Cdh4*	0.0

Data are average FPKM (fragments per kilobase of exon per million fragments mapped) from three independent pooled samples of ventricular zone from embryonic day 17 (E17) and adult rats. Genes with FPKM expression < 1.0 were considered not expressed (underlined in Table).

Table 4 | Gene expression of junction related genes in embryonic ventricular zone and adult ventricular ependyma.

Gene ID	Fold change(E17/Adult)	Fold change(Adult/E17)
ACTINS		
Actb	6.96	0.14
Actg1	Present in embryo only	
Actl6b	Present in embryo only	
Actn4	No difference between ages	
Actr10	2.32	0.43
Actr1a	3.79	0.26
Actr1b	0.32	3.17
Actr2	2.36	0.42
Actr3	3.94	0.25
Actr3b	Present in adult only	
CADHERINS		
Cdh13	Present in embryo only	
Cdh2	12.53	0.08
CLAUDINS		
Cldn11	Present in adult only	
Cldn5	Present in embryo only	
CATENINS		
Ctnna1	No difference between ages	
Ctnna2	3.54	0.28
Ctnnb1	3.95	0.25
Ctnnbip1	Present in embryo only	
Ctnnbl1	Present in embryo only	
Ctnnd2	No difference between ages	
GAP JUNCTION PROTEINS		
Gja1	Present in adult only	
Gjb1	Present in adult only	
Gjc3	Present in adult only	
JUNCTIONAL ADHESION MOLECULES		
Jam2	Present in adult only	
Jam3	Present in adult only	
PROTOCADHERIN		
Pcdhgc3	3.49	0.29
PLAKOPHILIN		
Pkp4	Present in adult only	

Average fold change in FPKM (fragments per kilobase of exon per million fragments mapped) from three independent pooled samples of ventricular zone from embryonic day 17 (E17) and ependyma from adult rats.

Expression Omnibus (http://www.ncbi.nlm.nih.gov/geo/) under accession code GSE44072.

Statistical analysis

Where applicable, data are expressed as mean ± SEM, or as a single mean value (RNA sequencing data). Where no SEM is provided the data are either a single value or a mean of two.

RESULTS

This study aimed to characterize the permeability properties of the CSF–brain interface during mouse development and to correlate it with changes in the expression of identified junctional proteins and cellular distribution of their protein products.

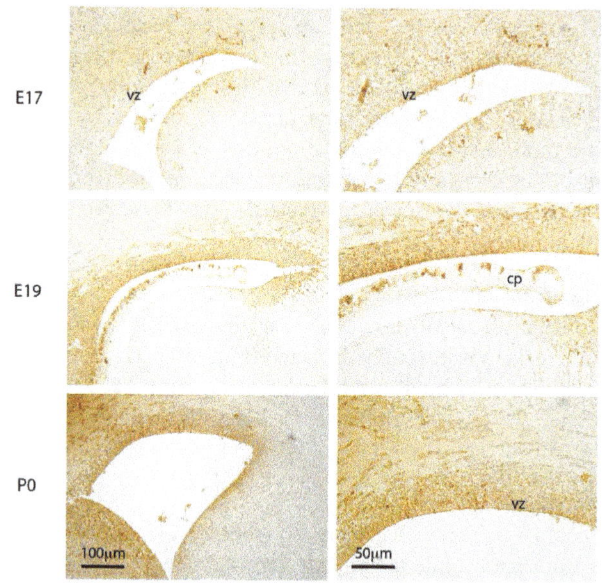

FIGURE 2 | Distribution of Biotin Ethylene Diamine (BED). Coronal sections (paraffin embedded) through cortical wall surrounding lateral ventricles of E17, E19, and P0 mouse brain after BED injection into the contralateral ventricle. Developed with DAB reaction. Note that at E17 there is cellular uptake of BED in some regions of the ventricular zone, but none appears to have penetrated into the brain extracellular space. At E19 and P0 there is both cellular uptake and diffusion into the extracellular space of the brain, especially into the ventral side of the ventricle. Much less staining is detected in the medial wall at all three ages. VZ, ventricular zone; CP, choroid plexus. Scale bar 100 µm in left panels and 50 µm in right panels.

PERMEABILITY PROPERTIES OF THE CSF-BRAIN BARRIER IN DEVELOPMENT

The permeability characteristics of the CSF–brain barrier were investigated using three different sized biotinylated dextran amines conjugated with rhodamine: 3, 10, and 70 kDa. In addition a small marker of 268 Da (BED) was used in fetal animals at E17, E19, and in P0. All animals, from E17 to adult, received an injection of 25 mg ml^{-1} of marker in sterile saline into one lateral ventricle as described in the Materials and Methods. Vibratome and paraffin-embedded microtome-cut sections from the ventricle contralateral to the injected side were analyzed. Results are illustrated in **Figures 2, 3** and summarized in **Figure 4.**

268DA BIOTIN ETHYLENEDIAMINE (BED)

Following injections into the lateral ventricle of E17 mice, BED was detected in many cells lining the ventricular system but not in at all aspects of the ventricular lining. BED reaction product was also faintly visible in the extracellular space of the ventricular zone between the cells (**Figure 2**). By E19 and P0, cellular uptake of BED was visible at all aspects of the ventricular lining and the extracellular staining in the brain parenchyma was clearly positive (illustrated in **Figure 3**). The results from fetal animals indicated that at these ages there is limited diffusion of molecules as small as 286 Da BED, between radial glial cells lining the CSF-brain interface. Uptake by individual ventricular cells was also present (**Figure 2**).

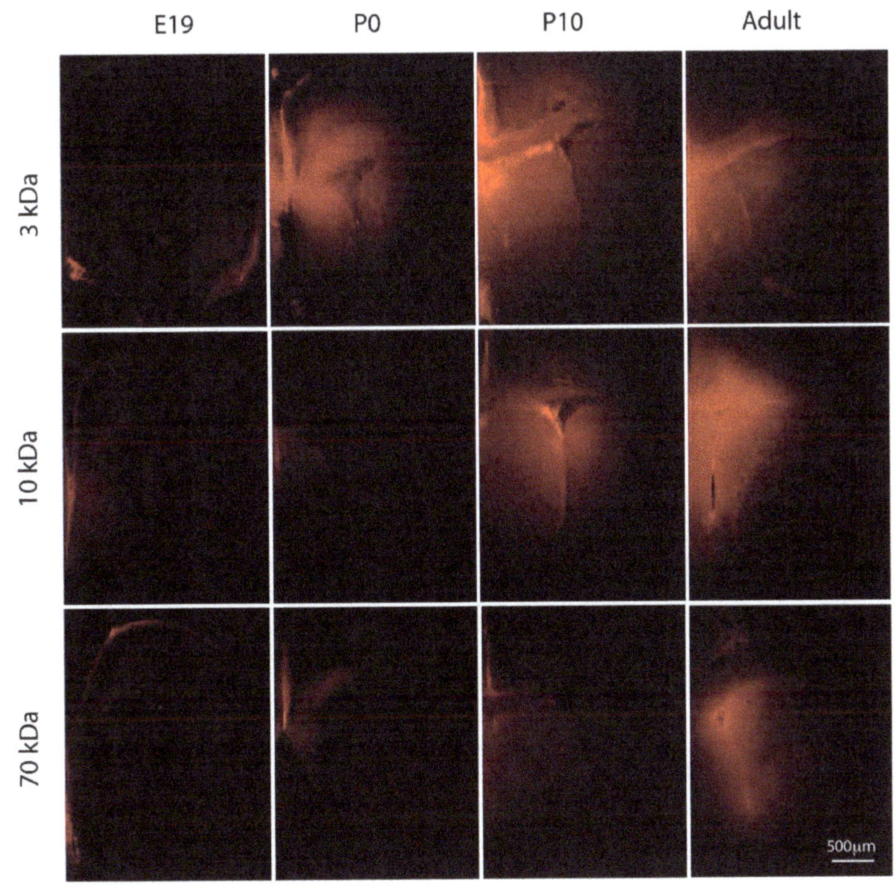

FIGURE 3 | Diffusion of different sized rhodamine labeled biotinylated dextrans (BDA) into postnatal mouse brain. Vibratome coronal sections (80 μm thick) through cortex of mice injected with different sized BDAs (3, 10, and 70 kDa). Markers were injected into the contralateral ventricle and left to diffuse for 2–3 min at E19 and P0, 5 min at P10 and 10 min in the adult. Note that none of the dextrans entered the brain at E19. In older brains there was a progressive increase in penetration depending on the size of the dextran. By adulthood all three dextrans were entering the brain to a similar extent. Apparent diffusion distances shown in **Figure 4**. Distribution of BED (286 Da) is illustrated in **Figure 2** for comparison. E, embryonic day; P, postnatal day. Scale bar 500 μm.

3 KDA RHODAMINE BDA (BDA3 KDA)

Following injections of BDA3 kDa into fetal (E17 and E19) lateral ventricles BDA3 kDa was detected in some cells lining the ventricular zone (**Figure 3**) but was not detected in the extracellular space of the brain, indicating that at these ages the diffusion of molecules of at least 3 kDa across the CSF-brain barrier was limited. It is possible that the specialized cellular uptake of small molecules may be the primary mechanism allowing their access to the early developing brain.

The earliest age at which diffuse labeling in the extracellular space of the brain was detected was in newborn pups (P0). At that age more BDA3 kDa appeared to diffuse into the medial aspect of the ventricle (as shown by a greater intensity of fluorescent marker, **Figure 3**) and indicates that the permeability of the inner CSF–brain barrier allows unhindered diffusion of a 3 kDa molecule from about the time of birth in mice (**Figures 3, 4**).

10 kDa RHODAMINE BDA (BDA10 kDa)

Diffusion of BDA10 kDa into the brain around the whole ventricular zone interface was prevented in E17 and E19 mice, as no fluorescent labeling was visible at either age in the brain (see **Figure 3**). At P0 results for BDA10 kDa were variable—a small amount of the marker (not measurable) was detected diffusing into the extracellular space of the ventricular zone in one pup from one litter, while in 2 other pups no diffusion was observed. This may indicate that at this stage of development there is a change in the permeability properties of the CSF–brain interface and a small difference (hours) in the age of the pups could explain the observed results. At older ages (P10 to adult) BDA10 kDa was found in brains from all animals including some intercellular presence in the ependymal layer. Thus, the permeability of the CSF–brain barrier changes between P0 and P10 to allow the diffusion of molecules up to 10 kDa (**Figures 3, 4**).

70 kDa RHODAMINE BDA (BDA70 kDa)

The earliest age at which BDA70 kDa was observed to diffuse into the brain was in P10 animals (**Figure 3**); however, this was only detected in the medial and lateral aspects of the ventricle. At P20 results were variable. In one litter, where two pups received an injection of 70 kDa, diffusion into the ventricular zone was apparent in one brain but not in the other. In pups from a second litter ($n = 2$), diffusion was not observed in the brain of either

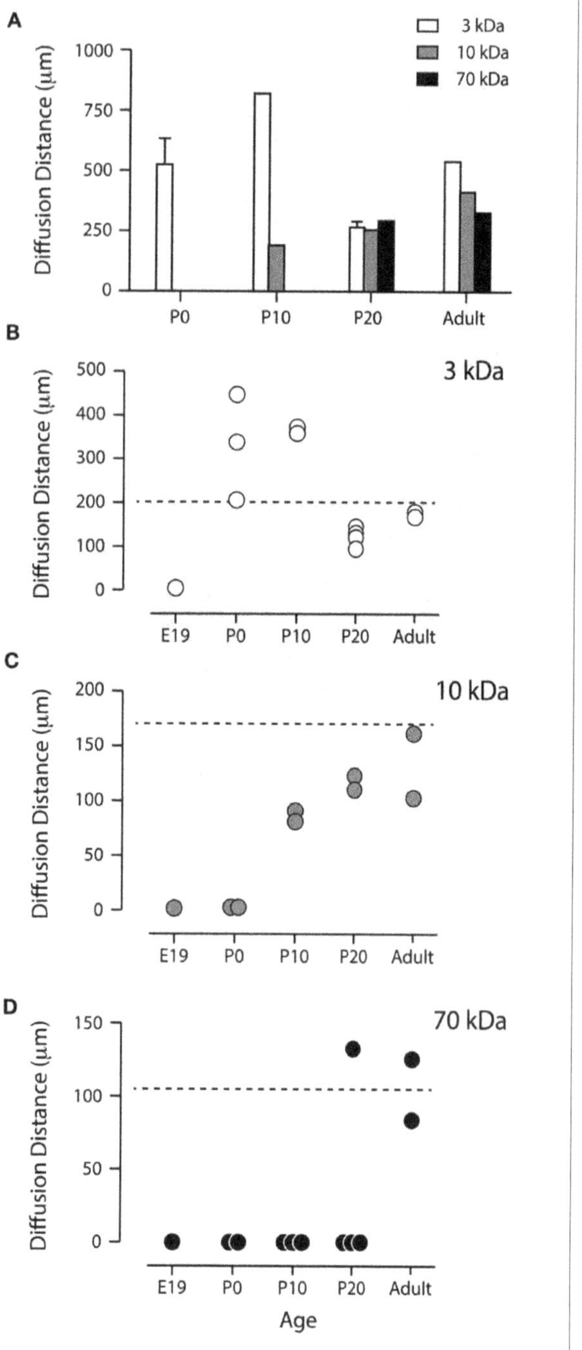

FIGURE 4 | (A) Apparent diffusion distance for three different sized biotinylated dextrans. The values were obtained by measuring the distance to which each marker penetrated into the dorso-lateral wall of the lateral ventricle after injections were made in the contralateral side. Mean ± SEM (only if $n > 2$), values from individual experiments are illustrated as circles in **(B–D)**. P, postnatal day. Note that none of the dextrans penetrated at E19 (see **B–D** and **Figure 3**). **(B,C)** Standardized apparent diffusion distances compared to theoretical values. Apparent diffusion distances were standardized by estimating the apparent diffusion distance at 1 min after intraventricular injection of each dextran at each age using Fick's second law of diffusion as different sized dextrans were left to diffuse for different periods of time (see Materials and Methods). The broken lines represent the calculated theoretical diffusion distance at 1 min. Each circle represents *(Continued)*

FIGURE 4 | Continued
a value obtained from individual pups. **(B)** BDA3 kDa appeared to diffuse without restraint from P0. There was no diffusion at E17 or E19 (only E19 illustrated). **(C)** BDA10 kDa did not enter the ventricular zone at P0 and appeared to diffuse less than the theoretical distance at P10 and P20. **(D)** BDA70 kDa only penetrated the ependyma at P20 in one pup out or four and in the adult. E, embryonic; P, postnatal.

animal. In the adult brain ($n = 2$) diffusion of the probe was observed from the ventricle into the brain in both animals. These results indicate that after the age of weaning (>P20) in the mouse there is no longer any size related diffusion restraint present at the CSF-brain interface for molecules up to 70 kDa (**Figures 3, 4**).

TOTAL PROTEIN CONCENTRATION IN CSF AND PLASMA OF MICE FROM E15 UNTIL ADULT

In order to establish if there is a correlation between changes in the permeability properties of the inner CSF–brain barrier and protein concentration in the CSF during brain development, total protein concentration in plasma and CSF of mice from E17 to adult was measured using the Bradford method (Bradford, 1976 see Materials and Methods). Results are shown in **Figure 5**. For completeness values obtained from a previous study (Liddelow et al., 2012) from E15 mice are also included.

As can be seen from **Figure 5A** the concentration of total protein in the CSF was higher in younger than in adult animals. There was no statistically significant difference between late fetal (E17 and E19) and P0 protein concentrations in CSF with values ranging from 227 ± 1.7 mg 100 ml^{-1} at E17 to 259 ± 23.7 mg 100 ml^{-1} at P0. However, there was a statistically significant difference between protein concentrations in the CSF at P0 (259 ± 23.7 mg 100 ml^{-1}) and P2 (201 ± 6.9; $p = 0.02$). After P2 there was a decline until adult levels were reached (26 ± 1.5 mg 100 ml^{-1}). In contrast, total protein concentration in plasma was lowest at E15 (465 ± 32.4 mg 100 ml^{-1}) and increased to 6188 ± 51.5 mg 100 ml^{-1} in adult plasma (**Figure 5B**). When these results are compared with the results obtained from permeability studies, it appears that the CSF–brain interface becomes less size-restricted for molecular diffusion at the time when the CSF protein levels begin to decline (i.e., after P0).

RNA SEQUENCING ANALYSIS OF EMBRYONIC VENTRICULAR ZONE AND ADULT EPENDYMA

In order to understand the molecular structure of strap junctions present between adjacent neuroepithelial ventricular zone cells in mouse fetal brain we employed RNA Sequencing analysis of lateral ventricular zone tissue from E17/18 embryos and ependyma from adult mice. Only the dorsolateral part of the lateral ventricular wall was sampled (see Materials and Methods). In this paper we focus only on genes that are thought to play a role in intercellular junctional structures. However, a more comprehensive analysis of the full RNA-Seq dataset dealing with the general development of the ventricular zone will be published elsewhere.

Table 3 lists the junction-related genes that were identified in embryonic ventricular zone (A) and adult ependyma (B). The Table also lists numerous genes known to be associated with tight junctions that were below the detection threshold of the method.

In the embryonic ventricular zone only 19 junction-related genes were present with FPKM (fragments per kilobase of exon per million fragments mapped) values above the cut off of 1.0. In the adult ependyma there were 23 detectable junction-related genes. In the embryonic ventricular zone 9 genes belonging to the actins were represented, 6 belonged to catenin gene family, 3 were cadherins and one was a claudin (*Cldn5*). No detectable levels of genes coding for gap junction proteins were observed. In the adult ependyma three genes for gap junction proteins were detected, eight genes were from the actin family, four were catenins and there was only one cadherin. Claudin-11 (*Cldn11*) was the gene expressed at the highest level in the adult ependyma (**Table 3**). Genes from this first pass analysis were subsequently grouped by their molecular categories and represented as differentially regulated between the two ages (i.e., the fold differences between E17 and adult). These are summarized in **Table 4**. In addition, genes that did not show age-related expression differences are also listed. Some genes were only present in the embryo in detectable copy numbers whereas others were present only in the adult. The largest single category was actin and actin-related genes—two (*Actg1*, *Actl6b*) were present only in the embryo; one (*Actr3b*) was present only in the adult. Another five were expressed at a higher level in the embryo than in the adult (*Actb, Actr3, Actr1a, Actr2, Actr10*) in the range 2.3–7.0-fold enrichment. In adult ependyma only one actin-related gene (*Actr1b*) was expressed at a higher level than in the embryo. The cadherin, *Cdh13* was only present in the embryo, while *Cdh2* was expressed at both ages but 13-fold higher in embryos than in the adult. Two claudins were detected, *Cldn5* only in the embryo and *Cldn11* only in the adult. Four catenins showed age-related differences in expression, all at a higher level in embryos. Two were present only in the embryo (*Ctnnbip1*, *Ctnnbl1*) and 2 were expressed at a higher level in the embryo (*Ctnna2*, 3.5-fold and *Ctnnb1*, 3.9-fold); the one protocadherin detected (*Pcdhgc3*) was also expressed only in the embryo. The gap junction (*Gja1*, *Gjb1*, *Gjc3*), junctional adhesion molecules (*Jam3*, *Jam3*) and one plakophilin (*Pkp4*) were all only expressed in the adult ependyma.

A summary of genes that were only present in embryonic ventricular zone or adult ependyma is listed in **Table 5**, together with genes that were expressed at similar levels at both ages.

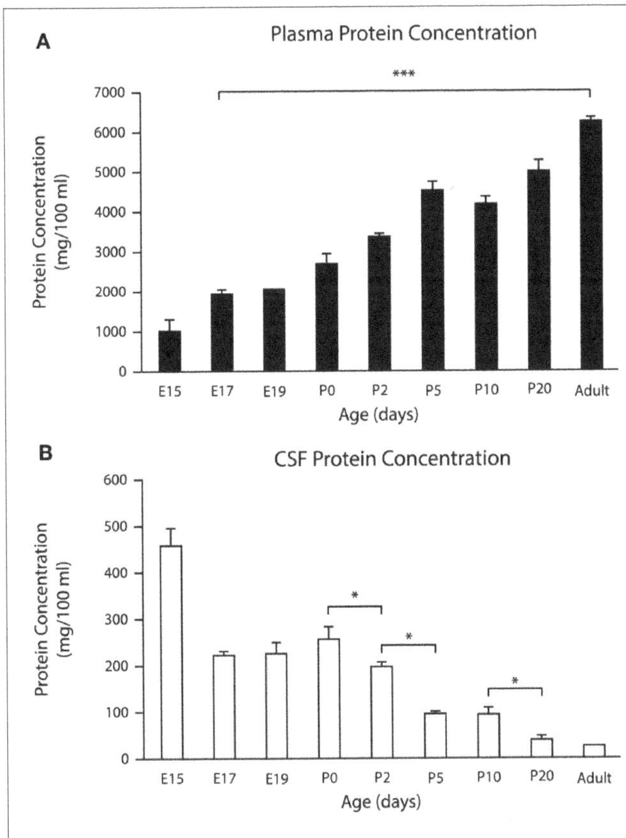

FIGURE 5 | Total protein concentration in (A) and in CSF (B) during development in the mouse. Mean ± SEM ($n = 3$–4). $^*p < 0.05$ compared with previous age group. E15 data from Liddelow et al. (2014). In CSF, maximum concentration was in the youngest embryos examined (E15). The lowest concentration was in adults. In plasma the lowest protein concentration was at E15 with a progressive increase to adulthood. $^{***}p < 0.001$. E, embryonic day; P, postnatal day.

DISTRIBUTION OF JUNCTIONAL PROTEINS AT THE INNER CSF-BRAIN INTERFACE

The overall distribution and cellular localization of the adherens junctional proteins N-cadherin (product of gene *Cdh2*), α- and β-catenin (*Ctnna1* and *Ctnnb1*) and of the tight junctional proteins claudin-5 and -11, (*Cldn5* and *Cldn11*), were investigated

Table 5 | Junction-associated genes present only at E17 or adult or not different at these ages in mouse ventricular zone/ependyma.

Gene ID	E17(AVE FPKM)	Adult(AVE FPKM)
PRESENT AT E17 ONLY		
Actl6b	7.7	0.9
Actg1	2.0	0.2
Ctnnbip1	1.6	0.3
Ctnnbl1	1.3	0.2
Cdh13	1.2	0.5
Cldn5	1.0	0.3
PRESENT IN ADULT ONLY		
Cldn11	0.0	304.7
Gja1	0.3	35.9
Pkp4	0.6	31.2
Gjc3	0.0	5.5
Jam3	0.2	3.5
Gjb1	0.0	1.9
Actr3b	0.7	1.1
NO CHANGE IN EXPRESSION		
Ctnnd	3.8	2.0
Actn4	1.3	2.2
Ctnna1	1.4	2.6

Data are FPKM (fragments per kilobase of exon per million fragments mapped) from three independent pooled samples of ventricular zone/ependyma from embryonic day 17 (E17) and adult mice. Full gene lists were truncated to remove transcripts with FPKM < 1.00. A fold change was considered significant if it was greater than 2.00.

using immunohistochemistry in paraffin embedded sections of mouse brains from E15/16 to adult. These protein candidates were chosen based on the transcriptomic analysis of the dataset as described above (see **Tables 3–5**). N-cadherin (*Cdh2*) and both catenin genes (*Ctnna1* and *Ctnnb1*) were expressed at levels that were higher in the fetal brains. *Cldn5* was only detected in the fetal ventricular zone while *Cldn11* was only detected in the adult. Although transcriptomic analysis was performed on samples dissected out from only the lateral wall of the lateral ventricles and most of the permeability data were also calculated from this area, results from immunohistochemical staining are described for all areas lining the ventricles and are illustrated in **Figures 6–8**.

Overall distribution

Immunostaining at E15/16 for junctional proteins identified in the transciptomic analysis as those expressed differentially between fetal and adult ages showed a weak surface staining for claudin-5 (between the two arrows in **Figure 6A**) in contrast to a much stronger reactivity for α-catenin, N-cadherin and β–catenin, which lined the entire lateral ventricular zone surface including the ganglionic eminence (**Figures 6B,C**). N–cadherin immunoreactivity was similar to that of α-catenin and β–catenin although it appeared stronger and also clearly included the surface of the ganglionic eminence (**Figure 6C**). All three adherens junctional proteins showed increased staining of the borders of the ganglionic eminence, at the bottom of the septal fork of the lateral ventricle and the pallio-subpallial boundary (arrows in **Figure 6C**).

Cellular distribution

A comparison of immunostaining for junctional proteins of E15/16 and P20/adult lateral telencephalic wall at high magnification (**Figure 7** from boxed areas in **Figures 6A–D**) showed a prominent claudin-5 reactivity in endothelial cells of the sinusoid blood vessels in the subventricular zone but also a distinct staining corresponding to the apical-most radial glial cell membranes (**Figure 7A**). In contrast the ventricular-facing surface of the ependymal cell lining in lateral ventricle of adult brain was devoid of claudin-5 reactivity (**Figure 7A1**), whereas the endothelial cells of fenestrated blood vessels of the choroid plexus were positive. Immunostaining for α-catenin, N-cadherin and β-catenin outlined the apical and apico-lateral most part of the ventricular zone cells in the lateral ventricular zone (**Figures 7B–D**). N-cadherin and β-catenin immunoreactivity included the cytoplasm of the radial glial cells (**Figures 7C,D** arrowheads). In the adult immunoreactivity for α-catenin was not observed in telencephalic wall, ependymal cells nor in choroid plexus (**Figure 7B1**). The apical ependymal surface was strongly stained for N-cadherin (**Figure 7C1**) but virtually no reactivity was found for β-catenin in the P20/adult forebrain in either the ependyma or in the subependymal zone (**Figure 7D1**).

Since *Cldn11* was only detected in the adult mouse telencephalic wall we compared immunostaining for claudin-11/OSP of E16 and P15 mouse forebrain (**Figures 8A,B**). The early developing forebrain showed a lack of reactivity in the entire telencephalic wall. Thus, the apical surface of ventricular zone (VZ) facing the lateral ventricle (LV) was completely devoid of claudin-11 immunoreactivity. The developing arachnoid barrier layer (*arrowheads*) was clearly claudin-11-positive. Leptomeningeal cells in the subarachnoidal space and on the outer surface of the telencephalic wall were not stained (**Figure 8A**). At P15 the ependymal and the subependymal zone of the lateral ventricle (LV) was unstained in marked contrast to the strongly stained myelinated early subependymal oligodendrocytes (**Figure 8B**, *arrows*).

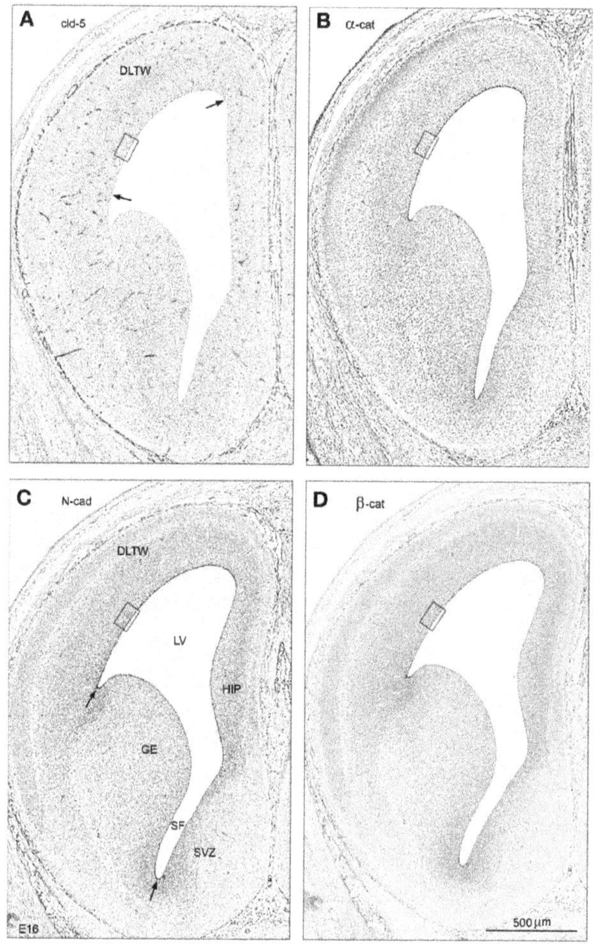

FIGURE 6 | Tight and adherens junctional proteins in embryonic mouse brain. An overall view of tight and adherens junctional proteins in the ventricular zone of early mouse CSF-brain interface at low magnification in coronal sections of E16 brain showing immunostaining for claudin-5 **(A)**, α-catenin **(B)**, N-cadherin **(C)**, and β–catenin **(D)**. Note the differences in distribution of immunopositive staining between different regions of the surface of the ventricular zone with strongest staining of the dorsolateral telencephalic wall (DLTW) and a weak or lacking immunoreactivity of the ganglionic eminence (GE). Arrows in A point to the border of faint claudin-5 reactivity of the ventricular surface of the dorsolateral wall, and in **(C)** to the increased staining of the dorsolateral and ventral borders of the ganglionic eminence. The boxed areas in **(A–D)** are shown in higher magnification in **Figure 7**. HIP, hippocampus; LV, lateral ventricle; SF, septal fork of the lateral ventricle; SVZ, septal ventricular zone. **(A–D)** Same magnification, scale bar 500 μm.

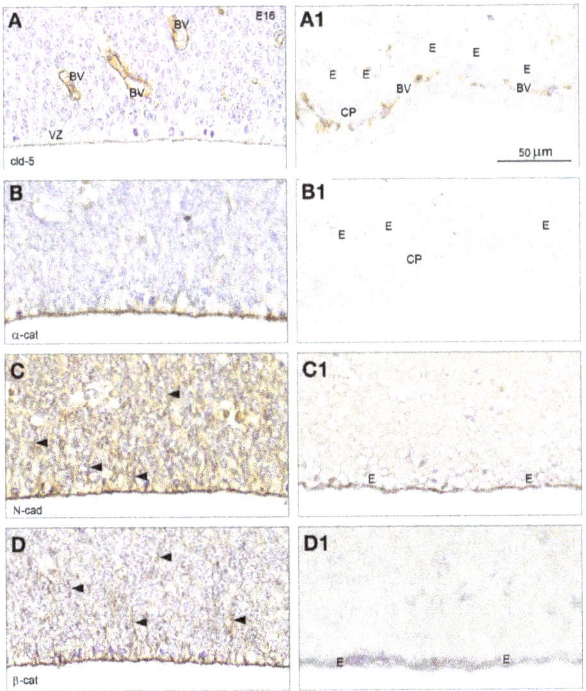

FIGURE 7 | Cellular distribution of adherens and tight junctional proteins at the lateral CSF-brain interface. High magnification coronal sections of E16 **(A–D)** from *boxed areas* in **Figure 6** and of adult **(A1–C1)** and P20 **(D1)** forebrain immunostained for claudin-5 **(A,A1)**, α-catenin **(B,B1)**, N-cadherin **(C,C1)**, and for β–catenin **(D,D1)**. **(A)** At E16 claudin-5 reactivity is prominent in endothelial cells of blood vessels (BV), but a distinct staining is also present corresponding to the apical-most part of the ventricular zone cells (VZ). **(A1)** In the adult forebrain ependymal cells (E) show no claudin-5 immunoreactivity in marked contrast to the positively stained endothelial cells of fenestrated blood vessels of the choroid plexus (CP). **(B–D)** At E16 immunostaining for α-catenin **(B)**, N-cadherin **(C)** and β-catenin **(D)** outlines the apical and apico-lateral most part of the ventricular zone cells,—compare **(A)** (apical) and **(D)** (apical and apico-lateral staining). N-cadherin and β-catenin immunostaining extends into the cytoplasm of the ventricular zone cells (*arrowheads* in **C,D**). **(B1)** Immunoreactivity for α-catenin is not present in adult forebrain, neither in ependymal cells (E) nor in the choroid plexus (CHP). **(C1,D1)** The surface of the ependymal cells (E) is strongly stained for N-cadherin but only little reactivity is observed after staining for β-catenin in the adult forebrain and virtually no reactivity is observed in the subependymal zone. Same magnification in **(A–D)** and **(A1–D1)**. Scale bar 50 μm.

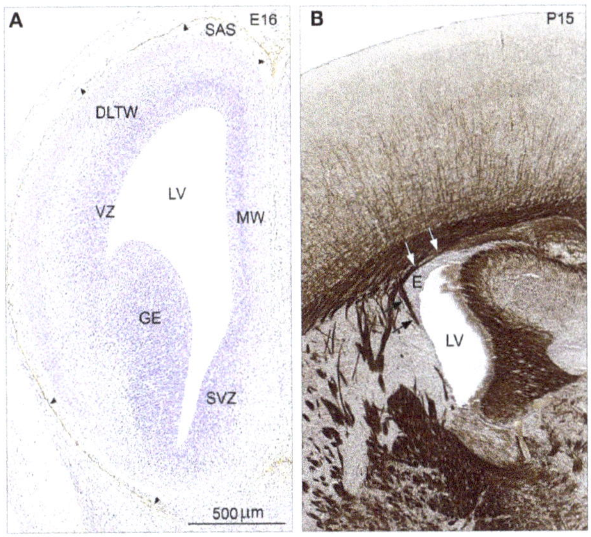

FIGURE 8 | Distribution of claudin-11/OSP immunoreactivity in coronal sections of E16 (A) and P15 (B) mouse forebrain. (A) Immunostaining for claudin-11/OSP of the early developing forebrain at E16 demonstrates a lack of reactivity in the entire telencephalic wall. Thus, the apical surface of ventricular zone (VZ) facing the lateral ventricle (LV) is devoid of immunostaining in all subregions— DLTW, dorsolateral telencephalic wall; MW, medial wall; SVZ, septal ventricular zone and GE, ganglionic eminence. The developing arachnoid barrier layer (*arrowheads*) is however, claudin-11/OSP positive. Leptomeningeal cells in the subarachnoidal space (SAS) and on the outer surface of the telencephalic wall are not stained. **(B)**. At P15 the ependymal zone (E) of lateral ventricle (LV) is unstained in marked contrast to the strongly stained tight junctions of myelin sheaths in early subependymal oligodendrocytes (*arrows*). Same magnification in **(A,B)**, scale bar 200 μm.

DISCUSSION

The brain develops within a well-defined environment that is controlled by a set of mechanisms present at the blood–brain barriers, which determine the exchange of molecules between the brain and the periphery (Saunders et al., 2012). The molecular exchange between the brain interstitial fluid, peripheral circulation and the CSF occurs across the interfaces between the brain, the blood and the CSF (Saunders et al., 2012). Properties of two of these barriers, the blood–brain barrier proper (between the brain and the blood) and the blood–CSF barrier (between the blood and the CSF) have been extensively studied, including during development (for review see Saunders et al., 2012) but the inner CSF–brain barrier, the last frontier together with the outer CSF-brain barrier as it were (see Brøchner et al., in preparation), is not well understood.

PERMEABILITY OF THE INNER CSF-BRAIN BARRIER

Here we have presented a study to investigate systematically the permeability properties of this inner barrier during development. Only one study has previously attempted to do so and also found that there was a size restriction at earlier ages compared to free diffusion at later stages of brain maturation (Fossan et al., 1985). However, in the study of Fossan et al. (1985) only one sized marker (HRP, 40 kDa) was used and only two developmental stages in fetal sheep were compared. The only other studies of ventricular zone in embryos appear to be those of Chang and Sive (2012a,b) in zebrafish. As in the present report, these authors used a series of different molecular sized dextrans (10–400 kDa FITC-conjugated) injected into the cerebral ventricles of zebrafish embryos as early as 22 h post fertilization. In 24 h post fertilization embryos the smallest 10 kDa dextran "leaked almost immediately into the neuroepithelium, whereas the 70 kDa dextrans moved only slowly into that tissue and 2000 kDa not at all." This contrasts with our results in mouse embryos (**Figures 2, 3**) in which even the smallest marker barely penetrated between the cells of the ventricular zone at E17-E19. This difference in permeability of the ventricular zone in the two studies could be due to the difference in species or to the stages of development examined.

Results presented here demonstrate that at early stages of fetal mouse brain development the CSF–brain interchange of inert lipid insoluble molecules is restricted for ones as small as 286 Da BED (**Figure 2**). The 3 kDa probe was not detected in the brain extracellular spaces until P0 (**Figure 3**). The size restriction for free diffusion appeared to progressively relax and after P20, the CSF–brain barrier no longer hindered diffusion of protein–sized molecules such as BDA70 kDa (**Figure 3**). However, both BED and BDA3 kDa were detected intracellular in the brain ventricular zone in some cells lining the lateral ventricles (**Figure 2**). This indicates that the primary mechanism involved in the potential penetration of lipid insoluble molecules, including larger compounds such as proteins (Cavanagh and Warren, 1985), into the early developing brain is restricted to specific cellular uptake and does not occur by non-specific intercellular diffusion.

In the present study the distance to which each sized probe diffused at each stage of brain development was estimated. However, in such an approach, penetration of a probe *in vivo* does not occur in an entirely free, unrestricted diffusion pattern. Values calculated in the present study were mostly less than the calculated theoretical rate using Fick's second law (a mathematical representation of free diffusion) even after allowing longer times for larger molecules to diffuse into the brain. The difference is most likely to be due to (i) CSF flow, (ii) the ventricular surface barrier, (iii) the cellular architecture of the brain into which the probes diffuse, and (iv) bulk flow of the interstitial fluid of the brain. Nevertheless, the results obtained from such calculations indicated that by adulthood the passive diffusion of molecules as large as 70 kDa was unrestricted while earlier in development the size restriction was progressively relaxed as the brain matured (**Figure 4**).

There is little information available about the rate of CSF flow in immature brains (Saunders, 1992) but the flow of brain interstitial fluid was studied previously by Cserr and her colleagues (e.g., Cserr et al., 1981; Szentistványi et al., 1984; Cserr, 1988). Their findings have been followed up recently using 2-photon microscopy (Iliff and Nedergaard, 2013; Thrane et al., 2013). The brain does not appear to possess a true lymphatic system like the rest of the body, although drainage from brain interstitial fluid into the cervical lymphatics has been demonstrated by studies over more than the past 100 years (see Abbott, 2004). Iliff and Nedergaard (2013) have coined the term, the glymphatic system to describe this drainage of the bulk flow of solutes. Fluid first flows via the para–arterial space—or Virchow–Robin space—and diffuses into the interstitial fluid. The interstitial fluid and solutes then diffuse into the brain parenchyma facilitated by astrocytes that possess aquaporin–4 (AQP–4) which assist in water transport. AQP–4 is expressed on the endfeet of astrocytes that line the para–arterial and para–venous spaces. Interstitial fluid and solutes are then drained via the para–venous spaces, which surround major drainage veins (Iliff and Nedergaard, 2013; Thrane et al., 2013; Xie et al., 2013).

In this study BDA probes of all three sizes were visible in the brain within many blood vessels but on closer inspection under the microscope it became apparent that these molecules were confined to the para–vascular (Virchow–Robin) spaces. This is illustrated in **Figure 9** where an example of large vessels in the adult brain after an intraventricular injection of BDA70 kDa or BDA10 kDa is shown.

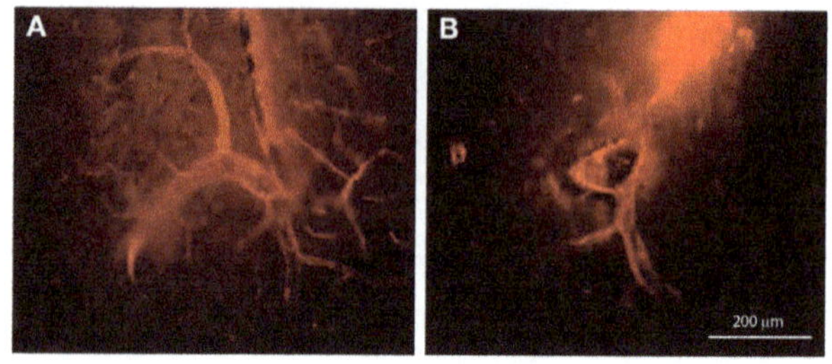

FIGURE 9 | Paravascular distribution of biotin dextrans, following intraventricular injection. Coronal sections of adult brains following intraventricular injection of BDA70K (A) or BDA10K (B). Note that most of the tracer is present in the paravascular or Virchow-Robin space and not in the lumen of blood vessels. Scale bar 200 μm.

The importance of our findings lies primarily in the observation of the impermeability of the CSF-brain interface early in development and its gradual opening up to progressively larger molecules in the postnatal period in the mouse. These permeability changes and those describer earlier in fetal sheep (Fossan et al., 1985) correlate with the presence of strap junctions in the ventricular zone of the developing brain and their subsequent disappearance at later stages of development (Møllgård et al., 1987).

CSF AND PLASMA PROTEIN CONCENTRATION

Part of the hypothesis of this study was that changes in the permeability of the CSF–brain barrier could be related to changes in protein concentration in the CSF (see Introduction). Results showed that the CSF protein concentration in the mouse embryo was highest at E15 followed by E17 and E19. There was a decline in protein concentration from P0 to P20. This drop in CSF protein concentration between P0 and P10 seems to coincide with the appearance of unhindered diffusion of BDA3 kDa and BDA10 kDa into the brain. The unrestricted diffusion of BDA70 kDa coincides with the drop in protein concentration between P10 and P20. By adulthood all three probes were visible in the brain extracellular space lining the ventricular system and the CSF protein concentration was at a minimum (**Figure 5B**).

Previous studies have shown that the premature infiltration of protein into the brain during development is closely linked with altered neurogenesis (Stolp et al., 2011b). Neurogenesis begins in the mouse ventricular zone at approximately E13.5 and astrogliogenesis begins to occur in the brain between the approximate ages of E16 and E18 (Götz and Huttner, 2005; Stolp et al., 2011a,b). This is around the age when the CSF protein concentration began to drop, the permeability properties of the barrier were transforming, and when progressive remodeling of the barrier with respect to junctional proteins was beginning to occur (see below).

MOLECULAR MAKE-UP OF STRAP JUNCTIONS

Strap junctions between cells lining the ventricular zone have only been described in embryonic brains (Møllgård et al., 1987). Their molecular structure is not known but freeze fracture images show cell-cell junctional interactions that are thought to exclude intercellular passage of molecules between CSF and the brain (Fossan et al., 1985; Møllgård et al., 1987). Permeability studies described in the present study identified changes in the size of molecules able to diffuse across this interface. This is the first study in which an attempt was made to describe possible molecular make up of strap junctional complexes.

Because the molecular structure of strap junctions is not known it seems reasonable to suggest that genes that are expressed exclusively in the embryonic ventricular zone, or at least at a higher level than in the adult, will be involved in their formation. By the same token it would seem unlikely that genes expressed only or at a higher level in the adult would be involved in strap junction structure. However, the genes that are expressed at both ages, but not differentially so, could not be ruled out as contributing to strap junction structure. In fact only three such genes were identified (*Actn4*, *Ctnna1*, and *Ctnnd2*, **Table 5**).

A striking finding was that very few of the genes known to be involved in intercellular tight junction formation (see Bauer et al., 2011; Van Itallie and Anderson, 2014) appear to be expressed in the ventricular zone of the lateral wall of the lateral ventricle in mouse embryos. Claudin-5 has been associated with cerebral endothelial tight junctions (Nitta et al., 2003). In this study its gene was only detected in the embryo, albeit at a rather low level (FPKM—1.00, the lowest level of detection using this method). Our immunohistochemical results showed prominent staining for claudin-5 in endothelial cells of blood vessels in the subventricular zone at this age; but there was also some distinctive immunostaining of the apical-most part of the ventricular zone cells (**Figures 6, 7**). Claudin-5 has also been demonstrated in the ventricular zone of zebrafish embryos (Zhang et al., 2010). These authors and others (e.g., Chang and Sive, 2012a) have interpreted this as indicating that the ventricular zone/neuroepithelial cells are joined by tight junctions. The transmission electron micrographs in Zhang et al. (2010) are too low resolution for identification of the nature of the intercellular junctions, but loss of claudin-5 resulted in disruption of these intercellular junctions and allowed passage of lanthanum. As shown by Møllgård et al. (1987) it requires freeze fracture to identify these junctions as strap junctions. Otherwise in our data set transcripts for traditionally important tight junction protein genes such as occludin, MAGUK-like proteins, including ZOs, tricellulin (MarvelD2), JAMs, ESAM, were not detectable. This is in spite of their presence, as detected by immunohistochemistry, as early as E12 mouse (Møllgård et al., unpublished observations) and immunostaining for ZO-1 in zebrafish embryonic neuroepithelium (Zhang et al., 2010). The expression of *Cldn5* (**Table 4**) and its presence demonstrated by immunohistochemistry (see **Figure 7A**) together with lack of expression of many other tight junction genes suggests strongly that claudin-5 may be a component of strap junctions in the embryonic ventricular zone. In addition, representatives of all three of the key gene families involved in cell adhesion in epithelia (Adams et al., 1996) were present and expressed either exclusively or at a higher level in the embryo (**Table 4**). These were seven actin or actin-related genes, two cadherins, one protocadherin and four catenins. It has been thought for a long time (Adams et al., 1996) that the actin cytoskeleton stabilizes epithelial intercellular junctions by attachment to cadherins (Hirano et al., 1987; Matsuzaki et al., 1990) via cytoplasmic interactions with catenins (Nagafuchi and Takeichi, 1988; Ozawa and Kemler, 1992). However, more recently this concept has been challenged and it appears that the linkage between the cadherin-catenin complex and actin filaments may be more dynamic than previously thought (Drees et al., 2005; Yamada et al., 2005; Weis and Nelson, 2006). Zhang et al. (2010) illustrate quite widespread immunostaining for actin in 30 h post fertilization zebrafish embryos but do not mention which antibodies were used.

In epithelia of metazoans specialized cell-cell adhesion proteins comprise the classical cadherin/β-catenin/α-catenin complex and it is the cadherins that provide the link between adjacent cells and catenins that link the cadherins to the underlying actin cytoskeleton (Miller et al., 2013). Our current RNA-Seq data shows that all of the key components of intercellular adhesion junctions are present in the ventricular zone of mouse embryo lateral ventricles although some of the specific genes are different from those usually identified in adherens junctions of mammalian epithelia. The expression of these adherens junctional genes in the ventricular zone of the embryonic mouse brain is consistent with previous ultrastructural studies of the ventricular zone in the developing sheep and human brain showing the presence of well-formed adherens junctions between the cells in this region (Saunders and Møllgård, 1984; Møllgård and Saunders, 1986).

The ultrastructural information available shows that the ventricular zone junctions have a particular configuration of a single strand in freeze fracture, which has an orientation perpendicular to the CSF surface of the cells rather than a circumferential "belt-like" configuration typical of tight and adherens junctions; although in thin-section electron microscopy these junctions have been described as having tight junction and adhesion-like elements (Møllgård et al., 1987). The typical intercellular junctions in the adult ependyma are prominent gap junctions, whereas only few and small gap junctions associated with the strap junctional elements are present in the embryonic ventricular zone (see Figure 9A in Møllgård et al., 1987). In marked contrast to this, strap junctions are only present in the ventricular zone of the early developing brain (Møllgård et al., 1987). It is noteworthy that in the current study it was only in the adult that gap junction genes were identified (*Gja1*, *Gjb1*, *Gjc3*, see **Table 4**). Also in adult ependyma only one actin-related gene was expressed at a higher level (*Actr1b*); in addition, one claudin (*Cldn11*), two Jams (*Jam2* and *Jam3*) and one plakophilin (*Pkp4*) were expressed at a higher level. Two catenin genes were present in adult ependyma but expressed at a much lower level than in the embryo, whereas another was expressed at the same level at the two ages. Thus, it is quite clear that the gene profile of junction-related genes is quite different in embryonic ventricular zone and in adult ependyma.

Actins, particularly β-actin are also important for a variety of other cellular functions some of which may be related to their presence in the ventricular zone of embryonic brain. β-actin has been suggested to comprise between a half to two thirds of mammalian brain actin (Choo and Bray, 1978; Otey et al., 1987) although in a β-actin knock out actin levels were maintained by upregulation of γ- and α-smooth muscle actin; however there was about 70% perinatal lethality (Cheever et al., 2012). β-actin is involved in a range of cellular functions during development including migration (Ayala et al., 2007) and growth cone guidance (Dent and Gertler, 2003). These functions may be important for the differentiation and migration of ventricular zone cells, which contribute to the formation of the layered neocortex (Molnár and Clowry, 2012). It does seem therefore that the main families of proteins involved in strap junction formation are likely to be actins, cadherins, catenins and claudin-5. Some of these proteins were also investigated by immunohistochemistry to establish their cellular distribution (see below).

LIMITATIONS OF THE STUDY

Permeability

A number of factors may have affected the outcomes of the permeability experiments. During development the volume of the lateral ventricles changes and the distance between the ventricles and from the cerebral surface to the interior of the ventricles increases (Liddelow et al., 2011) as does the flow of CSF (Saunders, 1992). Thus, the likelihood of a successfully injected probe reaching the contralateral ventricle can be variable. In order to overcome these limitations, the volume of dextran that was injected was increased with age and the time allowed for the dextran to diffuse into the contralateral ventricle was also increased. These limitations appear to be more significant in the older ages and this was reflected in the reduced number of successful injections in P20 and adult animals.

Great care was taken to inject the same volume into each ventricle at each age, but it was difficult to determine how much of this diffused into the contralateral ventricle. This limited the ability to properly measure the diffusion distances and then accurately compare them between animals. Intraperitoneal injections of these probes would at first appear to be the solution to this problem; however, with age, the amount of probe that needed to be introduced would have to be increased dramatically to offset the loss through renal excretion. Obstruction of the renal system has been used to restrict such losses thus retaining higher concentrations of marker in blood, but may represent an unphysiological state and was deemed unnecessarily stressful for the animals (Habgood et al., 1993). The most consistent approach to such experiments is an *in vivo* ventricular perfusion (as was done in fetal sheep, Fossan et al., 1985). This is impracticable in mice due to their very small size, especially at fetal stages.

Animal ages, numbers and injection route

The small size and vulnerability of exposed fetuses meant that numbers of fetal animals with successful injections ranged between one and three experimental animals per age, mostly two separate litters. For each probe all postnatal experiments were conducted on pups from a minimum of two different litters.

Morphology

For the permeability studies brains were embedded in agar and cut into 100 μm sections using the vibratome (Leica). This method allowed for clearer observation of the diffusion of molecules into the brain. Some brains were embedded in paraffin and cut into 5 μm thick coronal sections. This method better indicated the cellular uptake of the probes.

Cellular distribution of junctional proteins

There is no information available about the molecular composition of strap junctions limiting the ability to use immunohistochemistry to detect cellular changes at this interface. Immunohistochemistry of candidate proteins was based on the RNA-Seq results. It is possible that some other junctional proteins, that were either below the detection levels or were simply not identified in the transcriptomic analysis, could also be involved. We are preparing a more comprehensive immunohistochemical study of strap junctions using all available antibodies to junctional proteins (Møllgård et al., unpublished observations).

Sampling of the lateral wall of the lateral ventricles and RNA-Seq analysis

The lateral wall of both lateral ventricles was carefully dissected out under a dissecting microscope. However, it is inevitable that some tissue from the sub-ventricular layer was also obtained. This probably explains the finding of a high level of *cldn11* in adult mice. Tight junctions of myelin sheaths in developing subependymal oligodendrocytes were strongly positive for claudin-11/OSP (oligodendrocyte-specific protein, **Figure 8B**) after P10 and the developing claudin-11 positive arachnoid barrier layer present in E16 (see, **Figure 8A**) was not within the dissected sample. The dissected samples from E17/18 lateral telencephalic wall would have included claudin-5 positive blood vessels in the subventricular zone (**Figure 7A**), but also in the adult subependymal layer. Claudin-5, occludin and ZO-1 are known to be present in the blood vessel tight junctions from their earliest development. In this study *Occl* and *Tjp1* (ZO-1) expression were not detected presumably because they were below the detection level. Small gap junctions also connect adjacent neuroepithelial cells in the ventricular zone but no gap junctional proteins were detected, i.e., were also below the detection level.

We avoided contamination by the choroid plexus and checked RNA-Seq datasets for choroid plexus specific genes such as transthyretin (Dickson et al., 1985; Thomas et al., 1988). Samples used in this study were transthyretin negative. Because of the unknown degree of possible contamination of the sample by underlying sub-ventricular zone cells, the datasets were only mined for known junctional proteins. This, in principle, limited our analysis to intercellular complexes mostly occurring in the ventricular zone/ependymal layer. It is possible that there are as yet unrecognized junctional genes in our data set that contribute to the structure of strap junctions.

CONCLUSION

We have studied the permeability properties and junctional-protein characteristics of the inner CSF-brain interface during mouse brain development. Permeability of this barrier gradually changed from highly restrictive (to molecules even as small as 286 Da size) in fetal ages to unrestricted diffusion (to molecules at least as large as 70 KDa) in the adult. Molecular characterization, using RNA Sequencing of the ventricular zone (fetus) and ependyma (adult), identified several genes of known junctional proteins that are expressed at this inner CSF-brain barrier in a developmentally regulated manner. It was also found that the age-dependent changes in permeability characteristics correlate with changes in the cellular distribution of junctional proteins: cadherins, catenins and claudin-5. We suggest that these junctional proteins are involved in the formation of strap junctions and in regulation of the changing diffusional properties of this barrier. Further work will be required to establish the scope of the control mechanisms in the CSF-brain interface during development and their significance for normal brain development.

REFERENCES

Abbott, N. J. (2004). Evidence for bulk flow of brain interstitial fluid: significance for physiology and pathology. *Neurochem. Int.* 45, 545–552. doi: 10.1016/j.neuint.2003.11.006

Adams, C. L., Nelson, W. J., and Smith, S. J. (1996). Quantitative analysis of cadherin-catenin-actin reorganization during development of cell-cell adhesion. *J. Cell Biol.* 135, 1899–1911.

Adinolfi, M. (1985). The development of the human blood-CSF-brain barrier. *Dev. Med. Child Neurol.* 27, 532–537.

Anders, S., Pyl, P. T., and Huber, W. (2015). HTSeq—a Python framework to work with high-throughput sequencing data. *Bioinformatics* 31, 166–169. doi: 10.1093/bioinformatics/btu638

Ayala, R., Shu, T., and Tsai, L.-H. (2007). Trekking across the brain: the journey of neuronal migration. *Cell* 128, 29–43. doi: 10.1016/j.cell.2006.12.021

Bauer, H. C., Traweger, A., Zweimueller-Mayer, J., Lehner, C., Tempfer, H., Krizbai, I., et al. (2011). New aspects of the molecular constituents of tissue barriers. *J. Neural. Transm.* 118, 7–21. doi: 10.1007/s00702-010-0484-6

Bradford, M. M. (1976). A rapid and sensitive method for the quantitation of microgram quantities of protein utilizing the principle of protein-dye binding. *Anal. Biochem.* 72, 248–254.

Brightman, M. W., and Reese, T. S. (1969). Junctions between intimately apposed cell membranes in the vertebrate brain. *J. Cell Biol.* 40, 648–677.

Cavanagh, M. E., and Warren, A. (1985). The distribution of native albumin and foreign albumin injected into lateral ventricles of prenatal and neonatal rat forebrains. *Anat. Embryol.* 172, 345–351.

Chang, J. T., and Sive, H. (2012a). An assay for permeability of the zebrafish embryonic neuroepithelium. *J. Vis. Exp.* e4242. doi: 10.3791/4242

Chang, J. T., and Sive, H. (2012b). Manual drainage of the zebrafish embryonic brain ventricles. *J. Vis. Exp.* e4243. doi: 10.3791/4243

Cheever, T. R., Li, B., and Ervasti, J. M. (2012). Restricted morphological and behavioral abnormalities following ablation of β-actin in the brain. *PLoS ONE* 7:e32970. doi: 10.1371/journal.pone.0032970

Choo, Q. L., and Bray, D. (1978). Two forms of neuronal actin. *J. Neurochem.* 31, 217–224.

Cserr, H. F. (1988). Role of secretion and bulk flow of brain interstitial fluid in brain volume regulation. *Ann. N.Y. Acad. Sci.* 529, 9–20.

Cserr, H. F., Cooper, D. N., Suri, P. K., and Patlak, C. S. (1981). Efflux of radiolabeled polyethylene glycols and albumin from rat brain. *Am. J. Physiol.* 240, F319–F328.

Dent, E. W., and Gertler, F. B. (2003). Cytoskeletal dynamics and transport in growth cone motility and axon guidance. *Neuron* 40, 209–227. doi: 10.1016/S0896-6273(03)00633-0

Desmond, M. E., and Jacobson, A. G. (1977). Embryonic brain enlargement requires cerebrospinal fluid pressure. *Dev. Biol.* 57, 188–198.

Dickson, P. W., Aldred, A. R., Marley, P. D., Tu, G. F., Howlett, G. J., and Schreiber, G. (1985). High prealbumin and transferrin mRNA levels in the choroid plexus of rat brain. *Biochem. Biophys. Res. Commun.* 127, 890–895.

Drees, F., Pokutta, S., Yamada, S., Nelson, W. J., and Weis, W. I. (2005). Alpha-catenin is a molecular switch that binds E-cadherin-beta-catenin and regulates actin-filament assembly. *Cell* 123, 903–915. doi: 10.1016/j.cell.2005.09.021

Duckett, S. (1968). The germinal layer of the growing human brain during early fetal life. *Anat. Rec.* 161, 231–245. doi: 10.1002/ar.1091610208

Dziegielewska, K. M., Evans, C. A., Lai, P. C., Lorscheider, F. L., Malinowska, D. H., Møllgård, K., et al. (1981). Proteins in cerebrospinal fluid and plasma of fetal rats during development. *Dev. Biol.* 83, 193–200.

Dziegielewska, K. M., Evans, C. A., Malinowska, D. H., Møllgård, K., Reynolds, J. M., Reynolds, M. L., et al. (1979). Studies of the development of brain barrier systems to lipid insoluble molecules in fetal sheep. *J. Physiol. (Lond).* 292, 207–231.

Dziegielewska, K. M., Evans, C. A., Malinowska, D. H., Møllgård, K., Reynolds, M. L., and Saunders, N. R. (1980). Blood-cerebrospinal fluid transfer of plasma proteins during fetal development in the sheep. *J. Physiol. (Lond).* 300, 457–465.

Dziegielewska, K. M., Habgood, M., Jones, S. E., Reader, M., and Saunders, N. R. (1989). Proteins in cerebrospinal fluid and plasma of postnatal Monodelphis domestica (grey short-tailed opossum). *Comp. Biochem. Physiol. B* 92, 569–576.

Dziegielewska, K. M., Hinds, L. A., Sarantis, M. E., Saunders, N. R., and Tyndale-Biscoe, C. H. (1986). Proteins in cerebrospinal fluid and plasma of the pouch young tammar wallaby (Macropus eugenii) during development. *Comp. Biochem. Physiol. B* 83, 561–567.

Dziegielewska, K. M., and Saunders, N. R. (1988). "The development of the blood-brain barrier: proteins in fetal and neonatal CSF, their nature and origins," in *Handbook of Human Growth and Developmental Biology,* Vol 1. *Neural, Sensory, Motor and Integrative Development,* eds E. Meisami and P. S. Timiras (Boca Raton: CRC Press), 169–191.

Dziegielewska, K. M., and Saunders, N. R. (2002). The ins and outs of brain-barrier mechanisms. *Trends Neurosci.* 25, 69–71. doi: 10.1016/S0166-2236(02)02068-4

Ek, C. J., Dziegielewska, K. M., Habgood, M. D., and Saunders, N. R. (2012). Barriers in the developing brain and neurotoxicology. *Neurotoxicology* 33, 586–604. doi: 10.1016/j.neuro.2011.12.009

Engelhardt, B., and Liebner, S. (2014). Novel insights into the development and maintenance of the blood-brain barrier. *Cell Tissue Res.* 355, 687–699. doi: 10.1007/s00441-014-1811-2

Fossan, G., Cavanagh, M. E., Evans, C. A., Malinowska, D. H., Møllgård, K., Reynolds, M. L., et al. (1985). CSF-brain permeability in the immature sheep fetus: a CSF-brain barrier. *Brain Res.* 350, 113–124.

Gentleman, R. C., Carey, V. J., Bates, D. M., Bolstad, B., Dettling, M., Dudoit, S., et al. (2004). Bioconductor: open software development for computational biology and bioinformatics. *Genome Biol.* 5:R80. doi: 10.1186/gb-2004-5-10-r80

Götz, M., and Huttner, W. B. (2005). The cell biology of neurogenesis. *Nat. Rev. Mol. Cell Biol.* 6, 777–788. doi: 10.1038/nrm1739

Habgood, M. D., Knott, G. W., Dziegielewska, K. M., and Saunders, N. R. (1993). The nature of the decrease in blood-cerebrospinal fluid barrier exchange during postnatal brain development in the rat. *J. Physiol. (Lond).* 468, 73–83.

Hirano, S., Nose, A., Hatta, K., Kawakami, A., and Takeichi, M. (1987). Calcium-dependent cell-cell adhesion molecules (cadherins): subclass specificities and possible involvement of actin bundles. *J. Cell Biol.* 105, 2501–2510.

Hubbard, T. J. P., Aken, B. L., Ayling, S., Ballester, B., Beal, K., Bragin, E., et al. (2009). Ensembl 2009. *Nucleic Acids Res.* 37, D690–D697. doi: 10.1093/nar/gkn828

Iliff, J. J., and Nedergaard, M. (2013). Is there a cerebral lymphatic system? *Stroke* 44, S93–S95. doi: 10.1161/STROKEAHA.112.678698

Iliff, J. J., Wang, M., Liao, Y., Plogg, B. A., Peng, W., Gundersen, G. A., et al. (2012). A paravascular pathway facilitates CSF flow through the brain parenchyma and the clearance of interstitial solutes, including amyloid β. *Sci. Transl. Med.* 4, 147ra111. doi: 10.1126/scitranslmed.3003748

Johansson, P. A., Dziegielewska, K. M., Liddelow, S. A., and Saunders, N. R. (2008). The blood-CSF barrier explained: when development is not immaturity. *Bioessays* 30, 237–248. doi: 10.1002/bies.20718

Langmead, B., Trapnell, C., Pop, M., and Salzberg, S. L. (2009). Ultrafast and memory-efficient alignment of short DNA sequences to the human genome. *Genome Biol.* 10:R25. doi: 10.1186/gb-2009-10-3-r25

Levitt, P., Cooper, M. L., and Rakic, P. (1981). Coexistence of neuronal and glial precursor cells in the cerebral ventricular zone of the fetal monkey: an ultrastructural immunoperoxidase analysis. *J. Neurosci.* 1, 27–39.

Liddelow, S. A., Dziegielewska, K. M., Ek, C. J., Habgood, M. D., Bauer, H., Bauer, H.-C., et al. (2013). Mechanisms that determine the internal environment of the developing brain: a transcriptomic, functional and ultrastructural approach. *PLoS ONE* 8:e65629. doi: 10.1371/journal.pone.0065629

Liddelow, S. A., Dziegielewska, K. M., Møllgård, K., Whish, S. C., Noor, N. M., Wheaton, B. J., et al. (2014). Cellular Specificity of the Blood-CSF Barrier for Albumin Transfer across the Choroid Plexus Epithelium. *PLoS ONE* 9:e106592. doi: 10.1371/journal.pone.0106592

Liddelow, S. A., Dziegielewska, K. M., Vandeberg, J. L., Noor, N. M., Potter, A. M., and Saunders, N. R. (2011). Modification of protein transfer across blood/cerebrospinal fluid barrier in response to altered plasma protein composition during development. *Eur. J. Neurosci.* 33, 391–400. doi: 10.1111/j.1460-9568.2010.07509.x

Liddelow, S. A., Temple, S., Møllgård, K., Gehwolf, R., Wagner, A., Bauer, H., et al. (2012). Molecular characterisation of transport mechanisms at the developing mouse blood-CSF interface: a transcriptome approach. *PLoS ONE* 7:e33554. doi: 10.1371/journal.pone.0033554

Matsuzaki, F., Mège, R. M., Jaffe, S. H., Friedlander, D. R., Gallin, W. J., Goldberg, J. I., et al. (1990). cDNAs of cell adhesion molecules of different specificity induce changes in cell shape and border formation in cultured S180 cells. *J. Cell Biol.* 110, 1239–1252.

Miller, P. W., Clarke, D. N., Weis, W. I., Lowe, C. J., and Nelson, W. J. (2013). The evolutionary origin of epithelial cell-cell adhesion mechanisms. *Curr. Top. Membr.* 72, 267–311. doi: 10.1016/B978-0-12-417027-8.00008-8

Mishra, P. K., and Teale, J. M. (2012). Transcriptome analysis of the ependymal barrier during murine neurocysticercosis. *J. Neuroinflammation* 9, 141. doi: 10.1186/1742-2094-9-141

Møllgård, K., Balslev, Y., Lauritzen, B., and Saunders, N. R. (1987). Cell junctions and membrane specializations in the ventricular zone (germinal matrix) of the developing sheep brain: a CSF-brain barrier. *J. Neurocytol.* 16, 433–444.

Møllgård, K., and Saunders, N. R. (1986). The development of the human blood-brain and blood-CSF barriers. *Neuropathol. Appl. Neurobiol.* 12, 337–358.

Molnár, Z., and Clowry, G. (2012). Cerebral cortical development in rodents and primates. *Prog. Brain Res.* 195, 45–70. doi: 10.1016/B978-0-444-53860-4.00003-9

Nagafuchi, A., and Takeichi, M. (1988). Cell binding function of E-cadherin is regulated by the cytoplasmic domain. *EMBO J.* 7, 3679–3684.

Nitta, T., Hata, M., Gotoh, S., Seo, Y., Sasaki, H., Hashimoto, N., et al. (2003). Size-selective loosening of the blood-brain barrier in claudin-5-deficient mice. *J. Cell Biol.* 161, 653–660. doi: 10.1083/jcb.200302070

Otey, C. A., Kalnoski, M. H., and Bulinski, J. C. (1987). Identification and quantification of actin isoforms in vertebrate cells and tissues. *J. Cell. Biochem.* 34, 113–124. doi: 10.1002/jcb.240340205

Ozawa, M., and Kemler, R. (1992). Molecular organization of the uvomorulin-catenin complex. *J. Cell Biol.* 116, 989–996.

Robinson, M. D., McCarthy, D. J., and Smyth, D. K. (2010). edgeR: a bioconductor package for differential expression analysis of digital gene expression data. *Bioinformatics* 26, 139–140. doi: 10.1093/bioinformatics/btp616

Saunders, N. R. (1992). "Ontogenetic development of brain barrier mechanisms," in *Physiology and Pharmacology of the Blood-Brain Barrier,* Vol. 103, *Handbook of Experimental Pharmacology,* ed M. W. Bradbury (Berlin; Heidelberg: Springer Berlin Heidelberg), 327–369.

Saunders, N. R., Habgood, M. D., and Dziegielewska, K. M. (1999). Barrier mechanisms in the brain, II. Immature brain. *Clin. Exp. Pharmacol. Physiol.* 26, 85–91.

Saunders, N. R., Knott, G. W., and Dziegielewska, K. M. (2000). Barriers in the immature brain. *Cell. Mol. Neurobiol.* 20, 29–40. doi: 10.1023/A:1006991809927

Saunders, N. R., Liddelow, S. A., and Dziegielewska, K. M. (2012). Barrier mechanisms in the developing brain. *Front. Pharmacol.* 3:46. doi: 10.3389/fphar.2012.00046

Saunders, N. R., and Møllgård, K. (1984). Development of the blood-brain barrier. *J. Dev. Physiol.* 6, 45–57.

Stolp, H. B. (2013). Neuropoietic cytokines in normal brain development and neurodevelopmental disorders. *Mol. Cell. Neurosci.* 53, 63–68. doi: 10.1016/j.mcn.2012.08.009

Stolp, H. B., Johansson, P. A., Habgood, M. D., Dziegielewska, K. M., Saunders, N. R., and Ek, C. J. (2011a). Effects of neonatal systemic inflammation on blood-brain barrier permeability and behaviour in juvenile and adult rats. *Cardiovasc. Psychiatry Neurol.* 2011:469046. doi: 10.1155/2011/469046

Stolp, H. B., Liddelow, S. A., Sá-Pereira, I., Dziegielewska, K. M., and Saunders, N. R. (2013). Immune responses at brain barriers and implications for brain development and neurological function in later life. *Front. Integr. Neurosci.* 7:61. doi: 10.3389/fnint.2013.00061

Stolp, H. B., Turnquist, C., Dziegielewska, K. M., Saunders, N. R., Anthony, D. C., and Molnár, Z. (2011b). Reduced ventricular proliferation in the foetal cortex following maternal inflammation in the mouse. *Brain* 134, 3236–3248. doi: 10.1093/brain/awr237

Szentistványi, I., Patlak, C. S., Ellis, R. A., and Cserr, H. F. (1984). Drainage of interstitial fluid from different regions of rat brain. *Am. J. Physiol.* 246, F835–F844.

Tennyson, V., and Pappas, G. (1962). An electron microscope study of ependymal cells of the fetal, early postnatal and adult rabbit. *Z. Zellforsch. Mikrosk. Anat.* 56, 595–618.

Thomas, T., Power, B., Hudson, P., Schreiber, G., and Dziadek, M. (1988). The expression of transthyretin mRNA in the developing rat brain. *Dev. Biol.* 128, 415–427.

Thrane, A. S., Takano, T., Rangroo Thrane, V., Wang, F., Peng, W., Ottersen, O. P., et al. (2013). *In vivo* NADH fluorescence imaging indicates effect of aquaporin-4 deletion on oxygen microdistribution in cortical spreading depression. *J. Cereb. Blood Flow Metab.* 33, 996–999. doi: 10.1038/jcbfm.2013.63

Van Itallie, C. M., and Anderson, J. M. (2014). Architecture of tight junctions and principles of molecular composition. *Semin. Cell Dev. Biol.* 36, 157–165. doi: 10.1016/j.semcdb.2014.08.011

Weis, W. I., and Nelson, W. J. (2006). Re-solving the cadherin-catenin-actin conundrum. *J. Biol. Chem.* 281, 35593–35597. doi: 10.1074/jbc.R600027200

Xie, L., Kang, H., Xu, Q., Chen, M. J., Liao, Y., Thiyagarajan, M., et al. (2013). Sleep drives metabolite clearance from the adult brain. *Science* 342, 373–377. doi: 10.1126/science.1241224

Yamada, S., Pokutta, S., Drees, F., Weis, W. I., and Nelson, W. J. (2005). Deconstructing the cadherin-catenin-actin complex. *Cell* 123, 889–901. doi: 10.1016/j.cell.2005.09.020

Zhang, J., Piontek, J., Wolburg, H., Piehl, C., Liss, M., Otten, C., et al. (2010). Establishment of a neuroepithelial barrier by Claudin5a is essential for zebrafish brain ventricular lumen expansion. *Proc. Natl. Acad. Sci. U.S.A.* 107, 1425–1430. doi: 10.1073/pnas.0911996107

8

Functional and genetic analysis of choroid plexus development in zebrafish

Hannah E. Henson[1,2†‡], Chaithanyarani Parupalli[1‡], Bensheng Ju[1] and Michael R. Taylor[1,3]*

[1] Chemical Biology and Therapeutics, St. Jude Children's Research Hospital, Memphis, TN, USA
[2] Integrated Program in Biomedical Sciences, College of Graduate Health Sciences, University of Tennessee Health Science Center, Memphis, TN, USA
[3] Pharmaceutical Sciences Division, School of Pharmacy, University of Wisconsin-Madison, Madison, WI, USA

***Correspondence:**
Michael R. Taylor, Pharmaceutical Sciences Division, School of Pharmacy, University of Wisconsin-Madison, 777 Highland Avenue, Madison, WI 53705-2222, USA
e-mail: michael.taylor@wisc.edu

† Present address:
Hannah E. Henson, Department of Biology, University of Kentucky, Lexington, USA

‡ These authors have contributed equally to this work.

The choroid plexus, an epithelial-based structure localized in the brain ventricle, is the major component of the blood-cerebrospinal fluid barrier. The choroid plexus produces the cerebrospinal fluid and regulates the components of the cerebrospinal fluid. Abnormal choroid plexus function is associated with neurodegenerative diseases, tumor formation in the choroid plexus epithelium, and hydrocephaly. In this study, we used zebrafish (*Danio rerio*) as a model system to understand the genetic components of choroid plexus development. We generated an enhancer trap line, *Et(cp:EGFP)*^{sj2}, that expresses enhanced green fluorescent protein (EGFP) in the choroid plexus epithelium. Using immunohistochemistry and fluorescent tracers, we demonstrated that the zebrafish choroid plexus possesses brain barrier properties such as tight junctions and transporter activity. Thus, we have established zebrafish as a functionally relevant model to study choroid plexus development. Using an unbiased approach, we performed a forward genetic dissection of the choroid plexus to identify genes essential for its formation and function. Using *Et(cp:EGFP)*^{sj2}, we isolated 10 recessive mutant lines with choroid plexus abnormalities, which were grouped into five classes based on GFP intensity, epithelial localization, and overall choroid plexus morphology. We also mapped the mutation for two mutant lines to chromosomes 4 and 21, respectively. The mutants generated in this study can be used to elucidate specific genes and signaling pathways essential for choroid plexus development, function, and/or maintenance and will provide important insights into how these genetic mutations contribute to disease.

Keywords: choroid plexus, zebrafish, forward genetic screen, Claudin 5, transporters, fluorescein, genetic mapping

INTRODUCTION

The choroid plexus consists of polarized epithelial cells projecting into the brain ventricle to create a blood-cerebrospinal fluid barrier between fenestrated capillaries and the cerebrospinal fluid (Wolburg and Paulus, 2010). These epithelial cells are modified ependymal cells derived from embryonic neuroepithelial cells that form intercellular tight junctions and express multiple families of transporters that create both a physical and chemical barrier. The choroid plexus also plays an important role in the production and secretion of the cerebrospinal fluid and the regulation of central nervous system homeostasis. Although the choroid plexus of the lateral brain ventricles was documented by Herophilus, an ancient Greek physician (Dohrmann, 1970; Dziegielewska et al., 2001), there has been little research aimed toward identifying the genetic pathways essential for choroid plexus formation and function. Previous studies have classified choroid plexus development by observing modifications in cell morphology, measuring glycogen content as it matures, and examining gene expression (Dohrmann, 1970; Strazielle and Ghersi-Egea, 2000; Dziegielewska et al., 2001; Kratzer et al., 2012, 2013; Liddelow et al., 2014). Signaling pathways such as Sonic hedgehog (Huang et al., 2009; Nielsen and Dymecki, 2010), BMP (Currle et al., 2005), and Notch (Irvin et al., 2004) have been found to contribute to choroid plexus formation. However, how these pathways interact with one another to generate the choroid plexus and the downstream components involved in its development, function, and maintenance are unknown. Understanding normal development and function in the choroid plexus is crucial to unraveling how these mechanisms become altered in diseases. The choroid plexus has been associated with various disease conditions, including choroid plexus tumors (Wolburg and Paulus, 2010), hydrocephalus (Wodarczyk et al., 2009), and neurodegenerative diseases such as Alzheimer's disease (Alvira-Botero and Carro, 2010) and multiple sclerosis (Vercellino et al., 2008). Identifying altered genes and signaling pathways in the choroid plexus that cause disease initiation or progression can help determine potential therapeutic targets for treatment.

Abbreviations: Cldn5, Claudin 5; CNS, central nervous system; CP, choroid plexus; CPe, choroid plexus epithelium; CSF, cerebrospinal fluid; dpf, days post-fertilization; dCP, diencephalic choroid plexus; EGFP, enhanced green fluorescent protein; *Et(cp:EGFP)*^{sj2}, *Enhancer trap(choroid plexus:enhanced green fluorescent protein)*^{sj2}; hpf, hours post-fertilization; mCP, myelencephalic choroid plexus; MDR1, Multidrug Resistance Transporter 1; MRP1, Multidrug Resistance-Associated Protein 1; OAT3, Organic Anion Transporter 3; PTU, N-Phenylthiourea.

Models used to study the choroid plexus have included (1) mice, because of their similarity to the human choroid plexus in gene expression patterns (Janssen et al., 2013); (2) marsupials, because post-natal lateral ventricle development occurs outside of the womb (Liddelow et al., 2010); and (3) *in vitro* cell culture systems to study choroid plexus transport (Monnot and Zheng, 2013). However, these models do not provide real-time, *in vivo* developmental information. We propose, as have others (Bill et al., 2008; Garcia-Lecea et al., 2008), that zebrafish are a suitable vertebrate model to analyze and genetically dissect choroid plexus development and function *in vivo*, as they offer several advantages such as having central nervous system structures similar to those in mammals, rapid *ex utero* development, transparency, large numbers of offspring, and genetic tractability (Goldsmith and Jobin, 2012).

Previous studies have examined the role of Shh and Notch signaling in choroid plexus development using zebrafish (Bill et al., 2008; Garcia-Lecea et al., 2008). However, these studies did not examine functional choroid plexus barrier properties such as tight junctions and transporters. Here, we generated an enhancer trap line, *Et(cp:EGFP)*^{sj2}, that expresses enhanced green fluorescent protein (EGFP) in epithelial cells of the diencephalic choroid plexus and myelencephalic choroid plexus. We used this enhancer trap line to visualize choroid plexus development *in vivo* and demonstrated that several components of the zebrafish choroid plexus are comparable to human. We also performed a small-scale ENU-mutagenesis screen and identified 10 recessive mutant lines. These mutants were classified into five categories on the basis of EGFP expression and choroid plexus morphology. We also genetically mapped the mutations from two mutant lines using bulked-segregant analysis. The cloning and characterization of these mutants will provide important insights into the genetic pathways that regulate formation and function of the choroid plexus in health and disease.

MATERIALS AND METHODS

FISH LINES AND MAINTENANCE

Zebrafish were maintained at 28.5° on a 14 h light/dark cycle. Embryos used for imaging or for screening F_3 larvae were collected in egg water (0.03% Instant Ocean) containing 0.02% methylene blue and treated at 24 h post-fertilization (hpf) with 0.003% 1-phenyl-2-thiourea (PTU) (Sigma) to prevent pigment formation. Zebrafish were maintained in accordance with established protocols and all experiments were approved by the St. Jude Children's Research Hospital Institutional Animal Care and Use Committee.

GENERATION OF THE *Et(cp:EGFP)*^{sj2} LINE

To generate the *Et(cp:EGFP)*^{sj2} line, EGFP was released from the pEGFP-N1 vector (Clontech) by *Bam*HI and *Not*I digestion and inserted into the pTRE-Tight vector (Clontech). The *TRE-tight:EGFP* fragment was released by *Xho*I and *Cla*I digestion and inserted into the pT2AL200R150G vector (Urasaki et al., 2006). Approximately 30 pg of the resulting T2 (*TRE-tight:EGFP)* plasmid DNA was co-injected with 30 pg of *in vitro* transcribed Tol2 transposase mRNA into single-cell embryos of the AB strain. The embryos were raised to adults and screened for germline transmission by examining their offspring for EGFP expression.

IMMUNOHISTOCHEMISTRY (IHC)

Larvae were anesthetized in 0.02% tricaine and fixed in 4% paraformaldehyde (PFA) (Electron Microscopy Sciences) at 4° overnight and washed the next day in 1× phosphate buffered serum (PBS) (Calbiochem). Samples were sunk in 30% sucrose/PBS at 4° overnight. Larval 1-month-old brain tissues, and adult brains were embedded in Optimal Cutting Temperature (O.C.T.) Compound (Tissue-Tek), frozen on dry ice, and stored at −80°. Tissues were sectioned using a Leica CM 1950 cryostat. Sections were washed in PBS for 5 min followed by three 5 min washes in PBST [PBS/0.03% Triton X-100 (Sigma)]. Sections were incubated in blocking buffer [PBST with 5% goat serum (Gibco) and 1% BSA (Sigma)] for 3 h at room temperature. Primary antibodies were incubated at 4° overnight followed by secondary antibody incubation for 2 h at room temperature. Sections were washed in PBST four times for 15 min after primary and secondary antibody incubations. Primary antibodies included rabbit anti-GFP (1:500; Invitrogen) and mouse anti-Zpr1 (1:100; ZIRC). Secondary antibodies included Alexa Fluor goat anti-rabbit 488 (1:200; Invitrogen) and Alexa Fluor goat anti-mouse 555 (1:200; Invitrogen). Antibody dilutions were prepared in blocking buffer. Sections were counterstained with 1 μg/mL DAPI (Roche) for 1 min, rinsed briefly in PBS, and mounted with Fluoromount (Electron Microscopy Sciences). Images were taken on a Nikon AZ100 microscope and analyzed using NIS-Elements AR 3.2 software.

WHOLE-MOUNT IHC

Embryos were incubated in egg water with 0.003% PTU to prevent pigment formation. At 4 and 6 days post-fertilization (dpf), larvae were anesthetized in 0.02% tricaine and fixed in 4% PFA overnight. The next day, samples were washed in 1× PBS followed by 1× PBST and treated with 20 μg/mL Proteinase K (New England Biolabs) for 15 min. The reaction was stopped by adding 10% lamb serum (Gibco) followed by additional washes in PBST. Samples were blocked with 10% lamb serum for 1–4 h and incubated in primary antibody at 4° overnight. Samples were washed the next day in PBST and incubated in secondary antibody at 4° overnight. Antibodies used included rabbit anti-GFP (1:100; Invitrogen), mouse anti-Zpr1 (1:50; ZIRC), mouse anti-Cldn5 (1:100; Invitrogen), Alexa Fluor goat anti-rabbit 488 (1:200; Invitrogen), and Alexa Fluor goat anti-mouse 555 (1:200; Invitrogen). Additional washes in PBST were done the following day and stored in 1× PBS. Samples were embedded in 0.8% low-melting point agarose (Invitrogen) made in 1× PBS and imaged on Nikon C1Si laser scanning confocal microscope. Z-stacks were compiled to create maximum intensity projection images using Nikon NIS-Elements 3.1 imaging software.

FLUORESCENT TRACER INJECTIONS

To observe transporter activity in the choroid plexus, *Et(cp:EGFP)*^{sj2} larvae at 4 dpf were anesthetized in 0.02% tricaine and injected intravenously into the common cardinal vein with approximately 1–2 nL of 100 μM rhodamine 123

(Sigma-Aldrich) using a micromanipulator and a pneumatic picopump (World Precision Instruments). The total blood volume of zebrafish embryos at 2 dpf has been estimated to be 60 nL (Craig et al., 2012), so the blood volume is not significantly altered upon injection. Immediately after the injections, larvae were embedded in 1.2% low-melting-point agarose (Invitrogen) made in egg water. Larvae were imaged on a Nikon C1Si confocal microscope and analyzed using Nikon EZC1 3.91 software.

To study choroid plexus function, Casper larvae (lacking melanocytes and iridophores) (White et al., 2008) were anesthetized in 0.02% tricaine and intravenously injected into the common cardinal vein with approximately 0.3–2 nL of 10 mg/mL rhodamine- and fluorescein-labeled dextrans at 2, 3, and 4 dpf. Fluorescent tracers included a 3-kDa fluorescein dextran, a 10-kDa rhodamine dextran, and a 40-kDa anionic fluorescein dextran (Invitrogen). Immediately after the injections, larvae were laterally embedded in 1.2% low-melting-point agarose made in egg water. To observe tracer permeability into the brain ventricle, time-lapse images were collected every 2 min for 1 h with a Nikon AZ100 microscope equipped with a shutter (Sutter Instruments) and analyzed with Nikon NIS-Elements 3.2 software. *Et(cp:EGFP)*^{sj2} larvae were also injected intravenously with the 10-kDa rhodamine dextran at 2 and 4 dpf and imaged on a Nikon C1Si confocal microscope with Nikon EZC1 3.91 software.

To visualize brain ventricle morphology in wild-type and mutant *Et(cp:EGFP)*^{sj2}, PTU-treated larvae at 4 dpf were anesthetized and intraventricularly injected with approximately 2 nL of 40-kDa fluorescein-labeled dextran as described previously (Gutzman and Sive, 2009). Larvae were imaged immediately after the injection using a Nikon SMZ1500 epifluorescence stereomicroscope and analyzed with Nikon NIS-Elements 3.1 software. Ventricular injections of rhodamine 123 and fluorescein were performed as described previously (Gutzman and Sive, 2009) in Casper larvae at 4 dpf and imaged on a Nikon C1Si confocal microscope with Nikon EZC1 3.91 software.

FLUORESCEIN TREATMENT

Casper and *Et(cp:EGFP)*^{sj2} larvae were incubated for 4 h in the dark with 50 μM fluorescein (Fluka). Larvae were briefly rinsed 12 times in egg water, anesthetized in 0.02% tricaine, and embedded in 1.2% low-melting-point agarose. After 30 min, larvae were imaged using a Nikon SMZ1500 epifluorescence stereomicroscope and analyzed with Nikon NIS-Elements 3.1 software.

STATISTICAL ANALYSIS OF TRACER PERMEABILITY

The ratio of the fluorescence intensity in the ventricle to that in the heart was calculated at the 30-min timepoint when the leakiest tracer reached saturation. The ratio was then normalized against the tracer having the greatest mean intensity in the ventricle at 30 min. A One-Way ANOVA test was performed in Microsoft Excel to determine whether there was a significant difference in fluorescent intensity between the tracers and developmental timepoints. A Tukey's *post-hoc* test was performed to determine which tracers were statistically significant to one another at each developmental timepoint. A significance value of $\alpha = 0.05$ was used, and *P*-values were calculated using the GraphPad software *P*-value calculator. Error bars were based on the mean of 7 observations using standard error.

N-ETHYL-N-NITROSOUREA (ENU) MUTAGENESIS AND FORWARD GENETIC SCREENING

Twenty *Et(cp:EGFP)*^{sj2} males were treated three times with 3 mM ENU (Sigma) for 1 h each at weekly intervals as described previously (Driever et al., 1996). After 1 month, ENU-treated males were mated to *Et(cp:EGFP)*^{sj2} females to produce the F_1 generation. F_1 pairwise crosses were performed to produce F_2 families. F_2 families that did not contain at least 4 male/female pairs were sacrificed. Pairwise crosses for each F_2 family were done at least six times if possible to identify F3 offspring with homozygous recessive mutations. F_2 pairs deemed heterozygous for a recessive mutation were maintained in miniboxes for use in genetic mapping experiments. To screen for choroid plexus mutants, F_3 larvae at 4 dpf were anesthetized and visualized using a Nikon SMZ1500 epifluorescence stereomicroscope to identify abnormal GFP expression or patterning in the choroid plexus. A mutant line was confirmed if approximately 25% of the total offspring displayed a choroid plexus phenotype.

GENOMIC DNA ISOLATION

Adult zebrafish were anesthetized in 0.02% tricaine (Sigma-Aldrich) and tail clipped. As the fish recovered in system water, the tail clip was immediately immersed into 50 μL digest buffer (0.2 M NaCl, 10 mM Tris 8.0, 5 mM EDTA, 0.1% SDS, 0.1 mg/ml Proteinase K). Samples were incubated overnight at 50°. After brief centrifugation, 450 μL of 100% ethanol (EtOH) added. Samples were centrifuged at 21,130 *g* for 10 min, the supernatant was removed, and 500 μL of 70% EtOH added to wash the pellet. Samples were centrifuged at 21,130 *g* or 15,000 rpm for 5 min. After removing the supernatant, the samples were stored at room temperature for about 30 min to evaporate excess EtOH. The DNA pellets were resuspended with 50 μL of TE buffer (10 mM Tris and 1 mM EDTA, pH 8.0).

For zebrafish larvae, wild-type and mutants were anesthetized, separated into 1.5 mL eppendorf tubes, and immersed in 1 mL 100% methanol (MeOH) (Sigma-Aldrich). Samples were stored at −20° overnight. The following day, individual wild-type and mutant larvae were transferred into 0.5 mL tubes and the excess MeOH removed. Once all the MeOH evaporated, 10 μL of digest buffer (same as above) was added to each tube. Samples were incubated overnight at 50°. DNA was isolated as described above for adults except the volume of 100% EtOH and 70% EtOH was 180 μL and the volume of TE buffer was 25 μL.

GENETIC MAPPING

After identifying a mutant line, the *Et(cp:EGFP)*^{sj2} F_2 heterozygous parents were each outcrossed to the polymorphic TL strain. From this outcross, we identified AB/TL hybrids heterozygous for the recessive mutation by screening their offspring. The wild-type and mutant offspring from these heterozygous hybrids were collected and their DNA was extracted (see above). A genome scan using 192 polymorphic Z-markers was performed with DNA pooled from 30 wild-type and 30 mutant larvae as previously described (Muto et al., 2005). Wild-type and mutant

DNA was amplified using the Accuprime Taq DNA Polymerase System (Invitrogen). The resulting PCR products were analyzed for genetic linkage by agarose gel electrophoresis. For fine genetic mapping, individual wild-type and mutant DNA was amplified using Platinum PCR Supermix (Invitrogen). Z-markers used for genetic mapping were acquired from the zebrafish genome database at www.ensembl.org. Additional markers were designed by examining the Ensembl genome browser for polymorphic regions in the genome.

LIVE CONFOCAL IMAGING AND TIME-LAPSE MOVIES

Confocal imaging was performed on a Nikon C1Si confocal microscope and analyzed using Nikon EZC1 3.91 software. Scans of DIC and GFP images were acquired using a 20× objective at 4 μm intervals to create a z-stack maximum intensity projection image. To observe choroid plexus development, larvae were collected at ~30 hpf and prepared for imaging as described above. Z-stack images were acquired every 30 min over a 65 h period. Using NIS-Elements AR 4.0 software, images were smoothed and z-stacks were compiled to create an enhanced depth of focus (EDF) image. To compare choroid plexus development, wild-type and mutant larvae were imaged beginning at 54 hpf with images acquired every 30 min over a 48 h period. Supplemental movies run for the 48 h period except for Supplemental movie 6 which runs for 42 h.

RESULTS

GENERATION AND CHARACTERIZATION OF THE ZEBRAFISH CHOROID PLEXUS ENHANCER TRAP LINE *Et(cp:EGFP)^{sj2}*

In the process of producing a tetracycline-inducible transgenic line, we fortuitously generated the zebrafish choroid plexus line by an enhancer trap effect where EGFP became "trapped" within the genome and is now regulated by an enhancer. To generate this line, we co-injected a TRE-EGFP construct with *Tol2* transposase mRNA into single-cell zebrafish embryos. The TRE-EGFP construct was integrated into an enhancer region that regulates gene expression in the choroid plexus. Using Southern blot analysis, we identified a single TRE-EGFP insertion on chromosome 13 (data not shown). By sequencing genes within this region, we identified the TRE-GFP transgene between two genes *TATA box binding protein* (*tbp*) and *asparaginase-like1* (*asrgl1*), both of which according to zfin.org are not spatially restricted in their mRNA expression patterns. After performing *in situ* hybridization on *asrgl1*, we did not observe expression within the choroid plexus (data not shown). Because we were unable to identify choroid plexus specific genes along this region of Chromosome 13, we concluded that the GFP expression in the choroid plexus is the result of an enhancer trap affect where an enhancer localized upstream or downstream of GFP is regulating GFP expression. The insertion was transmitted to subsequent generations, thereby creating a stable line termed *Et(cp:EGFP)^{sj2}*.

GFP expression was specifically localized to the diencephalic choroid plexus in the third ventricle and the myelencephalic choroid plexus in the fourth ventricle at 3 dpf corresponding to the mammalian choroid plexus in third and fourth ventricles, respectively (**Figure 1A**). We identified that this integration resulted in EGFP expression in the diencephalic choroid plexus and myelencephalic choroid plexus based on two previously published papers also identifying GFP expression in the diencephalic choroid plexus and myelencephalic choroid plexus of zebrafish (Bill et al., 2008; Garcia-Lecea et al., 2008). Unlike mammals, the zebrafish choroid plexus is dorsal to the brain allowing for easy visualization of choroid plexus development. As mentioned in the two previous zebrafish choroid plexus studies, the myelencephalic choroid plexus in teleosts exists as a layer of GFP positive cells on the dorsal surface of the fourth ventricle and ventral to the outer skin epithelium, while the diencephalic choroid plexus is at the most dorsal portion of the third ventricle (Bill et al., 2008; Garcia-Lecea et al., 2008). This allows choroid plexus development to be easily visualized in the zebrafish because it is not buried inside the brain as in other vertebrates. Similarly as described in the dogfish shark, the myelencephalic choroid plexus lies over the brain ventricle rather than obstructed between the medulla and cerebellum (Villalobos et al., 2002). Other studies on zebrafish brain development describe how the development of the telencephalon folds outward with the proliferating cells on the outside rather than inward as seen in other vertebrates (Schmidt et al., 2013), suggesting the zebrafish has more of an "inside out" morphology. This type of development in zebrafish, termed the eversion model, begins with brain ventricular formation followed by the movement of surrounding neural tissue migrating into the ventricle space and results in an overlying ventricle surrounding the brain tissue (Folgueira et al., 2012). Because brain ventricular formation occurs prior to choroid plexus development, the eversion process may be responsible for this "inside out" morphology.

To gain further insight into the location of the choroid plexus in relation to other central nervous system structures, we used whole-mount immunohistochemistry (IHC) to stain *Et(cp:EGFP)^{sj2}* larvae with a Zpr-1 antibody labeling cone photoreceptors of the eye and the pineal gland. In other teleosts and mammals, the pineal gland directly interacts with the choroid plexus of the third ventricle (Omura et al., 1985; Skinner and Malpaux, 1999). Although the diencephalic choroid plexus is distinct from the pineal gland, we found a close association between the two structures, where the diencephalic choroid plexus was found anterior to the pineal gland (**Figure 1B**). Transverse sections showed the diencephalic choroid plexus positioned beneath the pineal gland (**Figure 1C**). Additional transverse sections through the myelencephalic choroid plexus showed a cluster of GFP-positive epithelial cells directly beneath the skin surface (**Figure 1D**). GFP expression in the diencephalic choroid plexus and myelencephalic choroid plexus was retained throughout development and at later stages, as shown in a 1-month-old *Et(cp:EGFP)^{sj2}* (**Figures 1E,F**).

To further demonstrate that this is indeed the choroid plexus, we cut sections from adult brains and showed expression of GFP in a structure historically referred to as the saccus dorsalis (**Figure 2**). This structure is homologous to the mammalian choroid plexus of the third ventricle. The saccus dorsalis in rainbow trout (*Salmo gairdneri*), has been described as a folded monolayer of epithelium that develops out of the diencephalic roof plate (Jansen et al., 1976). Because the saccus dorsalis has also been described to partially cover the pineal stalk (Tsuneki, 1986), similar to what we show in **Figure 1B**, we conclude that this is the

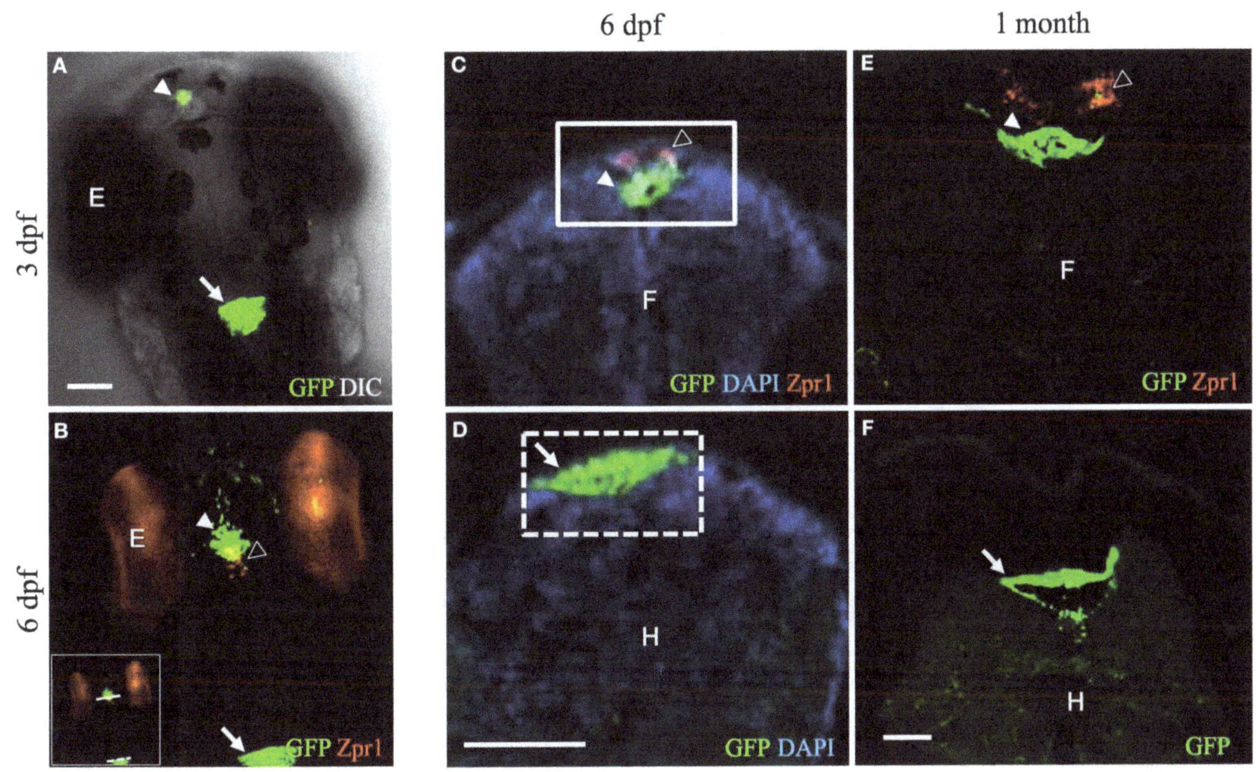

FIGURE 1 | The *Et(cp:EGFP)*^{sj2} line expresses GFP in the diencephalic choroid plexus and myelencephalic choroid plexus. **(A)** Confocal image showing the dorsal view of the head of 3 dpf *Et(cp:EGFP)*^{sj2} larvae expressing GFP in the diencephalic choroid plexus and myelencephalic choroid plexus. **(B)** Whole-mount immunohistochemical staining of *Et(cp:EGFP)*^{sj2} larvae at 6 dpf. GFP in green labels the diencephalic choroid plexus and myelencephalic choroid plexus, and Zpr-1 shown in red labels the pineal gland and photoreceptors. The yellow overlay demonstrates the interaction between the pineal gland and diencephalic choroid plexus. The solid and dashed lines across the diencephalic choroid plexus and myelencephalic choroid plexus in the inset image indicate approximate regions where sections were taken for **(C,D)**. **(C)** Transverse section through the diencephalic choroid plexus of 6 dpf *Et(cp:EGFP)*^{sj2} larvae stained with GFP, DAPI, and Zpr-1. **(D)** Transverse section through the myelencephalic choroid plexus of 6 dpf *Et(cp:EGFP)*^{sj2} larvae stained with GFP and DAPI. **(E)** Transverse section through the diencephalic choroid plexus of a 1-month-old *Et(cp:EGFP)*^{sj2} zebrafish stained with GFP and Zpr-1 to label the diencephalic choroid plexus and pineal gland, respectively. **(F)** Transverse section through the myelencephalic choroid plexus of a 1-month-old *Et(cp:EGFP)*^{sj2} zebrafish stained with GFP. Abbreviations: diencephalic CP, diencephalic choroid plexus; mCP, myelencephalic CP; GFP, green fluorescent protein; DAPI, 4′,6-diamidino-2-phenylindole; E, eye; F, forebrain; H, hindbrain. For all images: filled arrowhead, diencephalic choroid plexus; open arrowhead, pineal gland; arrow, myelencephalic choroid plexus. Scale bars are 50 μm.

choroid plexus of the third ventricle in zebrafish. We also detected GFP expression in the swimbladder (data not shown). The swimbladder consists of epithelial cells and has been compared to the mammalian lung (Winata et al., 2009). Using time-lapse confocal microscopy, GFP expression was detected in a subset of diencephalic choroid plexus cells as early as 30 hpf (see Supplemental Movie 1). We found that the myelencephalic choroid plexus epithelial cells migrated from the outer rhombomeres into the midbrain-hindbrain boundary as described previously (Garcia-Lecea et al., 2008) and also anteriorly from the developing spinal cord. These cells increase in GFP intensity as they coalesce to form a compact structure by approximately 72 hpf. There were no additional changes in choroid plexus morphology by 96 hpf.

ZEBRAFISH CHOROID PLEXUS EXPRESSES THE TIGHT JUNCTION PROTEIN CLAUDIN 5 AND POSSESSES TRANSPORTER ACTIVITY

The mammalian choroid plexus expresses many tight-junction proteins such as claudins (Lippoldt et al., 2000; Kratzer et al., 2012), occludin (Lagaraine et al., 2011), and junction adhesion molecules (Lagaraine et al., 2011). These tight junctions create a physical barrier between the blood and cerebrospinal fluid. To demonstrate that the zebrafish choroid plexus express tight junction protein similar to mammals, we studied Claudin 5 (Cldn5) expression because of the availability of an antibody that cross-reacts with zebrafish Cldn5 (Xie et al., 2010; Zhang et al., 2010). As predicted, whole-mount IHC analysis revealed Cldn5 expression at the cell membrane of zebrafish choroid plexus epithelium (**Figures 3A–C**). Cldn5 expression was also observed in the eyes, blood vessels, and neighboring ependymal cells (**Figures 3B,C**).

In mice, multidrug resistance transporters, such as MRP1, are expressed on the basolateral side of choroid plexus epithelium and regulate drug accumulation in the cerebrospinal fluid (Wijnholds et al., 2000). In addition to drug transport, MRP1 and MDR1, efflux fluorescent dyes such as rhodamine 123 (Saengkhae et al., 2003). To the best of our knowledge, no previous studies have demonstrated transporter function in zebrafish choroid

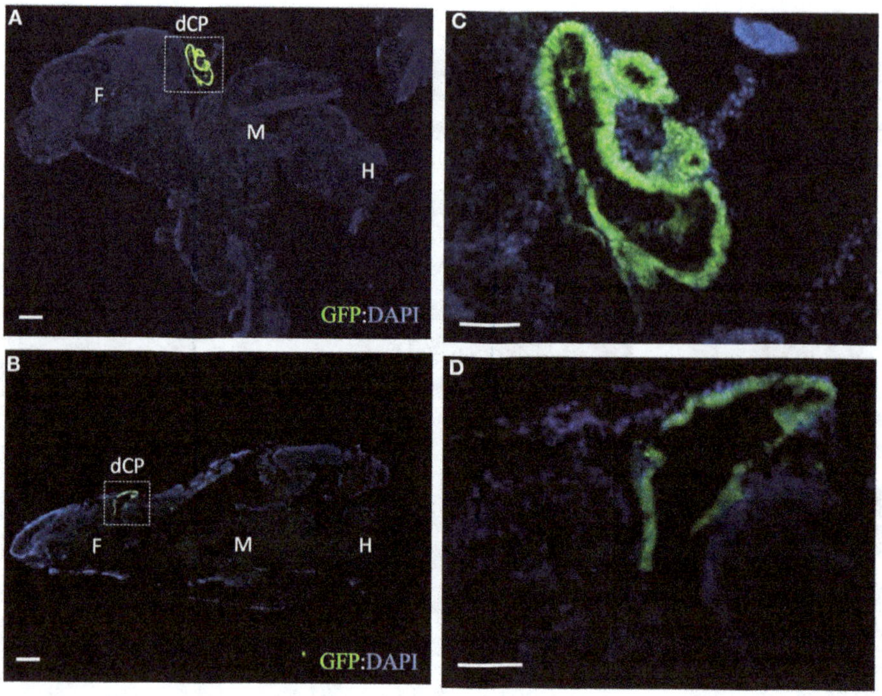

FIGURE 2 | The adult *Et(cp:EGFP)*^{sj2} expresses GFP in the saccus dorsalis. Sagital sections through adult brains were labeled with rabbit anti-GFP antibody (green) and counterstained with DAPI (blue). **(A,B)** shows GFP expression in the adult CP of the third ventricle taken through two different sagittal planes of the adult brain. Dashed-line boxes refer to magnified images shown in **(C,D)**. dCP: diencephalic CP; F: forebrain; M: midbrain; H: hindbrain. Scale bars are 100 μm.

plexus. To determine whether transporters contribute to the blood-cerebrospinal fluid barrier at the zebrafish choroid plexus, we intravenously injected rhodamine 123 into the *Et(cp:EGFP)*^{sj2} line at 4 dpf and observed its accumulation within the choroid plexus epithelium (**Figures 3D–F**). After injecting rhodamine 123 into the brain ventricle/cerebrospinal fluid, we also observed accumulation in the choroid plexus (**Figures 4A–D**), indicating that independent of what interface the rhodamine 123 resides (whether blood or cerebrospinal fluid), the dye is transported by the choroid plexus.

Another transporter that is highly expressed in the choroid plexus is organic anion transporter 3 (OAT3) (Keep and Smith, 2011). Fluorescein, a known substrate for OAT3, is taken up by the transporter on the apical side of the choroid plexus epithelium in a Na^+-dependent manner (Sykes et al., 2004). Because fluorescein is a low-molecular-weight green fluorescent dye, we soaked Casper zebrafish in 50 μM fluorescein to observe accumulation in the choroid plexus. The dye was ingested in the gut, entered the circulation, and concentrated in the diencephalic choroid plexus and myelencephalic choroid plexus (**Figures 3G,H**). Fluorescein injected into the brain ventricle had a similar pattern of accumulation in the myelencephalic choroid plexus and diencephalic choroid plexus (**Figures 4E–H**).

ZEBRAFISH CHOROID PLEXUS POSSESSES SIZE-SELECTIVE BARRIER PROPERTIES

To examine the function of the zebrafish choroid plexus in regulating passage from the bloodstream into the cerebrospinal fluid, we intravenously injected fluorescently labeled dextrans of various molecular weights into the transparent Casper line at 2, 3, and 4 dpf. Time-lapse imaging at 2 dpf, before the choroid plexus has fully developed, showed that 3-kDa fluorescein and 10-kDa rhodamine dextrans leaked from the bloodstream into the brain ventricle, whereas little to no 40-kDa fluorescein dextran escaped from the bloodstream into the ventricle (**Figure 5A**). By 3 dpf, there was still a significant difference with a *P*-value of < 0.0001 between the 3- and 10-kDa dextrans and the 40-kDa dextran; however, the overall permeability was lower at 3 dpf compared to 2 dpf (**Figure 5B**). By 4 dpf, when the choroid plexus was fully formed, there were no significant differences between the individual tracers (**Figure 5B**). Dorsal views of an intravenous injection of the 10-kDa dextran into *Et(cp:EGFP)*^{sj2} larvae at 2 dpf showed leakage into the brain ventricle as the choroid plexus continued to develop. Once formed by 4 dpf, dextran did not accumulate within the brain ventricle (**Figure 6A**). In addition, the 3- and 10-kDa dextrans were significantly more permeable at 2 dpf ($P < 0.0001$) compared to 3 and 4 dpf, but there was no significant difference in permeability for the 40-kDa dextran (**Figure 6B**).

IDENTIFICATION OF CHOROID PLEXUS MUTANTS

After demonstrating that the zebrafish choroid plexus develops and functions as the blood-cerebrospinal fluid barrier beginning at 3 dpf, we initiated a small-scale forward genetic screen to identify mutants with choroid plexus abnormalities. This screen focused primarily on myelencephalic choroid plexus defects.

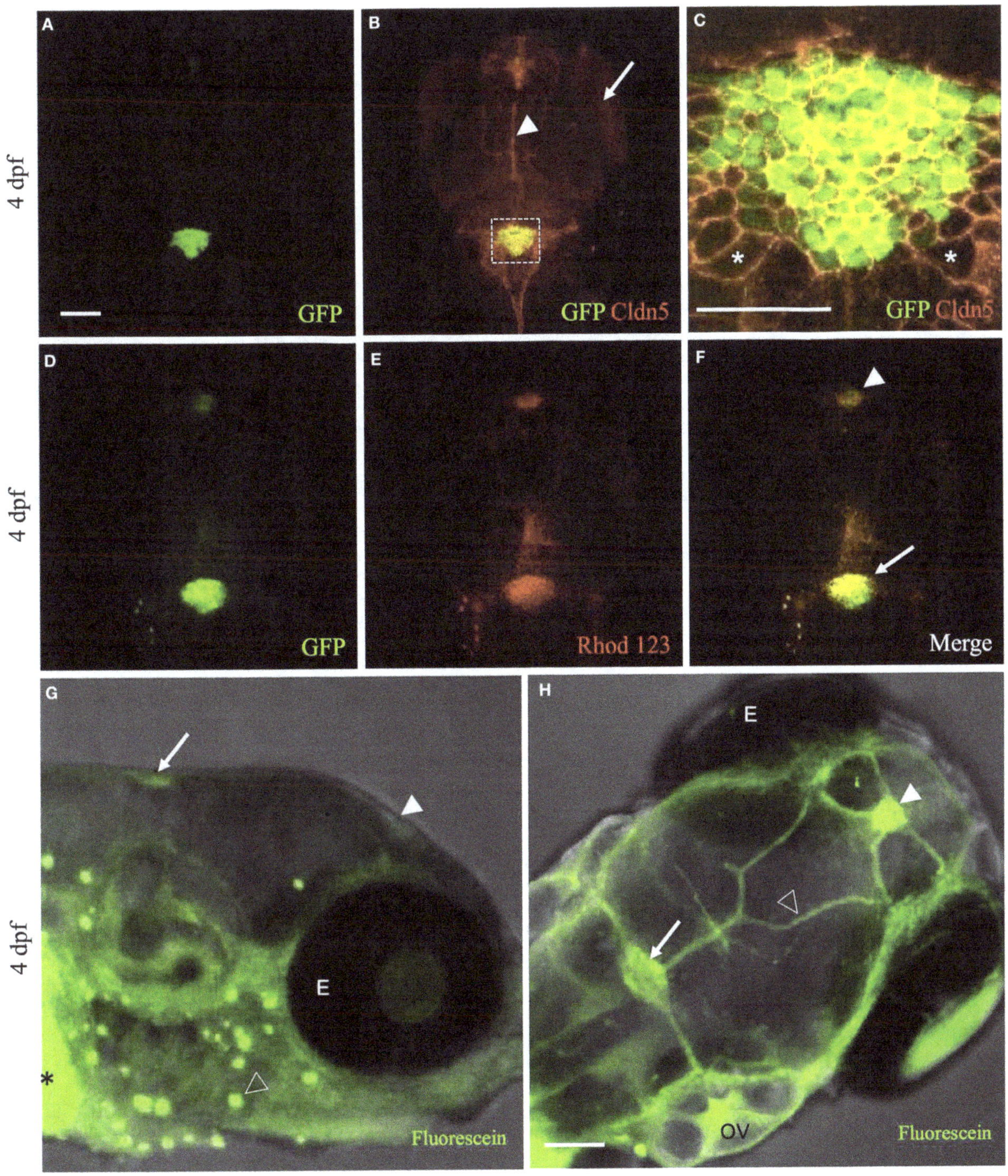

FIGURE 3 | The zebrafish CP possesses tight junction and transporter properties. (A) Whole-mount immunohistochemical staining of *Et(cp:EGFP)*[sj2] larvae at 4 dpf with GFP labeling the diencephalic choroid plexus and myelencephalic choroid plexus. **(B)** Whole-mount immunohistochemical staining with Claudin 5 antibody (red) showed expression in the eye (arrow), surface vessels (arrowhead), and CP. **(C)** Overlay of GFP and Claudin 5 staining revealed Claudin 5 expression surrounding the perimeter of CPe and ependymal cells. Examples of ependymal cells are shown with an asterisk (*). Images in **(A,B)** taken at 20× magnification and (C) at 40× magnification. **(D)** Live imaging of *Et(cp:EGFP)*[sj2] larvae at 4 dpf showed GFP expression in the CP. **(E,F)** Accumulation of rhodamine 123 in the diencephalic choroid plexus (arrowhead) and myelencephalic choroid plexus (arrow). **(G)** Side view of live Casper zebrafish treated at 4 dpf with 50 μM fluorescein for 4 h showed accumulation of fluorescein (represented in green) in the diencephalic choroid plexus (filled arrowhead) and myelencephalic choroid plexus (arrow) along with the gut (asterisk), and lateral line (open arrowhead). **(H)** Similar image as in **(G)** except for dorsal view showing accumulation in the diencephalic choroid plexus (filled arrowhead), myelencephalic choroid plexus (arrow), and overlying vasculature (open arrowhead). Abbreviations: dCP, diencephalic CP; mCP, myelencephalic CP; E, eye; OV; Otic vesicle. Scale bar in A and H is 50 μm. Scale bar in C is 20 μm.

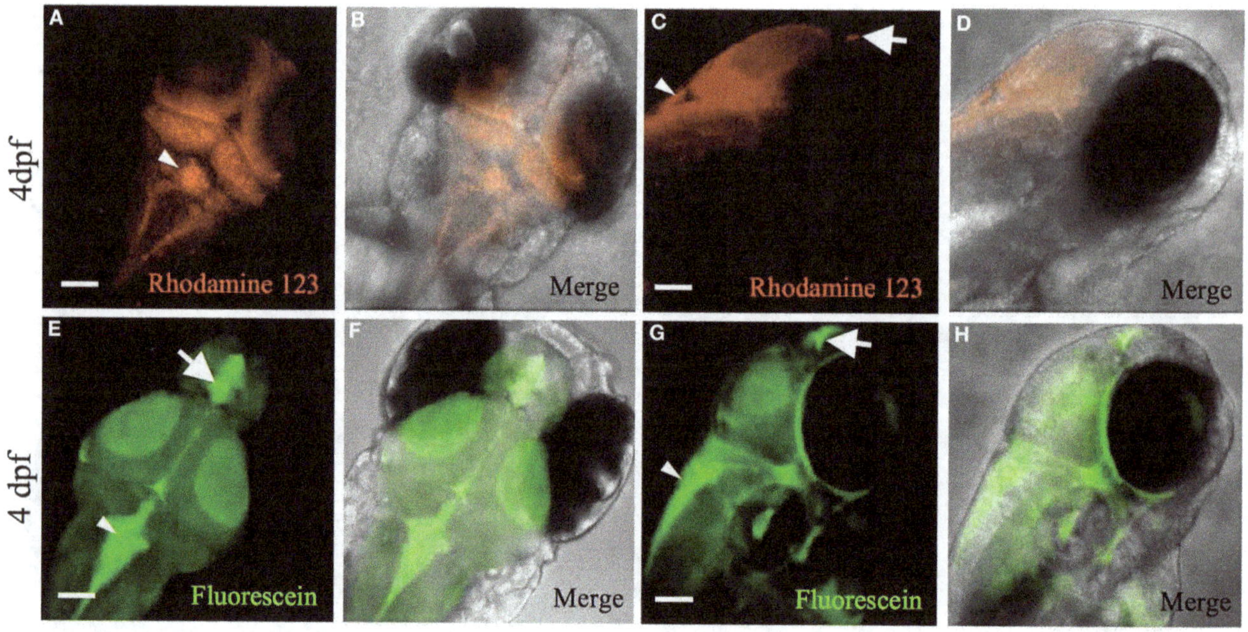

FIGURE 4 | Rhodamine 123 and fluorescein ventricle injection demonstrates transporter activity in the CP. Dorsal fluorescent **(A)** and merged (bright-field and Rhodamine 123) **(B)** confocal image of 4 dpf Casper larvae with Rhodamine 123 (red) injection into the brain ventricle. The rhodamine 123 concentrates within the myelencephalic choroid plexus (arrowhead). Rhodamine 123 also fluoresces green and co-localizes with red emission (not shown). Lateral fluorescent **(C)** and merged (bright-field and Rhodamine 123) **(D)** confocal image of 4 dpf Casper larvae with Rhodamine 123 (red) injection into the brain ventricle. The rhodamine 123 concentrates within the myelencephalic choroid plexus (arrowhead) and diencephalic choroid plexus (arrow). Dorsal fluorescent **(E)** and merged (bright-field and fluorescein) **(F)** confocal image of 4 dpf Casper larvae with fluorescein (green) injected into the brain ventricle. Fluorescein concentrates within the myelencephalic choroid plexus (arrowhead) and diencephalic choroid plexus (arrow). Lateral fluorescent **(G)** and merged(bright-field and fluorescein) **(H)** confocal image of 4 dpf Casper larvae with fluorescein (green) injected into the brain ventricle. Fluorescein concentrates within the myelencephalic choroid plexus (arrowhead) and diencephalic choroid plexus (arrow). Abbreviations: mCP, myelencephalic choroid plexus; dCP, diencephalic choroid plexus. Scale bar is 50 μm.

Table 1 shows the numbers of fish generated from this screen. Briefly, 20 F_0 *Et(cp:EGFP)*^{sj2} males were mutagenized with ENU. One month after treatment, ENU efficiency was tested by mating the males to Casper and screening for *nacre* or *roy* phenotypes. Approximately 1 in 250 (0.4%) larvae showed the *nacre* or *roy* phenotype. The mutagenized males were mated with *Et(cp:EGFP)*^{sj2} females to generate 409 F_1 fish. Adult F_1 pairs were mated together or with non-mutagenized *Et(cp:EGFP)*^{sj2} fish to produce 224 F_2 families. Of the F_2 families, 73 contained sufficient numbers to screen 4–6 pairs for mutants in the F_3 generation. We set up 1330 $F_2 \times F_2$ crosses (including re-crosses), with 421 crosses producing F_3 embryos. Larvae were screened at 4 dpf to identify choroid plexus defects based on GFP expression patterns. In total, we generated approximately16,339 F_3 embryos and screened approximately 12,196.

We identified 24 mutant lines with 10 recessive mutant lines having choroid plexus deformities. Time-lapse imaging showing choroid plexus development for wild-type and some mutants are demonstrated in Supplemental Movies 2–7. In addition to choroid plexus deformities, each of the10 recessive lines had other defects such as heart edema, small eyes, and small head. While several of the mutants exhibited brain cell death, many did not develop cell death until after the choroid plexus started to form. A description of the onset of brain cell death for each line is listed in **Table 2**. We also found spontaneous mutants that had normal morphology overall, but severely abnormal or no choroid plexus (data not shown). In addition, we found many mutants (some recessive and some spontaneous) with severe brain cell death and normal choroid plexus development (data not shown). The choroid plexus mutant lines were named based on the original F_2 family and pair number within that family. No mutants were adult viable and most did not survive past 4 dpf, except for *cp26.6* and *cp105.2,* which lived until 5 and 6 dpf, respectively. *cp27.5* and *cp44.10* mutants displayed similar phenotypes; however, complementation analysis showed that they were not in the same complementation group. On the basis of GFP intensity, epithelial localization, and overall choroid plexus morphology, we identified five classes: (I) mutants with reduced GFP expression, dispersed epithelial cells, and irregularly shaped choroid plexus; (II) mutants with normal GFP expression, small epithelial aggregates, and irregularly shaped choroid plexus; (III) mutants with normal GFP expression, small epithelial aggregates, and expanded choroid plexus; (IV) mutants with variable GFP expression, small epithelial aggregates, and expanded choroid plexus; and (V) mutants with normal GFP expression, compact epithelial cells, and enlarged choroid plexus. While complementation analysis was not performed between all of these mutants, we are fairly certain that these mutations are in different genes. However, we acknowledge that it is possible that different types of mutations in the same gene from different mutants could result in additional

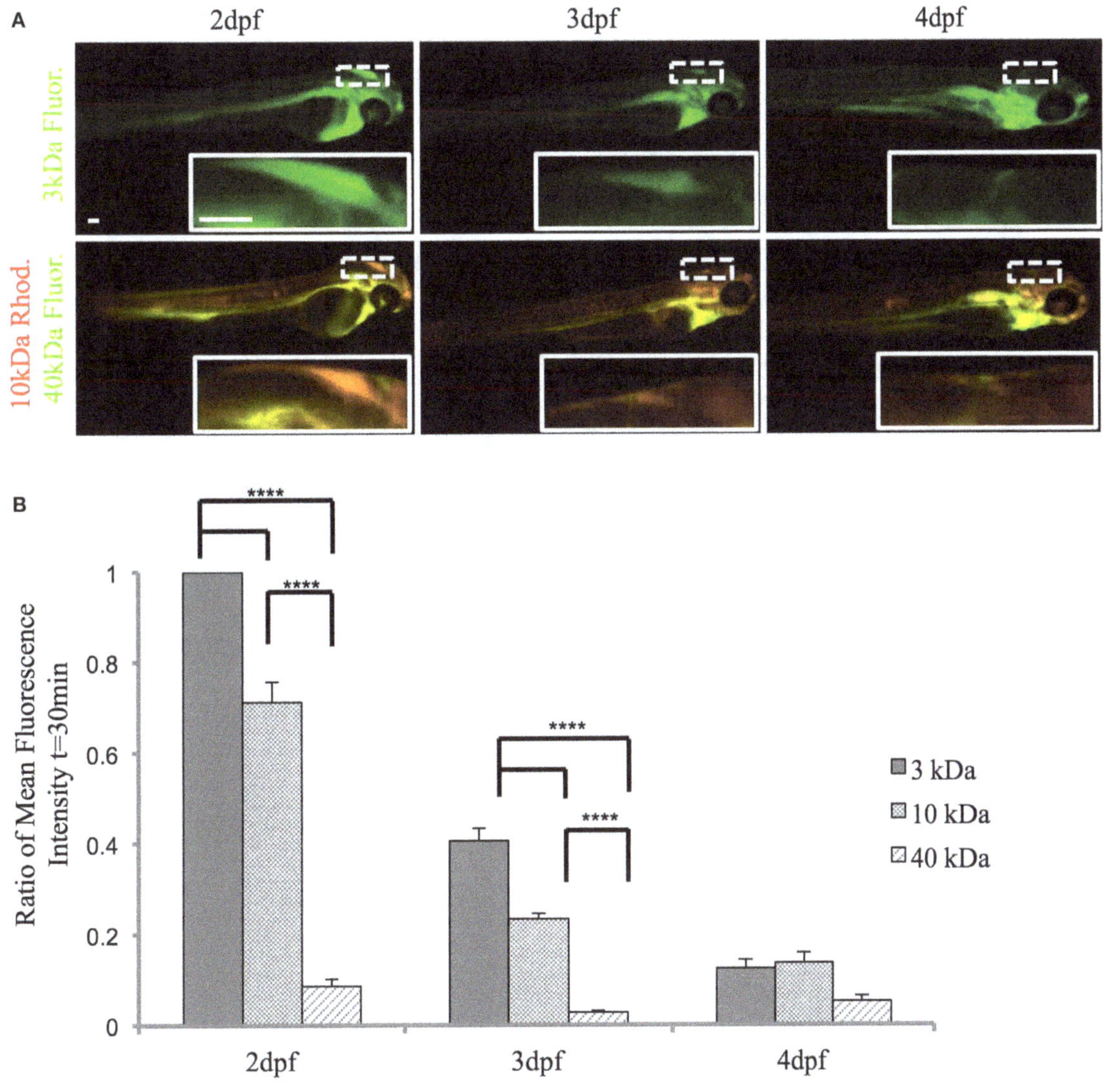

FIGURE 5 | The zebrafish CP is functional and possesses size-selective properties. Casper zebrafish were intravenously injected with fluorescent tracers at 2, 3, and 4 dpf to identify tracer leakage from blood into the cerebrospinal fluid. **(A)** The top panel shows severe leakage of the 3-kDa fluorescein dextran into the brain ventricle (inset) at 2 dpf, minor leakage at 3 dpf, and little, if any, dextran penetration at 4 dpf. The bottom panel shows permeability of the 10-kDa rhodamine dextran at 2 dpf (inset), which decreases by 4 dpf. The 40-kDa fluorescein dextran was the least permeable at each developmental timepoint. Images were taken at 1 h post-injection. **(B)** A ratio of fluorescence intensity in the brain ventricle relative to the heart was measured at 30 min post-injection as a readout for tracer leakage into the brain ventricle. A One-Way ANOVA shows that the 3-kDa fluorescein dextran and the 10-kDa rhodamine dextran are significantly more permeable (i.e., greater mean fluorescence intensity) than the 40-kDa fluorescein dextran at 2 and 3 dpf. By 4 dpf, there was no significant difference in fluorescence intensity. Measurements are expressed as mean ± *SE* for $n = 7$; $^{****}p < 0.0001$. Abbreviations: Rhod, rhodamine dextran; Flour: fluorescein dextran. Scale bar is 50 μm.

phenotypes. A description of these mutants and choroid plexus morphology are presented in **Table 2** and **Figure 7**, respectively. Wild-type *Et(cp:EGFP)*^{sj2} larvae at 3 and 4 dpf are shown in **Figures 7A–D′** as a reference to compare with mutant classes.

To further classify these mutants, we analyzed brain ventricle morphology and transporter activity in the choroid plexus. To examine brain ventricle morphology, we injected a 40-kDa fluorescein dextran into the ventricle of *Et(cp:EGFP)*^{sj2} mutants that were generated by outcrossing the mutant lines to the wild-type TL strain, were GFP negative, and selected based upon phenotypic traits. Descriptions of brain ventricles and their morphology are presented in **Table 2** and **Figure 7**, respectively. None of the mutants except *cp26.6* and *cp105.2* had normal ventricle morphology, While some mutants such as *cp79.6* and *cp79.8* had a third, fourth, and lateral ventricles, the shape or size of the ventricle differed from wild-type. None of the mutants except *cp26.6* and *cp105.2* had normal ventricle morphology. Severe cases having no defined ventricular boundaries were observed in mutants *cp9.6*, *cp27.5*, *cp44.10*, and *cp151.2*.

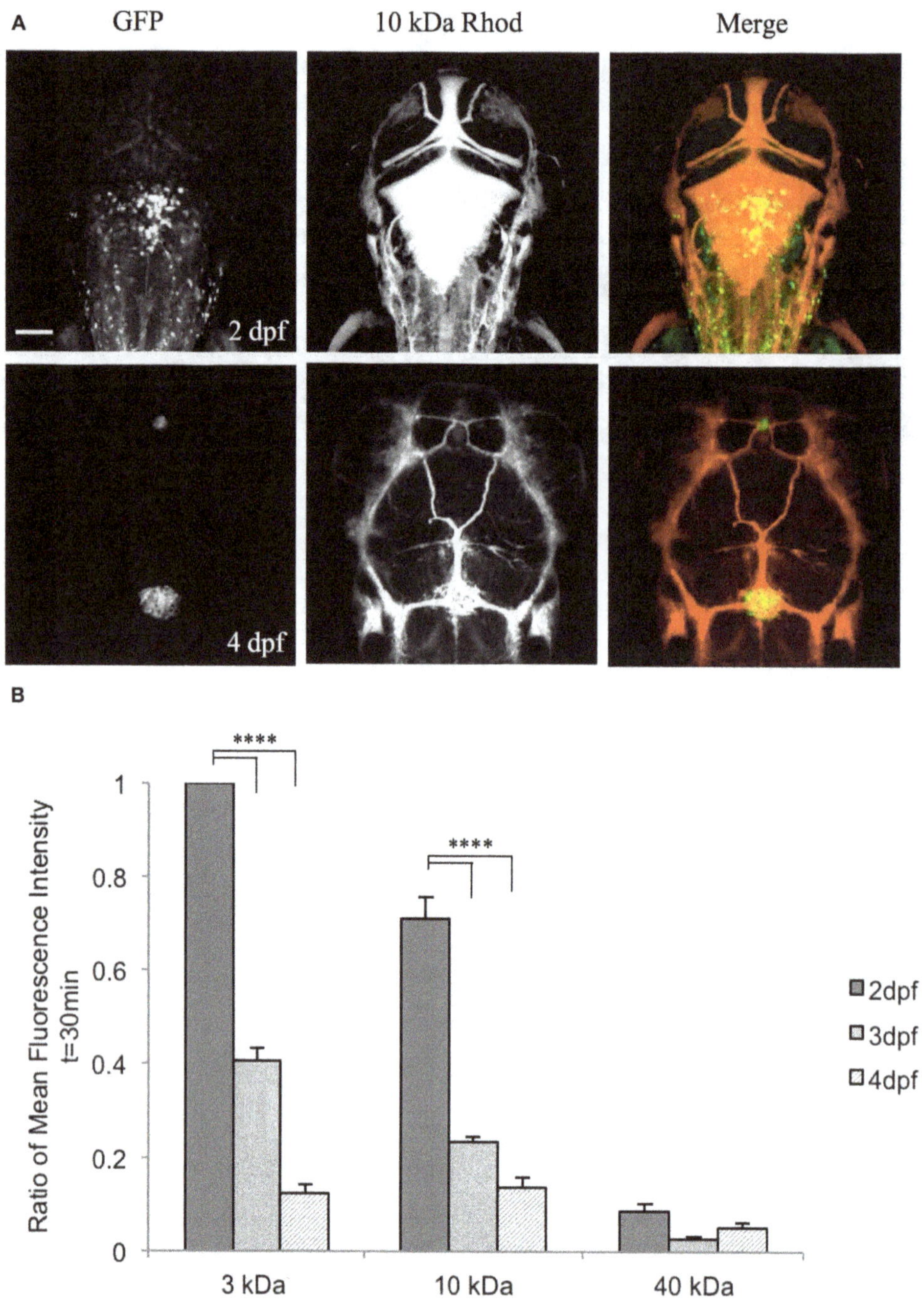

FIGURE 6 | The zebrafish CP becomes size-selective as it develops. **(A)** *Et(cp:EGFP)*^{sj2} larvae were intravenously injected with a 10 kDa rhodamine-dextran and the CP was imaged dorsally by confocal microscopy. At 2 dpf, the CP is not fully developed as observed by GFP expression and the 10 kDa rhodamine-dextran inundates the brain ventricle. By 4 dpf, the CP is fully formed and the 10 kDa rhodamine-dextran is retained within the vasculature and does not enter the brain ventricle. **(B)** A One-Way ANOVA analysis revealed that the 3 kDa fluorescein dextran and 10 kDa rhodamine dextran have a significantly higher fluorescent intensity in the brain ventricle (i.e., more permeable) at 2 dpf compared to 3 and 4 dpf. There is no significant difference between developmental time points for the 40 kDa fluorescein dextran. Measurements are means ± *SE* for $n = 7$; ****$p < 0.0001$. Scale bar is 50 μm.

FLUORESCEIN ASSAY TO DETERMINE CHOROID PLEXUS TRANSPORT

Fluorescein transport was used as a secondary assay to measure transporter activity in the choroid plexus and overall permeability (refer to **Figures 3G,H**). To determine if the choroid plexus could transport fluorescein in the mutants, larvae were treated at 3 dpf with 50 μM fluorescein as described above (**Figure 8**). In Class I mutants, *cp26.3* had fluorescein accumulation toward the anterior part of the brain and no fluorescein accumulated within the choroid plexus (**Figure 8E**). Fluorescein did not accumulate in the choroid plexus epithelium in the *cp140.2* mutant, but was

Table 1 | Number of zebrafish generated from the forward genetic screen.

Generation	Fish (*n*)
G_0 males mutagenized	20
G_0 males survived	9
F_1	409
F_2 families started	224
F_2 families screened	73
$F_2 \times F_2$ crosses	1330
F_2 families that spawned	421
F_3 embryos screened	12,196
Mutants lines identified	24
Mutant lines maintained	10

localized throughout the brain ventricle. These mutants also had a higher overall fluorescein uptake than wildtype. (**Figure 8M**).

In Class II mutants, *cp9.6* mutants also exhibited a higher overall uptake of fluorescein than wild-type and concentrated within the brain ventricle, gut, and heart. There was no distinct accumulation within the choroid plexus (**Figure 8F**). For *cp79.6*, the overall uptake of fluorescein was comparable to wild-type. We observed very faint punctate accumulate of fluorescein within the general area of the choroid plexus indicating possible transport (**Figure 8N**).

Class III mutants (*cp79.8* and *cp151.2*) had increased uptake of fluorescein compared to wild-type and both had accumulation within the brain ventricle, gut, and heart. No fluorescein accumulated within the choroid plexus epithelium (**Figures 8G–O**). A similar phenotype was observed in Class IV mutants (*cp27.5* and *cp44.10*) in that they also had increased uptake of fluorescein concentrated within the brain ventricle, gut, and heart, but no localization within choroid plexus epithelium (**Figures 8H–P**). We were not able conclude whether Class V mutants (*cp26.6* and *cp105.2*) demonstrated transport activity using this assay because of the inability to confidently identify GFP negative mutants at 3 and 4 dpf. Once we identified mutants by late 4–5 dpf, the fluorescein was rapidly cleared by the gut and was not distributed throughout the embryo (data not shown).

GENETIC MAPPING OF *cp9.6* AND *cp27.5*

To identify the mutated gene for lines *cp9.6* and *cp27.5*, which displayed hydrocephaly phenotypes, we performed genetic mapping using 192 polymorphic markers distributed evenly across the genome. By bulked segregant analysis, we found linkage to marker z3275 that mapped *cp9.6* to chromosome 4. With z3275, we tested 100 mutants and identified 4 recombinants in 200 meiotic events. The critical interval along the chromosome was defined by recombination analysis. We identified polymorphic markers on either side of z3275, z23802, and z15751; however, the lack of additional polymorphic markers within this region made it difficult to define a reasonable mapping distance.

For *cp27.5*, we identified markers z2363 and z15891 by bulked segregant analysis to map the mutation to chromosome 21. Within this critical interval, we identified the marker z9233 and found no recombinants out of 48 meioses. We then tested additional polymorphic markers and counted the number of recombinants on either side of z9233 to refine the critical interval. By testing polymorphic markers, BX530031.5 and BX530023.5, that we selected from the zebrafish genome published in Ensembl Zv9, we narrowed the region to ~0.4 Mb. In total, we analyzed 450 meioses. Future analysis will include testing candidate genes within this interval to identify the mutated gene.

DISCUSSION

The goal of our study was to establish zebrafish as a functionally relevant model to study choroid plexus development and as a screening tool to genetically dissect genes involved in choroid plexus formation, function, and maintenance. Although the choroid plexus has been studied in various *in vivo* and *in vitro* models (Dohrmann, 1970; Strazielle and Preston, 2003), the developmental and genetic aspects of this structure remain poorly understood largely due to the lack of innovative strategies and functionally relevant systems (Saunders et al., 2008). Also, current models do not easily allow for choroid plexus development to be visualized in real time. To overcome this limitation, we created an enhancer trap zebrafish line, $Et(cp{:}EGFP)^{sj2}$, which expresses EGFP within the diencephalic choroid plexus and myelencephalic choroid plexus. Using this line, choroid plexus development was easily observed in a live vertebrate by monitoring EGFP expression.

Previous studies have also generated enhancer trap lines in zebrafish expressing GFP in the choroid plexus (Bill et al., 2008; Garcia-Lecea et al., 2008). However, there are variations within these lines, including the subsets of cells expressing GFP. For example, in the Et^{Mn16} line (Bill et al., 2008), only a subset of cells of the myelencephalic choroid plexus express GFP. In addition, the *SqET33-E20* (Gateways) line has additional GFP expression in the rhombomeres (Garcia-Lecea et al., 2008). In our study, there was specific GFP expression in the diencephalic choroid plexus, myelencephalic choroid plexus, and swimbladder. In regards to GFP expression in the swimbladder, studies have shown that Sonic hedgehog (Shh) is expressed in the epithelial cells lining the swimbladder (Winata et al., 2009). Interestingly, the choroid plexus of other vertebrates has also been compared to the mammalian lung in a study by Nielsen and Dymecki (2010) demonstrating that Shh (also expressed in choroid plexus epithelia) is required for the synchronized outgrowth of the choroid plexus and fenestrated vasculature, similar to the need for Shh in coordinating the outgrowth of the lung (Nielsen and Dymecki, 2010). Since the zebrafish swimbladder has been compared to the mammalian lung (Winata et al., 2009), common underlying developmental pathways, such as Shh, required in both choroid plexus and swimbladder development, maybe be regulating GFP expression in these tissues. The variations in other enhancer trap lines may be due to transgenic DNA constructs integrating into different regions of the genome. Our PCR and Southern blot analysis revealed a single integration on chromosome 13. In contrast, the Gateways line has a single insertion on chromosome 24 (Garcia-Lecea et al., 2008), which likely accounts for the differences in expression patterns between lines. Similar to the previously published zebrafish choroid plexus papers (Bill et al., 2008; Garcia-Lecea et al., 2008), we were unable to identify the

Table 2 | Characterization of *Et(cp:EGFP)* mutants generated from the forward genetic screen.

Class	Allele	Map position	DPF	Other phenotypes(4 dpf)	Fluorescein transport	Onset of brain cell death (up to 4 dpf)	Initial circulation loss (up to 4 dpf)
I: reduced GFP expression, dispersed epithelia, and irregularly shaped CP	*cp26.3*[a]	ND	2–3	No swimbladder; brain and tail cell death; brain ventricle hemorrhaging; faint heartbeat; no circulation; no midbrain-hindbrain boundaries	Accumulates within third ventricle	3 dpf	3 dpf
	cp140.2	ND	2	Small head; small eyes; no swimbladder; heart edema; brain cell death; faint heartbeat and circulation; slightly larger third ventricle and wider lateral ventricles ventricle	Increased uptake; accumulates within brain ventricle	4 dpf	4 dpf
II: normal GFP expression, smaller epithelial aggregates, and irregularly shaped CP	*cp9.6*	LG 4	2	Small head; small eyes; no swimbladder; heart edema; occasional hydrocephalus; brain cell death; no circulation; no distinct third ventricle or lateral ventricles and severely reduced fourth ventricle	Increased uptake; accumulates within brain ventricle	2 dpf	4 dpf
	cp79.6	ND	2	Small head; small eyes; no swimbladder; heart edema; many still in chorion; brain cell death; hemorrhaging around heart; slow heartbeat; little to no circulation; wider lateral ventricles	Dispersed punctate staining on the dorsal ventricle surface	4 dpf	3 dpf
III: normal GFP expression, smaller epithelial aggregates, and expanded CP	*cp79.8*	ND	2	Small head; small eyes; no swimbladder; brain cell death; hemorrhaging around heart; decreased heartbeat and circulation; wider lateral ventricles	Increased uptake; accumulates within brain ventricle	4 dpf	3 dpf
	cp151.2	ND	2–3	Small head; small eyes; no swimbladder; brain cell death; minor swelling around head; occasional hemorrhaging around heart; smaller third ventricle and no defined lateral ventricles	Increased uptake; accumulates within brain ventricle	4 dpf	4 dpf
IV: variable GFP expression, smaller epithelial aggregates, and expanded CP	*cp27.5*	LG 21	2	Small head; small eyes; no swimbladder; brain cell death; heart edema; small arched body; curved tail; hydrocephalus; occasional hemorrhaging in brain ventricle; heartbeat, but little to no circulation; no defined ventricle boundaries	Increased uptake; accumulates within brain ventricle	2 dpf (localized to forebrain)	3 dpf

(Continued)

Table 2 | Continued

Class	Allele	Map position	DPF	Other phenotypes(4 dpf)	Fluorescein transport	Onset of brain cell death (up to 4 dpf)	Initial circulation loss (up to 4 dpf)
	cp44.10	ND	2	Small head; small eyes; no swimbladder; brain cell death; heart edema; small arched body; curved tail; hydrocephalus; occasional hemorrhaging around heart; heartbeat, but little to no circulation; no third ventricle or lateral ventricles and irregularly shaped fourth ventricle	Increased uptake; accumulates within brain ventricle	2 dpf (localized to forebrain)	4 dpf
V: normal GFP expression, compact epithelia, and enlarged CP	*cp26.6*[b]	ND	4	Rounded head, protruding lower jaw; no swimbladder; edema around heart, eyes, and gut; faint heartbeat and circulation; normal brain ventricle	N/A	N/A	4 dpf
	cp105.2[b]	ND	4–5	Rounded head, protruding lower jaw; no swimbladder; severe edema around heart, eyes, and gut; faint heartbeat and circulation; slightly smaller fourth ventricle	N/A	N/A	6 dpf

[a]*Observations recorded at 3 dpf;* [b]*observations recorded at 5 dpf; ND, not determined; N/A, not applicable.*

enhancer regulating GFP expression in the choroid plexus. This is often true with enhancer trap effects where is difficult to identify the enhancer if it acts at distances upstream or downstream of the reporter gene.

We have demonstrated blood-cerebrospinal fluid barrier properties in zebrafish by identifying tight junction proteins and transporter activity. We have shown Cldn5 expression within the choroid plexus and demonstrated that the zebrafish choroid plexus possess a chemical barrier that transports and concentrates rhodamine 123 and fluorescein in the choroid plexus epithelium. Rhodamine 123 directly interacts with MRP1 and MDR1 in an ATP-dependent manner (Shapiro and Ling, 1998; Daoud et al., 2000). Because previous studies have shown the specificity of rhodamine 123 to multidrug resistance proteins (MDRs), similar drug transporters are likely expressed in the zebrafish choroid plexus. Studies in mice have identified known transporters of rhodamine 123 such as MRP1 to be localized at the basolateral side of choroid plexus epithelium and have been shown to keep drugs such as etoposide out of the cerebrospinal fluid (Wijnholds et al., 2000; Keep and Smith, 2011). Our findings also confirm that transporters are present in the zebrafish choroid plexus by showing that: when coming from the bloodstream, rhodamine 123 accumulates within the choroid plexus and is prevented from entering the cerebrospinal fluid. When injected directly into the cerebrospinal fluid, the choroid plexus removed rhodamine 123 from the fluid as shown by dye accumulation within choroid plexus epithelium. Unfortunately, due to the lack of antibodies that cross-react with zebrafish proteins, we were unable to demonstrate the expression of specific transporters in the zebrafish choroid plexus. We tested an antibody against MDR1 (C219), but found expression only within brain endothelial cells of the blood-brain barrier (Umans and Taylor, 2012) and not the choroid plexus (data not shown). We also tested several commercially available antibodies against OAT3, but none cross-reacted with zebrafish. Additionally, while we did not observe Glut1 expression within the zebrafish choroid plexus, a recent review by Keep and Smith indicated that the BBB, not the blood-cerebrospinal fluid barrier, may be the major source of transporting glucose into the brain and that the choroid plexus may play a minor role in glucose transport (Keep and Smith, 2011).

We demonstrated barrier function in the zebrafish choroid plexus by injecting fluorescent tracers of different molecular weights and observing permeability across the choroid plexus epithelium into the cerebrospinal fluid. Once the choroid plexus fully formed by 4 dpf, the smallest tracer tested, a 3-kDa fluorescein dextran, was no longer permeable across the blood-cerebrospinal fluid barrier as it was in earlier developmental stages. This result indicated a tightening of the barrier as it develops. Although we did not distinguish between transcellular and paracellular transport, there appears to be a correlation between choroid plexus formation and decreased permeability, suggesting that a physical barrier is preventing molecule entry rather than being cleared by a cerebrospinal fluid drainage pathway. For

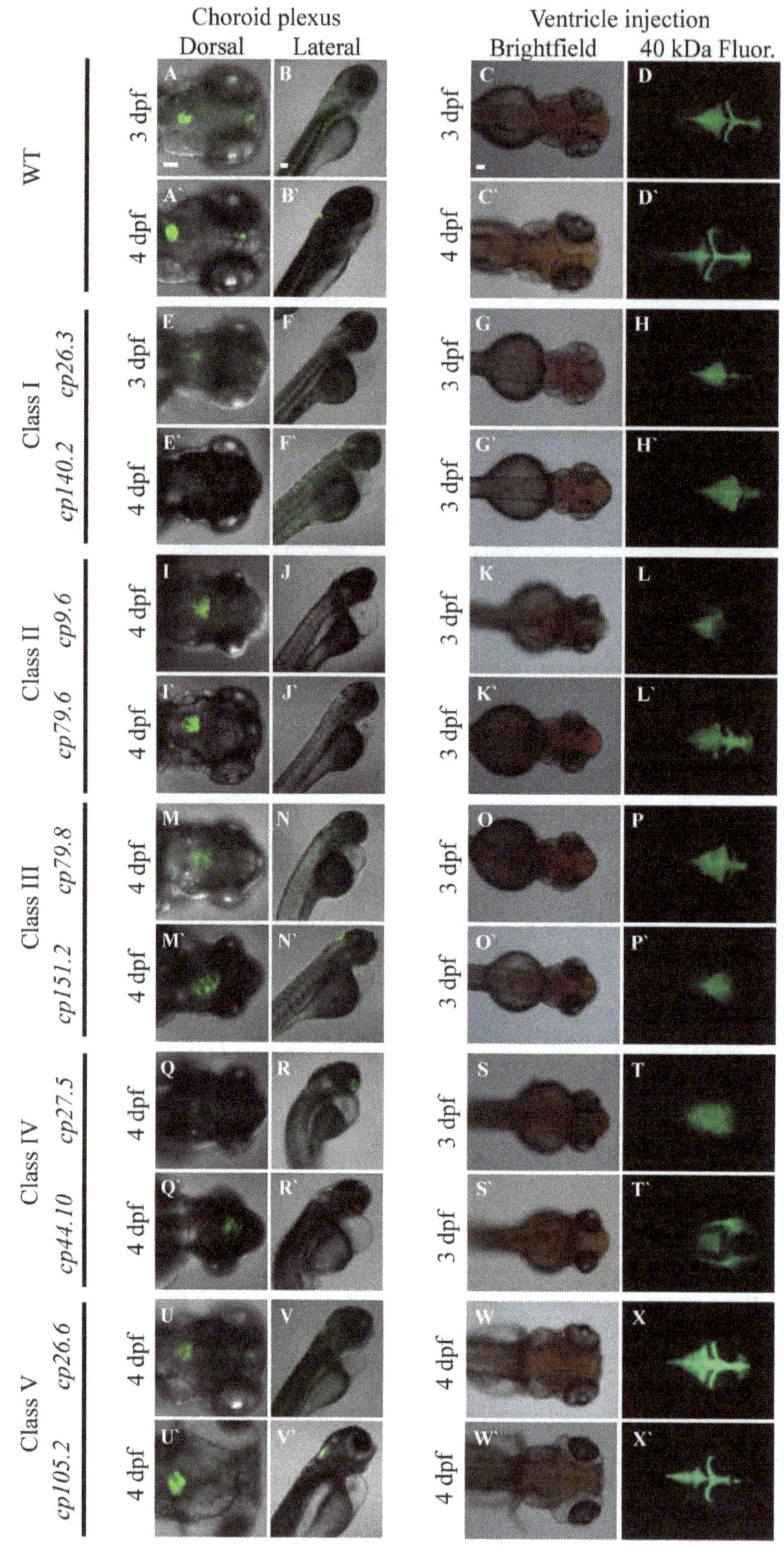

FIGURE 7 | Forward genetic screen identifies five classes of CP mutants. **(A–B′)** Wild-type *Et(cp:EGFP)*^{sj2} larvae at 3 dpf and 4 dpf. **(C–C′)** Bright field image of 3 and 4 dpf wild-type after ventricle injection of the 40-kDa fluorescein dextran. **(D–D′)** Fluorescent image of 3 and 4 dpf wild-type after ventricle injection of the 40-kDa fluorescein dextran. Class I: **(E,F)** *cp26.3* at 3 dpf. **(E′,F′)** *cp140.2* at 4 dpf. **(G)** Bright field image of *cp26.3* at 3 dpf after ventricle injection of the 40-kDa fluorescein dextran. **(G′)** Bright field

(Continued)

FIGURE 7 | Continued
image of *cp140.2* at 3 dpf after ventricle injection of the 40-kDa fluorescein dextran. **(H)** Fluorescent image of *cp26.3* at 3 dpf after ventricle injection of the 40-kDa fluorescein dextran. **(H′)** Fluorescent image of *cp140.2* at 3 dpf after ventricle injection of the 40-kDa fluorescein dextran. Class II: **(I,J)** *cp9.6* at 4 dpf. **(I′,J′)** *cp79.6* at 4 dpf. **(K)** Bright field image of *cp9.6* at 3 dpf after ventricle injection of the 40-kDa fluorescein dextran. **(K′)** Bright field image of *cp79.6* at 3 dpf after ventricle injection of the 40-kDa fluorescein dextran. **(L)** Fluorescent image of *cp9.6* at 3 dpf after ventricle injection of the 40-kDa fluorescein dextran. **(L′)** Fluorescent image of *cp79.6* at 3 dpf after ventricle injection of the 40-kDa fluorescein dextran. Class III: **(M,N)** *cp79.8* at 4 dpf. **(M′,N′)** *cp151.2* at 4 dpf. **(O)** Bright field image of *cp79.8* at 3 dpf after ventricle injection of the 40-kDa fluorescein dextran. **(O′)** Bright field image of *cp151.2* at 3 dpf after ventricle injection of the 40-kDa fluorescein dextran. **(P)** Fluorescent image of *cp79.8* at 3 dpf after ventricle injection of the 40-kDa fluorescein dextran. **(P′)** Fluorescent image of *cp151.2* at 3 dpf after ventricle injection of the 40-kDa fluorescein dextran. Class IV: **(Q,R)** *cp27.5* at 4dpf. **(Q′,R′)** *cp44.10* at 4 dpf. **(S)** Bright field image of *cp27.5* at 3 dpf after ventricle injection of the 40-kDa fluorescein dextran. **(S′)** Bright field image of *cp44.10* at 3 dpf after ventricle injection of the 40-kDa fluorescein dextran. **(T)** Fluorescent image of *cp27.5* at 3 dpf after ventricle injection of the 40-kDa fluorescein dextran. **(T′)** Fluorescent image of *cp44.10* at 3 dpf after ventricle injection of the 40-kDa fluorescein dextran. Class V: **(U,V)** *cp26.6* at 4 dpf. **(U′,V′)** *cp105.2* at 4 dpf. **(W)** Bright field image of *cp26.6* at 4 dpf after ventricle injection of the 40-kDa fluorescein dextran. **(W′)** Bright field image of *cp105.2* at 4 dpf after ventricle injection of the 40-kDa fluorescein dextran. **(X)** Fluorescent image of *cp26.6* at 4 dpf after ventricle injection of the 40-kDa fluorescein dextran. **(X′)** Fluorescent image of *cp105.2* at 4 dpf after ventricle injection of the 40-kDa fluorescein dextran. The first, third, and fourth panels for each class are dorsal views while the second panel is a lateral view. The first and second panels for each class were acquired by confocal microscopy. The third and fourth panels were acquired by fluorescent stereoscopy. The first panel for each class is at 20× magnification, the second panel is at 10× magnification, and the third and fourth panels are at 16× magnification. 40 kDa Fluor, 40 kDa Fluorescein Dextran. Scale bars in A, B, and C are 50 μm.

example, this is demonstrated when we injected the 40-kDa tracer into the bloodstream on day 4 and never observed tracer accumulation within the ventricle throughout the course of the timelapse. Rather than suggesting that the tracer is being cleared from the ventricle by cerebrospinal fluid flow, we observed that the tracer never entered the ventricle in the first place. This indicated to us that a physical barrier is preventing the dextran from crossing the barrier. Had we observed accumulation of the dextran within the cerebrospinal fluid/brain ventricle after injection, and then observed a decrease in the amount of tracer in the ventricle over time, then we would suggest that cerebrospinal fluid flow is the contributing factor and not a physical blockage of the dextran by the barrier as we observed. In immature brain barriers, it has been reported that the accumulation of molecules within the cerebrospinal fluid is not due to increased permeability of the barrier but reduced cerebrospinal fluid flow (Saunders et al., 2008). In contrast, more mature brain barriers have increased cerebrospinal fluid flow that limits the accumulation of molecules within the ventricular space (Saunders et al., 2008). Our study showed that after the formation of the choroid plexus there was no tracer penetration into the ventricle. Therefore, a decrease in tracer accumulation in the brain ventricle does not appear to be due to increased cerebrospinal fluid clearance, but due to physical barrier properties of the choroid plexus. The decrease in barrier permeability as the choroid plexus develops establishes the zebrafish choroid plexus as a functioning organ with size-selective barrier properties.

Forward genetic screens have been performed in various multicellular organisms such as plants (Meinke and Sussex, 1979), flies (Nusslein-Volhard and Wieschaus, 1980), worms (Sin et al., 2014), zebrafish (Driever et al., 1996), and mice (Nolan et al., 2000). These screens have been very successful in discovering genes involved in embryonic patterning, organ development, and behavior (Stemple et al., 1996; Horvitz, 1999; Muto et al., 2005). To characterize the mutants in our study, we examined not only GFP expression in the choroid plexus but also ventricle morphology and transporter activity. Previous studies have grouped zebrafish brain ventricle mutants into four categories: midline separation defects, reduced ventricle size, lateral ventricles and fourth ventricle abnormalities, and absence of lumen inflation (Lowery et al., 2009). Because none of our choroid plexus mutants exhibited a phenotype at 24 hpf, we did not expect to see defects in midline separation as described in Lowery et al. (2009). Choroid plexus mutants such as *cp79.6* and *cp140.2* have a brain ventricle that closely resembles normal larvae at 2 dpf (Lowery et al., 2007), indicating these mutants may have a developmental delay and not necessarily a brain ventricle defect. Also, *cp140.2* mutants at 3 dpf are similar to wild-type larvae at 2 dpf in that the fluorescein accumulated within the brain ventricle rather than concentrating within choroid plexus epithelium as it does normally on day 3. Many mutants exhibited an increased overall uptake of fluorescein, which may indicate defects in the skin epithelial barrier as well and increased permeability to absorb small molecules from their surroundings.

While mutants exhibit little to no heart beat and circulation when screened on day 4, as described in **Table 2**, the majority of mutants do have a strong heart beat and rapid circulation indistinguishable from wild-type prior to this timepoint. The initial onset of circulation loss describes when we first observed mutants with decreased or no circulation. Not all of the mutants had loss of circulation at the same time, but the onset describes when we observed the first mutant from a spawn having no circulation. Because most began to have decreased heartbeat and circulation at 4 dpf after the choroid plexus has already developed, we conclude that other factors are regulating choroid plexus development. However, we cannot rule out that circulation is required for choroid plexus maintenance. We also do not attribute the lack of blood flow to abnormal choroid plexus development, because we identified spontaneous mutants with a normal choroid plexus but no circulation (data not shown). After injecting single-cell embryos with a cardiac troponin morpholino to block heartbeat (Sehnert et al., 2002), we identified no choroid plexus defects resembling abnormalities of the five mutant classes (data not shown). Therefore, we conclude that if loss of circulation alone was the factor governing abnormal choroid plexus development in these mutants, we should see a choroid plexus that resembled that of troponin morphants. Because many mutants continued to have a heartbeat and circulation at 3 dpf, which is essential for brain ventricle expansion (Lowery and Sive, 2005), we also did not expect ventricle expansion defects in these mutants. While

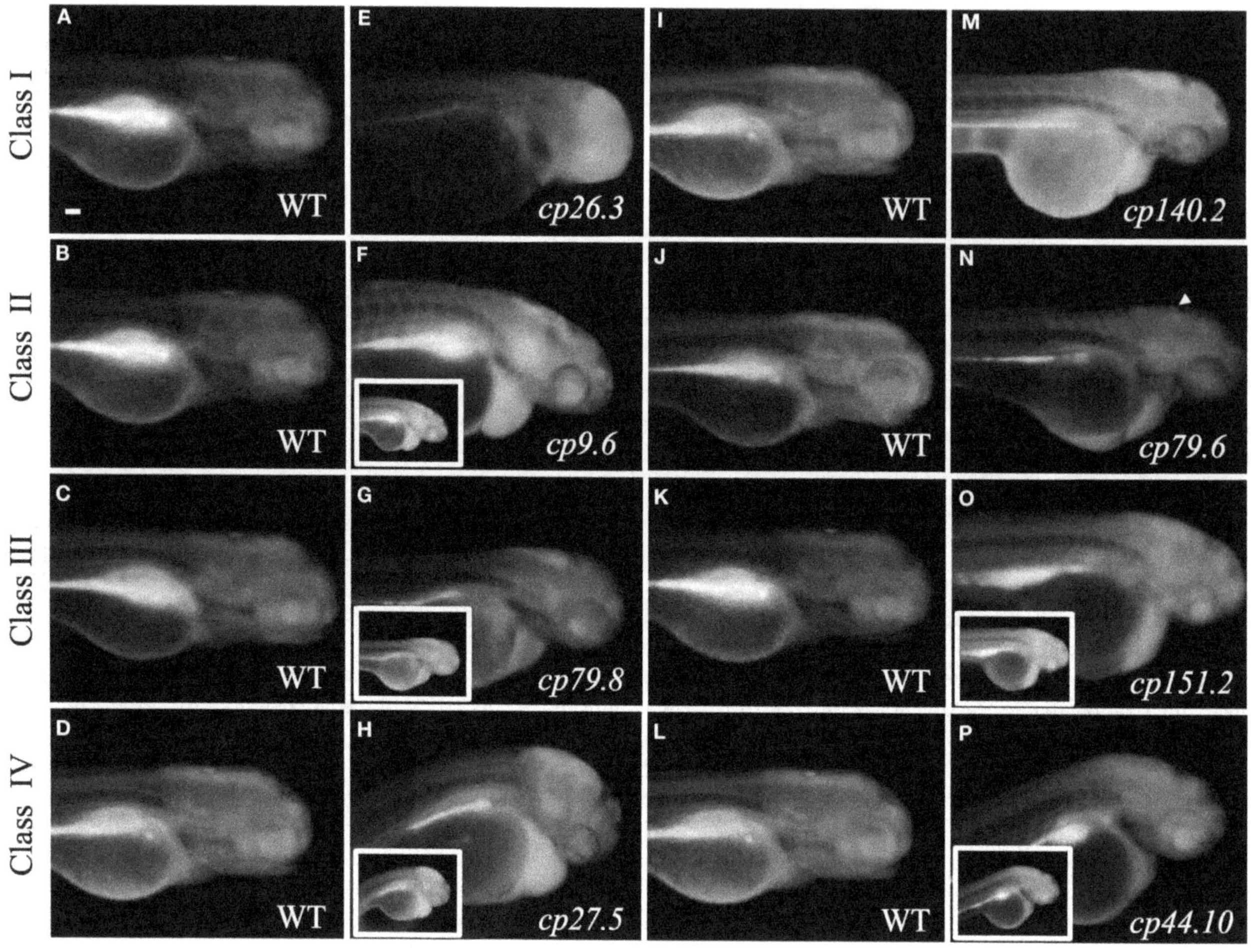

FIGURE 8 | Fluorescein assay determines CP transport activity in mutants. (A–D) and **(I–L)** Wild-type larvae treated at 3 dpf with 50 μM fluorescein. **(E)** *cp26.3* mutant at 3 dpf. **(F)** *cp9.6* mutant at 3 dpf. Inset image is acquired at the same exposure to the corresponding wild-type in **(B)**. **(G)** *cp79.8* mutant at 3 dpf. Inset image is acquired at the same exposure to the corresponding wild-type in **(C)**. **(H)** *cp27.5* mutant at 3 dpf. Inset image is acquired at the same exposure to the corresponding wild-type in **(D)**. **(M)** *cp140.2* mutant at 3 dpf. **(N)** *cp79.6* mutant at 3 dpf. Punctate accumulation of fluorescein in the brain ventricle is shown with an arrowhead. **(O)** *cp151.2* mutant at 3 dpf. Inset image is acquired at the same exposure to the corresponding wild-type in **(K)**. **(P)** *cp44.10* mutant at 3 dpf. Inset image is acquired at the same exposure to the corresponding wild-type in **(L)**. The larger images for **(F,G,H,O,P)** were taken at a lower exposure compared to the corresponding wild-type in order to visualize where the fluorescein was concentrating throughout the larvae. Scale bar is 50 μm.

ventricle morphology varied between mutants, all had expanded ventricles.

The mutants identified in our screen will provide the tools necessary to investigate several genes associated with choroid plexus development and barrier function. After isolating the defective genes from these mutants, we can define the correlation between the genes involved and the phenotypic abnormalities we observed. Although we identified mutants with brain cell death, we do not contribute cell death alone as a factor responsible for abnormal choroid plexus development and believe that the processes can be unrelated. This is supported by the identification of larvae with brain cell death developed a normal choroid plexus. Furthermore, for the mutants we characterized further, we did not observe the onset of cell death until after the choroid plexus had already started to develop for many of the lines, or if cell death was present, it was not near the choroid plexus itself. We also found larvae that had normal morphology overall, but abnormal or no choroid plexus indicating again that cell death is not the sole mechanism responsible for abnormal choroid plexus development and that specific pathways exist in regulation choroid plexus formation and function.

We expect some of the genes we identify will be specifically related to a choroid plexus defect rather than housekeeping genes causing an overall severely abnormal animal. Recent discoveries have shed light on the importance of the choroid plexus and its contribution to disease. For example, transcriptome analysis during early development revealed that the choroid plexus expresses numerous genes essential for choroid plexus function, including those for tight junctions, transporters, and metabolic function (Liddelow et al., 2012), protecting the brain from potentially harmful insults (Kratzer et al., 2013). Previous studies have also identified genetic components associated with choroid plexus dysfunction and disease. Genes involved in these pathologies include Polycystin-1 deficiency, which contributes to hydrocephaly (Wodarczyk et al., 2009). Because some types of hydrocephalus can be congenital, we plan to look at the mutant lines displaying hydrocephalus-like phenotypes with expanded ventricles (e.g., *cp27.5* and *cp9.6*) and determine whether we can find genetic linkage to this phenotype. In addition, mutations in Twist-related protein-1 and constitutively active Notch 3 promote proliferation and invasion in choroid plexus tumors (Wolburg and Paulus, 2010). Furthermore, disruption of the blood-cerebrospinal fluid barrier in multiple sclerosis can cause inflammation and leakage of T lymphocytes into the cerebrospinal fluid (Vercellino et al., 2008; Wolburg and Paulus, 2010). In patients with Alzheimer's disease, the choroid plexus has decreased function in amyloid beta plaque clearance (Alvira-Botero and Carro, 2010; Wolburg and Paulus, 2010). Since the mutations in the choroid plexus lines we identified are embryonic lethal, they may not be good representations to model later life diseases such as multiple sclerosis or Alzheimer's disease. However, we can investigate whether the choroid plexus is compromised in these mutants in regards to specific aspects of these diseases, such as an increased influx of immune cells into the cerebrospinal fluid characterized in multiple sclerosis, or reduced cerebrospinal fluid flow found in Alzheimer's disease patients. Identifying the genetic mutations that produce similar pathologies of these diseases may provide insight into the mechanisms that occur in the choroid plexus at later stages in life for these conditions.

The choroid plexus mutants identified in our study will be used to identify genes essential for maintaining epithelial barrier integrity as well as genes essential for initial barrier formation. Reverse genetic studies have shown that transcription factors such as *Otx2* aid in choroid plexus development and maintenance (Johansson et al., 2013). Also, augurin, a protein encoded by the esophageal cancer related gene-4 (*Ecrg4*) and thought to act as a tumor suppressor, has a higher expression in the choroid plexus than other tissues. Interestingly, morpholino knockdown of *Ecrg4* in zebrafish results in increased central nervous system cell proliferation and hydrocephaly (Gonzalez et al., 2011). Additional studies in zebrafish showed that the clusterin gene, which encodes a secreted glycoprotein that aids in aggregation and contributes to Alzheimer's disease by colocalizing with plaques (Thambisetty et al., 2010), is similar to its human counterpart and is expressed in the diencephalic choroid plexus and myelencephalic choroid plexus (Jiao et al., 2011). Demonstrating the similarity in gene expression in zebrafish and human choroid plexus is important when considering the use of zebrafish as a disease model for choroid plexus-related conditions. Our study provides evidence that the barrier properties and function of zebrafish choroid plexus are similar to those of mammalian choroid plexus. Ultimately, the genes discovered from our choroid plexus mutants will provide a better understanding of the genetic and molecular mechanisms involved in choroid plexus formation and function and new insights into how these normal processes become altered in disease.

AUTHOR CONTRIBUTIONS

Hannah E. Henson wrote the manuscript and Michael R. Taylor edited the manuscript. Hannah E. Henson performed the characterization study including Claudin 5 staining, transporter experiments, and fluorescent tracer experiments. Hannah E. Henson also performed the forward genetic screen, fluorescein assay, and genetic mapping. Chaithanyarani Parupalli performed the forward genetic screen. Chaithanyarani Parupalli and Hannah E. Henson performed the time-lapse imaging on wild-type and choroid plexus mutants. Bensheng Ju and Michael R. Taylor generated the $Et(cp:EGFP)^{sj2}$ line.

ACKNOWLEDGMENTS

We thank Jennifer Peters and Victoria Frohlich from the St. Jude Children's Research Hospital Cell and Tissue Imaging Center for their assistance with the confocal images. Images were acquired at the Cell & Tissue Imaging Center which is supported by St Jude Children's Research Hospital and NCI P30 CA021765-34. We thank Vani Shanker from St. Jude Children's Research Hospital Scientific Editing for editing the manuscript. We also thank members of the Taylor lab for assistance and support. This work was funded by The Hartwell Foundation, St. Jude Children's Research Hospital, and ALSAC.

REFERENCES

Alvira-Botero, X., and Carro, E. M. (2010). Clearance of amyloid-beta peptide across the choroid plexus in Alzheimer's disease. *Curr. Aging Sci.* 3, 219–229. doi: 10.2174/1874609811003030219

Bill, B. R., Balciunas, D., McCarra, J. A., Young, E. D., Xiong, T., Spahn, A. M., et al. (2008). Development and Notch signaling requirements of the zebrafish choroid plexus. *PLoS ONE* 3:e3114. doi: 10.1371/journal.pone.0003114

Craig, M. P., Gilday, S. D., Dabiri, D., and Hove, J. R. (2012). An optimized method for delivering flow tracer particles to intravital fluid environments in the developing zebrafish. *Zebrafish* 9, 108–119. doi: 10.1089/zeb.2012.0740

Currle, D. S., Cheng, X., Hsu, C. M., and Monuki, E. S. (2005). Direct and indirect roles of CNS dorsal midline cells in choroid plexus epithelia formation. *Development* 132, 3549–3559. doi: 10.1242/dev.01915

Daoud, R., Kast, C., Gros, P., and Georges, E. (2000). Rhodamine 123 binds to multiple sites in the multidrug resistance protein (MRP1). *Biochemistry* 39, 15344–15352. doi: 10.1021/bi0020574

Dohrmann, G. J. (1970). The choroid plexus: a historical review. *Brain Res.* 18, 197–218. doi: 10.1016/0006-8993(70)90324-0

Driever, W., Solnica-Krezel, L., Schier, A. F., Neuhauss, S. C., Malicki, J., Stemple, D. L., et al. (1996). A genetic screen for mutations affecting embryogenesis in zebrafish. *Development* 123, 37–46.

Dziegielewska, K. M., Ek, J., Habgood, M. D., and Saunders, N. R. (2001). Development of the choroid plexus. *Microsc. Res. Tech.* 52, 5–20. doi: 10.1002/1097-0029(20010101)52:1<5::AID-JEMT3>3.0.CO;2-J

Folgueira, M., Bayley, P., Navratilova, P., Becker, T. S., Wilson, S. W., and Clarke, J. D. (2012). Morphogenesis underlying the development of the everted teleost telencephalon. *Neural Dev.* 7, 32. doi: 10.1186/1749-8104-7-32

Garcia-Lecea, M., Kondrychyn, I., Fong, S. H., Ye, Z. R., and Korzh, V. (2008). *In vivo* analysis of choroid plexus morphogenesis in zebrafish. *PLoS ONE* 3:e3090. doi: 10.1371/journal.pone.0003090

Goldsmith, J. R., and Jobin, C. (2012). Think small: zebrafish as a model system of human pathology. *J. Biomed. Biotechnol.* 2012:817341. doi: 10.1155/2012/817341

Gonzalez, A. M., Podvin, S., Lin, S. Y., Miller, M. C., Botfield, H., Leadbeater, W. E., et al. (2011). Ecrg4 expression and its product augurin in the choroid plexus: impact on fetal brain development, cerebrospinal fluid homeostasis and neuroprogenitor cell response to CNS injury. *Fluids Barriers CNS* 8:6. doi: 10.1186/2045-8118-8-6

Gutzman, J. H., and Sive, H. (2009). Zebrafish brain ventricle injection. *J. Vis. Exp.* 26:e1218. doi: 10.3791/1218

Horvitz, H. R. (1999). Genetic control of programmed cell death in the nematode Caenorhabditis elegans. *Cancer Res.* 59, 1701s-1706s.

Huang, X., Ketova, T., Fleming, J. T., Wang, H., Dey, S. K., Litingtung, Y., et al. (2009). Sonic hedgehog signaling regulates a novel epithelial progenitor domain of the hindbrain choroid plexus. *Development* 136, 2535–2543. doi: 10.1242/dev.033795

Irvin, D. K., Nakano, I., Paucar, A., and Kornblum, H. I. (2004). Patterns of Jagged1, Jagged2, Delta-like 1 and Delta-like 3 expression during late embryonic and postnatal brain development suggest multiple functional roles in progenitors and differentiated cells. *J. Neurosci. Res.* 75, 330–343. doi: 10.1002/jnr.10843

Jansen, W. F., De Weger, R. A., Woutersen, R. A., Van Loveren, H., and Van De Kamer, J. C. (1976). The saccus dorsalis of the rainbow trout, Salmo gairdneri Richardson: histological, cytochemical, electron microscopical and autoradiographical observations. *Cell Tissue Res.* 167, 467–491. doi: 10.1007/BF00215179

Janssen, S. F., Van Der Spek, S. J., Ten Brink, J. B., Essing, A. H., Gorgels, T. G., Van Der Spek, P. J., et al. (2013). Gene expression and functional annotation of the human and mouse choroid plexus epithelium. *PLoS ONE* 8:e83345. doi: 10.1371/journal.pone.0083345

Jiao, S., Dai, W., Lu, L., Liu, Y., Zhou, J., Li, Y., et al. (2011). The conserved clusterin gene is expressed in the developing choroid plexus under the regulation of notch but not IGF signaling in zebrafish. *Endocrinology* 152, 1860–1871. doi: 10.1210/en.2010-1183

Johansson, P. A., Irmler, M., Acampora, D., Beckers, J., Simeone, A., and Gotz, M. (2013). The transcription factor Otx2 regulates choroid plexus development and function. *Development* 140, 1055–1066. doi: 10.1242/dev.090860

Keep, R. F., and Smith, D. E. (2011). Choroid plexus transport: gene deletion studies. *Fluids Barriers CNS* 8:26. doi: 10.1186/2045-8118-8-26

Kratzer, I., Liddelow, S. A., Saunders, N. R., Dziegielewska, K. M., Strazielle, N., and Ghersi-Egea, J. F. (2013). Developmental changes in the transcriptome of the rat choroid plexus in relation to neuroprotection. *Fluids Barriers CNS* 10:25. doi: 10.1186/2045-8118-10-25

Kratzer, I., Vasiljevic, A., Rey, C., Fevre-Montange, M., Saunders, N., Strazielle, N., et al. (2012). Complexity and developmental changes in the expression pattern of claudins at the blood-CSF barrier. *Histochem. Cell Biol.* 138, 861–879. doi: 10.1007/s00418-012-1001-9

Lagaraine, C., Skipor, J., Szczepkowska, A., Dufourny, L., and Thiery, J. C. (2011). Tight junction proteins vary in the choroid plexus of ewes according to photoperiod. *Brain Res.* 1393, 44–51. doi: 10.1016/j.brainres.2011.04.009

Liddelow, S. A., Dziegielewska, K. M., Mollgard, K., Whish, S. C., Noor, N. M., Wheaton, B. J., et al. (2014). Cellular Specificity of the Blood-CSF barrier for albumin transfer across the choroid plexus epithelium. *PLoS ONE* 9:e106592. doi: 10.1371/journal.pone.0106592

Liddelow, S. A., Dziegielewska, K. M., Vandeberg, J. L., and Saunders, N. R. (2010). Development of the lateral ventricular choroid plexus in a marsupial, monodelphis domestica. *Cerebrospinal Fluid Res.* 7:16. doi: 10.1186/1743-8454-7-16

Liddelow, S. A., Temple, S., Mollgard, K., Gehwolf, R., Wagner, A., Bauer, H., et al. (2012). Molecular characterisation of transport mechanisms at the developing mouse blood-CSF interface: a transcriptome approach. *PLoS ONE* 7:e33554. doi: 10.1371/annotation/2a9099a5-688b-4def-95a7-6ac13b10d096

Lippoldt, A., Liebner, S., Andbjer, B., Kalbacher, H., Wolburg, H., Haller, H., et al. (2000). Organization of choroid plexus epithelial and endothelial cell tight junctions and regulation of claudin-1, -2 and -5 expression by protein kinase C. *Neuroreport* 11, 1427–1431. doi: 10.1097/00001756-200005150-00015

Lowery, L. A., De Rienzo, G., Gutzman, J. H., and Sive, H. (2009). Characterization and classification of zebrafish brain morphology mutants. *Anat. Rec. (Hoboken)* 292, 94–106. doi: 10.1002/ar.20768

Lowery, L. A., Rubin, J., and Sive, H. (2007). Whitesnake/sfpq is required for cell survival and neuronal development in the zebrafish. *Dev. Dyn.* 236, 1347–1357. doi: 10.1002/dvdy.21132

Lowery, L. A., and Sive, H. (2005). Initial formation of zebrafish brain ventricles occurs independently of circulation and requires the nagie oko and snakehead/atp1a1a.1 gene products. *Development* 132, 2057–2067. doi: 10.1242/dev.01791

Meinke, D. W., and Sussex, I. M. (1979). Embryo-lethal mutants of Arabidopsis thaliana. A model system for genetic analysis of plant embryo development. *Dev. Biol.* 72, 50–61. doi: 10.1016/0012-1606(79)90097-6

Monnot, A. D., and Zheng, W. (2013). Culture of choroid plexus epithelial cells and *in vitro* model of blood-CSF barrier. *Methods Mol. Biol.* 945, 13–29. doi: 10.1007/978-1-62703-125-7_2

Muto, A., Orger, M. B., Wehman, A. M., Smear, M. C., Kay, J. N., Page-Mccaw, P. S., et al. (2005). Forward genetic analysis of visual behavior in zebrafish. *PLoS Genet.* 1:e66. doi: 10.1371/journal.pgen.0010066

Nielsen, C. M., and Dymecki, S. M. (2010). Sonic hedgehog is required for vascular outgrowth in the hindbrain choroid plexus. *Dev. Biol.* 340, 430–437. doi: 10.1016/j.ydbio.2010.01.032

Nolan, P. M., Peters, J., Strivens, M., Rogers, D., Hagan, J., Spurr, N., et al. (2000). A systematic, genome-wide, phenotype-driven mutagenesis programme for gene function studies in the mouse. *Nat. Genet.* 25, 440–443. doi: 10.1038/78140

Nusslein-Volhard, C., and Wieschaus, E. (1980). Mutations affecting segment number and polarity in Drosophila. *Nature* 287, 795–801. doi: 10.1038/287795a0

Omura, Y., Korf, H. W., and Oksche, A. (1985). Vascular permeability (problem of the blood-brain barrier) in the pineal organ of the rainbow trout, Salmo gairdneri. *Cell Tissue Res.* 239, 599–610. doi: 10.1007/BF00219238

Saengkhae, C., Loetchutinat, C., and Garnier-Suillerot, A. (2003). Kinetic analysis of rhodamines efflux mediated by the multidrug resistance protein (MRP1). *Biophys. J.* 85, 2006–2014. doi: 10.1016/S0006-3495(03)74628-1

Saunders, N. R., Ek, C. J., Habgood, M. D., and Dziegielewska, K. M. (2008). Barriers in the brain: a renaissance? *Trends Neurosci.* 31, 279–286. doi: 10.1016/j.tins.2008.03.003

Schmidt, R., Strahle, U., and Scholpp, S. (2013). Neurogenesis in zebrafish - from embryo to adult. *Neural Dev.* 8:3. doi: 10.1186/1749-8104-8-3

Sehnert, A. J., Huq, A., Weinstein, B. M., Walker, C., Fishman, M., and Stainier, D. Y. (2002). Cardiac troponin T is essential in sarcomere assembly and cardiac contractility. *Nat. Genet.* 31, 106–110. doi: 10.1038/ng875

Shapiro, A. B., and Ling, V. (1998). Stoichiometry of coupling of rhodamine 123 transport to ATP hydrolysis by P-glycoprotein. *Eur. J. Biochem.* 254, 189–193. doi: 10.1046/j.1432-1327.1998.2540189.x

Sin, O., Michels, H., and Nollen, E. A. (2014). Genetic screens in Caenorhabditis elegans models for neurodegenerative diseases. *Biochim. Biophys. Acta* 1842, 1951–1959. doi: 10.1016/j.bbadis.2014.01.015

Skinner, D. C., and Malpaux, B. (1999). High melatonin concentrations in third ventricular cerebrospinal fluid are not due to Galen vein blood recirculating through the choroid plexus. *Endocrinology* 140, 4399–4405.

Stemple, D. L., Solnica-Krezel, L., Zwartkruis, F., Neuhauss, S. C., Schier, A. F., Malicki, J., et al. (1996). Mutations affecting development of the notochord in zebrafish. *Development* 123, 117–128.

Strazielle, N., and Ghersi-Egea, J. F. (2000). Choroid plexus in the central nervous system: biology and physiopathology. *J. Neuropathol. Exp. Neurol.* 59, 561–574.

Strazielle, N., and Preston, J. E. (2003). Transport across the choroid plexuses *in vivo* and *in vitro*. *Methods Mol. Med.* 89, 291–304. doi: 10.1385/1-59259-419-0:291

Sykes, D., Sweet, D. H., Lowes, S., Nigam, S. K., Pritchard, J. B., and Miller, D. S. (2004). Organic anion transport in choroid plexus from wild-type and organic anion transporter 3 (Slc22a8)-null mice. *Am. J. Physiol. Renal Physiol.* 286, F972–F978. doi: 10.1152/ajprenal.00356.2003

Thambisetty, M., Simmons, A., Velayudhan, L., Hye, A., Campbell, J., Zhang, Y., et al. (2010). Association of plasma clusterin concentration with severity, pathology, and progression in Alzheimer disease. *Arch. Gen. Psychiatry* 67, 739–748. doi: 10.1001/archgenpsychiatry.2010.78

Tsuneki, K. (1986). A survey of occurrence of about seventeen circumventricular organs in brains of various vertebrates with special reference to lower groups. *J. Hirnforsch.* 27, 441–470.

Umans, R. A., and Taylor, M. R. (2012). Zebrafish as a model to study drug transporters at the blood-brain barrier. *Clin. Pharmacol. Ther.* 92, 567–570. doi: 10.1038/clpt.2012.168

Urasaki, A., Morvan, G., and Kawakami, K. (2006). Functional dissection of the *Tol2* transposable element identified the minimal *cis*-sequence and a highly repetitive sequence in the subterminal region essential for transposition. *Genetics* 174, 639–649. doi: 10.1534/genetics.106.060244

Vercellino, M., Votta, B., Condello, C., Piacentino, C., Romagnolo, A., Merola, A., et al. (2008). Involvement of the choroid plexus in multiple sclerosis autoimmune inflammation: a neuropathological study. *J. Neuroimmunol.* 199, 133–141. doi: 10.1016/j.jneuroim.2008.04.035

Villalobos, A. R., Miller, D. S., and Renfro, J. L. (2002). Transepithelial organic anion transport by shark choroid plexus. *Am. J. Physiol. Regul. Integr. Comp. Physiol.* 282, R1308–R1316. doi: 10.1152/ajpregu.00677.2001

White, R. M., Sessa, A., Burke, C., Bowman, T., Leblanc, J., Ceol, C., et al. (2008). Transparent adult zebrafish as a tool for *in vivo* transplantation analysis. *Cell Stem Cell* 2, 183–189. doi: 10.1016/j.stem.2007.11.002

Wijnholds, J., Delange, E. C., Scheffer, G. L., Van Den Berg, D. J., Mol, C. A., Van Der Valk, M., et al. (2000). Multidrug resistance protein 1 protects the choroid plexus epithelium and contributes to the blood-cerebrospinal fluid barrier. *J. Clin. Invest.* 105, 279–285. doi: 10.1172/JCI8267

Winata, C. L., Korzh, S., Kondrychyn, I., Zheng, W., Korzh, V., and Gong, Z. (2009). Development of zebrafish swimbladder: the requirement of Hedgehog signaling in specification and organization of the three tissue layers. *Dev. Biol.* 331, 222–236. doi: 10.1016/j.ydbio.2009.04.035

Wodarczyk, C., Rowe, I., Chiaravalli, M., Pema, M., Qian, F., and Boletta, A. (2009). A novel mouse model reveals that polycystin-1 deficiency in ependyma and choroid plexus results in dysfunctional cilia and hydrocephalus. *PLoS ONE* 4:e7137. doi: 10.1371/journal.pone.0007137

Wolburg, H., and Paulus, W. (2010). Choroid plexus: biology and pathology. *Acta Neuropathol.* 119, 75–88. doi: 10.1007/s00401-009-0627-8

Xie, J., Farage, E., Sugimoto, M., and Anand-Apte, B. (2010). A novel transgenic zebrafish model for blood-brain and blood-retinal barrier development. *BMC Dev. Biol.* 10:76. doi: 10.1186/1471-213X-10-76

Zhang, J., Piontek, J., Wolburg, H., Piehl, C., Liss, M., Otten, C., et al. (2010). Establishment of a neuroepithelial barrier by Claudin5a is essential for zebrafish brain ventricular lumen expansion. *Proc. Natl. Acad. Sci. U.S.A.* 107, 1425–1430. doi: 10.1073/pnas.0911996107

9

The contribution of CXCL12-expressing radial glia cells to neuro-vascular patterning during human cerebral cortex development

Mariella Errede*[†]*, Francesco Girolamo*[†]*, Marco Rizzi, Mirella Bertossi, Luisa Roncali and Daniela Virgintino* *

Department of Basic Medical Sciences, Neurosciences and Sensory Organs, University of Bari School of Medicine, Bari, Italy

****Correspondence:***
Daniela Virgintino, Human Anatomy and Histology Unit, Department of Basic Medical Sciences, Neurosciences, and Sensory Organs, Bari University Medical School, Piazza Giulio Cesare, Policlinico-70124 Bari, Italy
e-mail: daniela.virgintino@uniba.it

[†]These authors have contributed equally as first authors.

This study was conducted on human developing brain by laser confocal and transmission electron microscopy (TEM) to make a detailed analysis of important features of blood-brain barrier (BBB) microvessels and possible control mechanisms of vessel growth and differentiation during cerebral cortex vascularization. The BBB status of cortex microvessels was examined at a defined stage of cortex development, at the end of neuroblast waves of migration, and before cortex lamination, with BBB-endothelial cell markers, namely tight junction (TJ) proteins (occludin and claudin-5) and influx and efflux transporters (Glut-1 and P-glycoprotein), the latter supporting evidence for functional effectiveness of the fetal BBB. According to the well-known roles of astroglia cells on microvessel growth and differentiation, the early composition of astroglia/endothelial cell relationships was analyzed by detecting the appropriate astroglia, endothelial, and pericyte markers. GFAP, chemokine CXCL12, and connexin 43 (Cx43) were utilized as markers of radial glia cells, CD105 (endoglin) as a marker of angiogenically activated endothelial cells (ECs), and proteoglycan NG2 as a marker of immature pericytes. Immunolabeling for CXCL12 showed the highest level of the ligand in radial glial (RG) fibers in contact with the growing cortex microvessels. These specialized contacts, recognizable on both perforating radial vessels and growing collaterals, appeared as CXCL12-reactive *en passant, symmetrical* and *asymmetrical*, vessel-specific RG fiber swellings. At the highest confocal resolution, these RG varicosities showed a CXCL12-reactive dot-like content whose microvesicular nature was confirmed by ultrastructural observations. A further analysis of RG varicosities reveals colocalization of CXCL12 with Cx43, which is possibly implicated in vessel-specific chemokine signaling.

Keywords: neuroangiogenesis, blood-brain barrier, tight junctions, transporters, radial glia, chemokine CXCL12, connexin 43, human fetus

INTRODUCTION

Radial glial (RG) cells were first described in the developing CNS by Magini and Ramón y Cajal in the late 19th century (Bentivoglio and Mazzarello, 1999). Their function as scaffolding for neuroblast migration during cortical histogenesis was postulated and demonstrated by Rakic in the early 1970s (Rakic, 1971, 1972) and then, at the beginning of the new millennium, their role as neuronal and glial precursors in the developing CNS was definitively demonstrated (Malatesta et al., 2000; Malatesta and Götz, 2013). The evidence that RG cells fulfill many functions has attracted new attention to these cells and new discoveries about their diverse functions in the developing brain are rapidly accumulating.

Abbreviations: BBB, blood-brain barrier; CD105, endoglin; CNS, Central Nervous System; Coll IV, collagen type IV; Cx43, connexin 43; CXCL12, C-X-C motif chemokine 12; EC, endothelial cells; GFAP, glial fibrillary acidic protein; Glut-1, glucose transporter isoform 1; MVs, microvesicles; NG2, nerve/glial antigen 2; P-gp, P-glycoprotein; RG, radial glia; TJ, tight junction.

RG cells differ taxonomically in primates and other mammalian species due to differences in their involvement in neurogenesis, and the timing and region of their appearance, as regards the expression of typical RG immunomarkers (Howard et al., 2008; Xu et al., 2014). For example, in humans, the intermediate filament proteins, glial fibrillary acidic protein (GFAP), and vimentin, are expressed concomitantly in RG from the start of neurogenesis (Choi and Lapham, 1978; Virgintino et al., 1998; Howard et al., 2006). In contrast, in rodents, RG cells undergo a more protracted maturation and become GFAP-positive only at late fetal stages, after neurogenesis is complete, and vimentin is no longer detectable (Rickmann and Wolff, 1985). Moreover, in human telencephalon, due to the larger size of the cerebral cortex compared with the rodent cortex, a "mature" GFAP-expressing RG precociously develops long shafts that may reach a length of 3000–7000 μm and show early, special vascular relations (Rakic, 1972; Virgintino et al., 1998).

Pioneering studies have demonstrated that angiogenically formed microvessels invade the developing brain by perforating

Table 1 | Synopsis of CXCL12 and CXCR4/CXCR7 immunoreactivity in developing brain.

Cell type	CXCL12	CXCR4	CXCR7
Radial glia cells	cytoplasm^{high}	-	-
Perivascular astrocytes	cytoplasm^{high}	-	-
Neuroblasts	-	nucleus^{high}	nucleus^{high}
Endothelial cells	cytoplasm^{low}	-	-
Pericytes	-	cytoplasm^{high}	cytoplasm^{high}

Modified from Virgintino et al. (2013).

the basement membrane and penetrating through the external glial limiting membrane to supply the developing nervous tissue, under the control of a concentration gradient of soluble growth factors (Risau et al., 1988; Risau and Wolburg, 1990; Engelhardt and Risau, 1995). In humans the growing microvessels arrange themselves according to geometrically precise paths that parallel the RG arrangement, taking on a common radial pattern and forming mutual, multiple contacts (Bär, 1980; Marin-Padilla, 1985; Virgintino et al., 1998; Rakic, 2007; Marín-Padilla, 2012). In recent years it has become increasingly evident that the role of RG cells during brain vascularization may be more specific than was previously thought. In fact, besides a simple activity providing tracks for growing vessels, RG cells have been suggested to be the source of factors such as vascular endothelial growth factor (VEGF) and Wnt, that intertwine with each other and other angiogenic pathways to facilitate the guidance of penetrating microvessels, stimulate proliferation of endothelial cells (ECs) and sustain vessel stabilization (Liebner and Plate, 2010; Bussmann et al., 2011; Quaegebeur et al., 2011).

During human cerebral cortex vascularization, subsets of RG cells and perivascular astrocytes have been demonstrated, showing high levels of chemokine CXCL12 expression (Virgintino et al., 2013). This chemokine, also known as stromal-derived factor-1 (SDF-1), plays multiple roles in CNS development, its expression in the brain being involved in neural progenitor differentiation, and neuronal cell migration (Tiveron et al., 2006; Peng et al., 2007; Stumm and Höllt, 2007; Li et al., 2008; Tiveron and Cremer, 2008). Moreover, cells of neural crest origin, located in the developing, innermost layer of the meninges, have been demonstrated to be involved in neurogenesis, secreting molecular cues including chemokine CXCL12, that seem to regulate cortical interneuron settlement, and Cajal–Retzius cell tangential migration (Stumm et al., 2003; Borrell and Marín, 2006; Paredes et al., 2006; Li et al., 2008; Siegenthaler et al., 2009).

In addition, CXCL12 and its receptor CXCR4 (C-X-C chemokine receptor) belong to a restricted group of pro-angiogenic molecules that, albeit within a limited developmental window, display a neuro-specific angiogenic activity (Bussmann et al., 2011; Quaegebeur et al., 2011). Overall, these data are consistent with previous observations of human developing cerebral cortex, which have described CXCR4/CXCR7-reactive neuroblasts and subsets of CXCL12 RG cells and astrocytes in close association with CXCR4/CXCR7-reactive microvascular ECs and pericytes (Virgintino et al., 2013; see also **Table 1**). Accordingly, a model

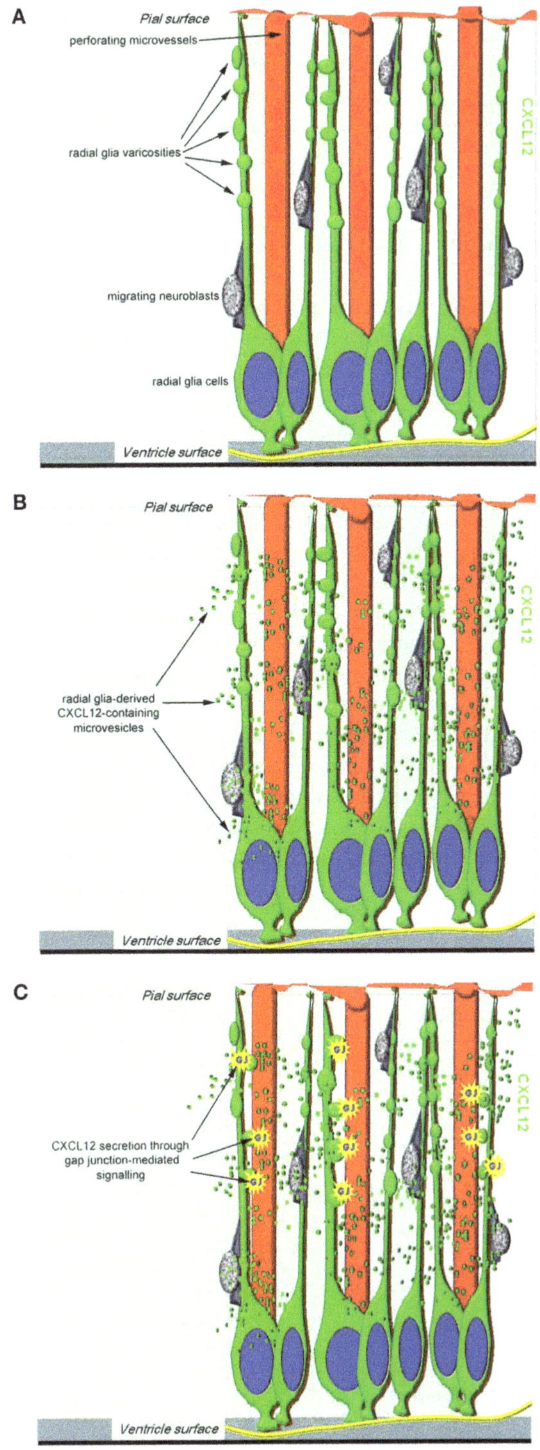

FIGURE 1 | A proposed model of RG-derived CXCL12 regulation of cerebral cortex development and vascularization. (A) In the working model, CXCL12 radial glia cells have a central role not only in neurogenesis and neuroblast migration but also in neuroangiogenesis, being ideally positioned to coordinate neuro-vascular cerebral cortex patterning. **(B)** Radial glia-derived CXCL12-containing microvesicles may convey their signal to the ECs of growing microvessels. **(C)** One potential mechanism by which CXCL12 secretion can be modulated in radial glia cells is through gap junction-mediated signaling.

of synchronized neuro-vascular patterning centered on CXCL12 RG cells has been proposed (**Figure 1**) and appears to be supported by the present results that have identified, by parallel laser confocal and electron microscopy analyses, RG-microvessel subcellular units shaped by RG varicosities containing CXCL12 microvesicles (MVs) and connexin 43 (Cx43) as a regulatory molecule.

MATERIALS AND METHODS

HISTOLOGY

Autopsy specimens of telencephalon were collected from 4 human fetuses spontaneously aborted due to preterm rupture of the placental membranes (22 weeks of gestation). The sampling and handling of human specimens conformed to the ethical rules of the Department of Pathology, Medical School, University of Bari, Italy, and approval was gained from the local Ethics Committee of the National Health System in compliance with the principles stated in the Declaration of Helsinki. The fetal age was estimated on the basis of the crown-rump length and/or pregnancy records (counting from the last menstrual period). At autopsy, the selected fetuses did not reveal macroscopic structural abnormalities and/or malformations of the central nervous system. The dorso-lateral wall of the telencephalic vesicles (future neocortex) was dissected and fixed for 2–3 h at 4°C by immersion in 2% paraformaldehyde plus 0.2% glutaraldehyde solution. Specimens were then washed in phosphate buffered saline (PBS, pH 7.6) and serially sectioned by a vibrating microtome. 20 μm sections were collected at regular intervals and processed for conventional histological analysis with toluidine blue staining to ascertain the absence of microscopic malformations; all the other sections were stored in PBS plus 0.02% paraformaldehyde for fluorescence immunolabeling.

IMMUNOFLUORESCENCE AND LASER CONFOCAL MICROSCOPY

Multiple immunostainings were carried out with the following polyclonal antisera (pAbs) and monoclonal antibodies (mAbs), all diluted in blocking buffer (1% bovine serum albumin and 2% fetal calf serum in PBS): rabbit pAb anti-Glut 1, mouse mAb anti-P-gp, mouse mAb anti-Claudin-5, rabbit pAb anti-Occludin, mouse mAb anti-CXCL12/SDF-1, rabbit pAb anti-CD105, rabbit pAb anti-NG2 (generous gift from W. B. Stallcup, The Burnham Institute for Medical Research, La Jolla, CA, USA), mouse mAb anti-GFAP, rat mAb anti-GFAP, rabbit pAb anti-collagen type IV (Coll IV), rabbit pAb anti-Cx43 (**Table 2**). After adhesion on polylysine slides (Menzel-Glaser, GmbH, Braunschweig, Germany) by drying for 10 min at room temperature, the sections were submitted to the following protocols: rehydration with PBS for 5 min at room temperature or microwave pretreatment in 0.01M citrate buffer (pH 6.0) for 15 min at 750W when required (**Table 2**); incubation with 0.5% Triton X-100 in PBS for 30 min at room temperature and with blocking buffer 30 min at room temperature, with single or combined primary antibodies overnight at 4°C, then with appropriate fluorophore-conjugated secondary antibodies (**Table 2**). Finally, the sections were washed for 10 min × 3 in PBS between each step, counterstained with either TO-PRO-3™ (1:10K dilution; Invitrogen Corporation, Carlsbad, CA, USA) or Sytox® Green (1:5K dilution; Invitrogen), mounted in Vectashield (Vector Laboratories, Inc. Burlingame, CA, USA), and finally sealed with nail varnish. Negative controls were prepared by using primary antibodies to

Table 2 | List of primary and secondary antibodies combined in multiple immunolabelings.

Primary antibodies	Host IgG	Dilution	Antigen retrieval	Producer	Code number
anti-Glut 1	rabbit IgG	1:100	–	Millipore[a]	07-1401
anti-P-gp	mouse IgG_{2a}	1:10	–	Signet[b]	8720-01 C494
anti-Claudin-5	mouse IgG_1	1:20	MW	Zymed[c]	18-7364 4C3C2
anti-Occludin	rabbit IgG	1:50	–	Zymed[c]	71-1500
anti-CXCL12/SDF-1	mouse IgG_1	1:10	MW	R&D Systems[d]	MAB350
anti-CD105	rabbit IgG	prediluted	MW	Abcam[e]	ab27422
anti-NG2	rabbit IgG	1:50	–	W.B. Stallcup	–
anti-GFAP	mouse IgG_1	1:50	–	Novocastra[f]	NCL-GFAP-GA5
anti-GFAP	rat IgG_{2a}	1:50	–	Invitrogen[g]	13-0300
anti-Coll IV	rabbit IgG	1:50	–	Acris[h]	R1041
anti-Cx43	rabbit IgG	1:50	MW	Millipore[a]	AB1728

Secondary antibodies	Dilution	Producer	Code number
1 goat anti-rabbit Alexa 555	1:300	Invitrogen[g]	A21429
2 goat anti-mouse Alexa 555	1:300	Invitrogen[g]	A21425
3 goat anti-mouse Alexa 488	1:300	Invitrogen[g]	A11001
4 goat anti-rabbit Alexa 488	1:300	Invitrogen[g]	A11070
5 goat anti-rat Alexa 555	1:300	Invitrogen[g]	A21434
6 goat anti-mouse Alexa 633	1:300	Invitrogen[g]	A21126

Glut 1/GFAP (revealed by 1, 3); Occludin/P-gp (1, 3); Occludin/Claudin-5 (1, 3); CD105/CXCL12 (4, 2); CXCL12/GFAP/Coll IV (6, 5, 4); CXCL12/Cx43 (3, 1). [a] Millipore-Chemicon; Billerica, MA, USA. [b] Signet Laboratories, Dedham, MA, USA. [c] Zymed Laboratories, Invitrogen Corporation, Carlsbad, CA, USA. [d] R&D Systems, Minneapolis, MN, USA. [e] Abcam, Cambridge, UK. [f] Vision Biosystem Novocastra, Newcastle upon Tyne, UK. [g] Invitrogen, Eugene, OR, USA. [h] Acris Antibodies GmbH; Herford, Germany. MW, high-temperature microwave pre-treatment of tissue sections.

stain inappropriate tissues, omitting the primary antibodies, pre-adsorbing the primary antibodies with an excess of antigen when available, or mismatching the secondary antibodies on appropriate preparations. When not ascertained in previous experiments, the specificity of primary antibodies was tested on tissue sections known to contain the antigen, as positive controls, and applying the same immunostaining protocols described above. Human adult brain sections were used to test the BBB-specific markers (Glut 1, P-gp, Claudin-5, Occludin), Cx43 antibody was tested on human and mouse brain sections and on mouse heart sections, while sections from human tonsils were useful for assessing CXCL12 and CD105, immunoreactivity (control sections were kindly provided by E. Maiorano, Department of Emergency and Organ Transplantation, Pathological Anatomy Unit, Faculty of Medicine, University of Bari, Bari, Italy). The sections were examined under the Leica TCS SP5 confocal laser-scanning microscope (Leica Microsystems, Mannheim, Germany) using a sequential scan procedure. Confocal images were taken at 250 nm intervals through the z-axis of the sections. Confocal images were taken with 40X and 63X oil lenses. Z-stacks of serial optical planes (projection images) and single optical planes were analyzed by Leica confocal software (Multicolor Package; Leica Microsystems). The size of RG varicosities and MVs was evaluated with LAS-AF SP5 software (Leica Microsystems) on 63X magnification fields zoomed 3 times. MVs diameter (nm) was measured on single optical planes from CXCL12-labeled sections ($n = 18$) for a total

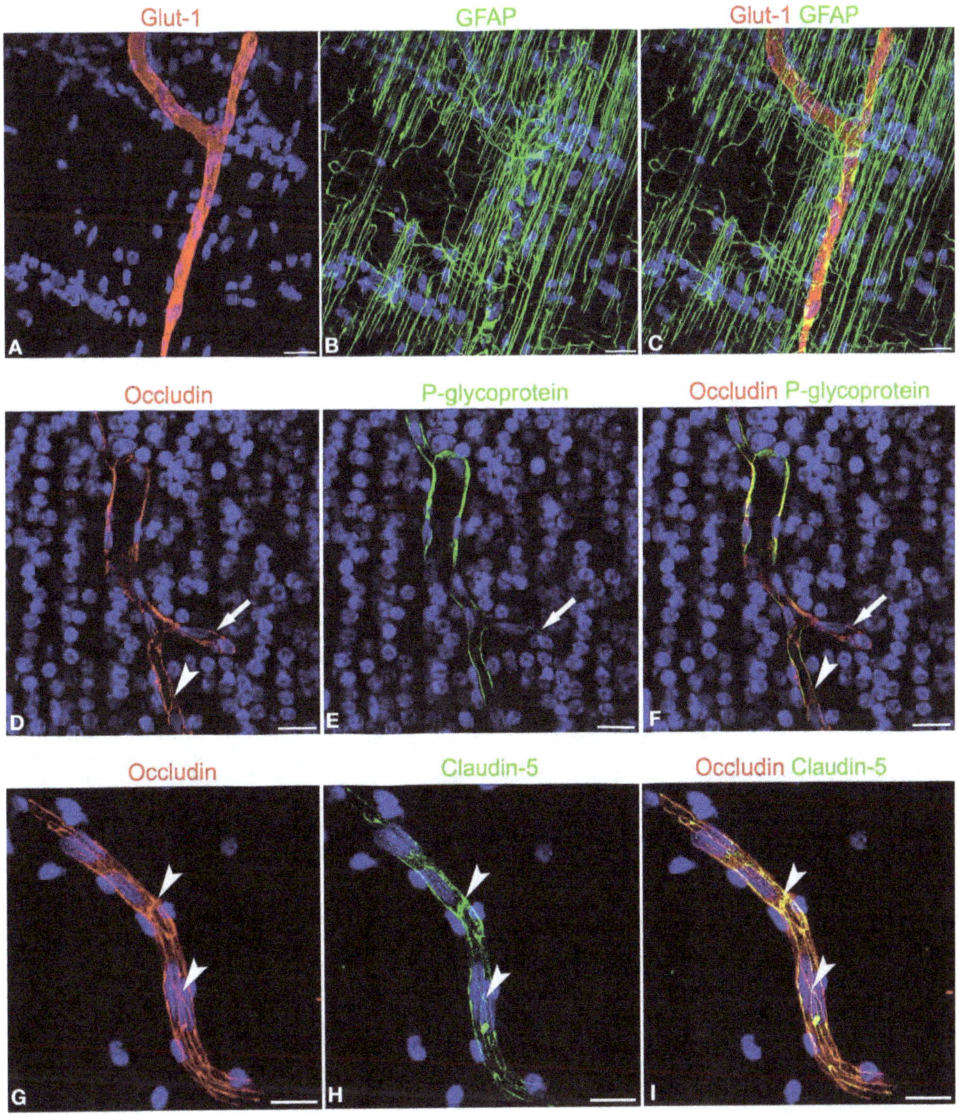

FIGURE 2 | Confocal images of human cerebral cortex at midgestation double labeled with Glut-1/GFAP, occludin/P-glycoprotein, and occludin/claudin-5. (A–C) A radial microvessel surrounded by GFAP-reactive RG fibers is revealed by the Glut-1 reactive endothelial cells. **(D–F)** On a stem vessel and its collateral (*arrow*) endothelial P-glycoprotein colocalize with occludin reactivity; note in **(E)** the lower levels of P-glycoprotein expression on the newly formed vessel branch (*arrow*) and in **(D)** and **(F)** the junctional linear pattern of occludin (*arrowhead*). **(G–I)** Occludin appears arranged according to a typical junctional pattern and colocalizes at points with claudin-5 (*arrowheads*). Bars: **A–C** and **D–F** 25 μm; **G–I** 30 μm.

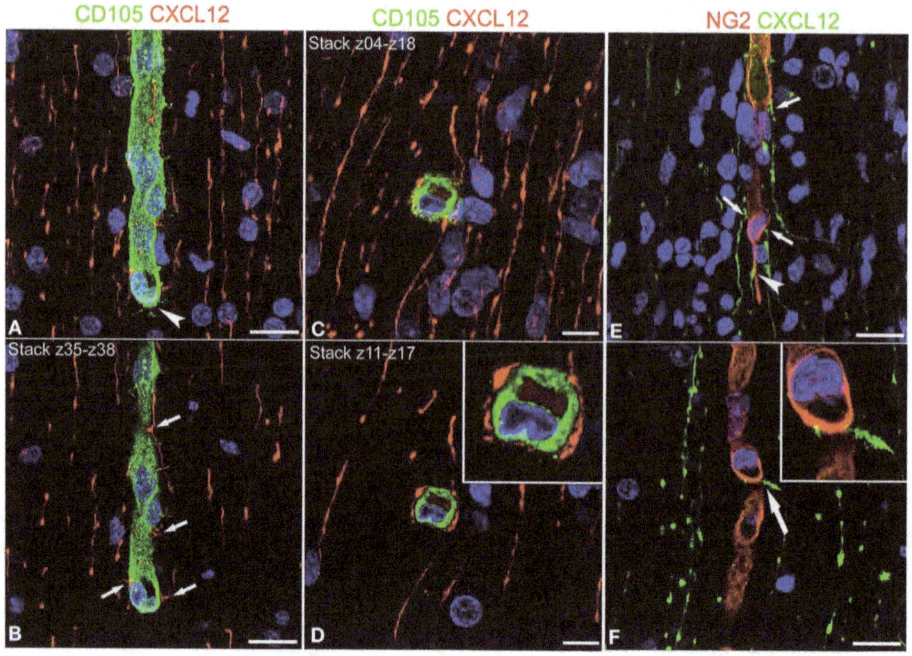

FIGURE 3 | Confocal images of human cerebral cortex at midgestation double labeled with CD105/CXCL12 (A–D) and NG2/CXCL12 (E,F). CXCL12-reactive RG fibers show evenly spaced varicosities **(A)** that make contacts at regular intervals (better recognizable on the selection of optical planes z35–z38; **B**, *arrows*) with a CD105 labeled, perforating cortex microvessel; note in **(A)** the tip endothelial cell on the growing vessel front (*arrowhead*). **(C,D)** Transverse view of a vascular branch completely surrounded by CXCL12 RG fibers, whose intimate relationships are better recognizable on a shorter stack of optical planes (z11–z17, **D**; *inset*). **(E)** Multiple CXCL12-reactive varicosities touching the NG2 pericyte cover (*arrows*) and a pericyte leading process (*arrowhead*); **(F)** One CXCL12-labeled varicosity bents to contact the vessel wall (*arrow* in **F**; *inset*). Bars: **A,B** 20 μm; **C,D** 10 μm; **E,F** 20 μm.

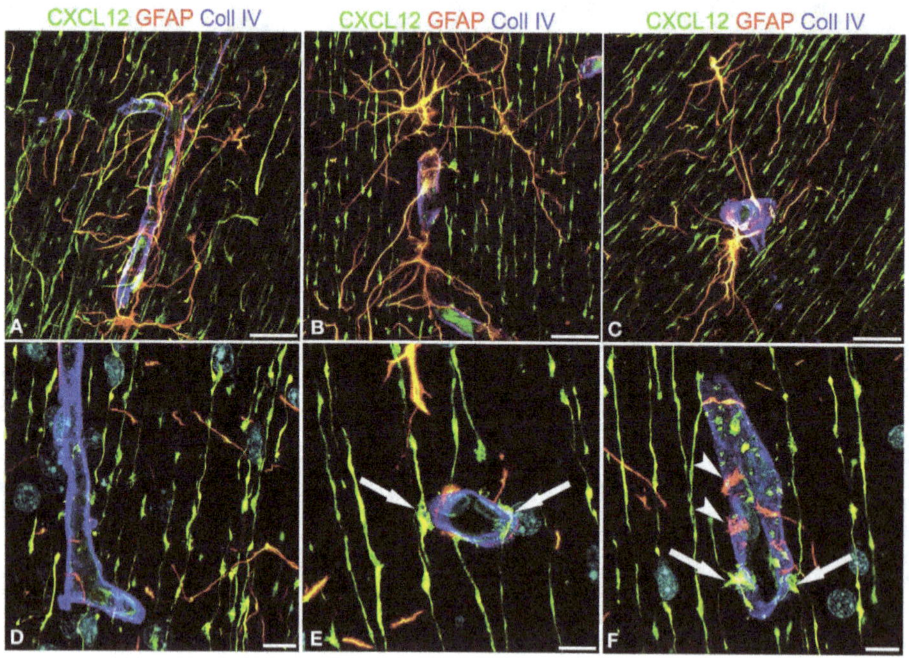

FIGURE 4 | Confocal images of human cerebral cortex at midgestation after multiple labeling with CXCL12, GFAP, and Coll IV. (A–C) GFAP-CXCL12-reactive perivascular astrocytes and CXCL12-reactive RG cells contributing perivascular endings to the microvessel wall revealed by collagen IV (*blue*). **(D–F)** On selected single optical planes the RG vascular contacts are distinguishable, two *en passant, symmetrical* varicosities on the vessel wall (**E**, *arrows*) and two omega-shaped *asymmetrical* varicosities on either sides of the vessel profile (**F**, *arrows*); note in **(F)** classical GFAP-labeled astrocyte end-feet (*arrowheads*). Bars: **A–C** 20 μm; **D–F** 10 μm.

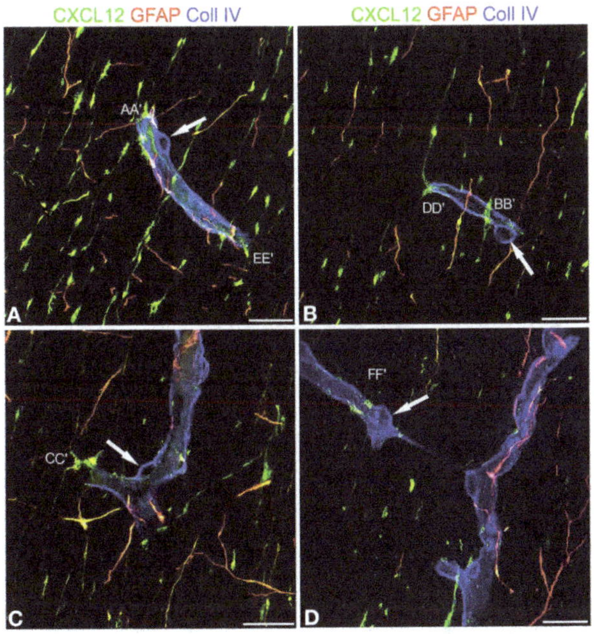

FIGURE 5 | Confocal images of human cerebral cortex at midgestation after multiple labeling with CXCL12, GFAP, and Coll IV. (A–D) A further collection of CXCL12-reactive RG varicosities in contact with the vessel wall, whose Coll IV staining also shows the bulging nuclei of pericytes (*arrows* in **A–D**). Single RG-vascular contacts are recognizable in these pictures **(AA′, BB′, CC′, DD′, EE′, and FF′)** and are shown as enlarged details in **Figure 6**. Bars: **A–D** 20 μm.

of 50 fields. The results were expressed as a "range" of size from a minimum to a maximum value.

TRANSMISSION ELECTRON MICROSCOPY

Small samples collected from the previously described telencephalon specimens were submitted to electron microscopy procedures. Briefly, samples were fixed in 0.1 M phosphate-buffered 3% glutaraldehyde, post-fixed in phosphate-buffered 1% OsO4, dehydrated in serial alcohols, and embedded in Epon 812. Ultrathin sections were cut with an LKB V ultramicrotome (LKB Bromma, Sollentuna, Sweden), stained with uranyl acetate and lead citrate, and observed under a CM 10 Philips electron microscope (Philips, Eindhoven, The Netherlands).

RESULTS

CEREBRAL CORTEX MICROVESSELS SHOW A BBB-SPECIFIC PHENOTYPE

The expression of blood-brain barrier (BBB)-specific markers was analyzed in microvessels that, at the end of neuronal migration and beginning of cortex lamination, in the fetal age of around midgestation, vascularize the cerebral cortex, radially invading the neural wall from the pial surface to the deeper subcortical layers. Their endothelial lining is characterized by a strong reactivity to fundamental metabolic and efflux barrier-specific transporters, such as the glucose transporter isoform 1, Glut-1, and to a member of the ABC (ATP-binding cassette) superfamily, the multidrug transporter P-glycoprotein (P-gp or ABCB1). On double staining with Glut-1 and the astroglia marker GFAP, radial vessels appear surrounded by a curtain of GFAP-reactive RG fibers and their ECs express high levels of Glut-1 (**Figures 2A–C**). Cortex stem microvessels appear aligned with rows of neuroblasts and are seen to form their first collaterals, stem vessels and branches being revealed by the endothelial expression of P-gp (**Figures 2E,F**). The presence of two BBB transporters indirectly implies that tight junction (TJ) formation is in progress in ECs and that the barrier is partially functional. In fact, on double staining with P-gp and the TJ protein occludin, the latter appears highly expressed on both stem vessels and collaterals, and shows a linear, junctional staining pattern (**Figures 2D–F**). Also on double staining with the TJ protein claudin-5, occludin displays a clearly junctional distribution, whereas a punctate cytoplasmic pattern still prevails for claudin-5 (**Figures 2G–I**). Overall, these data demonstrate an ongoing process of BBB differentiation in human cerebral cortex microvessels at midgestation.

VESSEL-SPECIFIC CONTACTS OCCUR BETWEEN CXCL12-REACTIVE RG FIBERS AND CORTEX MICROVESSELS

Cerebral cortex microvessels are also revealed by the endothelial marker CD105, which also allows recognition of the growing front of the invading vessels, that is characterized by CD105-reactive endothelial tip cells (**Figures 3A,B**). On double immunostaining for CXCL12, CD105 labeled microvessels appear surrounded by palisades of CXCL12-reactive RG fibers and in direct contact with sequences of swellings characterizing the RG fibers (**Figures 3A,B**) that are also seen in close contact with radial vessel collaterals (**Figures 3C,D**). Double staining with proteoglycan NG2 antibody as a pericyte marker also demonstrates several points of apposition between regular sequences of RG vascular varicosities and the microvessel wall (**Figures 3E,F**).

These first observations were extended by triple immunostaining with GFAP and CXCL12, as a classical and a novel marker of RG cells, respectively, and with collagen type IV (Coll IV) as a marker of the vascular basal lamina (**Figures 4A–F**). By this staining, in the subcortical layers, where the earliest astrocytes become recognizable, the microvessels appear surrounded by a perivascular subset of astrocytes that express high levels of both GFAP and CXCL12 (see also Virgintino et al., 2013) (**Figures 4A,B**). On the same sections, RG fibers reveal a lower GFAP immunostaining and a higher staining of CXCL12 (**Figures 4A–C**). The two markers colocalize on RG vessel-specific varicosities that make *en passant* contacts maintaining a symmetrical profile, denoted as *symmetrical* varicosities, or assume an omega-like shape and are therefore indicated as *asymmetrical* varicosities (**Figures 4D–F**). In favorable conditions of tissue and antigenicity preservation, and with the opportune setting of laser potency and confocal parameters, the described RG *symmetrical* and *asymmetrical* varicosities appear filled by CXCL12-labeled dot-like structures that sometimes display a microvesicular nature (**Figures 5A–D, 6A–F,A′,F′**). The CXCL12 MVs are densely packed within varicosities measuring about 1–1.5 μm and show a diameter of 100–200 nm (**Figures 5A–D, 6A–F,A′–F′**). At sites of vascular contact, CXCL12 densities

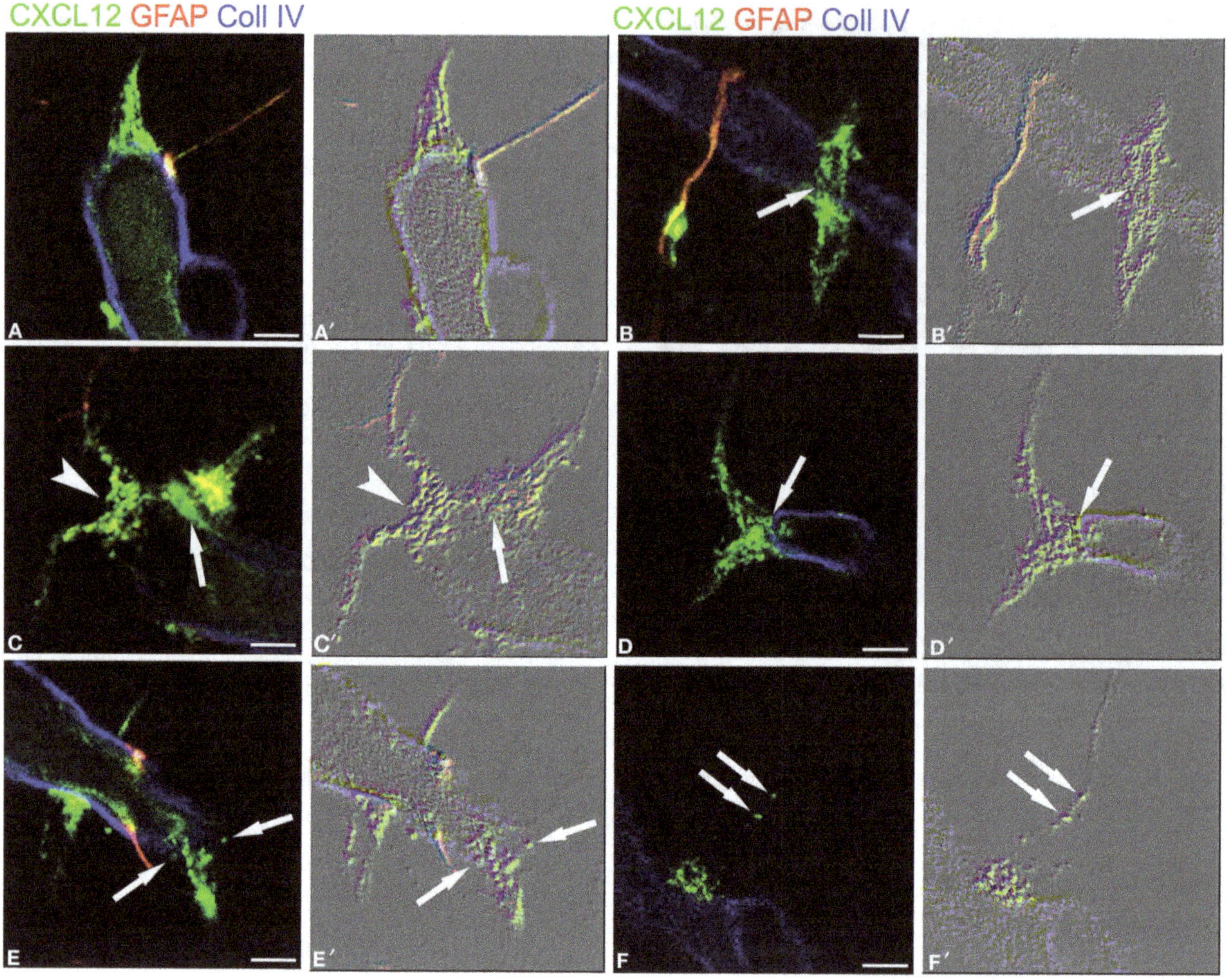

FIGURE 6 | RG-vascular contacts shown in Figure 5, (A–F) and the same pictures rendered with an embossed image filter (A′–F′). The profile in relief of MV-like subcellular structures is amplified and well-recognizable on the flat surface; note in **(A,A′)** gathered MVs, in **(B,B′)** an *en passant, symmetrical* varicosity (*arrow*), in **(C,C′)** an *asymmetrical* varicosity (*arrowhead*) and an endothelial CXCL12-reactive density faced by a RG contact (*arrow*), in **(D,D′)** a clearly recognizable MV (*arrow*), in **(E,E′)** released MVs (*arrows*), and in **(F,F′)** MVs within the RG fiber (*arrows*). Bars: **A–F** 2.5 μm.

are also recognizable beneath the Coll IV basal membrane (**Figure 6C**).

RG VARICOSITY AND MVs ARE CLEARLY REVEALED BY TRANSMISSION ELECTRON MICROSCOPY

When comparing confocal images of radial microvessels, after triple immunostaining for CXCL12, GFAP, and Coll IV (**Figures 7A,B**), with similar fields studied by transmission electron microscopy (TEM), some details, appreciated in the former, become clearly defined by ultrastructural observations (**Figures 7C,D**). The vesicular nature of the subcellular structures observed by confocal microscopy after CXCL12 immunolabeling is confirmed (**Figures 7A–D**), while RG varicosities and the vascular basal membrane are seen in close contact at several points of the vessel wall (**Figures 7C,D**). MVs appear homogeneous in size and aligned against the varicosity membrane facing the vessel contact site (**Figures 7C,D**).

GAP JUNCTION PROTEIN Cx43 COLOCALIZES WITH CHEMOKINE CXCL12 IN RG VARICOSITIES

The presence of Cx43 was revealed in double immunostaining for CXCL12 and Cx43, the rationale for this approach being sustained by data on Cx43 involvement in RG-guided neuronal migration (Elias et al., 2007; Matsuuchi and Naus, 2013) and by studies on Cx43 in RG cells (Virgintino et al., 2001; Errede et al., 2002). Cx43 plaques are revealed along the RG fibers and concentrate in vessel-contacting RG varicosities, where Cx43 extensively colocalizes with CXCL12 (**Figures 8A–D**).

DISCUSSION

RADIAL GLIAL CELL VARICOSITIES AND CXCL12 MVs INVOLVED IN CEREBRAL CORTEX VASCULARIZATION

In 1887, when Giuseppe Magini utilized for the first time the Golgi impregnation technique on mammalian developing cerebral cortex, he described "neuroglial cells with very long

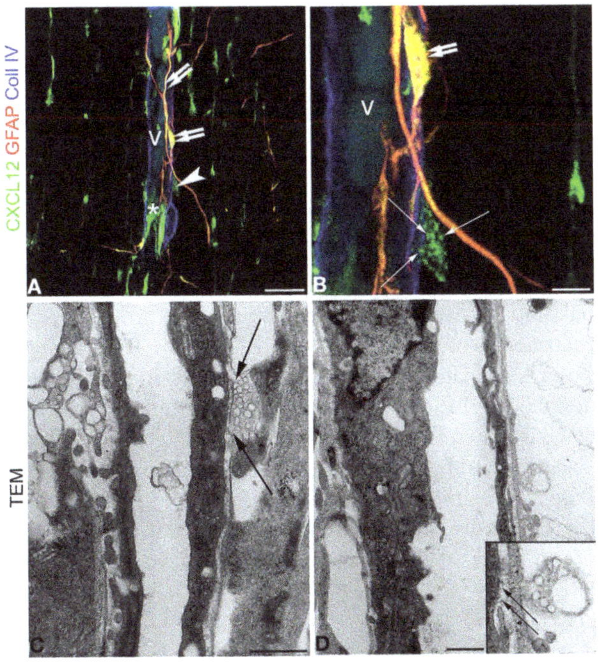

FIGURE 7 | Confocal images (A,B) and transmission electron microscopy (C,D) of human cerebral cortex at midgestation. (A,B) Triple labeling with CXCL12, GFAP, and Coll IV shows the profile of a radial vessel (v) contacted by GFAP/CXCL12-reactive perivascular astrocyte processes (*double arrows*) and CXCL12-reactive RG fibers (*asterisk*); a RG varicosity (*arrowhead*) in contact with the vessel wall is enlarged in **(B)** and appears filled by CXCL12 labeled MVs (*arrows*). **(C,D)** At ultrastructural level, perivascular RG varicosities show their content of membrane-bound MVs regularly aligned with the vessel contact side (**C** and *inset* in **D**; *arrows*). Bars: **A** 20 μm; **B** 5 μm; **C,D** 5 μm.

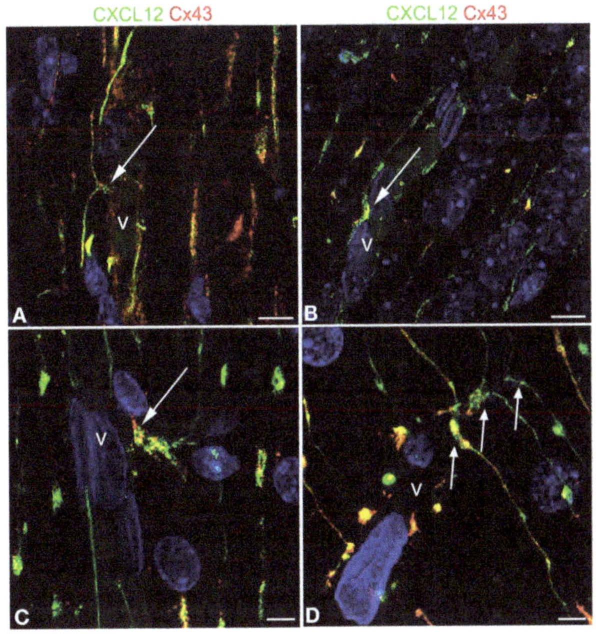

FIGURE 8 | Confocal images of human cerebral cortex at midgestation double labeled with CXCL12 and Cx43. (A–D) Examples of *omega-shaped/asymmetrical* varicosities (*arrows*) in contact with the vessel wall (v) characterized by CXCL12/Cx43 colocalization; note in **(D)** the regular sequence of deflected RG fibers forming asymmetrical contacts (*arrows*). Bars: **A,B** 10 μm; **C,D** 5 μm.

and thin filaments bearing numerous varicosities or swellings" (Bentivoglio and Mazzarello, 1999). Subsequently, in 1904, Cajal confirmed the existence of radiating fibers and extended Magini's work, definitely describing "swelling intercalated along the radial glia fibers protoplasmic accumulation" (Ramón y Cajal, 1904). In recent studies on neurogenic RG in rat embryos, DiI-labeled RG cells have shown a "Golgi-like" morphology, including the small varicosities, that have been described as points of cytoplasm accumulation in the flux and reflux of fluid through the cell during mitosis (Weissman et al., 2003; Kriegstein and Alvarez-Buylla, 2009). Surprisingly, CXCL12, a chemokine that accumulates in RG fibers, can show these cellular structures in detail, going beyond the mere profile of cytoplasmic swelling, and instead suggesting a role as specialized cellular sites. RG cells, like cerebellar Bergmann glia and retinal Müller cells, both examples of RG-like glial cells in adult CNS, may display a differential distribution of organelles and membrane domains along their length (Fedoroff and Vernadakis, 1986). The described RG varicosities can be regarded as special compartments of the cell devoted to closely adjoining the vessel wall to form specific vascular contacts.

CXCL12-bearing MVs, as cell-derived MVs (diameter ranging from 0.1 to 1 μm) involved in cell-to-cell communication, may directly bud from the plasma membrane to convey their membrane-associated bioactive molecule to the target cells (György et al., 2011; Frühbeis et al., 2012; Kalra et al., 2012). It has been demonstrated that cultured astrocytes shed MVs from cell domains interpreted as astrocyte end-feet, which contain angiogenic factors, FGF-2, and VEGF, and membrane associated ß1-integrin (Proia et al., 2008), MVs can, therefore, participate in angiogenic events, transferring pro-angiogenic factors to ECs (Boulanger and Tedgui, 2005; Muralidharan-Chari et al., 2010; Martinez and Andriantsitohaina, 2011). Moreover, it has also been shown that tumor-derived MVs released by tumor ECs can be taken up by normal ECs through endocytosis, and promote motility and tube formation, conferring proangiogenic properties to quiescent ECs (Kawamoto et al., 2012). It has been demonstrated that in zebrafish brain and in rat developing retina, chemokine CXCL12 signaling specifically controls the correct pathfinding of newly formed microvessels (Strasser et al., 2010; Unoki et al., 2010; Bussmann et al., 2011; Fujita et al., 2011). Our findings support these roles, suggesting that the chemokine can become available, through the shedding of MVs from RG varicosities, for ligand/receptor interactions on ECs or, alternatively, after MVs endocytosis, for direct EC activation.

CXCL12 VESSEL-SPECIFIC ACTIVITY REGULATED BY Cx43 NON-CHANNEL ROLES

The preliminary results that show a CXCL12/Cx43 colocalization in RG glio-vascular contacts suggest that the release of

CXCL12 can be regulated by the activation of Cx43 hemichannels, non-junctional structures that can be involved in the release of signaling molecules, and that are a common attribute of cells during development, forming functional hexameric rings before proper gap junctions appear (Nagy et al., 2004; Nielsen et al., 2012; Stehberg et al., 2012; Giaume et al., 2013; Zhou and Jiang, 2014). In fact, during cerebral cortex development, Cx43 displays channel-independent roles also when regulating neuroblast migration (Matsuuchi and Naus, 2013). Moreover, as demonstrated for human bone marrow stromal cells, the secretion of functional CXCL12 by RG cells could be mediated by Cx43 (Schajnovitz et al., 2011), and Cx43 has been found to regulate CXCL12-mediated Rap1 EC spreading "*in vitro*" (Machtaler et al., 2011).

ACTIVATION AND COOPERATION OF MULTIPLE PRO-ANGIO-MORPHOGENETIC PATHWAYS

The emergence of the chemokine system as a key signal during CNS development and vascularization raises the issue of a possible functional interaction with other pro-angiogenic pathways such as the canonical Wnt/β-catenin pathway, whose involvement in regulating vascular morphogenesis has already been described, together with a CNS-specific angiogenic, and barriergenesis function in concert with other signaling pathways (Daneman et al., 2009; Dejana, 2010; Reis and Liebner, 2013). As suggested by studies on the effect of RG cells ablation, a cooperative effect of CXCL12/CXCR4–Wnt/β-catenin exists during brain vascularization. In fact, in absence of RG cells, a significant reduction has been observed of cortical thickness, and the regression of nascent brain vessels, *via* the inhibition of EC Wnt signaling in a contact and stage-dependent manner (Ma et al., 2013). Moreover, the interaction between Wnt/β-catenin signaling and the chemokine receptors CXCR4 and CXCR7 leads to a coordinated cell migration *via* differential receptor regulation (Aman and Piotrowski, 2008); this same cooperation may generate localized molecular cues, inducing differentiation of BBB properties and cortex microvessel maturation (Engelhardt and Liebner, 2014).

In conclusion, this study, carried out during human cerebral cortex development, supports the concept of an involvement of RG cells in the synchronized regulation of neuro-vascular patterning and early BBB differentiation. According to our model (**Figures 1A–C**), this may take place thanks to the unique, spatial distribution of RG cells, the varicosity/MV/CXCL12/Cx43 machinery, and the help of an overlapping repertoire of signaling molecules (Carmeliet and Tessier-Lavigne, 2005; Vasudevan and Bhide, 2008; Tam and Watts, 2010).

AUTHOR CONTRIBUTIONS

Mariella Errede Substantial contribution to the design of the work, acquisition, electron microscopy analysis, interpretation of data. Francesco Girolamo Substantial contribution to the design of the work; acquisition, confocal microscopy analysis, interpretation of data. Marco Rizzi Substantial contribution to acquisition and confocal microscopy analysis, interpretation of data. Mirella Bertossi Substantial contribution to interpretation of electron microscopy data and revising the work critically for important intellectual content. Luisa Roncali Substantial contribution in revising the work critically for important intellectual content and final approval of the version to be published. Daniela Virgintino Substantial contributions to the conception of the work, drafting the work and revising it critically; final approval of the version to be published.

ACKNOWLEDGMENTS

We are indebted to W. B. Stallcup (The Sanford-Burnham Institute for Molecular Medicine, La Jolla, CA, USA) for polyclonal anti-NG2/CSPG4 D2 antiserum and to E. Maiorano (Department of Emergency and Organ Transplantation, Pathological Anatomy Unit, Faculty of Medicine, University of Bari, Bari, Italy) for histological, control sections. Mary Victoria Pragnell is gratefully acknowledged for language help. This work has been funded by grants from Fondazione Cassa di Risparmio di Puglia to Daniela Virgintino and from the Italian Ministry of the University and Scientific Research (MIUR), Progetto di Ricerca d'Interesse Nazionale to Luisa Roncali.

REFERENCES

Aman, A., and Piotrowski, T. (2008). Wnt/beta-catenin and Fgf signaling control collective cell migration by restricting chemokine receptor expression. *Dev. Cell* 15, 749–761. doi: 10.1016/j.devcel.2008.10.002

Bär, T. (1980). The vascular system of the cerebral cortex. *Adv. Anat. Embryol. Cell Biol.* 59, 1–62. doi: 10.1007/978-3-642-67432-7_1

Bentivoglio, M., and Mazzarello, P. (1999). The history of radial glia. *Brain Res. Bull.* 49, 305–315. doi: 10.1016/S0361-9230(99)00065-9

Borrell, V., and Marín, O. (2006). Meninges control tangential migration of hem-derived Cajal-Retzius cells via CXCL12/CXCR4 signaling. *Nat. Neurosci.* 9, 1284–1293. doi: 10.1038/nn1764

Boulanger, C. M., and Tedgui, A. (2005). Dying for attention: microparticles and angiogenesis. *Cardiovasc. Res.* 67, 1–3. doi: 10.1016/j.cardiores.2005.05.001

Bussmann, J., Wolfe, S. A., and Siekmannm, A. F. (2011). Arterial-venous network formation during brain vascularization involves hemodynamic regulation of chemokine signaling. *Development* 138, 1717–1726. doi: 10.1242/dev.059881

Carmeliet, P., and Tessier-Lavigne, M. (2005). Common mechanisms of nerve and blood vessel wiring. *Nature* 436, 193–200. doi: 10.1038/nature03875

Choi, S. H., and Lapham, L. W. (1978). Radial glia In the human letal cerebrum a combined Golgi, immunofluorescent and electron microscopic study. *Brain Res.* 148, 295–311. doi: 10.1016/0006-8993(78)90721-7

Daneman, R., Agallin, D., Zhou, L., Kubnert, F., Kuo, J. C., and Barres, B. A. (2009). Wnt/β-catenin signaling is required for CNS, but not non-CNS angiogenesis. *Proc. Natl. Acad. Sci. U.S.A.* 106, 641–646. doi: 10.1073/pnas.0805165106

Dejana, E. (2010). The role of wnt signaling in physiological and pathological angiogenesis. *Circ. Res.* 107, 943–952. doi: 10.1161/CIRCRESAHA.110.223750

Elias, L. A., Wang, D. D., and Kriegstein, A. R. (2007). Gap junction adhesion is necessary for radial migration in the neocortex. *Nature* 448, 901–907. doi: 10.1038/nature06063

Engelhardt, B., and Liebner, S. (2014). Novel insights into the development and maintenance of the blood-brain barrier. *Cell Tiss. Res.* 355, 687–699. doi: 10.1007/s00441-014-1811-2

Engelhardt, B., and Risau, W. (1995). "The development of the blood-brain barrier" in *The Development of the Blood-Brain Barrier*, eds J. Greenwood, D. Begley, M. Segal (London: Plenum), 10–100.

Errede, M., Benagiano, V., Girolamo, F., Flace, P., Bertossi, M., Roncali, L., et al. (2002). Differential expression of connexin43 in foetal, adult and tumour-associated human brain endothelial cells. *Histochem. J.* 34, 265–271. doi: 10.1023/A:1023344106815

Fedoroff, S., and Vernadakis, A. (1986). *Astrocytes. Development, Morphology and Regional Specialization of Astrocytes.* London: Academic Press.

Frühbeis, C., Fröhlich, D., and Krämer-Albers, E. M. (2012). Emerging roles of exosomes in neuron-glia communication. *Front. Physiol.* 3:119. doi: 10.3389/fphys.2012.00119

Fujita, M., Cha, Y. R., Pham, V. N., Sakurai, A., Roman, B. L., Gutkind, J. S., et al. (2011). Assembly and patterning of the vascular network of the vertebrate hindbrain. *Development* 138, 1705–1715. doi: 10.1242/dev.058776

Giaume, C., Leybaert, L., Naus, C. C., and Sáez, J. C. (2013). Connexin and pannexin hemichannels in brain glial cells: properties, pharmacology, and roles. *Front. Pharmacol.* 4:88. doi: 10.3389/fphar.2013.00088

György, B., Szabó, T. G., Pásztói, M., Pál, Z., Misják, P., Aradi, B., et al. (2011). Membrane vesicles, current state-of-the-art: emerging role of extracellular vesicles. *Cell. Mol. Life Sci.* 68, 2667–2688. doi: 10.1007/s00018-011-0689-3

Howard, B., Chen, Y., and Zecevic, N. (2006). Cortical progenitor cells in the developing human telencephalon. *Glia* 53, 57–66. doi: 10.1002/glia.20259

Howard, B. M., Mo, Z., Filipovic, R., Moore, A. R., Antic, S. D., and Zecevic, D. (2008). Radial glia cells in the developing human brain. *Neuroscientist* 14, 459–473. doi: 10.1177/1073858407313512

Kalra, H., Simpson, R. J., Ji, H., Aikawa, E., Altevogt, P., Askenase, P., et al. (2012). Vesiclepedia: a compendium for extracellular vesicles with continuous community annotation. *PLoS Biol.* 10:e1001450. doi: 10.1371/journal.pbio.1001450

Kawamoto, T., Ohga, N., Akiyama, K., Hirata, N., Kitahara, S., Maishi, N., et al. (2012). Tumor-derived microvesicles induce proangiogenic phenotype in endothelial cells via endocytosis. *PLoS ONE* 7:e34045. doi: 10.1371/journal.pone.0034045

Kriegstein, A., and Alvarez-Buylla, A. (2009). The glial nature of embryonic and adult neural stem cells. *Annu. Rev. Neurosci.* 32, 149–184. doi: 10.1146/annurev.neuro.051508.135600

Li, G., Adesnik, H., Li, J., Long, J., Nicoll, R. A., Rubenstein, J. L., et al. (2008). Regional distribution of cortical interneurons and development of inhibitory tone are regulated by Cxcl12/Cxcr4 signaling. *J. Neurosci.* 28, 1085–1098. doi: 10.1523/JNEUROSCI.4602-07.2008

Liebner, S., and Plate, K. H. (2010). Differentiation of the brain vasculature: the answer came blowing by the Wnt. *J. Angiogenesis Res.* 2, 1–10. doi: 10.1186/2040-2384-2-1

Ma, S., Kwon, H. J., Johng, H., Zang, K., and Huang, Z. (2013). Radial glial neural progenitors regulate nascent brain vascular network stabilization via inhibition of Wnt signaling. *PLoS Biol.* 11:e1001469. doi: 10.1371/journal.pbio.1001469

Machtaler, S., Dang-Lawson, M., Choi, K., Jang, C., Naus, C. C., and Matsuuchi, L. (2011). The gap junction protein Cx43 regulates B-lymphocyte spreading and adhesion. *J. Cell Sci.* 124, 2611–2621. doi: 10.1242/jcs.089532

Malatesta, P., and Götz, M. (2013). Radial glia – from boring cables to stem cell stars. *Development* 140, 483–486. doi: 10.1242/dev.085852

Malatesta, P., Hartfuss, E., and Götz, M. (2000). Isolation of radial glial cells by fluorescent-activated cell sorting reveals a neuronal lineage. *Development* 127, 5253–5263.

Marin-Padilla, M. (1985). Early vascularization of the embryonic cerebral cortex: Golgi and electron microscopic studies. *J. Comp. Neurol.* 241, 237–249. doi: 10.1002/cne.902410210

Marín-Padilla, M. (2012). The human brain intracerebral microvascular system: development and structure. *Front. Neuroanat.* 6:38. doi: 10.3389/fnana.2012.00038

Martinez, M. C., and Andriantsitohaina, R. (2011). Microparticles in angiogenesis: therapeutic potential. *Circ. Res.* 109, 110–119. doi: 10.1161/CIRCRESAHA.110.233049

Matsuuchi, L., and Naus, C. C. (2013). Gap junction proteins on the move: connexins, the cytoskeleton and migration. *Biochim. Biophys. Acta* 1828, 94–108. doi: 10.1016/j.bbamem.2012.05.014

Muralidharan-Chari, V., Clancy, J. W., Sedgwick, A., and D'Souza-Schorey, C. (2010). Microvesicles: mediators of extracellular communication during cancer progression. *J. Cell Sci.* 123, 1603–1611. doi: 10.1242/jcs.064386

Nagy, J. I., Dudek, F. E., and Rash, J. E. (2004). Update on connexins and gap junctions in neurons and glia in the mammalian nervous system. *Brain Res. Brain Res. Rev.* 47, 191–215. doi: 10.1016/j.brainresrev.2004.05.005

Nielsen, M. S., Nygaard Axelsen, L., Sorgen, P. L., Verma, V., Delmar, M., and Holstein-Rathlou, N. H. (2012). Gap junctions. *Compr. Physiol.* 2, 1981–2035. doi: 10.1002/cphy.c110051

Paredes, M. F., Li, G. N., Berger, O., Baraban, S. C., and Pleasure, S. J. (2006). Stromal-derived factor-1 (CXCL12) regulates laminar position of Cajal-Retzius cells in normal and dysplastic brains. *J. Neurosci.* 26, 9404–9412. doi: 10.1523/JNEUROSCI.2575-06.2006

Peng, H., Kolb, R., and Kennedy, J. E. (2007). Differential expression of CXCL12 and CXCR4 during human fetal neural progenitor cell differentiation. *J. Neuroimmun. Pharmacol.* 2, 251–258. doi: 10.1007/s11481-007-9081-3

Proia, P., Schiera, G., Mineo, M., Ingrassia, A. M., Santoro, G., Savettieri, G., et al. (2008). Astrocytes shed extracellular vesicles that contain fibroblast growth factor-2 and vascular endothelial growth factor. *Int. J. Mol. Med.* 21, 63–67. doi: 10.3892/ijmm.21.1.63

Quaegebeur, A., Lange, C., and Carmeliet, P. (2011). The neurovascular link in health and disease: molecular mechanisms and therapeutic implications. *Neuron* 71, 406–424. doi: 10.1016/j.neuron.2011.07.013

Rakic, P. (1971). Neuron-glia relationship during granule cell migration in developing cerebellar cortex. A Golgi and electronmicroscopic study in *Macacus Rhesus. J. Comp. Neurol.* 141, 283–312. doi: 10.1002/cne.901410303

Rakic, P. (1972). Mode of cell migration to the superficial layers of fetal monkey neocortex. *J. Comp. Neurol.* 145, 61–83. doi: 10.1002/cne.901450105

Rakic, P. (2007). The radial edifice of cortical architecture. *Brain Res. Rev.* 55, 204–219. doi: 10.1016/j.brainresrev.2007.02.010

Ramón y Cajal, S. (1904). *Textura del Sistema Nervioso del Hombre y de los Vertebrados.* Madrid: Moya.

Reis, M., and Liebner, S. (2013). Wnt signaling in the vasculature. *Exp. Cell Res.* 319, 1317–1323. doi: 10.1016/j.yexcr.2012.12.023

Rickmann, M., and Wolff, J. R. (1985). Prenatal gliogenesis in the neopallium of the rat. *Adv. Anat. Embryol. Cell Biol.* 93, 37–66.

Risau, W., Gautschi-Sova, P., and Bohlen, P. (1988). Endothelial cell growth factors in embryonic and adult chick brain are related to human acidic fibroblast growth factor. *EMBO J.* 7, 959–962.

Risau, W., and Wolburg, H. (1990). Development of the blood-brain barrier. *Trends Neurosci.* 13, 174–178. doi: 10.1016/0166-2236(90)90043-A

Schajnovitz, A., Itkin, T., D'Uva, G., Kalinkovich, A., Golan, K., Ludin, A., et al. (2011). CXCL12 secretion by bone marrow stromal cells is dependent on cell contact and mediated by connexin-43 and connexin-45 gap junctions. *Nat. Immunol.* 12, 391–398. doi: 10.1038/ni.2017

Siegenthaler, J. A., Ashique, A. M., Zarbalis, K., Patterson, K. P., Hecht, J. H., Kane, M. A., et al. (2009). Retinoic acid from the meninges regulates cortical neuron generation. *Cell* 139, 597–609. doi: 10.1016/j.cell.2009.10.004

Stehberg, J., Moraga-Amaro, R., Salazar, C., Becerra, A., Echeverría, C., Orellana, J. A., et al. (2012). Release of gliotransmitters through astroglial connexin 43 hemichannels is necessary for fear memory consolidation in the basolateral amygdala. *FASEB J.* 26, 3649–3657. doi: 10.1096/fj.11-198416

Strasser, G. A., Kaminker, J. S., and Tessier-Lavigne, M. (2010). Microarray analysis of retinal endothelial tip cells identifies CXCR4 as a mediator of tip cell morphology and branching. *Blood* 115, 5102–5110. doi: 10.1182/blood-2009-07-230284

Stumm, R., and Höllt, V. (2007). CXC chemokine receptor 4 regulates neuronal migration and axonal pathfinding in the developing nervous system: implications for neuronal regeneration in the adult brain. *J. Mol. Endocrinol.* 38, 377–382. doi: 10.1677/JME-06-0032

Stumm, R. K., Zhou, C., Ara, T., Lazarini, F., Dubois-Dalcq, M., Nagasawa, T., et al. (2003). CXCR4 regulates interneuron migration in the developing neocortex. *J. Neurosci.* 23, 5123–5130.

Tam, S. J., and Watts, R. J. (2010). Connecting vascular and nervous system development: angiogenesis and the blood-brain barrier. *Annu. Rev. Neurosci.* 33, 379–408. doi: 10.1146/annurev-neuro-060909-152829

Tiveron, M. C., and Cremer, H. (2008). CXCL12/CXCR4 signalling in neuronal cell migration. *Curr. Opin. Neurobiol.* 18, 237–244. doi: 10.1016/j.conb.2008.06.004

Tiveron, M. C., Rossel, M., Moepps, B., Zhang, Y. L., Seidenfaden, R., and Favor, J., et al (2006). Molecular interaction between projection neuron precursors and invading interneurons via stromal-derived factor 1 (CXCL12)/CXCR4 signaling in the cortical subventricular zone/intermediate zone. *J. Neurosci.* 26, 13273–13278. doi: 10.1523/JNEUROSCI.4162-06.2006

Unoki, N., Murakami, T., Nishijima, K., Ogino, K., van Rooijen, N., and Yoshimura, N. (2010). SDF-1/CXCR4 contributes to the activation of tip cells and microglia in retinal angiogenesis. *Invest. Ophthalmol. Vis. Sci.* 51, 3362–3371. doi: 10.1167/iovs.09-4978

Vasudevan, A., and Bhide, P. G. (2008). Angiogenesis in the embryonic CNS: a new twist on an old tale. *Cell Adh. Migr.* 2, 167–169. doi: 10.4161/cam.2.3.6485

Virgintino, D., Errede, M., Rizzi, M., Girolamo, F., Strippoli, M., Wälchli, T., et al. (2013). The CXCL12/CXCR4/CXCR7 ligand-receptor system regulates neuro-glio-vascular interactions and vessel growth during human brain development. *J. Inherit. Metab. Dis.* 36, 455–466. doi: 10.1007/s10545-012-9574-y

Virgintino, D., Maiorano, E., Errede, M., Vimercati, A., Greco, P., Selvaggi, L., et al. (1998). Astroglia-microvessel relationship in the developing human telencephalon. *Int. J. Dev. Biol.* 42, 1165–1168.

Virgintino, D., Robertson, D., Errede, M., Benagiano, V., Bertossi, M., Ambrosi, G., et al. (2001). Expression of the gap junction protein connexin43 in human telencephalon microvessels. *Microvasc. Res.* 62, 435–439. doi: 10.1006/mvre.2001.2345

Weissman, T., Noctor, S. C., Clinton, B. K., Honig, L. S., and Kriegstein, A. R. (2003). Neurogenic radial glial cells in reptile, rodent and human: from mitosis to migration. *Cereb. Cortex* 13, 550–559. doi: 10.1093/cercor/13.6.550

Xu, L., Tang, X., Wang, Y., Xu, H., and Fan, X. (2014). Radial glia, the keystone of the development of the hippocampal dentate gyrus. *Mol. Neurobiol.* doi: 10.1007/s12035-014-8692-y. [Epub ahead of print].

Zhou, J. Z., and Jiang, J. X. (2014). Gap junction and hemichannel-independent actions of connexins on cell and tissue functions - An update. *FEBS Lett.* 588, 1186–1192. doi: 10.1016/j.febslet.2014.01.001

10

Transport of thyroid hormones via the choroid plexus into the brain: the roles of transthyretin and thyroid hormone transmembrane transporters

Samantha J. Richardson[1]*, Roshen C. Wijayagunaratne[1], Damian G. D'Souza[1], Veerle M. Darras[2] and Stijn L. J. Van Herck[2]

[1] *School of Medical Sciences, RMIT University, Bundoora, VIC, Australia*
[2] *Laboratory of Comparative Endocrinology, Biology Department, KU Leuven, Leuven, Belgium*

***Correspondence:**
Samantha J. Richardson, School of Medical Sciences, RMIT University, Plenty Road, PO Box 71, Bundoora, VIC 3083, Australia
e-mail: samantha.richardson@rmit.edu.au

Thyroid hormones are key players in regulating brain development. Thus, transfer of appropriate quantities of thyroid hormones from the blood into the brain at specific stages of development is critical. The choroid plexus forms the blood-cerebrospinal fluid barrier. In reptiles, birds and mammals, the main protein synthesized and secreted by the choroid plexus is a thyroid hormone distributor protein: transthyretin. This transthyretin is secreted into the cerebrospinal fluid and moves thyroid hormones from the blood into the cerebrospinal fluid. Maximal transthyretin synthesis in the choroid plexus occurs just prior to the period of rapid brain growth, suggesting that choroid plexus-derived transthyretin moves thyroid hormones from blood into cerebrospinal fluid just prior to when thyroid hormones are required for rapid brain growth. The structure of transthyretin has been highly conserved, implying strong selection pressure and an important function. In mammals, transthyretin binds T4 (precursor form of thyroid hormone) with higher affinity than T3 (active form of thyroid hormone). In all other vertebrates, transthyretin binds T3 with higher affinity than T4. As mammals are the exception, we should not base our thinking about the role of transthyretin in the choroid plexus solely on mammalian data. Thyroid hormone transmembrane transporters are involved in moving thyroid hormones into and out of cells and have been identified in many tissues, including the choroid plexus. Thyroid hormones enter the choroid plexus via thyroid hormone transmembrane transporters and leave the choroid plexus to enter the cerebrospinal fluid via either thyroid hormone transmembrane transporters or via choroid plexus-derived transthyretin secreted into the cerebrospinal fluid. The quantitative contribution of each route during development remains to be elucidated. This is part of a review series on ontogeny and phylogeny of brain barrier mechanisms.

Keywords: blood-cerebrospinal fluid barrier, brain, choroid plexus, development, evolution, thyroid hormones, transthyretin, thyroid hormone transporters

THYROID HORMONES

Thyroid hormones (THs) are key players in regulating development of the brain. Insufficient THs during prenatal development in humans can lead to cretinism and mental retardation, whereas insufficient THs in adult life can result in fatigue, lethargy, mental impairment, weight gain, cold intolerance and in severe cases, clinical depression. THs act mainly by regulating transcription of specific genes. THs are synthesized in the thyroid gland and are secreted into the blood. Most of the TH secreted from the thyroid gland is the precursor form (T4). About 80% of the active form (T3) is generated by deiodination of T4 to T3 in target tissues. In the blood, >99% of TH is bound to specific plasma proteins known as TH distributor proteins. Because THs are lipophilic they partition between the lipid phase and the aqueous phase with a ratio of 20,000:1 (Dickson et al., 1987). The binding of THs to TH distributor proteins prevents avid partitioning of THs into the lipid membranes of cells and ensures that there is a sufficiently large pool of TH circulating in the blood (Mendel et al., 1987). In humans, the main TH distributor proteins are albumin, transthyretin (TTR) and thyroxine-binding globulin (TBG), all of which are synthesized by the liver. In addition, a small fraction is distributed by lipoproteins including ApoB100 (Benvenga et al., 1989). The free hormone hypothesis states that it is the free hormone in blood (not the protein-bound hormone) that is important for biological activity (Mendel, 1989). Thus, THs must dissociate from the distributor proteins before they can exert their effects.

In human blood 99.97% of T4 and 99.70% of T3 is bound to the TH distributor proteins (Mendel, 1989). Of these, TBG has the highest affinity for T4 and T3 (1.0×10^{10} M^{-1} and 4.6×10^{8} M^{-1}, respectively), TTR has intermediate affinity (7.0×10^{7} M^{-1} and 1.4×10^{7} M^{-1}, respectively) and albumin has the lowest affinity (7.0×10^5 M^{-1} and 1.0×10^5 M^{-1}, respectively). Together, these three TH distributor proteins form a buffering network for free T4 in blood, which could help to protect against hypothyroidism (abnormally low levels of free TH in blood) or hyperthyroidism (abnormally high levels of free TH in blood) (Schreiber and Richardson, 1997). The older literature and some modern text books state that the role of TH distributor proteins in blood is to overcome low TH solubility. However, the concentration of free T4 in human blood is about 25 pM and the maximum solubility of T4 in physiological saline is 2.3 μM, i.e., about 100,000 times the concentration of free T4 (Schreiber and Richardson, 1997). Therefore, TH distributor proteins must play a role other than to aid the solubility of THs in the blood and CSF.

The concentrations of each of the TH distributor proteins in adult human blood varies greatly: TBG at 0.015 g/l, TTR at 0.25 g/l and albumin at 42 g/l. Traditionally it has been believed that in blood, TBG distributes about 75% of thyroid hormones, TTR distributes 15% and albumin transports about 10%. Because TBG binds about 75%, it is sometimes referred to as the "most important" thyroid hormone distributor. However, this is too simplistic, as the biological importance is related to the delivery of THs to cells, which is dependent on the dissociation rates of T3 and T4 from the distributor proteins and capillary transit times. To determine which of the three TH distributor proteins contributes most effectively to hormone delivery to tissues, the dissociation rates and the capillary transit times have to be considered. In brief, the dissociation rates for T4 and T3 from TBG are 0.018 and 0.16 s^{-1}, respectively; from TTR are 0.094 and 0.69 s^{-1}, respectively and from albumin are 1.3 and 2.2 s^{-1}, respectively (Mendel and Weisiger, 1990). Thus, given the capillary transit times for various tissues (Mendel et al., 1989), TTR is responsible for much of the immediate delivery of THs to tissues (Robbins, 2000).

THs have multiple mechanisms of action which can be grouped into "genomic" and "non-genomic" mechanisms of action. Non-genomic mechanisms include membrane-initiated mechanisms via binding to specific integrins (Davis et al., 2005, 2011; Lin et al., 2012); cytosolic kinase-initiated interactions which have non-genomic effects on glucose metabolism (Moeller et al., 2006, 2011) and rapid activation of kinases in signaling cascades in mitochondria resulting in altered fatty acid metabolism (Sayre and Lechleiter, 2012). The genomic pathway, which is generally better known and studied, involves thyroid hormone receptors (TRs). Free (unbound) THs enter target cells via the TH transmembrane transporters (Hennemann et al., 2001), which are responsible for influx and efflux of THs from cells. For genomic actions of THs within the cell nucleus, T4 can be deiodinated to T3 (considered the "active" form of TH). The family of deiodinases can either activate (e.g., T4 to T3) or inactivate (e.g., T3 to T2; T4 to rT3) THs within the cell (Darras et al., 2015). T3 exerts genomic effects by binding to TRs which are nuclear transcription factors. T3 can bind TRs either in the cytoplasm and translocate into the nucleus, or bind TRs in the nucleus. T3 binding to TR hetero-dimer complexes on thyroid response elements in the promotor of specific genes causes dissociation of co-repressor proteins and association of co-activator proteins. The resulting complex then initiates transcription of genes that are positively regulated by THs. Some genes are negatively regulated by THs, whereby binding of T3 induces the opposite changes and turns off transcription. Thus, it is crucial that the appropriate concentration of THs is present in the critical regions of the brain at each stage of development, to ensure normal brain maturation. This requires that sufficient (but not excess) THs move from the blood into the brain at critical stages of development. There are several pathways for THs to move from the blood into the CSF, but this review will focus on the route via the choroid plexus i.e., the blood-CSF barrier.

THE CHOROID PLEXUS

The choroid plexus is a villous structure located in the lateral, third and fourth ventricles of the brain and is the site of the blood-CSF barrier. The structure of the choroid plexus is similar in all vertebrates studied to date (Ek et al., 2005). The blood supply to the choroid plexus comes from two posterior choroidal arteries, which branch from the internal carotid arteries. The rate of blood flow to the choroid plexus has been estimated to be about 3.5 faster than that to the rest of the brain (Zheng, 2005). The choroid plexus epithelial cells are joined by tight junctions, giving the tissue its barrier properties (Ek et al., 2005). The choroid plexus produces about 70% of the CSF, and thus has a major influence on its composition (Cserr, 1971). In humans the total CSF is replaced about four times per day (Brown et al., 2005). In comparison to the blood, which mixes, the CSF has a pipeline type of flow which does not mix. Consequently, the composition of the CSF can vary depending on the site from which it is sampled (Cserr, 1971). The choroid plexus barrier ensures that the composition of the CSF is very different to that of the blood. For example, in adult mammals, the CSF has only about 0.5% total protein concentration compared to that in the blood (Brown et al., 2005) and the relative ratios of proteins in the blood compared to the CSF differ markedly. However, the total protein concentration in the CSF changes during development, peaking early in development and then gradually decreasing to adult levels (Saunders, 1992). For a comprehensive summary of the development of the choroid plexus (see Ek et al., 2005).

TTR SYNTHESIS BY THE CHOROID PLEXUS

The first description of TTR synthesis in the brain was in 1985 (Soprano et al., 1985). Soon after, Schreiber's group identified TTR mRNA as being located only in the choroid plexus of the brain (Dickson et al., 1985) and then specifically in the choroid plexus epithelial cells (Stauder et al., 1986). The first experiments suggesting that TTR synthesis by the choroid plexus was involved in the movement of TH from the blood into the CSF were published in 1987. ^{125}I-T4 was injected into the blood of rats and was detected in various brain structures: initially it accumulated in the choroid plexus to ~250% the level in blood. Thereafter, ^{125}I-T4 accumulated in the CSF, after which it began to appear in the cortex and striatum of the brain. However, when the analogous experiment was repeated using ^{125}I-T3, there was no specific accumulation of ^{125}I-T3 in the choroid plexus. This was interpreted as TTR synthesis by the choroid plexus being involved in the movement of T4 but not T3, from the blood across the choroid plexus into the CSF (Dickson et al., 1987). TTR synthesized by the choroid plexus was shown to be secreted into the CSF and not into the blood (Schreiber et al., 1990; Duan et al., 1991) i.e., unidirectional secretion of TTR by the choroid plexus 100% into the CSF. Then Köhrle's group demonstrated that the TTR-T4 complex from the blood is not transported as such into the CSF; and the movement of T4 from the blood into the CSF is dependent on the concentration of free T4 in the serum and on T4 binding to choroid plexus-derived TTR i.e., if the TH binding capacity of TTR was disrupted, then TH did not cross the choroid plexus (Chanoine et al., 1992). Schreiber's group showed that if protein synthesis was blocked in a choroid plexus epithelial monolayer cell culture system, then T4 did not accumulate in the apical chamber (Southwell et al., 1993). Furthermore, the concentration of free T4 is higher in CSF than in the blood, thus, the unidirectional secretion of TTR (or TTR-T4) was moving T4 against the free T4 gradient (Southwell et al., 1993). These were the key experiments suggesting that the synthesis and secretion of TTR by the choroid plexus was involved in movement of T4 from the blood into the CSF.

The choroid plexus is the tissue with the highest concentration of TTR mRNA per gram tissue weight. The adult rat choroid plexus has an 11 times higher concentration of TTR mRNA compared to the liver (4.4 vs. 0.39 μg TTR mRNA per gram wet weight) (Schreiber et al., 1990). In chickens, the adult choroid plexus has a 22 times higher concentration of TTR mRNA compared to the liver (7.2 vs. 0.33 μg TTR mRNA per gram wet) (Duan et al., 1991). Furthermore, at the protein level, TTR is the major protein synthesized and secreted by the choroid plexus of eutherians, marsupials, monotremes, birds, and reptiles (Harms et al., 1991). The common ancestor of those animals whose choroid plexus specializes in TTR synthesis and secretion are the stem-reptiles, whose brains showed the first traces of neocortex (Kent, 1987). As THs are lipophilic, the increase in lipid volume of the brain could have been a selection pressure in turning on TTR synthesis in the choroid plexus and secreting it into the CSF, to act as a TH-binding protein in the CSF, thereby reducing the partitioning of THs into the lipid membranes and allowing a greater distribution of TH throughout the CSF (Schreiber and Richardson, 1997). Thus, the onset of TTR synthesis in the choroid plexus is suggested to have occurred at the stage of the stem-reptiles, about 300 million years ago (Schreiber and Richardson, 1997). TTR is synthesized in the liver of amphibians and fish during specific stages of development (see Richardson, 2007), but until now synthesis of TTR in the choroid plexus of amphibians and fish has not been described [although TTR mRNA has been detected in whole brain of sea bream (Santos and Power, 1999)]. The main protein synthesized and secreted by amphibian choroid plexus is a lipocalin (Achen et al., 1992), which could be the functional precursor of choroid plexus-derived TTR, as lipocalins are known to bind small hydrophobic molecules. That the choroid plexus specializes in the synthesis and secretion of TTR in such a great range of vertebrates is also suggestive of an important function. Furthermore, the amino acid sequence of TTRs across all vertebrates is so highly conserved, that it forms a single motif (Hennebry et al., 2006). Such high conservation of primary structure can be explained by extremely strong selection pressures during the past 500 million years.

ALTRICIAL vs. PRECOCIAL BRAIN DEVELOPMENT AND TTR SYNTHESIS BY THE CHOROID PLEXUS

The brain develops at different rates in different vertebrate species. At the time of birth, the brain of precocial animals (e.g., chickens, sheep) is significantly further developed than the brains of altricial animals (e.g., rats, mice). Therefore, it is of interest to compare the ontogeny of TTR synthesis in the choroid plexus of altricial animals compared with precocial animals.

In rats (23 days gestation), TTR mRNA was first detected in the choroid plexus at E12.5 in the 4th ventricle, at E13.5 in the lateral ventricles, and at E17.5 in the third ventricle. The proportion of TTR mRNA in total RNA increased 40-fold from E12.5 until birth (Fung et al., 1988). Because the choroid plexus develops faster than many other parts of the brain (Sturrock, 1979), part of this 40-fold increase in TTR mRNA could have been due to the increase in size of the choroid plexus with respect to the size of the brain. The peak of TTR mRNA as a proportion of total brain mRNA (about 140% the level in adults) occurred 2 days before birth, just prior to the period of fastest brain growth. By 8 days after birth, TTR mRNA levels had decreased to adult levels (Fung et al., 1988).

In sheep (155 days gestation), TTR mRNA was detected in choroid plexus from very early embryos (Tu et al., 1990). In sheep, the maximum increase in size of the choroid plexus (E70) occurred before that of the rest of the brain (E105). At E40 the proportion of TTR mRNA in total mRNA was 34% of that in adult choroid plexus. By E90, this had increased to 70% of the adult value, and stayed constant at this level during the remainder of gestation (Tu et al., 1990).

In sheep (precocial), the maximal increase in brain weight occurred 50 days *before* birth (Tu et al., 1990), whereas in rats (altricial), the maximal increase in brain weight was about 9 days *after* birth (Fung et al., 1988). The ratio of choroid plexus weight to total brain weight in sheep decreased to a stable value about 20 days *before* birth (Tu et al., 1990), whereas that for rats occurred about 15 days *after* birth (Fung et al., 1988). For both species, the choroid plexus had its maximal growth rate prior to that of the rest of the brain.

The critical period of brain development which is dependent on THs is earlier for precocial animals than for altricial animals (Fisher and Polk, 1989). The maximum TTR mRNA level in the choroid plexus of sheep (precocial) occurred during the first half of gestation, whereas in rats (altricial), it occurred only 2 days prior to birth. If TTR is involved in moving THs across the choroid plexus into the brain, and if this TTR then has a role in TH distribution within the CSF, the timing of the maximal synthesis of TTR by the choroid plexus is highly appropriate.

In summary, in the 1990s it was proposed that T4 bound to a TH distributor protein in blood, is in equilibrium with free T4 which is lipophilic, so partitions into the choroid plexus. Within the choroid plexus, the newly synthesized TTR by the epithelial cells binds to the T4 that entered the choroid plexus from the blood. Choroid plexus-derived TTR is 100% secreted into the CSF (not into the blood), so the TTR-T4 complex would be secreted into the CSF, followed by its distribution via the CSF to the brain tissue. Thus, the TTR synthesized by the choroid plexus is involved in moving T4 from the blood into the CSF, against the free T4 gradient (Chanoine et al., 1992; Southwell et al., 1993; Schreiber and Richardson, 1997). We now know some of these concepts to be outdated (see below).

HUMANS LACKING TTR HAVE NOT BEEN REPORTED

Cases of humans lacking either of the other two TH distributor proteins: albumin (Minchiotti et al., 2013) or thyroxine-binding globulin (Refetoff, 1989) have been described. Such people are apparently healthy and without overt clinical symptoms. However, no humans lacking TTR have been reported. In the 1990s the hypothesis was that because TTR is the only TH distributor protein synthesized in the brain, is secreted unidirectionally across the apical surface of the choroid plexus epithelial cells into the CSF, its role in the movement of TH from the blood into the CSF, its intermediate affinity for T4 (between those of albumin and thyroxine-binding globulin), and its role is being the most effective at distributing T4 to cells (see above), that it was thought to be crucial for survival, most probably due to the requirement of adequate amounts of TH for normal CNS development (Harms et al., 1991).

There are cases of humans with mutations in TTR resulting in higher affinity for THs, including Gly6Ser (~12% of the population), Thr119Met, Ala109Thr, and Ala109Val (Refetoff et al., 1996 and references therein). Of these four variants, only Ala109Thr resulted in affected individuals consistently having elevated serum T4 levels (Moses et al., 1982) [although Ala109Val individuals had elevated rT3 levels (Refetoff et al., 1996)]. More than 100 point mutations in human TTR result in TTR amyloidosis (familial amyloidotic polyneuropathy) (Benson, 2009). Whilst the variant TTRs can have differing affinities for T4 (Rosen et al., 1993) the patients are generally euthyroid (no publications indicating otherwise; and personal communication from Merrill Benson). This is possibly because in the blood, only about 1 in 200 TTRs have a TH bound. Therefore, if some of this TTR is deposited as amyloid then it might not affect overall TH distribution. The point being made here is that whilst there are diseases associated with TTR, there are no humans without TTR, whereas there are healthy humans without either albumin or thyroxine-binding globulin.

However, the function of TTR synthesized by the choroid plexus has been debated. Some believe it to be involved with the movement of T4 from the blood into the CSF (based on the functional, developmental and evolutionary data presented above), whilst others dispute this (read below). The controversy arose when TTR null mice were created and were essentially without an overt phenotype.

TTR NULL MICE

The production of TTR null mice (Episkopou et al., 1993) that were viable and fertile threw the above hypothesis on the role of choroid plexus-derived TTR into debate. TTR null mice had reduced levels of total T4, total T3, retinol, and retinol-binding protein in their blood, but did not show any overt phenotype. Consequently, some concluded that TTR was not important for THs to reach the brain e.g., (Palha et al., 1994, 1997, 2000). One study concluded that there were no differences in the distribution of the THs to tissues of TTR null mice compared with wild-type mice, except in the choroid plexus, where the T4 level was 14% in the TTR null mice compared to wild-type mice (Palha et al., 2000). A semi-quantitative morphological study suggested that wildtype and TTR null mice that had been injected intravenously with ^{125}I-T4 or ^{125}I-T3 did not show any difference in TH distribution throughout their brains (Palha et al., 2002). This bolstered the interpretation that TTR is not an important TH distributor and that TTR null mice should be considered euthyroid (Palha et al., 1994, 2000; Palha, 2002). However, this did not appear to correspond to the earlier data showing that choroid plexus-derived TTR was involved with movement of T4 from the blood into the brain (Dickson et al., 1987; Schreiber et al., 1990; Chanoine et al., 1992; Southwell et al., 1993).

Soon thereafter, the regulation of neural stem cell cycle in the subventricular zone of adult rodent brain was shown to be dependent on TRα/TH by influencing both cell proliferation and apoptosis (Lemkine et al., 2005). Consequently, it was hypothesized that if TTR was involved in the delivery of THs to the neural stem cell niche, then this population of cells in TTR null mice would be affected. Indeed, TTR null mice were shown to have reduced apoptosis of neural stem cells in the subventricular zone compared to wildtype mice. Furthermore, the level of apoptosis was similar to that of hypothyroid wildtype mice, implying a significant reduction of TH delivery to neural stem cells in this niche (Richardson et al., 2007). It was suggested that because the dissociation rate of T4 from albumin differs so significantly to that of T4 from TTR, and because the concentration of albumin in the CSF is significantly lower than that in the blood, that in the absence of TTR, albumin would be unlikely to distribute significant amounts of TH beyond the ependymal layer of the brain, resulting in the reduction of TH reaching the subventricular zone dur to a shallower TH gradient (Richardson et al., 2007). This study highlighted the importance of TTR in delivering THs to at least one of the two populations of neural stem cells in adult mammalian brain.

Until then, all studies involving TTR null mice had been focussed on adult mice. However, it is well known that THs affect growth and development, particularly of the CNS (Morreale de Escobar et al., 1987). In severe cases, TH deficiency in human babies during gestation results in stunted growth and mental retardation. Therefore, several aspects of growth known to be influenced by TH were examined during post-natal development in TTR null mice. The absence of TTR resulted in delays in several TH-regulated events including bone growth, CNS maturation, intestine and muscle development and in weaning (Monk et al., 2013). Furthermore, there was no specific accumulation of ^{125}I-T4 in the choroid plexus of adult TTR null mice, following intravenous injection. This was in stark contrast to the accumulation of ^{125}I-T4 in the choroid plexus of adult wildtype mice, following intravenous injection (Monk, 2006). This delay in TH-regulated events in the CNS of TTR null mice indicated that TTR has a role in TH delivery in the CNS during development.

In summary, there was strong evolutionary and developmental evidence that choroid plexus-derived TTR was important for moving THs into the brain, but this was not backed-up by analyses of TTR null mice. Therefore, there had to be another mechanism for THs to enter the brain and presumably the choroid plexus.

TH TRANSMEMBRANE TRANSPORTERS

The first publication on TH transport that indicated an energy-dependent process for TH uptake into cells was in 1954 (Christensen et al., 1954) but was "lost" in the literature for decades. In the 1970s Rao demonstrated that TH entry into cells was temperature-dependent, saturable, high-affinity, and low-capacity, ligand specific, could transport against a gradient and required metabolic energy (Rao, 1981). Yet some researchers missed these publications and believed that because THs could avidly partition into cell membranes, they could diffuse across the membrane as a mode of entry into cells. For a history of hypotheses about TH entry into cells, see (Hennemann et al., 2001). Currently, it is known that THs enter cells via TH transmembrane transporters, which participate in the influx and efflux of THs into and out of cells. Several classes of TH transmembrane transporter proteins that belong to the family of solute carrier (Slc) transporters have been identified e.g. organic anion transporting polypeptides (OATPs), monocarboxylate transporters (MCTs) and L-type amino acid transporters (LATs), and actively participate in entry and exit of THs into and out of cells (Visser et al., 2011).

Several TH transmembrane transporters have been localized to the choroid plexus (Mayerl et al., 2012) and their distribution in the choroid plexus differs between species (Wirth et al., 2014). Most TH transmembrane transporters identified to date are promiscuous with respect to the range of metabolites they transport. Only MCT8 has been identified as being specific to transport of THs and their derivatives (Kinne et al., 2010). Intriguingly, there exists dramatic species-specificity in TH transmembrane transporters deficiency phenotypes. For example, human males with MCT8 mutations present with mental retardation (IQ <40), speech deficits and severe neurological abnormalities (known as the Allan-Herndon-Dudley syndrome), whereas MCT8 null mice are without an overt neurological phenotype (Kersseboom and Visser, 2011). The discovery of the suite of TH transmembrane transporters, particularly in the choroid plexus, was important in understanding how TTR null mice were without an overt phenotype. The difference in phenotype between MCT8 variant human males and MCT8 null mice, could point toward elucidating why TTR null mice are viable, yet no human lacking TTR has been reported. Possibly, this could be due to different combinations of TH transmembrane transporters in the choroid plexus and at the blood-brain barrier, thereby partially compensating for the lack of choroid plexus-derived TTR in mice (but equivalent mechanisms lacking in humans). For example, Lat2 is synthesized in the choroid plexus of mice but not in the choroid plexus of humans (Wirth et al., 2009) or chickens (Darras et al., 2015). This may be an explanation for the mild phenotype of TTR null mice, yet the apparent absence of humans lacking TTR. For a more detailed discussion on the role of TH transmembrane transporters, deiodinases and the establishment of TH gradients across membranes, see a comprehensive review by Schweizer and Kohrle (2013).

The majority of current information on TH transmembrane transporters has been derived from only human and rodent data. A recent, comprehensive review on expression of TH transmembrane transporters during development in zebrafish, *Xenopus tropicalis*, chicken, and mouse (Darras et al., 2015) highlights how much is still unknown. Whilst the developing choroid plexus has only been analyzed for TH transmembrane transporters in a few species, interesting differences are emerging. For example, zebrafish choroid plexus does not synthesize MCT8, which contrasts with MCT8 synthesis in the choroid plexus of chickens and rodents. Furthermore, Lat2 is synthesized in the choroid plexus of mice but not humans (Wirth et al., 2009) and appears to be totally absent in chickens (Darras et al., 2015).

From an evolutionary perspective, we need to elucidate the developmental expression profiles for each of the TH transmembrane transporters in the choroid plexus from a variety of vertebrates representing each of the vertebrate classes. In particular, a comparison of expression of TH transmembrane transporters in the choroid plexus of animals who synthesize TTR in their choroid plexus (reptiles, birds, and mammals) with those who do not synthesize TTR in their choroid plexus (fish and amphibians) should be made. Furthermore, comparisons of TH transmembrane transporter expression profiles in the choroid plexus between precocial and altricial species would be intriguing. A comparison of the expression profiles of TH transmembrane transporters in mammalian choroid plexus vs. those in choroid plexus from non- mammals should be made, as mammalian TTRs are the exception in having higher affinity for T4 than T3. TTRs from all other vertebrates have higher affinity for T3 than for T4 (see below). Such studies could shed light on the relative roles of each of the TH transmembrane transporters and choroid plexus-derived TTR in the overall movement of THs from the blood into the CSF during development.

MAMMALIAN TTRs ARE THE EXCEPTION

In all studied species of fish, amphibians, reptiles and birds, TTR has higher affinity for T3 than T4, whereas in mammals TTR has higher affinity for T4 than for T3 (Richardson, 2007). Thus, mammals are the exception in this regard. Is it possible that whilst TTR made by the choroid plexus of mammals moves T4 into the brain, TTR from other animals moves T3 into the brain? What could have been the selection pressure for the change to TTR from distributing T3 to distributing T4? One possibility could be a greater level of control, requiring an additional level of regulation (i.e., deiodination of T4 to T3) at the target site. For example, different regions of the brain generate different proportions of T3 by local deiodination (van Doorn et al., 1985). Two features that distinguish mammalian brains from non-mammalian brains that are regulated (at least in part) by thyroid hormones are the corpus callosum which is heavily myelinated, and the highly developed cortex. The point here is that mammals may be the exception rather than the rule, when it comes to modes of TH entry into the CNS, so we should not just consider mammalian data. Furthermore, we have seen examples between eutherian species, of significant differences in TH transmembrane transporters (e.g., Lat2).

The literature is often skewed toward data on mammals, especially humans (due to our self-centerd interests in medicine/disease) and mice (due to the ease of working with them: inbred strains, short generation times, knock-in/out genetic manipulations etc), so we should be careful in analysing data from humans and rodents or eutherian mammals and drawing generalized conclusions, which may not be applicable to all mammals, let alone to all vertebrates. Furthermore, data from knock-out mice can sometimes raise more questions than they answer.

CONFUSION ARISING FROM MOUSE KO MODELS OF TH MOVEMENT INTO THE BRAIN

TTR null mice have 36% T4 levels in their brain compared to wildtype mice (Palha et al., 1997). This implies that TTR is responsible for the other 64% of T4 moving into the brain. However, Mct8/Oatp1c1 double knock-out mice are cited as having only 10% TH concentration in their brains compared to wildtype mice (Muller and Heuer, 2014). However, careful analysis of the original paper reveals that only the forebrain (and not the entire brain) was analyzed for TH content (Mayerl et al., 2014). Furthermore, if TH transmembrane transporters are responsible for moving significant amounts of TH into and out of the choroid plexus, then why do TTR null mice have only 14% T4 in their choroid plexus compared with wildtype mice? How do these data from TH transmembrane transporter and TTR null mice correlate with the data from Chanoine et al. (1992)? The quantitative contributions of the various mechanisms for TH moving across the blood-CSF barrier (the choroid plexus) and across the blood-brain barrier need to be investigated in greater detail.

CURRENT HYPOTHESIS FOR TH MOVEMENT FROM BLOOD VIA THE CHOROID PLEXUS TO THE CSF

Our current hypothesis for the movement of TH from the blood via the choroid plexus is depicted in **Figure 1**. In this Figure, T4 (major form of TH secreted by the thyroid gland) is depicted.

1. T4 dissociates from TH distributor proteins in the blood.
2. T4 enters the choroid plexus via TH transporters.
3. TTR is synthesized by the choroid plexus epithelial cells.
4. Some T4 will bind TTR synthesized in the choroid plexus epithelial cells.
5. T4 moves out of the choroid plexus into the CSF via either secretion of the T4-TTR complex; or via TH transmembrane transporters.

It is worth noting that there is a higher concentration free T4 in CSF than in blood, so net movement of TH from the blood to the CSF is against this gradient. Therefore, it would not be surprising if several mechanisms for moving TH from the blood via the choroid plexus (and the blood-brain barrier) had evolved.

CONCLUSION

From the above controversy regarding the importance of TTR synthesis by the choroid plexus, several points support the

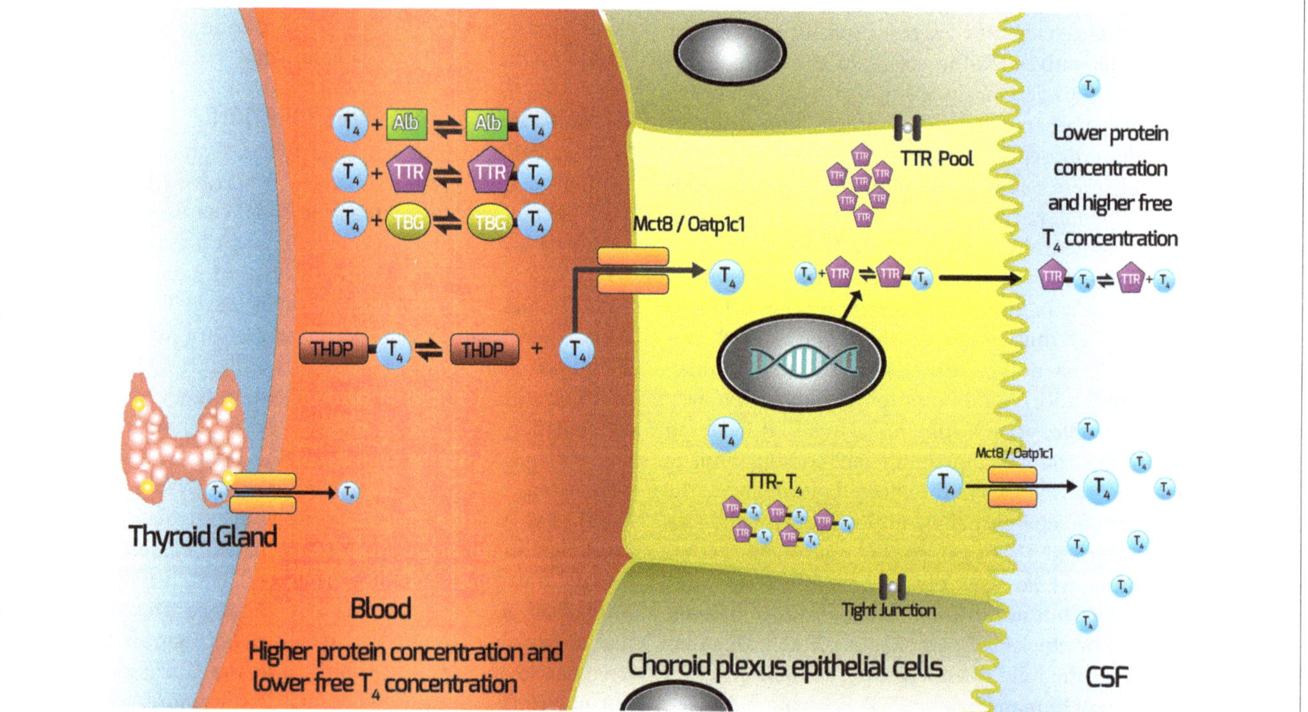

FIGURE 1 | Current hypothesis of mechanisms involved with TH movement from the blood across the choroid plexus into the CSF. THs are synthesized in the thyroid gland and secreted into the blood, where >99% are bound by the TH distributor proteins (THDPs) which include albumin (Alb), transthyretin (TTR), thyroxine-binding globulin (TBG) and to a lesser extent by specific lipoproteins, depending on the species and the stage of development. The main form of TH released from the thyroid gland is T4, so T4 is used as the example in this schematic. T4 dissociates from TH distributor proteins in the blood and enters the choroid plexus via TH transmembrane transporters (which may include Mct8 and Oatp1c1, depending on the species). TTR is synthesized by the choroid plexus epithelial cells and is secreted into the CSF. Some T4 binds TTR synthesized in the choroid plexus epithelial cells. T4 moves out of the choroid plexus into the CSF via either secretion of the T4-TTR complex or via TH transmembrane transporters.

hypothesis that choroid plexus-derived TTR plays a role in the movement of THs from the blood to the brain and in distributing THs in the blood and CSF. These points include evolutionary, developmental, molecular and functional data. Therefore, it would follow that TTR synthesized by the choroid plexus would appear to have an important regulatory role in determining the delivery of thyroid hormones into the CSF.

In conclusion, there is evidence for two mechanisms for THs to move out of the choroid plexus into the CSF: (i) secretion of TH bound to choroid plexus-derived TTR, and (ii) efflux of THs via TH transmembrane transporters. The relative quantitative contribution of each of these mechanisms during each stage of CNS development is currently unknown and should be investigated. Furthermore, perhaps the role played by choroid plexus-derived TTR is more significant in non-mammalian vertebrates than in mammals. It would be interesting to analyze the developmental profiles of TH transmembrane transporters in the choroid plexus (and in other blood-brain barrier structures) in non-mammalian vertebrates during development. The delivery of the requisite concentrations of THs to specific areas of the brain at each stage of CNS development is so important, that it would be understandable for evolution to have positively selected for more than one strategy for THs to enter the CNS.

REFERENCES

Achen, M. G., Harms, P. J., Thomas, T., Richardson, S. J., Wettenhall, R. E., and Schreiber, G. (1992). Protein synthesis at the blood-brain barrier. The major protein secreted by amphibian choroid plexus is a lipocalin. *J. Biol. Chem.* 267, 23170–23174.

Benson, M. D. (2009). "Genetics: clinical implications of TTR amyloidosis," in *Recent Advances in Transthyretin Evolution, Structure and Biological Functions*, eds S. J. Richardson and V. Cody (Berlin: Springer), 173–189. doi: 10.1007/978-3-642-00646-3_11

Benvenga, S., Cahnmann, H., Gregg, R., and Robbins, J. (1989). Binding of thyroxine to human plasma low density lipoprotein through specific interaction with apolipoprotein B (apoB-100). *Biochimie* 71, 263–268. doi: 10.1016/0300-9084(89)90063-1

Brown, P. D., Speake, T., Davies, S. L., and Millar, I. D. (2005). "Ion transporters and channels involved in csf formation," in *The Blood-Cerebrospinal Fluid Barrier*, ed W. A. C. A. Zheng (Boca Raton, FL: Taylor & Francis Group), 119–145.

Chanoine, J. P., Alex, S., Fang, S. L., Stone, S., Leonard, J. L., Korhle, J., et al. (1992). Role of transthyretin in the transport of thyroxine from the blood to the choroid plexus, the cerebrospinal fluid, and the brain. *Endocrinology* 130, 933–938.

Christensen, H. N., Hess, B., and Riggs, T. R. (1954). Concentration of taurine, beta-alanine, and triiodothyronine by ascites carcinoma cells. *Cancer Res.* 14, 124–127.

Cserr, H. F. (1971). Physiology of the choroid plexus. *Physiol. Rev.* 51, 273–311.

Darras, V. M., Houbrechts, A. M., and Van Herck, S. L. (2015). Intracellular thyroid hormone metabolism as a local regulator of nuclear thyroid hormone receptor-mediated impact on vertebrate development. *Biochim. Biophys. Acta.* 1849, 130–141. doi: 10.1016/j.bbagrm.2014.05.004

Davis, P. J., Davis, F. B., and Cody, V. (2005). Membrane receptors mediating thyroid hormone action. *Trends Endocrinol. Metab.* 16, 429–435. doi: 10.1016/j.tem.2005.09.007

Davis, P. J., Davis, F. B., Mousa, S. A., Luidens, M. K., and Lin, H. Y. (2011). Membrane receptor for thyroid hormone: physiologic and pharmacologic implications. *Annu. Rev. Pharmacol. Toxicol.* 51, 99–115. doi: 10.1146/annurev-pharmtox-010510-100512

Dickson, P. W., Aldred, A. R., Marley, P. D., TU, G. F., Howlett, G. J., and Schreiber, G. (1985). High prealbumin and transferrin messenger RNA levels in the choroid plexus of rat brain. *Biochem. Biophys. Res. Commun.* 127, 890–895. doi: 10.1016/S0006-291X(85)80027-9

Dickson, P. W., Aldred, A. R., Menting, J. G., Marley, P. D., Sawyer, W. H., and Schreiber, G. (1987). Thyroxine transport in choroid plexus. *J. Biol. Chem.* 262, 13907–13915.

Duan, W., Achen, M. G., Richardson, S. J., Lawrence, M. C., Wettenhall, R. E., Jaworowski, A., et al. (1991). Isolation, characterization, cDNA cloning and gene expression of an avian transthyretin. Implications for the evolution of structure and function of transthyretin in vertebrates. *Eur. J. Biochem.* 200, 679–687. doi: 10.1111/j.1432-1033.1991.tb16232.x

Ek, C. J., Dziegielewska, K. M., and Saunders, N. R. (2005). "Devlopment of the blood-cerebrospinal fluid barrier," in *The Blood-Cerebrospinal Fluid Barrier*, ed W. A. C. A. Zheng (Boca Raton, FL: Chapman & Hall/CR, Taylor & Francis Group), 3-23105–3-23120.

Episkopou, V., Maeda, S., Nishiguchi, S., Shimada, K., Gaitanaris, G. A., Gottesman, M. E., et al. (1993). Disruption of the transthyretin gene results in mice with depressed levels of plasma retinol and thyroid-hormone. *Proc. Natl. Acad. Sci. U.S.A.* 90, 2375–2379. doi: 10.1073/pnas.90.6.2375

Fisher, D. A., and Polk, D. H. (1989). Development of the thyroid. *Baillieres Clin. Endocrinol. Metab.* 3, 627–657. doi: 10.1016/S0950-351X(89)80046-1

Fung, W. P., Thomas, T., Dickson, P. W., Aldred, A. R., Milland, J., Dziadek, M., et al. (1988). Structure and expression of the rat transthyretin (prealbumin) gene. *J. Biol. Chem.* 263, 480–488.

Harms, P. J., Tu, G. F., Richardson, S. J., Aldred, A. R., Jaworowski, A., and Schreiber, G. (1991). Transthyretin (prealbumin) gene expression in choroid plexus is strongly conserved during evolution of vertebrates. *Comp. Biochem. Physiol. B* 99, 239–249. doi: 10.1016/0305-0491(91)90035-C

Hennebry, S. C., Wright, H. M., Likic, V. A., and Richardson, S. J. (2006). Structural and functional evolution of transthyretin and transthyretin-like proteins. *Proteins* 64, 1024–1045. doi: 10.1002/prot.21033

Hennemann, G., Docter, R., Friesema, E. C., de Jong, M., Krenning, E. P., and Visser, T. J. (2001). Plasma membrane transport of thyroid hormones and its role in thyroid hormone metabolism and bioavailability. *Endocr. Rev.* 22, 451–476. doi: 10.1210/edrv.22.4.0435

Kent, G. C. (1987). *Comparative Anatomy of the Vertebrates.* St. Louis, MO: Time Mirror/Mosby College.

Kersseboom, S., and Visser, T. J. (2011). Tissue-specific effects of mutations in the thyroid hormone transporter MCT8. *Arq. Bras. Endocrinol. Metabol.* 55, 1–5. doi: 10.1590/S0004-27302011000100001

Kinne, A., Kleinau, G., Hoefig, C. S., Gruters, A., Kohrle, J., Krause, G., et al. (2010). Essential molecular determinants for thyroid hormone transport and first structural implications for monocarboxylate transporter 8. *J. Biol. Chem.* 285, 28054–28063. doi: 10.1074/jbc.M110.129577

Lemkine, G. F., Raj, A., Alfama, G., Turque, N., Hassani, Z., Alegria-Prevot, O., et al. (2005). Adult neural stem cell cycling *in vivo* requires thyroid hormone and its alpha receptor. *FASEB J.* 19, 863–865. doi: 10.1096/fj.04-2916fje

Lin, H. Y., Tang, H. Y., Davis, F. B., Mousa, S. A., Incerpi, S., Luidens, M. K., et al. (2012). Nongenomic regulation by thyroid hormone of plasma membrane ion and small molecule pumps. *Discov. Med.* 14, 199–206.

Mayerl, S., Muller, J., Bauer, R., Richert, S., Kassmann, C. M., Darras, V. M., et al. (2014). Transporters MCT8 and OATP1C1 maintain murine brain thyroid hormone homeostasis. *J. Clin. Invest.* 124, 1987–1999. doi: 10.1172/JCI70324

Mayerl, S., Visser, T. J., Darras, V. M., Horn, S., and Heuer, H. (2012). Impact of Oatp1c1 deficiency on thyroid hormone metabolism and action in the mouse brain. *Endocrinology* 153, 1528–1537. doi: 10.1210/en.2011-1633

Mendel, C. M. (1989). The free hormone hypothesis: a physiologically based mathematical model. *Endocr. Rev.* 10, 232–274. doi: 10.1210/edrv-10-3-232

Mendel, C. M., Cavalieri, R. R., Gavin, L. A., Pettersson, T., and Inoue, M. (1989). Thyroxine transport and distribution in nagase analbuminemic rats. *J. Clin. Invest.* 83, 143–148. doi: 10.1172/JCI113851

Mendel, C. M., and Weisiger, R. A. (1990). Thyroxine uptake by perfused rat liver. No evidence for facilitation by five different thyroxine-binding proteins. *J. Clin. Invest.* 86, 1840–1847. doi: 10.1172/JCI114914

Mendel, C. M., Weisiger, R. A., Jones, A. L., and Cavalieri, R. R. (1987). Thyroid hormone binding proteins in plasma facilitate uniform distribution of thyroxine within tissues - a perfused rat liver study. *Endocrinology* 120, 1742–1749. doi: 10.1210/endo-120-5-1742

Minchiotti, L., Galliano, M., Caridi, G., Kragh-Hansen, U., and Peters, T. Jr. (2013). Congenital analbuminaemia: molecular defects and biochemical and clinical aspects. *Biochim. Biophys. Acta* 1830, 5494–5502. doi: 10.1016/j.bbagen.2013.04.019

Moeller, L. C., Cao, X., Dumitrescu, A. M., Seo, H., and Refetoff, S. (2006). Thyroid hormone mediated changes in gene expression can be initiated by cytosolic action of the thyroid hormone receptor beta through the phosphatidylinositol 3-kinase pathway. *Nucl. Recept. Signal.* 4:e020. doi: 10.1621/nrs.04020

Moeller, L. C., Haselhorst, N. E., Dumitrescu, A. M., Cao, X., Seo, H., Refetoff, S., et al. (2011). Stanniocalcin 1 induction by thyroid hormone depends on thyroid hormone receptor beta and phosphatidylinositol 3-kinase activation. *Exp. Clin. Endocrinol. Diabetes* 119, 81–85. doi: 10.1055/s-0030-1262860

Monk, J. A. (2006). *Thyroid Hormone Homeostasis in Developing and Adult Transthyretin Null Mice.* Ph.D., The University of Melbourne.

Monk, J. A., Sims, N. A., Dziegielewska, K. M., Weiss, R. E., Ramsay, R. G., and Richardson, S. J. (2013). Delayed development of specific thyroid hormone-regulated events in transthyretin null mice. *Am. J. Physiol. Endocrinol. Metab.* 304, E23–E31. doi: 10.1152/ajpendo.00216.2012

Morreale de Escobar, G., Obregon, M. J., and Escobar del Rey, F. (1987). Fetal and maternal thyroid hormones. *Horm. Res.* 26, 12–27. doi: 10.1159/000180681

Moses, A. C., Lawlor, J., Haddow, J., and Jackson, I. M. (1982). Familial euthyroid hyperthyroxinemia resulting from increased thyroxine binding to thyroxine-binding prealbumin. *N. Engl. J. Med.* 306, 966–969. doi: 10.1056/NEJM198204223061605

Muller, J., and Heuer, H. (2014). Expression pattern of thyroid hormone transporters in the postnatal mouse brain. *Front. Endocrinol. (Lausanne)* 5:92. doi: 10.3389/fendo.2014.00092

Palha, J. A. (2002). Transthyretin as a thyroid hormone carrier: function revisited. *Clin. Chem. Lab. Med.* 40, 1292–1300. doi: 10.1515/CCLM.2002.223

Palha, J. A., Episkopou, V., Maeda, S., Shimada, K., Gottesman, M. E., and Saraiva, M. J. M. (1994). Thyroid-hormone metabolism in a transthyretin-null mouse strain. *J. Biol. Chem.* 269, 33135–33139.

Palha, J. A., Fernandes, R., de Escobar, G. M., Episkopou, V., Gottesman, M., and Saraiva, M. J. (2000). Transthyretin regulates thyroid hormone levels in the choroid plexus, but not in the brain parenchyma: Study in a transthyretin-null mouse model. *Endocrinology* 141, 3267–3272. doi: 10.1210/endo.141.9.7659

Palha, J. A., Hays, M. T., Deescobar, G. M., Episkopou, V., Gottesman, M. E., and Saraiva, M. J. M. (1997). Transthyretin is not essential for thyroxine to reach the brain and other tissues in transthyretin-null mice. *Am. J. Physiol. Endocrinol. Metab.* 35, E485–E493.

Palha, J. A., Nissanov, J., Fernandes, R., Sousa, J. C., Bertrand, L., Dratman, M. B., et al. (2002). Thyroid hormone distribution in the mouse brain: the role of transthyretin. *Neuroscience* 113, 837–847. doi: 10.1016/S0306-4522(02)00228-2

Rao, G. S. (1981). MOde of entry of steroid and thyroid hormones into cells. *Mol. Cell. Endocrinol.* 21, 97–108. doi: 10.1016/0303-7207(81)90047-2

Refetoff, S. (1989). Inherited thyroxine-binding globulin abnormalities in man. *Endocr. Rev.* 10, 275–293. doi: 10.1210/edrv-10-3-275

Refetoff, S., Marinov, V. S., Tunca, H., Byrne, M. M., Sunthornthepvarakul, T., and Weiss, R. E. (1996). A new family with hyperthyroxinemia caused by transthyretin Val109 misdiagnosed as thyrotoxicosis and resistance to thyroid hormone–a clinical research center study. *J. Clin. Endocrinol. Metab.* 81, 3335–3340.

Richardson, S. J. (2007). Cell and molecular biology of transthyretin and thyroid hormones. *Int. Rev. Cytol.* 258, 137–193. doi: 10.1016/S0074-7696(07)58003-4

Richardson, S. J., Lemkine, G. F., Alfama, G., Hassani, Z., and Demeneix, B. A. (2007). Cell division and apoptosis in the adult neural stem cell niche are differentially affected in transthyretin null mice. *Neurosci. Lett.* 421, 234–238. doi: 10.1016/j.neulet.2007.05.040

Robbins, J. (2000). "Thyroid hormone transport proteins and the physiology of hormone binding," in *Werner and Ingbar's the Thyroid - A Fundamental and Clinical Text, 8th Edn.*, eds L. E. Braverman and R. D. Utiger (Philadelphia, PA: Lippincott Williams & Wilkins), 105–120.

Rosen, H. N., Moses, A. C., Murrell, J. R., Liepnieks, J. J., and Benson, M. D. (1993). Thyroxine interactions with transthyretin: a comparison of 10 different naturally occurring human transthyretin variants. *J. Clin. Endocrinol. Metab.* 77, 370–374.

Santos, C. R. A., and Power, D. M. (1999). Identification of transthyretin in fish (*Sparus aurata*): cDNA cloning and characterisation. *Endocrinology* 140, 2430–2433. doi: 10.1210/endo.140.5.6898

Saunders, N. R. (1992). "Ontogenetic development of brain barrier mechanisms," in *Handbook of Experimental Pharmacology, Vol. 103, Physiology and Pharmacology of the Blood-Brain Barrier*, ed M. W. B. Bradbury (Berlin, Heidelberg: Springer-Verlag), 327–369. doi: 10.1007/978-3-642-76894-1_14

Sayre, N. L., and Lechleiter, J. D. (2012). Fatty acid metabolism and thyroid hormones. *Curr. Trends Endocinol.* 6, 65–76.

Schreiber, G., Aldred, A. R., Jaworowski, A., Nilsson, C., Achen, M. G., and Segal, M. B. (1990). Thyroxine transport from blood to brain via transthyretin synthesis in choroid plexus. *Am. J. Physiol.* 258, R338–R345.

Schreiber, G., and Richardson, S. J. (1997). The evolution of gene expression, structure and function of transthyretin. *Comp. Biochem. Physiol B Biochem. Mol. Biol.* 116, 137–160. doi: 10.1016/S0305-0491(96)00212-X

Schweizer, U., and Kohrle, J. (2013). Function of thyroid hormone transporters in the central nervous system. *Biochim. Biophys. Acta* 1830, 3965–3973. doi: 10.1016/j.bbagen.2012.07.015

Soprano, D. R., Herbert, J., Soprano, K. J., Schon, E. A., and Goodman, D. S. (1985). Demonstration of transthyretin mRNA in the brain and other extrahepatic tissues in the rat. *J. Biol. Chem.* 260, 11793–11798.

Southwell, B. R., Duan, W., Alcorn, D., Brack, C., Richardson, S. J., Kohrle, J., et al. (1993). Thyroxine transport to the brain: role of protein synthesis by the choroid plexus. *Endocrinology* 133, 2116–2126.

Stauder, A. J., Dickson, P. W., Aldred, A. R., Schreiber, G., Mendelsohn, F. A., and Hudson, P. (1986). Synthesis of transthyretin (pre-albumin) mRNA in choroid plexus epithelial cells, localized by *in situ* hybridization in rat brain. *J. Histochem. Cytochem.* 34, 949–952. doi: 10.1177/34.7.3458812

Sturrock, R. R. (1979). A morphological study of the development of the mouse choroid plexus. *J. Anat.* 129, 777–793.

Tu, G. F., Cole, T., Southwell, B. R., and Schreiber, G. (1990). Expression of the genes for transthyretin, cystatin C and beta A4 amyloid precursor protein in sheep choroid plexus during development. *Brain Res. Dev. Brain Res.* 55, 203–208. doi: 10.1016/0165-3806(90)90201-9

van Doorn, J., Roelfsema, F., and van der Heide, D. (1985). Concentrations of thyroxine and 3,5,3'-triiodothyronine at 34 different sites in euthyroid rats as determined by an isotopic equilibrium technique. *Endocrinology* 117, 1201–1208. doi: 10.1210/endo-117-3-1201

Visser, W. E., Friesema, E. C., and Visser, T. J. (2011). Minireview: thyroid hormone transporters: the knowns and the unknowns. *Mol. Endocrinol.* 25, 1–14. doi: 10.1210/me.2010-0095

Wirth, E. K., Roth, S., Blechschmidt, C., Holter, S. M., Becker, L., Racz, I., et al. (2009). Neuronal 3',3,5-triiodothyronine (T3) uptake and behavioral phenotype of mice deficient in Mct8, the neuronal T3 transporter mutated in Allan-Herndon-Dudley syndrome. *J. Neurosci.* 29, 9439–9449. doi: 10.1523/JNEUROSCI.6055-08.2009

Wirth, E. K., Schweizer, U., and Kohrle, J. (2014). Transport of thyroid hormone in brain. *Front. Endocrinol. (Lausanne)* 5:98. doi: 10.3389/fendo.2014.00098

Zheng, W. (2005). *The Blood-Cereprospinal Fluid Barrier.* Boca Raton, FL: Taylor & Franscis Group.

11

Blood-brain barrier dysfunction in disorders of the developing brain

Raffaella Moretti[1,2,3,4], Julien Pansiot[1,2,3], Donatella Bettati[1,2,3], Nathalie Strazielle[5,6], Jean-François Ghersi-Egea[5], Giuseppe Damante[4], Bobbi Fleiss[1,2,3,7], Luigi Titomanlio[1,2,3,8] and Pierre Gressens[1,2,3,7]*

[1] *INSERM U1141, Robert Debre's Hospital, Paris, France*
[2] *Université Paris Diderot, Sorbonne Paris Cité, UMRS 1141-PROTECT, Paris, France*
[3] *PremUP, Paris, France*
[4] *S. Maria della Misericordia Hospital, Università degli Studi di Udine, Udine, Italy*
[5] *Lyon Neurosciences Research Center, INSERM U1028, CNRS UMR5292 – Lyon University, Lyon, France*
[6] *Brain-i, Lyon, France*
[7] *Department of Division of Imaging Sciences and Biomedical Engineering, Centre for the Developing Brain, St. Thomas' Hospital, London, UK*
[8] *Pediatric Emergency Department, APHP, Robert Debré Hospital, Paris, France*

***Correspondence:**
Pierre Gressens, INSERM U-1141, Robert Debré University Hospital, 48, Bld Sérurier - 75019 Paris, France
e-mail: pierre.gressens@inserm.fr

Disorders of the developing brain represent a major health problem. The neurological manifestations of brain lesions can range from severe clinical deficits to more subtle neurological signs or behavioral problems and learning disabilities, which often become evident many years after the initial damage. These long-term sequelae are due at least in part to central nervous system immaturity at the time of the insult. The blood-brain barrier (BBB) protects the brain and maintains homeostasis. BBB alterations are observed during both acute and chronic brain insults. After an insult, excitatory amino acid neurotransmitters are released, causing reactive oxygen species (ROS)-dependent changes in BBB permeability that allow immune cells to enter and stimulate an inflammatory response. The cytokines, chemokines and other molecules released as well as peripheral and local immune cells can activate an inflammatory cascade in the brain, leading to secondary neurodegeneration that can continue for months or even years and finally contribute to post-insult neuronal deficits. The role of the BBB in perinatal disorders is poorly understood. The inflammatory response, which can be either acute (e.g., perinatal stroke, traumatic brain injury) or chronic (e.g., perinatal infectious diseases) actively modulates the pathophysiological processes underlying brain injury. We present an overview of current knowledge about BBB dysfunction in the developing brain during acute and chronic insults, along with clinical and experimental data.

Keywords: WMD, TBI, BBB, stroke, hypoxia-ischemia, brain, developemental disorders

INTRODUCTION

The blood-brain barrier (BBB) is a physical barrier essential for the maintenance of a precisely regulated intracerebral microenvironment. Its characteristics limit paracellular diffusion while allowing the tightly controlled receptor-mediated endocytosis of larger molecules and the transporter-mediated intake of smaller nutrients like glucose, insulin and iron. Endothelial cells interact closely with other central nervous system (CNS) cells such as neurons, pericytes and astrocytes, through adherens junctions, influx and efflux transporters, metabolic enzymes, the extracellular matrix, astrocytic endfeet etc. All these structures together constitute the Neurovascular Unit (NVU), and are believed to be essential for the regulation of BBB permeability (Ballabh et al., 2004).

For a long time, the BBB was considered "incomplete" during fetal life. However, there is ample evidence to suggest that the BBB is already well developed (Ballabh et al., 2005). For instance, the formation of tight junctions (TJs) takes place at the same time as angiogenesis (Virgintino et al., 2004), and even the first vessels to invade the avascular neuroectoderm are impermeable to albumin and immunoglobulins. Nevertheless, fetal brain vessels exhibit different, and in some respects increased, transport properties for amino acids and other metabolites, reflecting the higher demand for nutrients in the developing CNS (Ek et al., 2001, 2006; Johansson et al., 2006, 2008; Saunders et al., 2012). Understanding the changes that occur in the BBB during normal development is critical, as it is not only a site of possible

Abbreviations: BBB, blood-brain barrier; CAV, caveolin; Cld5, claudin-5; CNS, central nervous system; GM-IVH, Intraventricular hemorrhage of the germinal matrix; HIE, hypoxic-ischemic encephalopathy; HIF, hypoxia-inducible factor; IL, interleukin; LPS, lipopolysaccharide; MMP, matrix metalloproteinase; NO, nitric oxide; NOS, nitric oxide synthase; NVU, neurovascular unit; Occl, occluding; P, postnatal day; ROS, reactive oxygen species; TBI, traumatic brain injury; TIMP, tissue inhibitor of metalloproteinases; TJ, tight junction; TNF, tumor necrosis factor; VEGF, vascular endothelial growth factor; WMD, white-matter damage; ZO, zonula occludens.

vulnerability to injury but also a potential therapeutic route for injuries occurring during the perinatal period. Perinatal brain damage is one of the leading causes of lifelong disability, including cerebral palsy, seizure disorders, sensory impairment, and cognitive limitations (Low, 2004). This brain damage could be due to inflammatory, hypoxic-ischemic, hemorrhagic or excitotoxic mechanisms, or a combination of these. The lifetime cost of the care of one child affected by cerebral palsy is about 1 million US dollars (CDC CfDCaP, 2004), highlighting the need to develop new strategies for treatment and prevention. The only treatment with proven efficacy for perinatal brain injury is hypothermia, but this can only be applied safely to term infants with hypoxic-ischemic encephalopathy. Hypothermia in these infants reduces brain injury, doubling the chances of survival without clinical deficits (Edwards et al., 2010). However, more efforts are needed to find novel neuroprotective treatments for perinatal brain damage, especially in preterm infants. Designing neuroprotective molecules requires a detailed knowledge of the pathophysiology of brain damage, including BBB damage, in this population. This will facilitate the delivery of neuroprotective molecules, whose efficacy is strictly dependent on their capacity to cross brain barriers.

Currently, translational research is increasingly focused on the broader functional aspects of the brain response to injury, shifting from cell-oriented studies to experimental research on physiological concepts such as BBB integrity. This is due to the fact that dysfunctions of the BBB, such as the impairment of TJ formation/function, are a contributing factor in a number of neurological diseases in adults and infants. In models of perinatal injuries in term infants, cerebrovascular endothelial cells can be damaged by hypoxic-ischemic insults, an activated excitotoxic cascade or traumatic brain injury, leading to impaired BBB function. The link between BBB dysfunction and injury due to the dysregulation of developmental processes, such as occurs to a greater extent in preterm infants, is less well studied.

The aim of this review is to describe current understanding of BBB dysfunction in the developing brain during the most common subtypes of injury, supported by clinical and experimental data.

BASICS OF BBB DEVELOPMENT AND AGE-RELATED DIFFERENCES IN FUNCTION

The specific barrier characteristics of BBB endothelial cells within the developing CNS are induced during angiogenesis by complex crosstalk with cellular and acellular elements. During development, the CNS is vascularized by the angiogenic sprouting of vascular networks from the surrounding mesoderm in a precise spatiotemporal manner that differs among species. Which cell type is responsible for BBB differentiation has not yet been clarified: astrocytes have long been considered as the main source of BBB-inducing signals, but barrier induction most likely takes place well before astrocyte differentiation, so there is a probable influence of neuroblast cells or pericytes (Bauer and Bauer, 2000; Armulik et al., 2010; Daneman et al., 2010a). These different structures and cells have different maturation rates across species and across developmental stages, so animal models are not always representative of the human situation in every respect.

With regard to the developmental changes in the BBB, the presence of TJs in cerebral blood vessels and the expression of influx and efflux transporters is even higher at mid-gestation than in adulthood; for instance, TJs appear as early as 8 weeks of gestation in humans, at 13 days in mice and at postnatal day (P) 5 in *Monodelphis* opossums, which is when the first vessels appear in the neocortex (Ek et al., 2012). These TJ proteins are functional, as recent ultrastructural studies have demonstrated that the TJs of both endothelial cells in cerebral blood vessels and choroidal epithelial cells in embryos and neonates restrict the passage of low-molecular-weight molecules (Ek et al., 2003, 2006; Johansson et al., 2006). However, as these blood vessels do not display the properties of mature vessels with respect to pericyte coverage or junctional organization, it is probable that their BBB properties are not yet fully mature. This has been confirmed in part by a recent study showing that several hundreds of genes are differentially expressed between early postnatal and adult brain endothelial cells, indicating differences in molecular and probably physiological properties (Daneman et al., 2010b). However, the implication of these differences in the BBB across developmental stages for brain health remains unknown (Engelhardt and Liebner, 2014).

PRINCIPAL INSULTS TO THE DEVELOPING BRAIN AND THEIR ANIMAL MODELS

GERMINAL MATRIX HEMORRHAGE

Intraventricular hemorrhage of the germinal matrix (GM-IVH) causes very substantial and permanent injury, and is the leading cause of hydrocephalus in children. GM-IVH occurs when a hemorrhage in the GM breaks through the ependyma and into the lateral ventricles (see **Figure 1**). About 12,000 premature infants develop IVH every year in the United States alone (Vohr et al., 1999; Ballabh, 2010), with the incidence in extremely premature infants being approximately 45% (Wilson-Costello et al., 2005). Infants with a history of IVH have a higher incidence of seizures, neurodevelopmental delays, cerebral palsy and death. The incidence of IVH in very low birth weight infants (<1500 g) declined from 40% in the early 1980s to 20% in the late 1980s (Philip et al., 1989). However, because of the sharply increased survival of extremely premature infants, in the last two decades, the incidence of IVH has remained stable (Jain et al., 2009). Thus, IVH continues to be one of the major problems faced by premature infants in modern neonatal intensive care units worldwide. The etiopathogenesis of GM hemorrhage is multifactorial, with a combination of vascular and intravascular factors considered to be responsible. It is necessary to understand the reason for the vulnerability of GM microvessels to hemorrhage in order to develop therapeutic strategies.

GM-IVH has been modeled in several animal species including the dog, rabbit, sheep, rat, mouse and pig, either by directly injecting blood into the ventricles or by changing hemodynamic properties, such as blood pressure, the volume of blood circulating, serum glycerol, carbon dioxide, osmolarity or oxygenation levels (Goddard et al., 1980; Yoshioka et al., 1989; Balasubramaniam and Del Bigio, 2006; Georgiadis et al., 2008; Tosun et al., 2013). The two most-used animals models of IVH are the intracerebral injection of sterile collagenase, a hemorrhage-inducing agent

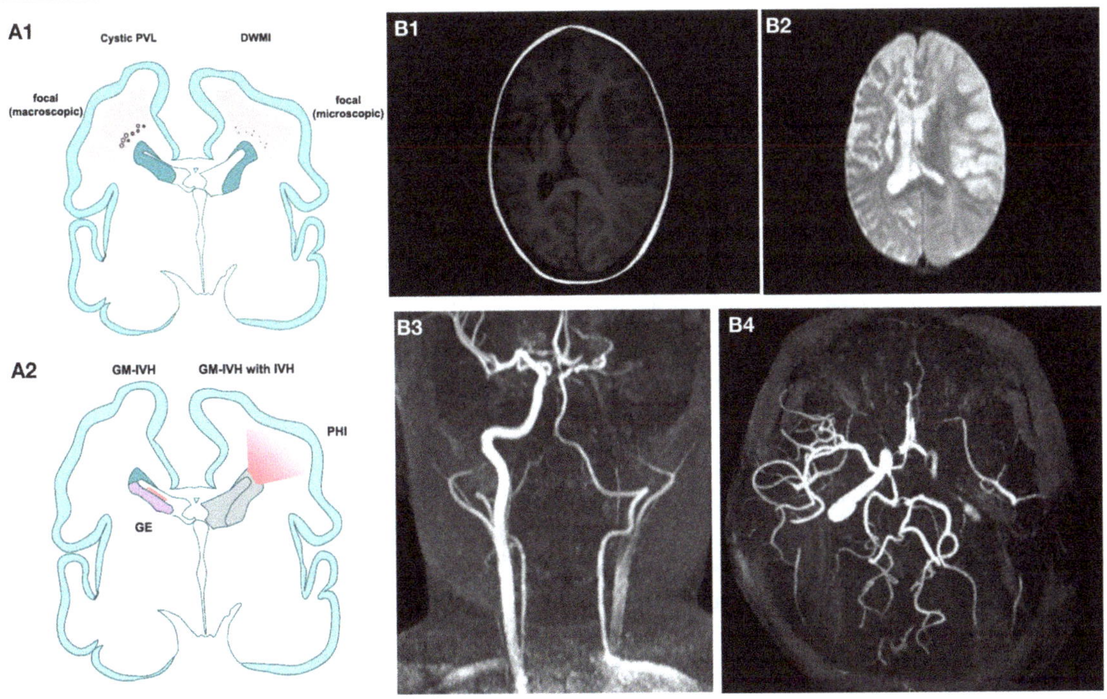

FIGURE 1 | (A) Modified by J. Volpe, Lancet Neurology 2009. **(A1)** Cystic Periventricular Leucomalacia (PVL) and Diffuse White Matter Injury (DWMI) and **(A2)** germinal matrix haemorrage-intraventricular Haemorrage (GMH-IVH) and GMH-IVH with periventricular Haemorrage infarction (PHI). Schematic coronal sections from the brain of a 28-week-old premature infant. Color key: Focal necrotic lesions in cystic PVL (small circles), focal necrotic lesions in DWMI (black dots), diffuse cellular changes in both cystic PVL and DWMI (pink), hemorrhage into ganglionic eminence (red) that results in IVH in the ependymal (left) or PHI (right). **(B,B1)** T1 weighted image illustrating an acute right ischemic stroke is a sickle cell disease children previously affected by a left ischemic stroke. **(B2)** Brain diffusion-weighted imaging (DWI) sequence of the same patient. **(B3,B4)** a 3D time-of-flight magnetic resonance angiography (MRA) suggesting dissection of the left internal carotid (**B2**: coronal view, **B3** transverse view).

(Krafft et al., 2012; Lekic et al., 2012), in mice, and the intracerebroventricular injection of fresh homologs blood in adult Sprague-Dawley rats or in piglets at 9–22 h of life (Aquilina et al., 2007, 2012). The appropriate model is selected based on the pathophysiology of hemorrhage induction and injury progression. The blood injection model mimics a rapidly progressing hemorrhage, whereas collagenase enzymatically disrupts the basal lamina of brain capillaries, causing an active bleed that generally evolves over several hours. The effects of GM-IVH on the BBB have not been extensively assessed in any of these models.

WHITE MATTER DAMAGE

White matter damage (WMD) is a characteristic injury of preterm infants, involving destructive microcystic lesions within the white matter, the disrupted maturation of oligodendrocytes and hypomyelination (Degos et al., 2010a) (see **Figure 1**). Although WMD is also observed in term infants, the relative contributions of direct injury to oligodendrocytes/myelin and secondary injury due to gray matter damage are still being defined. WMD is a healthcare priority, as it is the main cause of neurological handicap in preterm infants and the principal cause of cerebral palsy (Tahraoui et al., 2001). On a pathophysiological level, based on strong clinical evidence and a wealth of studies in animal models, the hypothesis of a purely hypoxic-ischemic cause of injury has been replaced by a multifactorial hypothesis. The central role of inflammation is now appreciated, given its contribution in terms of excess cytokines, free radicals, increased excitatory amino acid release (excitotoxicity), and trophic factor imbalance (Lipton and Rosenberg, 1994; Evrard et al., 1997; Yoon et al., 1997; Back et al., 1998). Clinical spectroscopy data do support a role for hypoxia-ischemia in the pathophysiology of WMD, but it is increasingly evident that inflammation-induced endothelial cell dysfunction and changes in glial metabolism may contribute substantially to these effects (Schuhmann et al., 2003; Lodygensky et al., 2014). The multifactorial hypothesis includes the concept of sensitization, whereby vulnerability to hypoxia-ischemia or excitotoxicity is enhanced by the preexistence of inflammation (Hagberg and Mallard, 2005; Favrais et al., 2007, 2011), which in the clinical setting is reported to occur in at least 40% of preterm infants.

Experimental paradigms that have addressed the pathophysiology of WMD include models in the mouse, rat and sheep using inflammation, excitotoxicity and hypoxia-ischemia (Tahraoui et al., 2001) (see **Table 1**). A well-characterized murine model of perinatal excitotoxic-induced WMD consists of the i.c. injection of the glutamate analog ibotenate, a potent neurotoxin that activates the N-methyl-D-aspartate receptor, in 5-day-old mouse pups (Marret et al., 1995). Ibotenate is commonly used to induce brain lesions in both the hippocampus and the white matter, in which it stimulates these receptors present on oligodendrocytes and microglia (Degos et al., 2010b), leading to microcysts similar

Table 1 | Some of the principal animal models mentioned in this review with correlate references.

Human pathologic condition	Animal used and age of the animal	Type of damage "inflicted"	References
GMH-IVH	Rabbit 29 day-gestation	Glycerol administration 3 h post-delivery	Ballabh et al., 2005
	Dog (terme beagle pups)	Phenilephrine hydrocloride i.v. injection	Baud et al., 2004
	Sprague-Dawley Rat P7	Intracerebral injection of glibenclamide	Bauer and Bauer, 2000
	Pregnant Wistar Dam	Intrauterine injection of glibenclamide	Bednarek et al., 2012
	CD-1 mice	Intrastriatal double injection of autologous whole blood, Intrastriatal injection of bacterial collagenase	Biran et al., 2008
	Piglet	i.c.v. injection of fresh homologs blood	Bolton et al., 1998; Blond et al., 2002
Diffuse white matter injury	Cat pregnant	LPS injections	Briones et al., 2011
	Rabbit pregnant	*E. coli* injections	Briones et al., 2011
	Dog (beagle) P14	Bilateral carotid occlusion	Briones et al., 2011
	Swiss Mouse P5	Interacerebral ibotenate injections	Briones et al., 2011
	Long Evans Mouse P7	Unilateral carotid ligation+ hypoxia	
H-I	P7 Wistar rats	Permanent occlusion of the Middle Cerebral Artery (MCA), pMCAo + O2 8%	Evrard et al., 1997
	Rice's model adapted to other rat's ages	"	Favrais et al., 2007, 2011
	Mouse P7	Blockade of the past External Carotid Artery-Internal Carotid Artery (ECA-ICA) bifurcation	Feng et al., 2008
		External-internal carotid artery	Favrais et al., 2011
	Mouse P8	Permanent occlusion of the Middle Cerebral Artery (MCA), pMCAo + O2 8%	Feng et al., 2008
	Mouse P10	"	Feng et al., 2008
	Mouse P12	"	Feng et al., 2008
Stroke	Wistar Rat P7	pMCAo +bilateral transient Common Carotid Artery (tCCAo) occlusion	Feng et al., 2008
	Wistar Rat P10	"	Feng et al., 2008
	CB17 mouse P12	pMCAO	Favrais et al., 2011
TBI			
Fluid percussion injury (FPI) models			
Middle	Rat	Fluid-percussion brain injury of graded severity	Labus et al., 2014
	Cat	Fluid-percussion injury (3.5 atm.)	Labus et al., 2014
	Rabbit	Pressure wave produced by a fluid-percussion device	
	Sheep		Labus et al., 2014
	Dog		
Lateral	Rat	Fluid-percussion brain injury of graded severity	Labus et al., 2014
	C57BL/6 Mouse	Right-sided parasagittal FPI	Labus et al., 2014
	Newborn pig	Lateral FPI moderate severity (1.9–2.1 atm)	Labus et al., 2014

(Continued)

Table 1 | Continued

Human pathologic condition	Animal used and age of the animal	Type of dommage "inflicted"	References
Weight-drop models	Rat	Impact injuries in the hindpaw cortical area segmented brass weight free-falling through a Plexiglas guide tube free-falling weight with a final impact of 0.01 J	Labus et al., 2014
	Rat adult		Labus et al., 2014
	C57BL/6 Mouse (10–16 weeks)		Labus et al., 2014
Controlled cortical impact injury Models	Ferret	stroke-constrained pneumatic impactor varying magnitudes of controlled cortical impact	Labus et al., 2014
	Mouse	pneumatic impactor	Labus et al., 2014
	Rat	CCI of velocity 3.5 m/s and dwell time 400 ms CCI + hypothermia	Labus et al., 2014
	Yorkshire Swine		Labus et al., 2014
	Monkey		Labus et al., 2014
	Cat	Cerebral wound made with a steel sphere with a velocity of 240–300 m/s (0.9–1.4 J)	Labus et al., 2014
Penetrating Ballistic-like injury model	Sprague-Dawley rats	Simulated ballistic wound to the right frontal hemisphere implemented by an inflatable penetrating probe	Labus et al., 2014
	C57Bl/6 Mouse pregnant (15 days of gestation)	LPS intrauterine injections	Labus et al., 2014

to those seen on post-mortem examination in preterm infants (Verney et al., 2012). In this model, vulnerability to WMD is increased by systemic inflammation (Dommergues et al., 2003; Favrais et al., 2007; Aden et al., 2010), and the BBB is slightly affected.

Animal models of preterm brain injury have also conclusively shown that exposure to inflammation alone, even at low levels, is sufficient to induce WMD similar to that seen clinically (Rousset et al., 2006; Bednarek et al., 2012). In addition to WMD, the exposure of fetal sheep to low-dose endotoxin leads to increased BBB permeability, as assessed by staining for plasma albumin extravasation (Yan et al., 2004). This effect has been noted in the cortical white and gray matter and the thalamus, but not the cerebellum. WMD comparable to that seen in preterm infants can also be induced in the mouse or rat brain by the Vannucci hypoxia-ischemia method at P3 or P5 or by chronic exposure to hypoxia (P3–P11) (Hagberg et al., 2002). There is very little information regarding the BBB in these models of preterm WMD.

HYPOXIC-ISCHEMIC ENCEPHALOPATHY

Hypoxic-ischemic encephalopathy (HIE) is considered a major cause of brain injury in term neonates. At present, there are no specific serum biomarkers or other tools to easily assess neurological injury at birth, either in terms of its severity or the prediction of neurodevelopmental outcome. Because of this knowledge gap, all newborns with moderate or severe encephalopathy are treated with hypothermia in an identical fashion. Randomized controlled trials of therapeutic hypothermia have demonstrated a reduction in death or severe disability at 18 months, but death and disability continue to occur in 30–70% of infants with severe to moderate HIE despite cooling therapy (Shankaran et al., 2005; Azzopardi et al., 2009; Tagin et al., 2012). The criteria used to identify neonates with so-called HIE are (1) a pH ≤ 7 or base deficit $\geq$16 mEq/L in umbilical cord arterial plasma, and (2) a history of an acute perinatal event or non-availability of arterial blood gas or a pH or base deficit in the borderline range associated with a 10-min APGAR score $\leq$5 or assisted ventilation at birth. An understanding of the neuropathological process that leads to HIE could lead to the identification of new markers of neuronal injury that correlate with disease and neurodevelopmental outcome, and thus facilitate a more targeted therapeutic approach using adjunctive therapies (Chalak et al., 2014).

To study the effects of oxygen and nutrient deprivation on the developing brain, the species most commonly used are sheep, rabbits, piglets and, most of all, rodents. Differences in temporal phases of development between human and animal brain structures make the choice of a specific species and the determination of a precise correlation between developmental stages in the animal model and the corresponding stage in neonatal brain development very complex. Based on several experimental studies evaluating the developmental profile of the main neural cells of interest, the scientific community has established that a reasonable comparison can be drawn between P3/5 rodents and preterm infants, and P7/10 rodents and term infants (Kinney and Volpe, 2012).

Across the wide range of species used to model HIE, the relative contribution of vessels supplying blood to the brain is variable (Purves, 1972). In rodents, brain ischemia induced by the occlusion of a single carotid artery is not always consistent, and injury is typically induced by combining this with systemic hypotension. This combination of insults in the P7 rat, known as the Rice-Vannucci model, was originally developed in 1981 and is considered the pioneering model of HIE (Rice et al., 1981). It has since been adapted to many postnatal ages and transferred to the mouse (Derugin et al., 1998; Sheldon et al., 1998; Ohshima et al., 2012; Tsuji et al., 2013). The brain's response to global hypoxia-ischemia is a multistep process. Within the first few hours, regionally specific increases of cerebral blood flow occur followed by decreases due to regional vasoconstriction or the collapse of cardiac output, with the subsequent onset of excitotoxicity, energy depletion and the generation of free radicals, leading to apoptotic and necrotic cell death and the generation of edema (Ferrari et al., 2010a). This phase is followed within a few hours/days by a second phase consisting of a neuroinflammatory response, mitochondrial permeabilization, reperfusion and loss of cerebral autoregulation, and the production of free radicals (Hamrick and Ferriero, 2003; McLean and Ferriero, 2004). Recent hypotheses describe a tertiary phase that occurs days or even years after the injury and that contributes to the persistence of inflammation and reduced efficacy of brain repair (Fleiss and Gressens, 2012).

The effects of hypoxia-ischemia on the adult BBB include the disruption of TJ proteins (in particular claudin-5 (Cld5), occludin (Occl), zonula occludens (ZO) -1 and -2 (Bolton et al., 1998; Fischer et al., 2002; Mark and Davis, 2002; Witt et al., 2003; Sandoval and Witt, 2008; Zehendner et al., 2013) and increased BBB permeability in *in vitro* studies (Fischer et al., 2000; Zhang et al., 2000; Mark and Davis, 2002). These events are mediated by proinflammatory cytokines such as tumor necrosis factor (TNF) α, interleukin (IL)-1β, IL-8, monocyte chemoattractant protein-1, intercellular adhesion molecule-1, vascular endothelial growth factor (VEGF) and nitric oxide (NO), and astrocytes seems to play a protective role (for a review, see Ballabh et al., 2004). However, differences between the mature and developing brain limit the possibility of extrapolating data from adult studies to neonates.

Concerning developmental age, there are few comparative studies between barriers in the adult and developing brain in this specific model, and the results are not always concordant; in fact, studies in sheep show that the BBB becomes less susceptible to hyperosmolar stress with age (Stonestreet et al., 2006), and in rodents, it seems to be more vulnerable to hypoxia-ischemia at early stages of development (Muramatsu et al., 1997). Studies in rodent models of neonatal hypoxia-ischemia have indicated that the integrity of brain barriers is compromised (Muramatsu et al., 1997; Ferrari et al., 2010b; Tu et al., 2011; Yang et al., 2013a), a finding confirmed by a study of cerebrospinal fluid (CSF) samples from HIE infants showing that the ratio of the albumin concentration in the CSF to that in the plasma is 5 times higher than normal, suggesting leaky brain barriers in these infants (Kumar et al., 2008). Most of these studies, however, precede more recent knowledge of BBB characteristics suggesting that the BBB is more resistant during the developmental period than after maturation (Johansson et al., 2008; Ek et al., 2012; Saunders et al., 2012). Additionally, these early studies did not examine specific TJ disruptions or undertake a qualitative evaluation of the passage of substance and molecules, assessing only immunoglobulin (Ig) G labeling at different time points. Further investigations are needed to better understand BBB behavior in this model.

STROKE

Ischemic stroke occurs when cerebral blood flow is locally interrupted due to a clot within a vessel (Davis and Donnan, 2012) (see **Figure 1**). Perinatal stroke is defined as a cerebrovascular event that occurs between 28 weeks of gestation and a postnatal age of 28 days. Its incidence is similar to that in the elderly, approximately 1 in 4000 live births (Lynch et al., 2002), and it is associated with cerebral palsy [which is correlated with infarct size (Lee et al., 2005)], epilepsy, language delays and behavioral abnormalities. Classically associated with hypoxia, recent animal models have used permanent middle cerebral artery occlusion in association with transient bilateral common carotid artery occlusion to mimic an isolated acute ischemic event followed by reperfusion on resuscitation. Currently, more reproducible models are the 1998 Renolleau model in P7 Wistar rats and the 2013 Tsuji model in P9 CB-17 mice (Charriaut-Marlangue et al., 2013). After stroke in adults, BBB leakage/disruption can occur either transiently, in two distinct phases (Belayev et al., 1996; Rosenberg et al., 1998), or continuously (McColl et al., 2008; Kuntz et al., 2014). Although the basic mechanisms of neurodegeneration after stroke are shared across age groups, immaturity critically affects brain susceptibility and response to ischemia-related insults, including modes of neuronal death, inflammation, leukocyte-mediated injury and susceptibility to reactive oxygen species (ROS) (Benjelloun et al., 1999).

TRAUMATIC BRAIN INJURY

Traumatic Brain Injury (TBI) in children can cause more severe cognitive and behavioral deficits than comparable injuries in mature brains, and is one of the most common reasons for the development of significant lifelong disability in a child (Anderson et al., 2005; Rivara et al., 2012; Stanley et al., 2012; Roozenbeek et al., 2013). This is particularly important if we consider that children under the age of 4 years more frequently undergo TBI than any other age group (Koepsell et al., 2011) and that injured infants under the age of 12 months are at high risk of requiring intensive care support (Keenan et al., 2003). A similar developmental sensitivity to TBI can be seen in a rodent model of TBI, in which TBI inflicted at P7 causes the maximum damage. In addition, during the first 3 weeks of life, rodents display high sensitivity to excitotoxicity, as seen during the developmental period in human brains (i.e., maximal brain growth, synaptogenesis, and myelination). Thus, P7 is considered the period of maximal sensitivity and the best age to evaluate effects of TBI in rodents (Bittigau et al., 1999).

TBI can be simulated in different ways in various animal models: in the 1980s, a variety of species including cats, dogs, pigs and non-human primates were used (Xiong et al., 2013), but since the 1990s the use of rodents has predominated thanks to the ease with which experiments can be carried out and managed, and the limited costs. In addition, the ability to genetically modify mice has confirmed their position as the most-used species in laboratory research (Longhi et al., 2001; Duhaime, 2006). Models of focal TBI are the most common, induced by the impact of an object on the head (contusion) or the sudden arrest of the head during motion (deceleration) not necessarily requiring contact with an object. The most common modes of contusion trauma induction are lateral fluid percussion injury (Thompson et al., 2005), controlled cortical impact injury (Dixon et al., 1991; Cernak, 2005; Ajao et al., 2012; Pop et al., 2013) and focal TBI through a closed skull (Chen et al., 1996). The primary injury process in TBI is mechanical damage (vascular damage and bleeding caused by shear forces), immediately followed by mast cell degranulation (Stokely and Orr, 2008), and a secondary pathological phase characterized by excitotoxicity, ischemia, mitochondrial dysfunction and apoptosis (Xiong et al., 2013). This phase leads to the activation of inflammatory processes, which are themselves neurotoxic (Hagberg et al., 2012) and mediated by immune cells resident in the brain as well as by the transmigration of systemic immune cells and BBB disruption (Ramlackhansingh et al., 2011).

An electron microscopic analysis of rat cerebral slices in an animal model of TBI (Dietrich et al., 1994) has revealed the presence of microscopic hemorrhagic contusions or petechia, especially in the white-gray matter interface underlying the somatosensory cortex and cisterna ambiens, demonstrating that primary shear-stress-induced vascular damage can be found distant from the initial injury site, indicating protein leakage and the extravasation of blood cells. The choroid plexus is also activated by TBI inflicted at a distance from the ventricles, leading not to blood-cerebrospinal fluid barrier disruption but to the homing of choroidal monocytes and neutrophils and the synthesis and secretion into the CSF of inflammatory chemokines (Szmydynger-Chodobska et al., 2009, 2012).

ROLE OF THE BBB IN THE PATHOPHYSIOLOGY OF DEVELOPMENTAL BRAIN INSULTS

It would be difficult to thoroughly analyze in this review the large amount of information available concerning the possible mechanisms that influence BBB disruption in the developing brain. We will therefore focus on a few selected factors.

EXCITOTOXICITY AND FREE RADICALS

NO is a weak free radical produced by the action of nitric oxide synthase (NOS). The direct effects of this molecule on the BBB during development have not been studied so far. However, studies in adult rats demonstrate that in a model of stress-induced neurodegeneration, the production of NO and related oxidative-nitrosative compounds via the expression of inducible NOS (iNOS) correlates with BBB disruption, as evaluated by $[^{14}C]$-sucrose uptake by brain tissue. The injection of the specific iNOS inhibitor 1400 W prevents this increase in BBB permeability. Since the developing brain is considered to be extremely vulnerable to free radical damage due to its high lipid content (O'Brien and Sampson, 1965), relatively high oxygen consumption and capacity for ROS generation, and low concentrations of the main antioxidant enzymes (Baud et al., 2004; Vannucci and Hagberg, 2004; Miller et al., 2012), a potential role of this free radical could be suspected.

Following neonatal hypoxia-ischemia, both neuronal (n) NOS and endothelial (e) NOS are up-regulated, but while nNOS knockout mice seem to be protected following neonatal hypoxia-ischemia (Ferriero et al., 1996), studies indicate that eNOS can play a neuroprotective role in the adult brain by influencing neural migration and outgrowth and acting as a downstream regulator of angiogenesis (Huang et al., 1996). Further studies are needed to clarify the different roles of specific NOS isoforms and their link with BBB disruption.

Concerning white matter insults, in the presence of an activated excitotoxic cascade, damage to cerebrovascular endothelial cells should cause alterations in BBB function that could exacerbate neuronal injury and death. Glutamic acid or glutamate the most important excitatory neurotransmitter in the CNS, also acts in the pathophysiology of neuronal damage. Excess glutamate is known to induce neuronal death through a process in which the overactivation of ionotropic and metabotropic glutamate receptors triggers several intracellular signaling pathways, leading to apoptosis, necrosis or both (Gudino-Cabrera et al., 2014). Glutamate agonists, such as ibotenate, are frequently used to reproduce excitotoxic insults in the CNS. However, there are, to our knowledge, no studies that directly evaluate the effects of excitotoxic insults on BBB permeability during development.

The pathophysiology of TBI can also be explained in part by free radical formation and the effects of these on the BBB. During TBI, the transmigration of circulating immune cells and local microglial activation leads to the production of NO, ROS and inflammatory mediators that are capable of interfering with the BBB (Perez-Asensio et al., 2005; Briones et al., 2011). For instance, the ROS-induced peroxidation of polyunsaturated fatty acids in cell membranes gives rise to active aldehydes, significantly increasing endothelial monolayer permeability in experimental studies (Chodobski et al., 2011). In addition, oxidative stress is associated with the endogenous antioxidant glutathione and the increased permeability of the BBB, although only to low-molecular-weight markers (Agarwal and Shukla, 1999), and hydrogen peroxide has been demonstrated to increase BBB permeability via the Extracellular-signal-regulated Kinase (ERK) signal transduction pathway, along with the redistribution of Occl and ZO-1 and -2 (Fischer et al., 2005).

ALTERATIONS OF THE BASAL LAMINA AND ENDOTHELIAL CELLS

One class of enzymes extensively studied for its role in the BBB is family of proteases known as the matrix metalloproteinases (MMPs). The MMPs cleave their protein substrates based on a conserved mechanism that involves the interaction of an active-site-bound water molecule with a Zn^{2+} ion. The MMPs participate not only in pathophysiological processes but also in many normal biological processes such as embryonic (including brain) development, organ morphogenesis, blastocyst implantation, bone remodeling and wound healing (Brew et al., 2000). Because of this dual nature of the MMPs, it would be interesting to uncover their role in the developing brain after neonatal hypoxia-ischemia and, more importantly, their long-term role in neurological function. MMPs disrupt the BBB by degrading TJ and basal lamina proteins, thereby leading to BBB leakage, leukocyte infiltration, brain edema and hemorrhage (Liu et al., 2012). The activity of the MMPs is regulated by a group of endogenous proteins called tissue inhibitors of metalloproteinases (TIMPs), which bind to active and alternative sites of activated MMPs.

MMPs have been implicated in cerebral ischemia, and several studies have revealed that plasma MMP-9 concentrations strongly correlate with stroke severity in patients and that MMP-9 inhibition attenuates early BBB disruption and cerebral edema while promoting the expression of TJ proteins and angiogenesis (Rosenberg et al., 1998; Liu et al., 2009; Gu et al., 2012; Yang et al., 2013b). For instance, in a mouse model of focal cerebral ischemia, the deletion of the TIMP-1 gene results in increased MMP-9 protein expression and gelatinolytic activity, and is accompanied by exacerbated BBB disruption, neuronal apoptosis and ischemic injury when compared to wild-type animals (Fujimoto et al., 2008). Correspondingly, BBB leakage is reduced by TIMP-1 overexpression, and 24 h infarct volumes are also reduced (Maier et al., 2006). MMP-9 has been shown to degrade TJ proteins (Cld-5, Occl, ZO-1) in animal models of focal cerebral ischemia (Yang and Rosenberg, 2011). Aberrant MMP-9 proteolytic activity degrades not only TJ proteins but also basal membrane proteins (e.g., fibronectin, laminin, collagen, and others). This degradation is associated with an increase in BBB permeability, resulting in brain infarction, edema and hypertension in both animal models (Lee et al., 2007; Rosenberg and Yang, 2007; Yang et al., 2007) and human patients (Gasche et al., 2001; Castellanos et al., 2003; Lo, 2008). In a study conducted in P7 rat pups, hypoxia-ischemia was induced by unilateral ligation of the right carotid artery followed by hypoxia, and a broad-spectrum MMP inhibitor was injected intraperitoneally (i.p.). This early MMP inhibition provided both acute and long-term neuroprotection by reducing TJ protein degradation, preserving BBB integrity and reducing brain edema after neonatal hypoxic-ischemic injury (Chen et al., 2009). In addition, IgG accumulation in the brain is reduced in neonatal MMP-9 knockout (KO) mice compared to wild-type mice 24 h after hypoxia-ischemia (Svedin et al., 2007; Vexler and Yenari, 2009), suggesting that MMP-9 contributes to the opening of the BBB shortly after hypoxia-ischemia. However, there are still several points that need to be clarified. Like many biological mediators, MMPs can be used for good or bad, and this seems to be the case in the brain too. In fact, although MMPs seem to be involved in damage early after stroke, other studies demonstrate that they take on another role later in the process, contributing to repair (Stolp et al., 2005). However, it has been noted that exogenous MMPs kill neurons in culture (Stonestreet et al., 2006; Stolp et al., 2011). This could be due to temporal variations in the action of MMP-9 and/or to the divergent functions of different subtypes of MMPs. These aspects are well reviewed in Lakhan et al. (2013). Briefly, whereas MMP-2 could play a role in the initial opening of the BBB, MMP-9 seems to be more important for the secondary, delayed, opening of the BBB after ischemia, which is necessary for vascular angiogenesis and neuronal regeneration.

A possible explanation for the action of the MMPs is mediation by caveolin-1 (Cav-1). ROS can stimulate MMP activation through the loss of caveolin-1, a protein encoded by the *cav1* gene and a critical determinant of BBB permeability (Gu et al., 2011). Recent studies have revealed that Cav-1 can prevent the degradation of TJ proteins and protect BBB integrity by inhibiting the production of reactive nitrogen species (RNS) and MMP activity. In addition, Cav-1 KO mice show higher rates of apoptotic cell death and larger infarct volumes than wild- in ischemic brains, and the production of NO induces the loss of Cav-1 in focal cerebral ischemia and reperfusion injury. The downregulation of Cav-1 is correlated with an increase in the activity of MMP-2 and -9, decreased ZO-1 expression and increased BBB permeability (Gu et al., 2012).

ANGIOGENESIS

Although hypoxia-induced angiogenesis is considered beneficial since it allows more oxygen delivery to ischemic regions, there are some associated aspects that are not necessarily positive. One of these aspects is BBB permeability. The main molecules implicated in this process of endothelial cell regression and regrowth are VEGF, placental growth factor, acidic fibroblast growth factor (FGF), TNFα, IL-8 and erythropoietin. The VEGF family has six homologs members, of which the most widely studied is VEGF-A, and 3 tyrosine kinase receptors. Of these, VEGF receptors -1 and -2, which bind VEGF-A, are involved in blood vessel growth, endothelial cell mitogenesis and vasodilatation (via NO-dependent pathways). VEGF is thus a key regulator of vasculogenesis, and endothelial cells that express VEGF also produce MMPs and plasminogen activators to initiate extracellular matrix degradation, the first step in angiogenesis. In response to hypoxia, hypoxia-inducible factor (HIF) -1 is stabilized, leading to the augmented expression of the angiogenic genes mentioned above (Semenza, 2010). Three HIF isoforms are known (HIF-1α, HIF-2α, and HIF-3α), of which HIF-2α is restricted to vascular endothelial cells (Skuli et al., 2009). It has been suggested that in endothelial cells, HIF-1α plays a role in metabolism, proliferation and survival, while HIF-2α is involved in cell migration, adhesion and vascular integrity. Following hypoxia in the neonatal brain, HIF-1α starts to accumulate in neurons, an effect that has been shown to be protective and antiapoptotic (Tahraoui et al., 2001; Tagin et al., 2012). However, in a study evaluating the role of HIF-1α in BBB permeability in a rat subarachnoid hemorrhage model, the elevated expression of HIF-1α in brain tissues temporally coincided with brain edema formation and BBB disruption. In addition, BBB disruption, as determined by the extravasation of Evans Blue (a standard ink tracer used in the CNS), was down-regulated by the inhibition of either HIF-1α or MMP-9. In the present study, the inhibition of HIF-1α reduced not only brain edema, but also the expression of aquaporin-4 (see Section on "Edema") and MMP-9, suggesting that HIF-1α may be a key protein in brain edema formation and BBB disruption, possibly through aquaporin-4 and MMP-9 regulation (Tcharmtchi et al., 2000). Whether the induction of HIF-1α is beneficial or harmful is thus still debatable. Some recent studies have reported that HIF-1α and its target genes may contribute to cell death, tissue destruction and the formation of brain edema, primarily in the acute phase after ischemic brain damage (Thibeault et al., 2001; Thompson et al., 2005). Therefore, inhibiting this molecule immediately following damage could be effective in improving neurological outcome by protecting the brain from secondary injury following edema and BBB disruption (Tcharmtchi et al., 2000).

VEGF also appears to have a dual response to hypoxia-ischemia depending on the time frame studied. Several studies conducted both in adults and, to a lesser extent, in the neonatal brain following hypoxia, show that the i.c. injection of VEGF results in reduced brain injury, with the reduction of brain edema and infarct volume, a decrease in apoptotic cells and BBB permeability (Kaya et al., 2005; Feng et al., 2008). In addition, the inhibition of VEGF receptor-2 decreases endothelial cell proliferation, increases cell death and worsens stroke injury in a neonatal rodent model (Shimotake et al., 2010). The most likely hypothesis is that the "early" upregulation of VEGF (between 1 and 3 h after MCAO) is associated with BBB permeability and contributes to ischemic injury, while conversely, the neuroprotective effects of VEGF, including neovascularization and neuronal protection, occur in the days (48 h) after hypoxia (Marti et al., 2000).

EDEMA

One of the most important complications of TBI is edema, which occurs more frequently in the pediatric than in the adult population. This is possibly due to the higher water content of the developing brain and also to the mechanism of regulation of water homeostasis. There are few *in vivo* studies of TBI and BBB disruption in neonates, with most focusing on juvenile rodents. The Badault group has recently evaluated the contribution of the aquaporins to the post-traumatic edema process in juvenile rats and mice (Badaut et al., 2011a,b, 2014; Fukuda et al., 2012, 2013). Pups treated with an inhibitor of aquaporin-4, siGLO siAQP4, show acute improvements in motor function (3 days after injury) and long-term improvements in spatial memory (60 days after injury) when compared with control animals. These improvements are associated with decreased edema formation, increased microglial activation, decreased BBB disruption, and reduced astrogliosis and neuronal death. The effectiveness of the treatment paradigm is associated with a 30% decrease in aquaporin-4 expression at the injection site. Thus, aquaporin's seems to be molecules significantly involved in post-TBI damage, and represent an interesting therapeutic target (Fukuda et al., 2013). Another study has revealed that the inhibition of a kinase involved in the development of brain edema, myosin light-chain kinase, by the administration of an inhibitor, ML-7, to P24 mice starting 4 h after TBI and every 24 h until sacrifice, significantly reduces BBB breakdown and the development of cerebral edema, and preserves neurological function (Rossi et al., 2013).

INFLAMMATORY RESPONSE

Neuroinflammation is a key pathological factor in most insults to the developing brain (Degos et al., 2010a). Neuroinflammation is induced by the invasion of pathogens or the release of damage-associated proteins by injured and dying cells. Inflammation includes the activation of microglia, astrocytes and endothelial cells, leading to the secretion of proinflammatory cytokines such as TNFα and IL-1β. There is an increased expression of endothelial adhesion molecules such as vascular cell adhesion molecule 1, intercellular adhesion molecule 1 and the selectins (Simi et al., 2007). Inflammatory processes are, moreover, associated with modifications of the molecular composition or functional state of TJs (Coisne and Engelhardt, 2011). Proinflammatory cytokines also influence the expression of MMPs, which increase BBB permeability by degrading TJs and extracellular matrix components in the endothelial basement membrane (Rosenberg, 2009). These events lead to barrier leakiness, which in turn allows pathogen and immune cell invasion (Labus et al., 2014).

Resident microglia are some of the first cells to respond to inflammatory stimuli. They can migrate, together with astrocytes, to the region of injury or infection, where they clean up cellular debris and produce proinflammatory cytokines such as IL-1β and IL-6. In the case of TBI and hypoxia-ischemia, mast cells also produce large quantities of proinflammatory mediators (Biran et al., 2008; Jin et al., 2009). With regard to the BBB, these cytokines lead to increased permeability and facilitate the entry of peripheral macrophages and cytokines from the systemic circulation. In the instance of inflammation following hypoxic-ischemic injury, this has the effect of exacerbating the excitotoxic cascade by further stimulating glutamate release and free radical and NO production (McLean and Ferriero, 2004). The importance of the mast cell response in causing brain damage after TBI is supported by post-insult treatment with cromoglycate, a mast cell stabilizer that inhibits mast cell degranulation and decreases BBB opening (Strbian et al., 2006), glial activation and neuronal death (Jin et al., 2007) sufficiently to provide long-term neuroprotection.

Leukocyte migration depends on strict interactions with the vascular endothelium, mediated by 3 groups of adhesion molecules: the selectins, the immunoglobulin superfamily (such as intercellular adhesion molecule 1) and the integrins. The pattern of recruitment of monocytes and macrophages is cytokine-specific: IL-1β leads to neutrophil recruitment while TNFα attracts monocytes (Blond et al., 2002). A comparative study in P7 and adult rats subjected to transient middle cerebral artery occlusion shows that Evans Blue extravasation, a measure of paracellular diffusion, the main method of entry for bulky proteins and leukocytes into the brain, remains low during the 24 h period following reperfusion in neonatal rats but is profoundly increased in adult rats. The largely unaltered paracellular diffusion in neonatal rats is associated with the increased expression of several TJ proteins (Vexler and Yenari, 2009) rather than with the decrease in their expression seen in adult rats after a similar injury. In contrast to stroke in adults, in P7 hypoxic-ischemic brains, the transmigration of neutrophils is far lower (Hudome et al., 1997). This may be related to the greater resistance of the BBB to hypoxia-ischemia-induced leaks at this age but also to the immaturity of both endothelial cells, which express less P-selectin (Lorant et al., 1999), and neutrophils, which are less capable of adhering to P-selectin (Tcharmtchi et al., 2000). The lower extent of leukocyte extravasation after ischemic injury in neonatal rats may contribute to the age difference in the structural and functional changes to the BBB after ischemia.

Specific studies have been carried out to examine the effects of inflammation on the functions of the developing BBB and how this influences the development of brain injury. A rather complex and unexpected effect of inflammatory stimuli on BBB integrity and leukocyte transmigration has been reported during the first 3 weeks of life in rats. A comparison of the extent of IgG infiltration in different brain regions following intrastriatal injections of IL-1 or TNFα in rats of different ages shows dramatically higher IgG accumulation in 21-day-old than in 2-h-old rat pups (Anthony et al., 1997, 1998; Schnell et al., 1999). These data demonstrate that at birth, the BBB is functional, and is in fact more resistant to inflammatory stress than in the juvenile brain.

Stolp et al. have conducted two studies of BBB behavior in neonatal, juvenile and adult rats in response to prolonged inflammatory stimuli, in particular the i.p. injection of 0.2 mg/kg lipopolysaccharide (LPS). They have demonstrated for the first time a possible link between changes in BBB permeability (evaluated by permeability to sucrose, inulin and plasma proteins and Cld-5 distribution) and behavioral alterations in animals exposed to the inflammatory stimulus early in development, i.e., on postnatal day (P) 0, P2, P4, P6, and P8. LPS treatment resulted in increased permeability only in adulthood, preceded by Cld-5 alterations in a few vessels at an earlier time point. However, due to the normally low permeability of cerebral blood vessels, it is probable that even a few vessels with altered permeability could significantly contribute to the overall properties of the BBB, and that these changes could explain the short-term changes seen in behavioral tests, in particular in the prepulse inhibition paradigm, that were distinguishable in juvenile animals but not in adult animals. Long-term changes in permeability, as shown by the sucrose permeability test, are correlated in adult rats with altered responses to the dark/light test, suggesting that the impact of inflammation could occur in several phases (short- and long-term) and that each phase could lead to different behavioral modifications (Stolp et al., 2005, 2011). A third study from the same group analyzes, in a similar model (using the opossum *Monodelphis domestica*), the ability of minocycline, a potent anti-inflammatory molecule, to modulate the inflammation-induced changes in BBB permeability and white matter damage following acute and prolonged inflammation during development. The effects of minocycline on inflammation were evaluated in terms of IL-1β mRNA levels in the spleen and brain, and of white blood cell counts in animals sacrificed 1.5 h after the first or fifth LPS injection (single or prolonged inflammatory stimuli). No differences in IL-1β levels were seen between groups, although white blood cells were significantly augmented in animals given prolonged LPS stimulation compared to non-treated animals. Interestingly minocycline significantly reduced this augmentation. The same results were obtained if permeability to ^{14}C-sucrose and plasma proteins were evaluated: animals that received a single injection of either LPS or LPS+minocycline showed no changes in BBB permeability to ^{14}C-sucrose or plasma proteins. Thus, the inclusion of minocycline probably did not prevent barrier permeability changes after a single LPS injection but prevented barrier permeability to proteins and ^{14}C-sucrose when administered during prolonged inflammation.

We have carried out further studies of the BBB in a model in which inflammation alone induces WMD, by the twice-daily i.p. injection of newborn rats or mice with IL-1 over 5 days (Favrais et al., 2011). We evaluated modifications in the expression of the most important choroid plexus TJ proteins at P2, the second day of injections, and 5 days after the beginning of the injections (Favrais et al., 2011; Riddle et al., 2011; Schang et al., 2014). Our results demonstrate that there is no significant non-specific disruption of BCSFB integrity, as assessed by paracellular permeability to tracers, and only a modest increase in Cld-3 expression in the choroidal tissue. In adult animal models of inflammation, the choroid plexus is known to be extremely sensitive to peripheral inflammatory stimuli, as demonstrated by the augmentation of cytokines and other inflammatory markers (Quan et al., 1999; Thibeault et al., 2001; Szmydynger-Chodobska et al., 2012), and the choroid plexus-CSF system appears to be crucial for immune cell trafficking into the CNS during neuroimmune surveillance as well as in the early stages of neuroinflammatory diseases (Reboldi et al., 2009; Schmitt et al., 2012). Thus, studies on the choroid plexus conducted in the context of moderate systemic perinatal inflammation occurring during a period approximating 28–35 weeks of gestation in humans, which alters the developmental program of the white matter, should focus more on the perturbation of specialized functions of the BCSFB, such as neuroimmune regulation, rather than on gross non-specific alterations of barrier integrity.

CONCLUSION

Inflammation, vascular reactivity and excitotoxicity are the main protagonists of perinatal diseases, and the BBB and NVU are certainly majorly implicated in these processes. As our knowledge of these processes increases, promising new targets for neuroprotection have been found. However, a lot of questions remain open, especially regarding differences between the behavior of young and adult brains. In addition, even though clinical studies are impossible for obvious ethical reasons, the use of animal models and/or *in vitro* studies impose great limitations in this domain, since the therapeutic options validated in these models are not always as effective when applied to humans. Funding research on the BBB, both in the pre-clinical and clinical domains, should be encouraged in order to better understand early cerebral development and develop effective therapeutic strategies.

ACKNOWLEDGMENTS

In vivo blood-CSF barrier assessment was carried out by the BIP platform, CRNL Inserm U1028, Lyon. A special thanks to Dr. S Rasika for her priceless proofreading and critical editing of the manuscript.

REFERENCES

Aden, U., Favrais, G., Plaisant, F., Winerdal, M., Felderhoff-Mueser, U., Lampa, J., et al. (2010). Systemic inflammation sensitizes the neonatal brain to excitotoxicity through a pro-/anti-inflammatory imbalance: key role of TNFalpha pathway and protection by etanercept. *Brain Behav. Immun.* 24, 747–758. doi: 10.1016/j.bbi.2009.10.010

Agarwal, R., and Shukla, G. S. (1999). Potential role of cerebral glutathione in the maintenance of blood-brain barrier integrity in rat. *Neurochem. Res.* 24, 1507–1514. doi: 10.1023/A:1021191729865

Ajao, D. O., Pop, V., Kamper, J. E., Adami, A., Rudobeck, E., Huang, L., et al. (2012). Traumatic brain injury in young rats leads to progressive behavioral deficits coincident with altered tissue properties in adulthood. *J. Neurotrauma* 29, 2060–2074. doi: 10.1089/neu.2011.1883

Anderson, V., Catroppa, C., Morse, S., Haritou, F., and Rosenfeld, J. (2005). Functional plasticity or vulnerability after early brain injury? *Pediatrics* 116, 1374–1382. doi: 10.1542/peds.2004-1728

Anthony, D. C., Bolton, S. J., Fearn, S., and Perry, V. H. (1997). Age-related effects of interleukin-1 beta on polymorphonuclear neutrophil-dependent increases in blood-brain barrier permeability in rats. *Brain* 120(Pt 3), 435–444. doi: 10.1093/brain/120.3.435

Anthony, D., Dempster, R., Fearn, S., Clements, J., Wells, G., Perry, V. H., et al. (1998). CXC chemokines generate age-related increases in neutrophil-mediated brain inflammation and blood-brain barrier breakdown. *Curr. Biol.* 8, 923–926. doi: 10.1016/S0960-9822(07)00373-9

Aquilina, K., Chakkarapani, E., and Thoresen, M. (2012). Early deterioration of cerebrospinal fluid dynamics in a neonatal piglet model of intraventricular hemorrhage and posthemorrhagic ventricular dilation. *J. Neurosurg. Pediatr.* 10, 529–537. doi: 10.3171/2012.8.PEDS11386

Aquilina, K., Hobbs, C., Cherian, S., Tucker, A., Porter, H., Whitelaw, A., et al. (2007). A neonatal piglet model of intraventricular hemorrhage and posthemorrhagic ventricular dilation. *J. Neurosurg.* 107, 126–136. doi: 10.3171/PED-07/08/126

Armulik, A., Genove, G., Mae, M., Nisancioglu, M. H., Wallgard, E., Niaudet, C., et al. (2010). Pericytes regulate the blood-brain barrier. *Nature* 468, 557–561. doi: 10.1038/nature09522

Azzopardi, D. V., Strohm, B., Edwards, A. D., Dyet, L., Halliday, H. L., Juszczak, E., et al. (2009). Moderate hypothermia to treat perinatal asphyxial encephalopathy. *N. Engl. J. Med.* 361, 1349–1358. doi: 10.1056/NEJMoa0900854

Back, S. A., Gan, X., Li, Y., Rosenberg, P. A., and Volpe, J. J. (1998). Maturation-dependent vulnerability of oligodendrocytes to oxidative stress-induced death caused by glutathione depletion. *J. Neurosci.* 18, 6241–6253.

Badaut, J., Ashwal, S., Adami, A., Tone, B., Recker, R., Spagnoli, D., et al. (2011b). Brain water mobility decreases after astrocytic aquaporin-4 inhibition using RNA interference. *J. Cereb. Blood Flow Metab.* 31, 819–831. doi: 10.1038/jcbfm.2010

Badaut, J., Ashwal, S., and Obenaus, A. (2011a). Aquaporins in cerebrovascular disease: a target for treatment of brain edema? *Cerebrovasc. Dis.* 31, 521–531. doi: 10.1159/000324328

Badaut, J., Fukuda, A. M., Jullienne, A., and Petry, K. G. (2014). Aquaporin and brain diseases. *Biochim. Biophys. Acta* 1840, 1554–1565. doi: 10.1016/j.bbagen.2013.10.032

Balasubramaniam, J., and Del Bigio, M. R. (2006). Animal models of germinal matrix hemorrhage. *J. Child Neurol.* 21, 365–371. doi: 10.1177/08830738060210050201

Ballabh, P. (2010). Intraventricular hemorrhage in premature infants: mechanism of disease. *Pediatr. Res.* 67, 1–8. doi: 10.1203/PDR.0b013e3181c1b176

Ballabh, P., Braun, A., and Nedergaard, M. (2004). The blood-brain barrier: an overview: structure, regulation, and clinical implications. *Neurobiol. Dis.* 16, 1–13. doi: 10.1016/j.nbd.2003.12.016

Ballabh, P., Hu, F., Kumarasiri, M., Braun, A., and Nedergaard, M. (2005). Development of tight junction molecules in blood vessels of germinal matrix, cerebral cortex, and white matter. *Pediatr. Res.* 58, 791–798. doi: 10.1203/01.PDR.0000180535.14093.FB

Baud, O., Li, J., Zhang, Y., Neve, R. L., Volpe, J. J., and Rosenberg, P. A. (2004). Nitric oxide-induced cell death in developing oligodendrocytes is associated with mitochondrial dysfunction and apoptosis-inducing factor translocation. *Eur. J. Neurosci.* 20, 1713–1726. doi: 10.1111/j.1460-9568.2004.03616.x

Bauer, H. C., and Bauer, H. (2000). Neural induction of the blood-brain barrier: still an enigma. *Cell. Mol. Neurobiol.* 20, 13–28. doi: 10.1023/A:1006939825857

Bednarek, N., Svedin, P., Garnotel, R., Favrais, G., Loron, G., Schwendiman, L., et al. (2012). Increased MMP-9 and TIMP-1 in mouse neonatal brain and plasma and in human neonatal plasma after hypoxia-ischemia: a potential marker of neonatal encephalopathy. *Pediatr. Res.* 71, 63–70. doi: 10.1038/pr.2011.3

Belayev, L., Busto, R., Zhao, W., and Ginsberg, M. D. (1996). Quantitative evaluation of blood-brain barrier permeability following middle cerebral artery occlusion in rats. *Brain Res.* 739, 88–96. doi: 10.1016/S0006-8993(96)00815-3

Benjelloun, N., Renolleau, S., Represa, A., Ben-Ari, Y., and Charriaut-Marlangue, C. (1999). Inflammatory responses in the cerebral cortex after ischemia in the P7 neonatal Rat. *Stroke* 30, 1916–1923. discussion: 1923–1914.

Biran, V., Cochois, V., Karroubi, A., Arrang, J. M., Charriaut-Marlangue, C., and Heron, A. (2008). Stroke induces histamine accumulation and mast cell degranulation in the neonatal rat brain. *Brain Pathol.* 18, 1–9. doi: 10.1111/j.1750-3639.2007.00092.x

Bittigau, P., Sifringer, M., Pohl, D., Stadthaus, D., Ishimaru, M., Shimizu, H., et al. (1999). Apoptotic neurodegeneration following trauma is markedly enhanced in the immature brain. *Ann. Neurol.* 45, 724–735.

Blond, D., Campbell, S. J., Butchart, A. G., Perry, V. H., and Anthony, D. C. (2002). Differential induction of interleukin-1beta and tumour necrosis factor-alpha may account for specific patterns of leukocyte recruitment in the brain. *Brain Res.* 958, 89–99. doi: 10.1016/S0006-8993(02)03473-X

Bolton, S. J., Anthony, D. C., and Perry, V. H. (1998). Loss of the tight junction proteins occludin and zonula occludens-1 from cerebral vascular endothelium during neutrophil-induced blood-brain barrier breakdown *in vivo*. *Neuroscience* 86, 1245–1257. doi: 10.1016/S0306-4522(98)00058-X

Brew, K., Dinakarpandian, D., and Nagase, H. (2000). Tissue inhibitors of metalloproteinases: evolution, structure and function. *Biochim. Biophys. Acta* 1477, 267–283. doi: 10.1016/S0167-4838(99)00279-4

Briones, T. L., Rogozinska, M., and Woods, J. (2011). Modulation of ischemia-induced NMDAR1 activation by environmental enrichment decreases oxidative damage. *J. Neurotrauma* 28, 2485–2492. doi: 10.1089/neu.2011.1842

Castellanos, M., Leira, R., Serena, J., Pumar, J. M., Lizasoain, I., Castillo, J., et al. (2003). Plasma metalloproteinase-9 concentration predicts hemorrhagic transformation in acute ischemic stroke. *Stroke* 34, 40–46. doi: 10.1161/01.STR.0000046764.57344.31

CDC CfDCaP. (2004). "Economic costs associated with mental retardation, cerbral palsy, hearing loss, and vision impairment: United States 2003," in *MMWWR Morb. Mortal. Wkly. Rep.* 53, (North Carolina), 57–59.

Cernak, I. (2005). Animal models of head trauma. *NeuroRx* 2, 410–422. doi: 10.1602/neurorx.2.3.410

Chalak, L. F., Sanchez, P. J., Adams-Huet, B., Laptook, A. R., Heyne, R. J., and Rosenfeld, C. R. (2014). Biomarkers for severity of neonatal hypoxic-ischemic encephalopathy and outcomes in newborns receiving hypothermia therapy. *J. Pediatr.* 164, 468–474 e461. doi: 10.1016/j.jpeds.2013.10.067

Charriaut-Marlangue, C., Bonnin, P., Leger, P. L., and Renolleau, S. (2013). Brief update on hemodynamic responses in animal models of neonatal stroke and hypoxia-ischemia. *Exp. Neurol.* 248, 316–320. doi: 10.1016/j.expneurol.2013.06.022

Chen, W., Hartman, R., Ayer, R., Marcantonio, S., Kamper, J., Tang, J., et al. (2009). Matrix metalloproteinases inhibition provides neuroprotection against hypoxia-ischemia in the developing brain. *J. Neurochem.* 111, 726–736. doi: 10.1111/j.1471-4159.2009.06362.x

Chen, Y., Constantini, S., Trembovler, V., Weinstock, M., and Shohami, E. (1996). An experimental model of closed head injury in mice: pathophysiology, histopathology, and cognitive deficits. *J. Neurotrauma* 13, 557–568.

Chodobski, A., Zink, B. J., and Szmydynger-Chodobska, J. (2011). Blood-brain barrier pathophysiology in traumatic brain injury. *Transl. Stroke Res.* 2, 492–516. doi: 10.1007/s12975-011-0125-x

Coisne, C., and Engelhardt, B. (2011). Tight junctions in brain barriers during central nervous system inflammation. *Antioxid. Redox Signal.* 15, 1285–1303. doi: 10.1089/ars.2011.3929

Daneman, R., Zhou, L., Agalliu, D., Cahoy, J. D., Kaushal, A., and Barres, B. A. (2010b). The mouse blood-brain barrier transcriptome: a new resource for understanding the development and function of brain endothelial cells. *PLoS ONE* 5:e13741. doi: 10.1371/journal.pone.0013741

Daneman, R., Zhou, L., Kebede, A. A., and Barres, B. A. (2010a). Pericytes are required for blood-brain barrier integrity during embryogenesis. *Nature* 468, 562–566. doi: 10.1038/nature09513

Davis, S. M., and Donnan, G. A. (2012). Clinical practice. Secondary prevention after ischemic stroke or transient ischemic attack. *N. Engl. J. Med.* 366, 1914–1922. doi: 10.1056/NEJMcp1107281

Degos, V., Favrais, G., Kaindl, A. M., Peineau, S., Guerrot, A. M., Verney, C., et al. (2010a). Inflammation processes in perinatal brain damage. *J. Neural. Transm.* 117, 1009–1017. doi: 10.1007/s00702-010-0411-x

Degos, V., Favrais, G., Kaindl, A. M., Peineau, S., Guerrot, A. M., Verney, C., et al. (2010b). Inflammation processes in perinatal brain damage. *J. Neural. Transm.* 117, 1009–1017. doi: 10.1007/s00702-010-0411-x

Derugin, N., Ferriero, D. M., and Vexler, Z. S. (1998). Neonatal reversible focal cerebral ischemia: a new model. *Neurosci. Res.* 32, 349–353. doi: 10.1016/S0168-0102(98)00096-0

Dietrich, W. D., Alonso, O., and Halley, M. (1994). Early microvascular and neuronal consequences of traumatic brain injury: a light and electron microscopic study in rats. *J. Neurotrauma* 11, 289–301. doi: 10.1089/neu.1994.11.289

Dixon, C. E., Clifton, G. L., Lighthall, J. W., Yaghmai, A. A., and Hayes, R. L. (1991). A controlled cortical impact model of traumatic brain injury in the rat. *J. Neurosci. Methods* 39, 253–262. doi: 10.1016/0165-0270(91)90104-8

Dommergues, M. A., Plaisant, F., Verney, C., and Gressens, P. (2003). Early microglial activation following neonatal excitotoxic brain damage in mice: a potential target for neuroprotection. *Neuroscience* 121, 619–628. doi: 10.1016/S0306-4522(03)00558-X

Duhaime, A. C. (2006). Large animal models of traumatic injury to the immature brain. *Dev. Neurosci.* 28, 380–387. doi: 10.1159/000094164

Edwards, A. D., Brocklehurst, P., Gunn, A. J., Halliday, H., Juszczak, E., Levene, M., et al. (2010). Neurological outcomes at 18 months of age after moderate hypothermia for perinatal hypoxic ischaemic encephalopathy: synthesis and meta-analysis of trial data. *BMJ* 340:c363. doi: 10.1136/bmj.c363

Ek, C. J., Dziegielewska, K. M., Habgood, M. D., and Saunders, N. R. (2012). Barriers in the developing brain and Neurotoxicology. *Neurotoxicology* 33, 586–604. doi: 10.1016/j.neuro.2011.12.009

Ek, C. J., Dziegielewska, K. M., Stolp, H., and Saunders, N. R. (2006). Functional effectiveness of the blood-brain barrier to small water-soluble molecules in developing and adult opossum (Monodelphis domestica). *J. Comp. Neurol.* 496, 13–26. doi: 10.1002/cne.20885

Ek, C. J., Habgood, M. D., Dziegielewska, K. M., Potter, A., and Saunders, N. R. (2001). Permeability and route of entry for lipid-insoluble molecules across brain barriers in developing Monodelphis domestica. *J. Physiol.* 536, 841–853. doi: 10.1111/j.1469-7793.2001.00841.x

Ek, C. J., Habgood, M. D., Dziegielewska, K. M., and Saunders, N. R. (2003). Structural characteristics and barrier properties of the choroid plexuses in developing brain of the opossum (Monodelphis Domestica). *J. Comp. Neurol.* 460, 451–464. doi: 10.1002/cne.10661

Engelhardt, B., and Liebner, S. (2014). Novel insights into the development and maintenance of the blood-brain barrier. *Cell Tissue Res.* 355, 687–699. doi: 10.1007/s00441-014-1811-2

Evrard, P., Marret, S., and Gressens, P. (1997). Environmental and genetic determinants of neural migration and postmigratory survival. *Acta Paediatr. Suppl.* 422, 20–26. doi: 10.1111/j.1651-2227.1997.tb18339.x

Favrais, G., Schwendimann, L., Gressens, P., and Lelievre, V. (2007). Cyclooxygenase-2 mediates the sensitizing effects of systemic IL-1-beta on excitotoxic brain lesions in newborn mice. *Neurobiol. Dis.* 25, 496–505. doi: 10.1016/j.nbd.2006.10.012

Favrais, G., van de Looij, Y., Fleiss, B., Ramanantsoa, N., Bonnin, P., Stoltenburg-Didinger, G., et al. (2011). Systemic inflammation disrupts the developmental program of white matter. *Ann. Neurol.* 70, 550–565. doi: 10.1002/ana.22489

Feng, Y., Rhodes, P. G., and Bhatt, A. J. (2008). Neuroprotective effects of vascular endothelial growth factor following hypoxic ischemic brain injury in neonatal rats. *Pediatr. Res.* 64, 370–374. doi: 10.1203/PDR.0b013e318180ebe6

Ferrari, D. C., Nesic, O. B., and Perez-Polo, J. R. (2010b). Oxygen resuscitation does not ameliorate neonatal hypoxia/ischemia-induced cerebral edema. *J. Neurosci. Res.* 88, 2056–2065. doi: 10.1002/jnr.22358

Ferrari, D. C., Nesic, O., and Perez-Polo, J. R. (2010a). Perspectives on neonatal hypoxia/ischemia-induced edema formation. *Neurochem. Res.* 35, 1957–1965. doi: 10.1007/s11064-010-0308-y

Ferriero, D. M., Holtzman, D. M., Black, S. M., and Sheldon, R. A. (1996). Neonatal mice lacking neuronal nitric oxide synthase are less vulnerable to hypoxic-ischemic injury. *Neurobiol. Dis.* 3, 64–71. doi: 10.1006/nbdi.1996.0006

Fischer, S., Wiesnet, M., Renz, D., and Schaper, W. (2005). H_2O_2 induces paracellular permeability of porcine brain-derived microvascular endothelial cells by activation of the p44/42 MAP kinase pathway. *Eur. J. Cell Biol.* 84, 687–697. doi: 10.1016/j.ejcb.2005.03.002

Fischer, S., Wobben, M., Kleinstuck, J., Renz, D., and Schaper, W. (2000). Effect of astroglial cells on hypoxia-induced permeability in PBMEC cells. *Am. J. Physiol. Cell Physiol.* 279, C935–C944.

Fischer, S., Wobben, M., Marti, H. H., Renz, D., and Schaper, W. (2002). Hypoxia-induced hyperpermeability in brain microvessel endothelial cells involves VEGF-mediated changes in the expression of zonula occludens-1. *Microvasc. Res.* 63, 70–80. doi: 10.1006/mvre.2001.2367

Fleiss, B., and Gressens, P. (2012). Tertiary mechanisms of brain damage: a new hope for treatment of cerebral palsy? *Lancet Neurol.* 11, 556–566. doi: 10.1016/S1474-4422(12)70058-3

Fujimoto, M., Takagi, Y., Aoki, T., Hayase, M., Marumo, T., Gomi, M., et al. (2008). Tissue inhibitor of metalloproteinases protect blood-brain barrier disruption in focal cerebral ischemia. *J. Cereb. Blood Flow Metab.* 28, 1674–1685. doi: 10.1038/jcbfm.2008.59

Fukuda, A. M., Adami, A., Pop, V., Bellone, J. A., Coats, J. S., Hartman, R. E., et al. (2013). Posttraumatic reduction of edema with aquaporin-4 RNA interference improves acute and chronic functional recovery. *J. Cereb. Blood Flow Metab.* 33, 1621–1632. doi: 10.1038/jcbfm.2013.118

Fukuda, A. M., Pop, V., Spagnoli, D., Ashwal, S., Obenaus, A., and Badaut, J. (2012). Delayed increase of astrocytic aquaporin 4 after juvenile traumatic brain injury: possible role in edema resolution? *Neuroscience* 222, 366–378. doi: 10.1016/j.neuroscience.2012.06.033

Gasche, Y., Copin, J. C., Sugawara, T., Fujimura, M., and Chan, P. H. (2001). Matrix metalloproteinase inhibition prevents oxidative stress-associated blood-brain barrier disruption after transient focal cerebral ischemia. *J. Cereb. Blood Flow Metab.* 21, 1393–1400. doi: 10.1097/00004647-200112000-00003

Georgiadis, P., Xu, H., Chua, C., Hu, F., Collins, L., Huynh, C., et al. (2008). Characterization of acute brain injuries and neurobehavioral profiles in a rabbit model of germinal matrix hemorrhage. *Stroke* 39, 3378–3388. doi: 10.1161/STROKEAHA.107.510883

Goddard, J., Lewis, R. M., Armstrong, D. L., and Zeller, R. S. (1980). Moderate, rapidly induced hypertension as a cause of intraventricular hemorrhage in the newborn beagle model. *J. Pediatr.* 96, 1057–1060. doi: 10.1016/S0022-3476(80)80641-X

Gu, Y., Dee, C. M., and Shen, J. (2011). Interaction of free radicals, matrix metalloproteinases and caveolin-1 impacts blood-brain barrier permeability. *Front. Biosci. (Schol. Ed).* 3, 1216–1231. doi: 10.2741/222

Gu, Y., Zheng, G., Xu, M., Li, Y., Chen, X., Zhu, W., et al. (2012). Caveolin-1 regulates nitric oxide-mediated matrix metalloproteinases activity and blood-brain barrier permeability in focal cerebral ischemia and reperfusion injury. *J. Neurochem.* 120, 147–156. doi: 10.1111/j.1471-4159.2011.07542.x

Gudino-Cabrera, G., Urena-Guerrero, M. E., Rivera-Cervantes, M. C., Feria-Velasco, A. I., and Beas-Zarate, C. (2014). Excitotoxicity triggered by neonatal monosodium glutamate treatment and blood-brain barrier function. *Archives Med. Res.* doi: 10.1016/j.arcmed.2014.11.014. [Epub ahead of print].

Hagberg, H., Gressens, P., and Mallard, C. (2012). Inflammation during fetal and neonatal life: implications for neurologic and neuropsychiatric disease in children and adults. *Ann. Neurol.* 71, 444–457. doi: 10.1002/ana.22620

Hagberg, H., Ichord, R., Palmer, C., Yager, J. Y., and Vannucci, S. J. (2002). Animal models of developmental brain injury: relevance to human disease. A summary of the panel discussion from the third hershey conference on developmental cerebral blood flow and metabolism. *Dev. Neurosci.* 24, 364–366. doi: 10.1159/000069040

Hagberg, H., and Mallard, C. (2005). Effect of inflammation on central nervous system development and vulnerability. *Curr. Opin. Neurol.* 18, 117–123. doi: 10.1097/01.wco.0000162851.44897.8f

Hamrick, S. E., and Ferriero, D. M. (2003). The injury response in the term newborn brain: can we neuroprotect? *Curr. Opin. Neurol.* 16, 147–154. doi: 10.1097/00019052-200304000-00005

Huang, Z., Huang, P. L., Ma, J., Meng, W., Ayata, C., Fishman, M. C., et al. (1996). Enlarged infarcts in endothelial nitric oxide synthase knockout mice are attenuated by nitro-L-arginine. *J. Cereb. Blood Flow Metab.* 16, 981–987. doi: 10.1097/00004647-199609000-00023

Hudome, S., Palmer, C., Roberts, R. L., Mauger, D., Housman, C., and Towfighi, J. (1997). The role of neutrophils in the production of hypoxic-ischemic brain injury in the neonatal rat. *Pediatr. Res.* 41, 607–616. doi: 10.1203/00006450-199705000-00002

Jain, N. J., Kruse, L. K., Demissie, K., and Khandelwal, M. (2009). Impact of mode of delivery on neonatal complications: trends between 1997 and 2005. *J. Mat. Fetal Neonat. Med.* 22, 491–500. doi: 10.1080/14767050902769982

Jin, Y., Silverman, A. J., and Vannucci, S. J. (2007). Mast cell stabilization limits hypoxic-ischemic brain damage in the immature rat. *Dev. Neurosci.* 29, 373–384. doi: 10.1159/000105478

Jin, Y., Silverman, A. J., and Vannucci, S. J. (2009). Mast cells are early responders after hypoxia-ischemia in immature rat brain. *Stroke* 40, 3107–3112. doi: 10.1161/STROKEAHA.109.549691

Johansson, P. A., Dziegielewska, K. M., Ek, C. J., Habgood, M. D., Liddelow, S. A., Potter, A. M., et al. (2006). Blood-CSF barrier function in the rat embryo. *Eur. J. Neurosci.* 24, 65–76. doi: 10.1111/j.1460-9568.2006.04904.x

Johansson, P. A., Dziegielewska, K. M., Liddelow, S. A., and Saunders, N. R. (2008). The blood-CSF barrier explained: when development is not immaturity. *Bioessays* 30, 237–248. doi: 10.1002/bies.20718

Kaya, D., Gursoy-Ozdemir, Y., Yemisci, M., Tuncer, N., Aktan, S., and Dalkara, T. (2005). VEGF protects brain against focal ischemia without increasing blood—brain permeability when administered intracerebroventricularly. *J. Cereb. Blood Flow Metab.* 25, 1111–1118. doi: 10.1038/sj.jcbfm.9600109

Keenan, H. T., Runyan, D. K., Marshall, S. W., Nocera, M. A., Merten, D. F., and Sinal, S. H. (2003). A population-based study of inflicted traumatic brain injury in young children. *JAMA* 290, 621–626. doi: 10.1001/jama.290.5.621

Kinney, H. C., and Volpe, J. J. (2012). Modeling the encephalopathy of prematurity in animals: the important role of translational research. *Neurol. Res. Int.* 2012:295389. doi: 10.1155/2012/295389

Koepsell, T. D., Rivara, F. P., Vavilala, M. S., Wang, J., Temkin, N., Jaffe, K. M., et al. (2011). Incidence and descriptive epidemiologic features of traumatic brain injury in King County, Washington. *Pediatrics* 128, 946–954. doi: 10.1542/peds.2010-2259

Krafft, P. R., Rolland, W. B., Duris, K., Lekic, T., Campbell, A., Tang, J., et al. (2012). Modeling intracerebral hemorrhage in mice: injection of autologous blood or bacterial collagenase. *J. Vis. Exp.* e4289. doi: 10.3791/4289

Kumar, A., Mittal, R., Khanna, H. D., and Basu, S. (2008). Free radical injury and blood-brain barrier permeability in hypoxic-ischemic encephalopathy. *Pediatrics* 122, e722–e727. doi: 10.1542/peds.2008-0269

Kuntz, M., Mysiorek, C., Petrault, O., Petrault, M., Uzbekov, R., Bordet, R., et al. (2014). Stroke-induced brain parenchymal injury drives blood-brain barrier early leakage kinetics: a combined *in vivo/in vitro* study. *J. Cereb. Blood Flow Metab.* 34, 95–107. doi: 10.1038/jcbfm.2013.169

Labus, J., Hackel, S., Lucka, L., and Danker, K. (2014). Interleukin-1beta induces an inflammatory response and the breakdown of the endothelial cell layer in an improved human THBMEC-based *in vitro* blood-brain barrier model. *J. Neurosci. Methods* 228, 35–45. doi: 10.1016/j.jneumeth.2014.03.002

Lakhan, S. E., Kirchgessner, A., Tepper, D., and Leonard, A. (2013). Matrix metalloproteinases and blood-brain barrier disruption in acute ischemic stroke. *Front. Neurol.* 4:32. doi: 10.3389/fneur.2013.00032

Lee, C. Z., Xue, Z., Zhu, Y., Yang, G. Y., and Young, W. L. (2007). Matrix metalloproteinase-9 inhibition attenuates vascular endothelial growth factor-induced intracerebral hemorrhage. *Stroke* 38, 2563–2568. doi: 10.1161/STROKEAHA.106.481515

Lee, J., Croen, L. A., Lindan, C., Nash, K. B., Yoshida, C. K., Ferriero, D. M., et al. (2005). Predictors of outcome in perinatal arterial stroke: a population-based study. *Ann. Neurol.* 58, 303–308. doi: 10.1002/ana.20557

Lekic, T., Manaenko, A., Rolland, W., Krafft, P. R., Peters, R., Hartman, R. E., et al. (2012). Rodent neonatal germinal matrix hemorrhage mimics the human brain injury, neurological consequences, and post-hemorrhagic hydrocephalus. *Exp. Neurol.* 236, 69–78. doi: 10.1016/j.expneurol.2012.04.003

Lipton, S. A., and Rosenberg, P. A. (1994). Excitatory amino acids as a final common pathway for neurologic disorders. *N. Engl. J. Med.* 330, 613–622. doi: 10.1056/NEJM199403033300907

Liu, J., Jin, X., Liu, K. J., and Liu, W. (2012). Matrix metalloproteinase-2-mediated claudin-5 redistribution contribute to blood brain barrier damage in early ischemic stroke stage. *J. Neurosci.* 9, 3044–3057. doi: 10.1523/JNEUROSCI.6409-11.2012

Liu, W., Hendren, J., Qin, X. J., Shen, J., and Liu, K. J. (2009). Normobaric hyperoxia attenuates early blood-brain barrier disruption by inhibiting MMP-9-mediated occludin degradation in focal cerebral ischemia. *J. Neurochem.* 108, 811–820. doi: 10.1111/j.1471-4159.2008.05821.x

Lo, E. H. (2008). A new penumbra: transitioning from injury into repair after stroke. *Nat. Med.* 14, 497–500. doi: 10.1038/nm1735

Lodygensky, G. A., Kunz, N., Perroud, E., Somm, E., Mlynarik, V., Huppi, P. S., et al. (2014). Definition and quantification of acute inflammatory white matter injury in the immature brain by MRI/MRS at high magnetic field. *Pediatr. Res.* 75, 415–423. doi: 10.1038/pr.2013.242

Longhi, L., Saatman, K. E., Raghupathi, R., Laurer, H. L., Lenzlinger, P. M., Riess, P., et al. (2001). A review and rationale for the use of genetically engineered animals in the study of traumatic brain injury. *J. Cereb. Blood Flow Metab.* 21, 1241–1258. doi: 10.1097/00004647-200111000-00001

Lorant, D. E., Li, W., Tabatabaei, N., Garver, M. K., and Albertine, K. H. (1999). P-selectin expression by endothelial cells is decreased in neonatal rats and human premature infants. *Blood* 94, 600–609.

Low, J. A. (2004). Determining the contribution of asphyxia to brain damage in the neonate. *J. Obstet. Gynaecol. Res.* 30, 276–286. doi: 10.1111/j.1447-0756.2004.00194.x

Lynch, J. K., Hirtz, D. G., DeVeber, G., and Nelson, K. B. (2002). Report of the National Institute of Neurological Disorders and Stroke workshop on perinatal and childhood stroke. *Pediatrics* 109, 116–123. doi: 10.1542/peds.109.1.116

Maier, C. M., Hsieh, L., Crandall, T., Narasimhan, P., and Chan, P. H. (2006). Evaluating therapeutic targets for reperfusion-related brain hemorrhage. *Ann. Neurol.* 59, 929–938. doi: 10.1002/ana.20850

Mark, K. S., and Davis, T. P. (2002). Cerebral microvascular changes in permeability and tight junctions induced by hypoxia-reoxygenation. *Am. J. Physiol. Heart Circ. Physiol.* 282, H1485–H1494. doi: 10.1152/ajpheart.00645.2001

Marret, S., Mukendi, R., Gadisseux, J. F., Gressens, P., and Evrard, P. (1995). Effect of ibotenate on brain development: an excitotoxic mouse model of microgyria and posthypoxic-like lesions. *J. Neuropathol. Exp. Neurol.* 54, 358–370. doi: 10.1097/00005072-199505000-00009

Marti, H. J., Bernaudin, M., Bellail, A., Schoch, H., Euler, M., Petit, E., et al. (2000). Hypoxia-induced vascular endothelial growth factor expression precedes neovascularization after cerebral ischemia. *Am. J. Pathol.* 156, 965–976. doi: 10.1016/S0002-9440(10)64964-4

McColl, B. W., Rothwell, N. J., and Allan, S. M. (2008). Systemic inflammation alters the kinetics of cerebrovascular tight junction disruption after experimental stroke in mice. *J. Neurosci.* 28, 9451–9462. doi: 10.1523/JNEUROSCI.2674-08.2008

McLean, C., and Ferriero, D. (2004). Mechanisms of hypoxic-ischemic injury in the term infant. *Semin. Perinatol.* 28, 425–432. doi: 10.1053/j.semperi.2004.10.005

Miller, S. L., Wallace, E. M., and Walker, D. W. (2012). Antioxidant therapies: a potential role in perinatal medicine. *Neuroendocrinology* 96, 13–23. doi: 10.1159/000336378

Muramatsu, K., Fukuda, A., Togari, H., Wada, Y., and Nishino, H. (1997). Vulnerability to cerebral hypoxic-ischemic insult in neonatal but not in adult rats is in parallel with disruption of the blood-brain barrier. *Stroke* 28, 2281–2288. discussion: 2288–2289. doi: 10.1161/01.STR.28.11.2281

O'Brien, J. S., and Sampson, E. L. (1965). Lipid composition of the normal human brain: gray matter, white matter, and myelin. *J. Lipid Res.* 6, 537–544.

Ohshima, M., Tsuji, M., Taguchi, A., Kasahara, Y., and Ikeda, T. (2012). Cerebral blood flow during reperfusion predicts later brain damage in a mouse and a rat model of neonatal hypoxic-ischemic encephalopathy. *Exp. Neurol.* 233, 481–489. doi: 10.1016/j.expneurol.2011.11.025

Perez-Asensio, F. J., Hurtado, O., Burguete, M. C., Moro, M. A., Salom, J. B., Lizasoain, I., et al. (2005). Inhibition of iNOS activity by 1400W decreases glutamate release and ameliorates stroke outcome after experimental ischemia. *Neurobiol. Dis.* 18, 375–384. doi: 10.1016/j.nbd.2004.10.018

Philip, A. G., Allan, W. C., Tito, A. M., and Wheeler, L. R. (1989). Intraventricular hemorrhage in preterm infants: declining incidence in the 1980s. *Pediatrics* 84, 797–801.

Pop, V., Sorensen, D. W., Kamper, J. E., Ajao, D. O., Murphy, M. P., Head, E., et al. (2013). Early brain injury alters the blood-brain barrier phenotype in parallel with beta-amyloid and cognitive changes in adulthood. *J. Cereb. Blood Flow Metab.* 33, 205–214. doi: 10.1038/jcbfm.2012.154

Purves, M. J. (1972). The physiology of the cerebral circulation. *Monogr. Physiol. Soc.* 1–414.

Quan, N., Stern, E. L., Whiteside, M. B., and Herkenham, M. (1999). Induction of pro-inflammatory cytokine mRNAs in the brain after peripheral injection of subseptic doses of lipopolysaccharide in the rat. *J. Neuroimmunol.* 93, 72–80. doi: 10.1016/S0165-5728(98)00193-3

Ramlackhansingh, A. F., Brooks, D. J., Greenwood, R. J., Bose, S. K., Turkheimer, F. E., Kinnunen, K. M., et al. (2011). Inflammation after trauma: microglial activation and traumatic brain injury. *Ann. Neurol.* 70, 374–383. doi: 10.1002/ana.22455

Reboldi, A., Coisne, C., Baumjohann, D., Benvenuto, F., Bottinelli, D., Lira, S., et al. (2009). C-C chemokine receptor 6-regulated entry of TH-17 cells into the CNS through the choroid plexus is required for the initiation of EAE. *Nat. Immunol.* 10, 514–523. doi: 10.1038/ni.1716

Rice, J. E. 3rd, Vannucci, R. C., and Brierley, J. B. (1981). The influence of immaturity on hypoxic-ischemic brain damage in the rat. *Ann. Neurol.* 9, 131–141. doi: 10.1002/ana.410090206

Riddle, A., Dean, J., Buser, J. R., Gong, X., Maire, J., Chen, K., et al. (2011). Histopathological correlates of magnetic resonance imaging-defined chronic perinatal white matter injury. *Ann. Neurol.* 70, 493–507. doi: 10.1002/ana.22501

Rivara, F. P., Vavilala, M. S., Durbin, D., Temkin, N., Wang, J., O'Connor, S. S., et al. (2012). Persistence of disability 24 to 36 months after pediatric traumatic brain injury: a cohort study. *J. Neurotrauma* 29, 2499–2504. doi: 10.1089/neu.2012.2434

Roozenbeek, B., Maas, A. I., and Menon, D. K. (2013). Changing patterns in the epidemiology of traumatic brain injury. *Nat. Rev. Neurol.* 9, 231–236. doi: 10.1038/nrneurol.2013.22

Rosenberg, G. A. (2009). Matrix metalloproteinases and their multiple roles in neurodegenerative diseases. *Lancet Neurol.* 8, 205–216. doi: 10.1016/S1474-4422(09)70016-X

Rosenberg, G. A., Estrada, E. Y., and Dencoff, J. E. (1998). Matrix metalloproteinases and TIMPs are associated with blood-brain barrier opening after reperfusion in rat brain. *Stroke* 29, 2189–2195. doi: 10.1161/01.STR.29.10.2189

Rosenberg, G. A., and Yang, Y. (2007). Vasogenic edema due to tight junction disruption by matrix metalloproteinases in cerebral ischemia. *Neurosurg. Focus* 22, E4. doi: 10.3171/foc.2007.22.5.5

Rossi, J. L., Todd, T., Bazan, N. G., and Belayev, L. (2013). Inhibition of Myosin light-chain kinase attenuates cerebral edema after traumatic brain injury in postnatal mice. *J. Neurotrauma* 30, 1672–1679. doi: 10.1089/neu.2013.2898

Rousset, C. I., Chalon, S., Cantagrel, S., Bodard, S., Andres, C., Gressens, P., et al. (2006). Maternal exposure to LPS induces hypomyelination in the internal capsule and programmed cell death in the deep gray matter in newborn rats. *Pediatr. Res.* 59, 428–433. doi: 10.1203/01.pdr.0000199905.08848.55

Sandoval, K. E., and Witt, K. A. (2008). Blood-brain barrier tight junction permeability and ischemic stroke. *Neurobiol. Dis.* 32, 200–219. doi: 10.1016/j.nbd.2008.08.005

Saunders, N. R., Liddelow, S. A., and Dziegielewska, K. M. (2012). Barrier mechanisms in the developing brain. *Front. Pharmacol.* 3:46. doi: 10.3389/fphar.2012.00046

Schang, A. L., Van Steenwinckel, J., Chevenne, D., Alkmark, M., Hagberg, H., Gressens, P., et al. (2014). Failure of thyroid hormone treatment to prevent inflammation-induced white matter injury in the immature brain. *Brain Behav. Immun.* 37, 95–102. doi: 10.1016/j.bbi.2013.11.005

Schmitt, C., Strazielle, N., and Ghersi-Egea, J. F. (2012). Brain leukocyte infiltration initiated by peripheral inflammation or experimental autoimmune encephalomyelitis occurs through pathways connected to the CSF-filled compartments of the forebrain and midbrain. *J. Neuroinflammation* 9, 187. doi: 10.1186/1742-2094-9-187

Schnell, L., Fearn, S., Schwab, M. E., Perry, V. H., and Anthony, D. C. (1999). Cytokine-induced acute inflammation in the brain and spinal cord. *J. Neuropathol. Exp. Neurol.* 58, 245–254. doi: 10.1097/00005072-199903000-00004

Schuhmann, M. U., Stiller, D., Skardelly, M., Bernarding, J., Klinge, P. M., Samii, A., et al. (2003). Metabolic changes in the vicinity of brain contusions: a proton magnetic resonance spectroscopy and histology study. *J. Neurotrauma* 20, 725–743. doi: 10.1089/089771503767869962

Semenza, G. L. (2010). Vascular responses to hypoxia and ischemia. *Arterioscler. Thromb. Vasc. Biol.* 30, 648–652. doi: 10.1161/ATVBAHA.108.181644

Shankaran, S., Laptook, A. R., Ehrenkranz, R. A., Tyson, J. E., McDonald, S. A., Donovan, E. F., et al. (2005). Whole-body hypothermia for neonates with hypoxic-ischemic encephalopathy. *N. Engl. J. Med.* 353, 1574–1584. doi: 10.1056/NEJMcps050929

Sheldon, R. A., Sedik, C., and Ferriero, D. M. (1998). Strain-related brain injury in neonatal mice subjected to hypoxia-ischemia. *Brain Res.* 810, 114–122. doi: 10.1016/S0006-8993(98)00892-0

Shimotake, J., Derugin, N., Wendland, M., Vexler, Z. S., and Ferriero, D. M. (2010). Vascular endothelial growth factor receptor-2 inhibition promotes cell death and limits endothelial cell proliferation in a neonatal rodent model of stroke. *Stroke* 41, 343–349. doi: 10.1161/STROKEAHA.109.564229

Simi, A., Tsakiri, N., Wang, P., and Rothwell, N. J. (2007). Interleukin-1 and inflammatory neurodegeneration. *Biochem. Soc. Trans.* 35, 1122–1126. doi: 10.1042/BST0351122

Skuli, N., Liu, L., Runge, A., Wang, T., Yuan, L., Patel, S., et al. (2009). Endothelial deletion of hypoxia-inducible factor-2alpha (HIF-2alpha) alters vascular function and tumor angiogenesis. *Blood* 114, 469–477. doi: 10.1182/blood-2008-12-193581

Stanley, R. M., Bonsu, B. K., Zhao, W., Ehrlich, P. F., Rogers, A. J., and Xiang, H. (2012). US estimates of hospitalized children with severe traumatic brain injury: implications for clinical trials. *Pediatrics* 129, e24–e30. doi: 10.1542/peds.2011-2074

Stokely, M. E., and Orr, E. L. (2008). Acute effects of calvarial damage on dural mast cells, pial vascular permeability, and cerebral cortical histamine levels in rats and mice. *J. Neurotrauma* 25, 52–61. doi: 10.1089/neu.2007.0397

Stolp, H. B., Dziegielewska, K. M., Ek, C. J., Potter, A. M., and Saunders, N. R. (2005). Long-term changes in blood-brain barrier permeability and white matter following prolonged systemic inflammation in early development in the rat. *Eur. J. Neurosci.* 22, 2805–2816. doi: 10.1111/j.1460-9568.2005.04483.x

Stolp, H. B., Johansson, P. A., Habgood, M. D., Dziegielewska, K. M., Saunders, N. R., and Ek, C. J. (2011). Effects of neonatal systemic inflammation on blood-brain barrier permeability and behaviour in juvenile and adult rats. *Cardiovasc. Psychiatry Neurol.* 2011:469046. doi: 10.1155/2011/469046

Stonestreet, B. S., Sadowska, G. B., Leeman, J., Hanumara, R. C., Petersson, K. H., and Patlak, C. S. (2006). Effects of acute hyperosmolality on blood-brain barrier function in ovine fetuses and lambs. *Am. J. Physiol. Regul. Integr. Comp. Physiol.* 291, R1031–R1039. doi: 10.1152/ajpregu.00883.2005

Strbian, D., Karjalainen-Lindsberg, M. L., Tatlisumak, T., and Lindsberg, P. J. (2006). Cerebral mast cells regulate early ischemic brain swelling and neutrophil accumulation. *J. Cereb. Blood Flow Metab.* 26, 605–612. doi: 10.1038/sj.jcbfm.9600228

Svedin, P., Hagberg, H., Savman, K., Zhu, C., and Mallard, C. (2007). Matrix metalloproteinase-9 gene knock-out protects the immature brain after cerebral hypoxia-ischemia. *J. Neurosci.* 27, 1511–1518. doi: 10.1523/JNEUROSCI.4391-06.2007

Szmydynger-Chodobska, J., Strazielle, N., Gandy, J. R., Keefe, T. H., Zink, B. J., Ghersi-Egea, J. F., et al. (2012). Posttraumatic invasion of monocytes across the blood-cerebrospinal fluid barrier. *J. Cereb. Blood Flow Metab.* 32, 93–104. doi: 10.1038/jcbfm.2011.111

Szmydynger-Chodobska, J., Strazielle, N., Zink, B. J., Ghersi-Egea, J. F., and Chodobski, A. (2009). The role of the choroid plexus in neutrophil invasion after traumatic brain injury. *J. Cereb. Blood Flow Metab.* 29, 1503–1516. doi: 10.1038/jcbfm.2009.71

Tagin, M. A., Woolcott, C. G., Vincer, M. J., Whyte, R. K., and Stinson, D. A. (2012). Hypothermia for neonatal hypoxic ischemic encephalopathy: an updated systematic review and meta-analysis. *Arch. Pediatr. Adolesc. Med.* 166, 558–566. doi: 10.1001/archpediatrics.2011.1772

Tahraoui, S. L., Marret, S., Bodenant, C., Leroux, P., Dommergues, M. A., Evrard, P., et al. (2001). Central role of microglia in neonatal excitotoxic lesions of the murine periventricular white matter. *Brain Pathol.* 11, 56–71. doi: 10.1111/j.1750-3639.2001.tb00381.x

Tcharmtchi, M. H., Smith, C. W., and Mariscalco, M. M. (2000). Neonatal neutrophil interaction with P-selectin: contribution of P-selectin glycoprotein ligand-1 and sialic acid. *J. Leukoc. Biol.* 67, 73–80.

Thibeault, I., Laflamme, N., and Rivest, S. (2001). Regulation of the gene encoding the monocyte chemoattractant protein 1 (MCP-1) in the mouse and rat brain in response to circulating LPS and proinflammatory cytokines. *J. Comp. Neurol.* 434, 461–477. doi: 10.1002/cne.1187

Thompson, H. J., Lifshitz, J., Marklund, N., Grady, M. S., Graham, D. I., Hovda, D. A., et al. (2005). Lateral fluid percussion brain injury: a 15-year review and evaluation. *J. Neurotrauma* 22, 42–75. doi: 10.1089/neu.2005.22.42

Tosun, C., Koltz, M. T., Kurland, D. B., Ijaz, H., Gurakar, M., Schwartzbauer, G., et al. (2013). The protective effect of glibenclamide in a model of hemorrhagic encephalopathy of prematurity. *Brain Sci.* 3, 215–238. doi: 10.3390/brainsci3010215

Tsuji, M., Ohshima, M., Taguchi, A., Kasahara, Y., Ikeda, T., and Matsuyama, T. (2013). A novel reproducible model of neonatal stroke in mice: comparison with a hypoxia-ischemia model. *Exp. Neurol.* 247, 218–225. doi: 10.1016/j.expneurol.2013.04.015

Tu, Y. F., Tsai, Y. S., Wang, L. W., Wu, H. C., Huang, C. C., and Ho, C. J. (2011). Overweight worsens apoptosis, neuroinflammation and blood-brain barrier damage after hypoxic ischemia in neonatal brain through JNK hyperactivation. *J. Neuroinflammation* 8:40. doi: 10.1186/1742-2094-8-40

Vannucci, S. J., and Hagberg, H. (2004). Hypoxia-ischemia in the immature brain. *J. Exp. Biol.* 207, 3149–3154. doi: 10.1242/jeb.01064

Verney, C., Pogledic, I., Biran, V., Adle-Biassette, H., Fallet-Bianco, C., and Gressens, P. (2012). Microglial reaction in axonal crossroads is a hallmark of noncystic periventricular white matter injury in very preterm infants. *J. Neuropathol. Exp. Neurol.* 71, 251–264. doi: 10.1097/NEN.0b013e3182496429

Vexler, Z. S., and Yenari, M. A. (2009). Does inflammation after stroke affect the developing brain differently than adult brain? *Dev. Neurosci.* 31, 378–393. doi: 10.1159/000232556

Virgintino, D., Errede, M., Robertson, D., Capobianco, C., Girolamo, F., Vimercati, A., et al. (2004). Immunolocalization of tight junction proteins in the adult and developing human brain. *Histochem. Cell Biol.* 122, 51–59. doi: 10.1007/s00418-004-0665-1

Vohr, B., Allan, W. C., Scott, D. T., Katz, K. H., Schneider, K. C., Makuch, R. W., et al. (1999). Early-onset intraventricular hemorrhage in preterm neonates: incidence of neurodevelopmental handicap. *Semin. Perinatol.* 23, 212–217. doi: 10.1016/S0146-0005(99)80065-2

Wilson-Costello, D., Friedman, H., Minich, N., Fanaroff, A. A., and Hack, M. (2005). Improved survival rates with increased neurodevelopmental disability for extremely low birth weight infants in the 1990s. *Pediatrics* 115, 997–1003. doi: 10.1542/peds.2004-0221

Witt, K. A., Mark, K. S., Hom, S., and Davis, T. P. (2003). Effects of hypoxia-reoxygenation on rat blood-brain barrier permeability and tight junctional protein expression. *Am. J. Physiol. Heart Circ. Physiol.* 285, H2820–H2831. doi: 10.1152/ajpheart.00589.2003

Xiong, Y., Mahmood, A., and Chopp, M. (2013). Animal models of traumatic brain injury. *Nat. Rev. Neurosci.* 14, 128–142. doi: 10.1038/nrn3407

Yan, E., Castillo-Melendez, M., Nicholls, T., Hirst, J., and Walker, D. (2004). Cerebrovascular responses in the fetal sheep brain to low-dose endotoxin. *Pediatr. Res.* 55, 855–863. doi: 10.1203/01.PDR.0000115681.95957.D4

Yang, D., Sun, Y. Y., Nemkul, N., Baumann, J. M., Shereen, A., Dunn, R. S., et al. (2013a). Plasminogen activator inhibitor-1 mitigates brain injury in a rat model of infection-sensitized neonatal hypoxia-ischemia. *Cereb. Cortex* 23, 1218–1229. doi: 10.1093/cercor/bhs115

Yang, Y., Estrada, E. Y., Thompson, J. F., Liu, W., and Rosenberg, G. A. (2007). Matrix metalloproteinase-mediated disruption of tight junction proteins in cerebral vessels is reversed by synthetic matrix metalloproteinase inhibitor in focal ischemia in rat. *J. Cereb. Blood Flow Metab.*27, 697–709. doi: 10.1038/sj.jcbfm.9600375

Yang, Y., and Rosenberg, G. A. (2011). MMP-mediated disruption of claudin-5 in the blood-brain barrier of rat brain after cerebral ischemia. *Methods Mol. Biol.* 762, 333–345. doi: 10.1007/978-1-61779-185-7_24

Yang, Y., Thompson, J. F., Taheri, S., Salayandia, V. M., McAvoy, T. A., Hill, J. W., et al. (2013b). Early inhibition of MMP activity in ischemic rat brain promotes expression of tight junction proteins and angiogenesis during recovery. *J. Cereb. Blood Flow Metab.* 33, 1104–1114. doi: 10.1038/jcbfm.2013.56

Yoon, B. H., Romero, R., Kim, C. J., Koo, J. N., Choe, G., Syn, H. C., et al. (1997). High expression of tumor necrosis factor-alpha and interleukin-6 in periventricular leukomalacia. *Am. J. Obstet. Gynecol.* 177, 406–411. doi: 10.1016/S0002-9378(97)70206-0

Yoshioka, H., Iino, S., Sato, N., Osamura, T., Hasegawa, K., Ochi, M., et al. (1989). New model of hemorrhagic hypoxic-ischemic encephalopathy in newborn mice. *Pediatr. Neurol.* 5, 221–225. doi: 10.1016/0887-8994(89)90079-9

Zehendner, C. M., Librizzi, L., Hedrich, J., Bauer, N. M., Angamo, E. A., de Curtis, M., et al. (2013). Moderate hypoxia followed by reoxygenation results in blood-brain barrier breakdown via oxidative stress-dependent tight-junction protein disruption. *PLoS ONE* 8:e82823. doi: 10.1371/journal.pone.0082823

Zhang, W., Smith, C., Howlett, C., and Stanimirovic, D. (2000). Inflammatory activation of human brain endothelial cells by hypoxic astrocytes *in vitro* is mediated by IL-1beta. *J. Cereb. Blood Flow Metab.* 20, 967–978. doi: 10.1097/00004647-200006000-00009

12

Dissecting gene expression at the blood-brain barrier

Melanie A. Huntley[1†], Nga Bien-Ly[2†], Richard Daneman[3*] and Ryan J. Watts[2*]

[1] Department of Bioinformatics and Computational Biology, Genentech Inc., South San Francisco, CA, USA
[2] Department of Neuroscience, Genentech Inc., South San Francisco, CA, USA
[3] Department of Pharmacology, University of California, San Diego, La Jolla, CA, USA

***Correspondence:**
*Richard Daneman, Department of Pharmacology, University of California San Diego, 9500 Gilman Drive 0636, La Jolla, 92093 CA, USA
e-mail: rdaneman@ucsd.edu;
Ryan J. Watts, Department of Neuroscience, Genentech Inc., 1 DNA Way, South San Francisco, 94080 CA, USA
e-mail: watts.ryan@gene.com*

†These authors have contributed equally to this work.

The availability of genome-wide expression data for the blood-brain barrier is an invaluable resource that has recently enabled the discovery of several genes and pathways involved in the development and maintenance of the blood-brain barrier, particularly in rodent models. The broad distribution of published data sets represents a viable starting point for the molecular dissection of the blood-brain barrier and will further direct the discovery of novel mechanisms of blood-brain barrier formation and function. Technical advances in purifying brain endothelial cells, the key cell that forms the critical barrier, have allowed for greater specificity in gene expression comparisons with other central nervous system cell types, and more systematic characterizations of the molecular composition of the blood-brain barrier. Nevertheless, our understanding of how the blood-brain barrier changes during aging and disease is underrepresented. Blood-brain barrier data sets from a wider range of experimental paradigms and species, including invertebrates and primates, would be invaluable for investigating the function and evolution of the blood-brain barrier. Newer technologies in gene expression profiling, such as RNA-sequencing, now allow for finer resolution of transcriptomic changes, including isoform specificity and RNA-editing. As our field continues to utilize more advanced expression profiling in its ongoing efforts to elucidate the blood-brain barrier, including in disease and drug delivery, we will continue to see rapid advances in our understanding of the molecular mediators of barrier biology. We predict that the recently published data sets, combined with forthcoming genomic and proteomic blood-brain barrier data sets, will continue to fuel the molecular genetic revolution of blood-brain barrier biology.

Keywords: blood-brain barrier, transcriptome, genomics, brain endothelial cells, expression profiling

1. HISTORICAL PERSPECTIVE ON DATASETS

In 1967 using exogenous peroxidase, Reese and Karnovsky demonstrated the subcellular localization of the blood-brain barrier (BBB) to be the endothelium forming the walls of vessels in the brain (Reese and Karnovsky, 1967). Two structural characteristics distinguished these endothelial cells from those in the heart and skeletal muscle: the presence of tight junctions, and the paucity of micropinocytotic vesicles. Early studies used microscopy and immunohistochemistry to visualize the presence and localization of a handful of known proteins within brain endothelial cells (BECs) (Risau et al., 1986), while *in situ* hybridization filled in the gaps for questions about expression patterns when antibodies were not available for specific targets. Nearly fifty years later, the underlying genes and developmental cascades that result in the unique traits of BECs are just beginning to be understood. Current critical advancements in our ability to both purify and culture BECs now allow for the study of their molecular mechanisms at an unprecedented level of breadth and depth.

Since the seminal discovery that brain endothelial cells limit the diffusion of blood-borne molecules, the following decades of work have made it clear that the BBB is not just a physical wall but a complex regulated physiology that allows the BECs to determine the movement of ions, molecules and cells between the blood and the neural tissue. At the heart of this physiology are molecular and structural specializations of BECs that differentiate them from endothelial cells in non-neural tissue. BECs are held together by tight junctions, which form a tight paracellular barrier that polarizes the cells into distinct luminal and abluminal membrane compartments. This tight paracellular junction coupled with the extremely low levels of transcytosis creates a physical barrier to hydrophilic molecules and allows cellular transport properties to determine movement of molecules between the blood and the brain. To regulate this movement, BECs express a series of different transporters that generally fall into two categories: efflux transporters and nutrient transporters (for an in depth review of BBB transporters see Saunders et al., 2013). Briefly, efflux transporters, such as ABCB1 (also known as p-glycoprotein, or Pgp), face the luminal surface and use energy generated from the hydrolysis of ATP to pump a wide

Abbreviations: ABC, ATP binding cassette; BBB, blood-brain barrier; BEC, brain endothelial cell; FACS, fluorescence activated cell sorting; HBMEC, human brain microvessel endothelial cell; hCMEC/D3, human cerebral microvascular endothelial cell line; HUVEC, human umbilical vein endothelial cell; LCM, laser capture microdissection; miRNA, microRNA.

array of lipophilic substrates up their concentrations gradients into the blood, thus limiting the passive diffusion of hydrophobic molecules into the brain. Nutrient transporters, such as Glut-1 (glucose transporter SLC2A1), Lat-1 (amino acid transporter light chain, SLC7A5) and Mct-1 (monocarboxylate transporter, SLC16A1), facilitate the movement of specific substrates down their concentration gradients, allowing specific molecules into or out of the brain. Thus, the BBB is not solely a physical barrier but it is a series of complex regulated physiological specializations of the BECs that control the microenvironment of the brain. Furthermore, work has demonstrated that many of these specializations of the BECs are not intrinsic, but regulated by interactions with neural cells including CNS pericytes and astrocytes, and immune cells including microglia and macrophages (Hudson et al., 2005; Armulik et al., 2011). Identifying the molecular signature of BECs and how they differ from ECs in other tissues, as well as key cell-cell signaling interactions in the neurovascular unit, are questions at the forefront in understanding the physiology of the BBB.

2. THE UTILITY OF DATASETS AS RESOURCES

High quality gene expression data has significantly impacted the direction of investigation by allowing for a better molecular understanding of BBB development, function, and dysfunction. Well-powered gene expression studies can validate hypothesis driven queries or open previously unexplored avenues of research in unbiased directions. Models of acute BBB dysfunction, such as stroke or ischemia, aid in elucidating mechanisms of impairment for development of therapeutics or preventative treatments. An understanding of BBB-specific transporter, receptor, and ion channel expression levels could benefit drug development efforts by aiding in the design of selective compounds for those that could evade efflux pumps (Pottiez et al., 2009) or utilize receptors to enhance therapeutic uptake in brain (Yu and Watts, 2013).

The variety of questions and issues that can be addressed related to BBB development and disease have vastly improved, thanks in part to genetic engineering approaches in rodents and other species, improved cellular isolation techniques, and the availability of bioinformatics software and experts that facilitate the mining of data sets for relevant genes worthy of further investigation. The combination of "big data" sets and molecular-genetic tools is beginning to elucidate biological mechanisms in many arenas, and our understanding of BBB biology is benefiting from this revolution.

2.1. KEY PARAMETERS FOR BBB GENOMIC STUDIES

The cellular complexity of the BBB presents a significant obstacle in the gathering of meaningful gene expression data. Brain endothelial cells are surrounded by the mural cells–pericytes and smooth muscle cells–and are further encapsulated by a basement membrane (see **Figure 1C**). The ensheathment of the vessels by astrocytic endfeet, likely receiving signals from neurons and microglia, serve to further regulate brain vascular function (Abbott, 2005). Therefore, these various cell types are intimately connected and unite in maintaining the integrity of the BBB. Thus a global analysis of BBB gene expression may necessitate the co-purification and co-analysis of these important non-BEC cell types along with BECs (Shusta, 2005). Early efforts to harvest brain vasculature for genomic analysis captured a majority of the cell types associated with BECs of the neurovascular unit. These earlier protocols relied on mechanical brain dissociation to isolate microvascular components, a technique known as vascular enrichment (Triguero et al., 1990; Boado and Pardridge, 1991), which uses a series of filtrations through nylon membranes or with glass beads followed with gradient centrifugation steps (Betz et al., 1979; Yousif et al., 2007). This contrasted with laser capture microdissection (LCM) methods for single capillary fragment isolation, which allows for highly localized sampling from specific human and mouse brain sections and could be restricted to diseased regions (Ball et al., 2002; Mojsilovic-Petrovic et al., 2004). Again, both methods do not specifically yield pure populations of BECs specifically, however, they do allow for a sampling of cells associated with the neurovascular unit and generally enrich for BECs for inferences to be drawn about CNS microvasculature.

Thus, several important considerations must be taken into account when designing genomic experiments to analyze the BBB. The most important parameter is to determine the desired cells or tissues to be analyzed and the method of purification. Because the key properties of the BBB are specializations of BECs, many studies have used methods to purify ECs from brain tissue, whereas others have used crude approaches to purify vessels (endothelial cells and pericytes) or entire fragments of the neurovascular unit (see **Figure 1**). In addition, the vasculature of the brain contains many different segments of the vascular tree including arteries, arterioles, capillaries, post-capillary venules, venules, and veins (Dorr et al., 2007), all of which contain barrier properties but each segment may have different transport, metabolic, signaling and cell adhesion properties. Gradient centrifugation has been used to specifically isolate microvessels (capillaries and post-capillary venules), whereas purification based on markers of ECs will contain BECs from all segments of the vascular tree. Also taken into consideration should be the species from which the samples are isolated, whether human, rodent or other model organism, and whether to examine acutely purified or cultured cells. The second parameter is the method of analysis. For transcriptomic generation of EST libraries, subtractive hybridization, microarrays and RNA sequencing are all common methods to examine RNA. Different methods of RNA extraction, including whole RNA, mRNA, small RNA, and tagged-ribosome isolation can highlight specific RNAs of interest. In addition, proteomics, metabolomics, lipidomics, epigenomics, and other "omics" analysis can give an even broader overview of the molecular composition of the BBB. The third parameter is the effective comparisons used for differential gene expression analysis. Identifying all the transcripts in a given cell can be challenging to decipher, however, generating a comparison of two cells that vary only for a given function can greatly narrow down the search for important genes. In the case of the BBB, several important comparisons have been made, including comparing BECs with whole brain extracts to identify EC specific genes, as well as comparing BECs with peripheral ECs to identify BBB-specific specializations (see **Table 1** for a summary of recent BBB expression profiling studies). The fourth important parameter to determine is the physiological setting in which to analyze the BBB. Much work has been done to identify

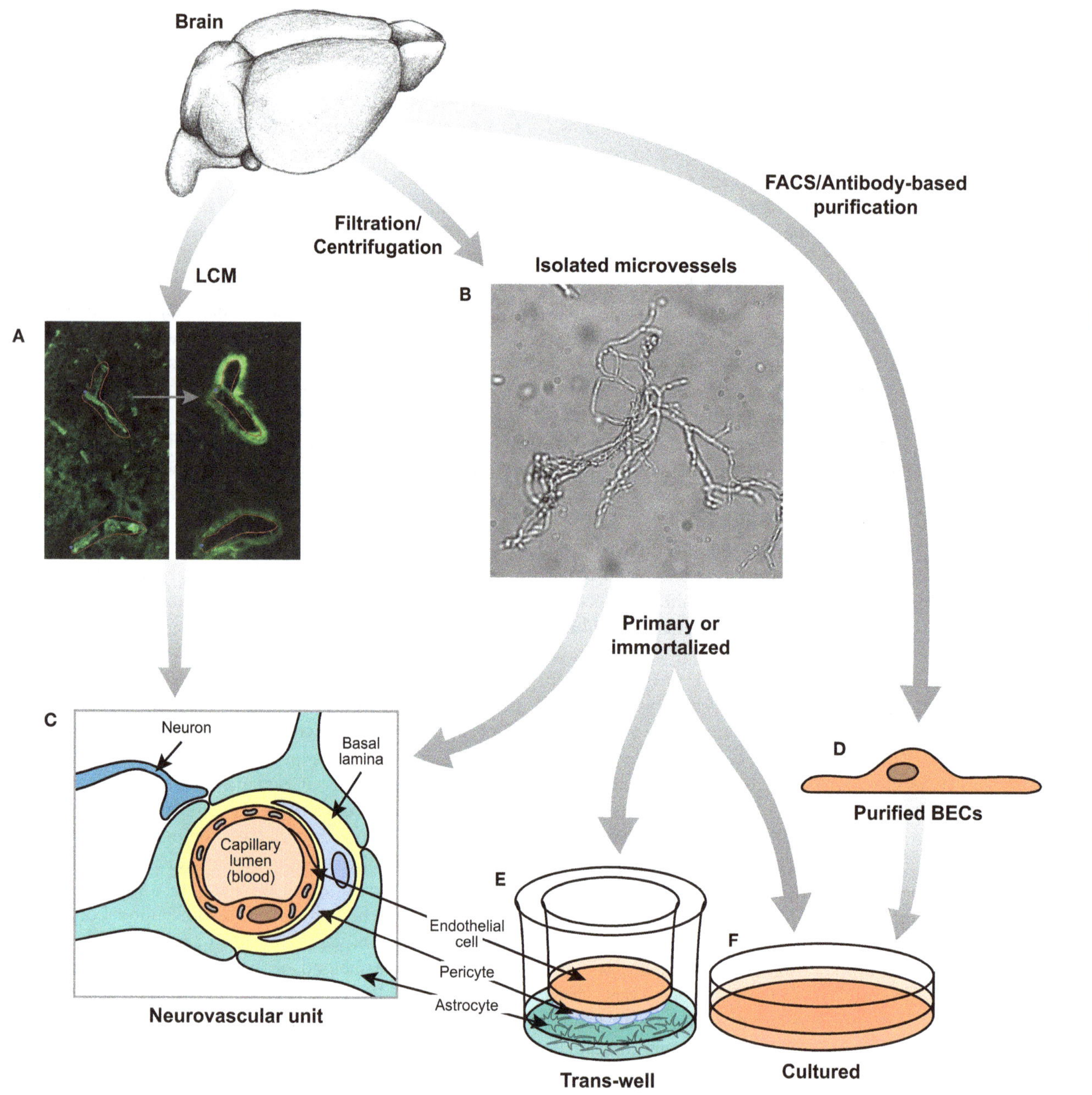

FIGURE 1 | Techniques for isolating BECs. (A) Laser capture microdissection or **(B)** mechanical filtration of brain microvessels can be used to isolate segments of the neurovascular unit **(C)**. FACS or other antibody based purification **(D)** can be performed to isolate BECs acutely. Isolated microvessels **(B)** and purified BECs **(D)** can be further cultured in a trans-well system **(E)** or other relevant *in vitro* culture systems **(F)**. Experiments based on the neurovascular unit **(C)**, purified primary BECs **(D)** and cultured BECs **(E,F)** will each provide valuable, but different insights into the biology of the BBB.

the gene expression signature of the BBB in a healthy adult animal, but studies have also examined the BBB during development, in different neurological disease settings, in mice with different mutations that affect BBB formation and function, or with the addition of different pharmacological agents. Each of these parameters will greatly influence the data set obtained and therefore careful consideration must be taken to ensure the best method of BEC purification and analysis.

2.2. METHODS OF ANALYSIS

Earlier transcriptomic approaches that yielded important initial insights on brain microvascular specific expression data included suppression subtractive hybridization and serial analysis of gene expression (SAGE) (Li et al., 2001; Shusta et al., 2002; Enerson and Drewes, 2006; Calabria and Shusta, 2008). For a detailed review on these techniques and early results, see Shusta (2005), Pottiez et al. (2009). A distinguishing aspect of the SAGE study of

Table 1 | Recent genomewide microarray expression data sets for the BBB.

Method of BBB isolation	Relevant study details	Species	*Dev study	Other tissues	Disease
ANTIBODY-BASED/FACS PURIFICATION					
Ben-Zvi et al., 2014	Tie2-GFP embryonic ECs from brain and lung	Mouse		+	
Tam et al., 2012	ECs from liver, lung, brain in embryo, pup, adult	Mouse	+	+	
Daneman et al., 2010a	Adult VCs from liver, lung, brain (+ postnatal), BECs and parenchyma	Mouse	+		
Daneman et al., 2010b	BECs from PDGFRb KO mice; BECs and pericytes from wild-type	Mouse	+		
Daneman et al., 2009	Tie2-GFP adult ECs from brain, liver and lung	Mouse		+	
Lyck et al., 2009	Primary PECAM+ BMECs, cultured b.End5 cells and BMECs	Mouse			
LCM					
Dieterich et al., 2012	Blood vessels associated with gliobastoma tumors	Human			+
Cunnea et al., 2010	Brain microvessels in multiple sclerosis patients	Human			+
Giger et al., 2010	Pyramidal neurons and vascular endothelium	Human			
Harris et al., 2008	Neurons and microvessels in schizophrenia patients	Human		+	+
FILTRATION/CENTRIFUGATION					
Wang et al., 2012a	BMVs from Alzheimer's patients and controls	Human			+
Armulik et al., 2010	BMVs from wild type, Tie2Cre, R26P+/0, pdgfb−/− (pericyte deficient)	Mouse	+		
He et al., 2011	BMVs from adult male rats	Rat			
CELL CULTURE					
Reijerkerk et al., 2013	Naive hCMEC/D3 cells with TNFα, IFNγ; astrocyte-media cultured	Human			
Lopez-Ramirez et al., 2013	hCMEC/D3 cells with TNFα and IFNγ	Human			+
Urich et al., 2012	hCMEC/D3 cells and human primary BECs	Human			
Barbier et al., 2011	HBECs with platelets ± TNF, plasmodium infected RBCs	Human			+
Himburg et al., 2010	BEC cultures and non-brain EC cultures	Human		+	
Li et al., 2008	HBMECs treated with amyloid-β	Human			+

**Developmental stages. BEC, brain endothelial cell; BMEC, brain microvascular endothelial cell; BMV, brain microvessel; HBEC, human brain endothelial cell; HBMEC, human brain microvessel endothelial cells; EC, endothelial cell; RBC, red blood cell; VC, vascular cell.*

rat brain microvessels was the comparison to rat neocortex and hippocampus tag catalogs and the resulting identification of 864 BBB enriched genes.

Today, expression microarrays offer a mature and commonly used platform to differentially compare gene expression between two samples. One of the earliest BBB gene expression studies using microarray established a protocol to profile human brain endothelial cells co-cultured with astrocytes under dynamic conditions with controlled intraluminal flow (Marroni et al., 2003). The authors observed that exposure to increased flow up-regulated cytoskeletal genes while also inhibiting cell cycling genes.

In the era of microarray data sets on the BBB (see **Table 1**), the number of genes that are queried on commercially available chips has increased several orders of magnitude, moving the field into truly high-throughput experiments and data. In addition, relatively small amounts of cells or tissue are now required for genome-wide transcriptomic approaches, thus facilitating a wide range of studies. Advancements and maturity of computational tools for this type of data analysis are now available allowing investigators to dive into these data sets and identify meaningful connections (Irizarry et al., 2003; Gentleman et al., 2004; Smyth, 2004; Falcon and Gentleman, 2007; Kauffmann et al., 2009). Online repositories, such as Gene Expression Omnibus and the European Nucleotide Archive, now allow researchers to deposit genome wide expression data sets to be queried and re-used by other groups. Indeed, many of the studies listed in **Table 1** have made use of previously published expression data sets from the BBB as an integral part of their analyses. The importance of continuing to expand the public availability of such data sets as an ongoing resource for the community cannot be overstated.

A discussion of newer techniques, such as next generation RNA-sequencing, will follow at the conclusion of this review.

3. EXPERIMENTAL PARADIGMS ANALYZED

Figure 1 summarizes the most common methods for isolation and purification used in BBB genome-wide expression studies. As many recent studies have shown, *in vitro* models of the BBB do not fully recapitulate the complexity of an intact organism. The use of newer techniques such as fluorescence activated cell sorting (FACS), immunopanning, magnetic bead immunoprecipitation, as well as advances to LCM may aid in acutely harvesting specifically BECs, or an enriched population of BECs, for downstream transcriptomic and proteomic studies. Navone et al. (2013) document recent protocols for the isolation of human and mouse brain microvascular endothelial cells. However, no technique or protocol is perfect as there are subtle considerations to be aware of which may factor largely into downstream data analysis. Even careful acute isolation and genomic profiling of BECs may be susceptible to general expression changes induced by mechanical shearing of brain parenchyma and/or microvessel tissue, enzymatic digestion, temperature fluctuations, etc. Careful pair-wise comparisons with the proper controls undergoing similar handling are critical to minimize bias in the data.

3.1. ACUTE ISOLATION AND PURIFICATION OF BRAIN MICROVASCULAR CELLS

The use of antibody-based techniques to isolate rodent brain endothelial cells has been reported in several recent studies. Magnetic beads coupled to murine or rat antibodies against CD31/PECAM allow for immunoprecipitation of endothelial cells from homogenates of brain (Lyck et al., 2009) and possibly other vascular organs for direct comparisons. Likewise, antibodies against CD31 can be immobilized onto culture plates for immunopanning enrichment of brain homogenates for acute isolation of BECs (Zhou et al., 2014a) or the use of other cell surface receptors such as anti-PDGFRβ for pericytes (Daneman et al., 2010b). This approach also allows for a negative selection step against microglia or pericytes to remove these non-BEC subtypes from the overall homogenate. A third BEC-specific antibody or antigen-selection technique utilizes fluorescence-activated cell sorting which would use either a fluorophore-coupled anti-BEC cellular marker (Daneman et al., 2010b; Tam et al., 2012) or transgenic mice that harbor BEC-specific promoters to direct expression of a fluorescent protein, such as Tie2-GFP mice (Daneman et al., 2009, 2010a; Ben-Zvi et al., 2014).

Moreover, LCM has experienced many improvements including the addition of immunostaining protocols and brighter, more specific dyes for identification of brain endothelia (Macdonald et al., 2008). Recent immuno-LCM studies have described differences in gene expression of brain capillaries vs. venules, and highlighted important roles for their heterogeneity (Macdonald et al., 2010). Increased antibody availability for other neurovascular unit cell types have also enabled cross comparison of gene expression as well as validation of cell type specificity of the data sets generated by mass spectrometry (Murugesan et al., 2011). Advances in equipment such as microscopes with automated stages, higher quality cameras, and sophisticated software have enabled more consistent tissue sampling and higher throughput.

3.2. *IN VITRO* BBB MODELS

Immortalized cell lines derived from rodent or human brain endothelial cells have been frequently used as a model system for gene expression studies despite their questionable physiological relevance. Cultured cells, especially those that can be passaged indefinitely, represent a key model system that allows for a high level of cellular homogeneity, consistency, and experimental reproducibility. Key components of the neurovascular unit can be reconstituted *in vitro* by growing BECs on filter inserts that sit above pericytes and/or astrocytes, allowing signaling mechanisms between these cell types to remain largely intact. Conversely, *in vitro* models may still lack the complex interactions between these cell types and the endogenous extracellular matrix, as well as surrounding neurons and microglia that exist *in vivo*. Complicated disease processes that are also in play *in vivo* are likely difficult to fully model in a transwell culture system and suffer from numerous drawbacks (Hawkins and Egleton, 2008; Pottiez et al., 2009). In other words, the neurovascular unit is essentially an organ system with numerous cellular interactions that make it virtually impossible to replicate outside of the organism. However, these culture paradigms also do enable investigators to determine what individual cell types can do in the absence of other cells, or with defined cellular interactions. For instance, culturing BECs alone can give an idea of which BBB properties are independent of signaling interactions within the neurovascular niche. Furthermore, by adding feeder layers of individual cells, such as astrocytes or pericytes, or signaling molecules or pharmacological agents, *in vitro* models can aid in determining how these factors directly influence BEC gene expression.

Primary BEC culture models obtained from bovine or rodent acutely isolated brain microvessels present another system for directed studies on BBB maintenance and function. Early efforts relied on isolation and enrichment of brain capillaries from rats followed by enzymatic digestion of the basement membrane to allow migration of endothelial cells for growth on an artificial substrate (Bowman et al., 1981). Bovine models have allowed for several benefits including greater amounts of starting material obtained from one animal, less variability between cultures from the same starting material, and importantly, retention of endothelial characteristics after serial passaging (Goetz et al., 1985).

The establishment of human cerebral microvessel cultures also yielded early, important insights into BBB function (Vinters et al., 1987). These culture systems were improved upon as tighter barriers were introduced with co-culture models containing astrocytes and by introducing intraluminal flow (Marroni et al., 2003). Human brain microvessel endothelial cells (HBMEC) have also been treated with amyloid-β to determine their gene expression changes using a cDNA array and identified a putative protective role for STC1 (Li et al., 2008).

3.3. COMPARISONS OF ACUTE VS. CULTURED BBB MODELS

Whether *in vitro* BBB models were derived from immortalized cell lines or acutely isolated from mouse or human brains, extensive efforts to characterize their gene expression signature have repeatedly revealed their limited approximation of *in vivo* complexity. Comparisons of BBB gene expression profiles from acutely isolated mouse brain endothelial cells vs. a period of brief culturing, or compared against a commonly used mouse brain endothelioma line (bEND5) revealed evidence of dedifferentiation of BEC qualities (i.e., reduced levels of tight junction proteins and amino acid transporters) induced by primary culture or immortalization (Lyck et al., 2009). A similar study which used suppression subtractive hybridization revealed that some transport-related brain endothelial genes were subsequently downregulated after BECs spent several days in culture compared to freshly isolated rat brain microvessels (Calabria and Shusta, 2008). The same study compared cultures containing puromycin (which decreases numbers of contaminating pericytes) for BEC expression and also the effect of hydrocortisone on cultures. More recently, transcriptome data from immortalized human BEC line hCMEC/D3 and primary human BEC (Urich et al., 2012) were compared with published data on acutely isolated mouse BECs (Daneman et al., 2010a) to highlight differences in levels of endothelial marker expression.

The authors found that although the human cells demonstrated expression of tight junction proteins, transporters and receptors, their levels were dramatically reduced compared to acutely isolated mouse BECs (Urich et al., 2012).

Nevertheless, using *in vitro* BBB models may yield some important initial insights into BEC response to external stimuli or stress. hCMEC/D3 cells have been recently profiled for their transcriptional response to TNFα and IFNγ and gene expression signatures identified span from factors involved in antigen presentation, cellular adhesion, cytokine-induced signaling pathways, to reduced transporter expression (Lopez-Ramirez et al., 2013). These data were compared to similar historical data sets that included TNFα-treated human umbilical vein (HUVEC) and primary human cerebral endothelial cell cells (Franzen et al., 2003).

3.4. MODELS OF BBB DEVELOPMENT

Wnt/β-catenin signaling has been implicated in driving CNS specific angiogenesis and regulating BBB formation and maintenance (Liebner et al., 2008; Stenman et al., 2008; Daneman et al., 2009; Wang et al., 2012b; Zhou et al., 2014b). Using microarray expression profiling comparing BECs with ECs from non-neural tissue, Daneman and colleagues identified that genes downstream of Wnt/β-catenin signaling were greatly enriched in endothelial cells of the brain but not liver or lung (Daneman et al., 2009, 2010a). Performing sophisticated genetic and functional experiments, the authors demonstrate that Wnt/β-catenin signaling is required to drive CNS-specific angiogenesis but not angiogenesis in other tissues. To identify if this CNS-specific angiogeneic program also induced BBB-specific gene expression in the endothelial cells, the authors utilized gene expression profiling of purified mouse brain endothelial cells cultured with and without Wnt ligands to find that Wnt induced the expression of BBB-specific nutrient transporters in the endothelial cells, and further showed that loss of Wnt signaling *in vivo* led to loss of Glut-1 expression in endothelial cells. More recently, Zhou et al. (2014b) demonstrated nearly identical canonical Wnt signaling mechanisms of development and maintenance between both the blood-brain and blood-retinal barriers.

The characterization of molecular cues and signaling pathways that guide both physiological and pathophysiological CNS angiogenesis may also stand to benefit greatly from expanded efforts at expression profiling of BECs within various parts of the neurovascular unit. Common guidance molecules that regulate both nerve and vascular remodeling such as Sema/Plex/Nrp, Slit/Robo, Netrin/Unc5, VEGF, and its tyrosine kinase receptors Flt-1 and Flk-1, have been extensively studied, however, the role of the canonical axon guidance molecules in CNS angiogenesis is less studied (Tam and Watts, 2010). Transcriptomics may also enable future studies on understanding the role of TGFb or EphB receptors and ligands in determining arteriovenous identity within the brain vasculature (Adams and Alitalo, 2007; Engelhardt and Liebner, 2014).

In addition to the involvement of Wnt signaling in BBB angiogenesis and barriergenesis, the role of growth factors and kinases beyond VEGF and Notch have also been further characterized. Mice deficient in PDGF-B lack microvascular pericytes and succumb to lethal microaneurisms during development due to incomplete brain vascularization (Lindahl et al., 1997). More recent studies on the importance of pericytes in barriergenesis and maintenance reported that significantly reduced pericyte coverage in PDGFRβ null fetal mice translated into increased permeability (Daneman et al., 2010b). Transcriptome signatures of BECs isolated from null mice were compared to wild type mice, which revealed increases in Angpt2, a Tie2 ligand involved in vascular permeability of peripheral endothelial cells but no downregulation of BBB-enriched genes. Thus pericytes may regulate the BBB by inhibiting the expression of genes that normally make endothelial cells leaky. In addition, the expression profile of pericytes acutely isolated from wild type mice was also generated, further providing a valuable data set for BBB neurovascular unit transcript comparisons (Daneman et al., 2010b).

For an in depth review on recent studies of developmental barriergenesis and repair, see Obermeier et al. (2013), Siegenthaler et al. (2013), Engelhardt and Liebner (2014).

3.5. EVOLUTIONARY STUDIES OF THE BBB

Two distinct cellular mechanisms of BECs appear to be evolutionarily conserved across all vertebrates and some invertebrates, including the fruit fly model organism, *Drosophila melanogaster*. These conserved traits include the tight junctions that prevent paracellular diffusion, and ATP binding cassette (ABC) transporters that efflux molecules back into the vascular luminal space. The *Drosophila* genome encodes proteins which are nearly identical in sequence to those that comprise vertebrate tight junctions (Wu and Beitel, 2004; Banerjee et al., 2006), and whose disruption leads to defects in humoral-CNS barrier function (Schwabe et al., 2005; Stork et al., 2008). Further, Mayer et al. (2009) established that the fly protein Mdr65 functions as an ABC transporter in the *Drosophila* hemolymph-brain barrier.

Validation of gene expression data in other species with a simplistic BBB may expedite the search for candidate genes that warrant further study in rodents or human tissue. For example, we recently profiled the rodent BBB at three developmental stages, used zebrafish to confirm the necessity of candidate genes in regulating angiogenesis, and followed with subsequent analysis of genetic interactions of two death receptors, DR6 and TROY, by returning to mice to confirm a role for these genes in rodent BBB development (Tam et al., 2012). As such, conserved pathways can be discovered in one species and further characterized in more tractable models. In fact, fruit fly, grasshopper, and zebrafish are gaining popularity as models for high throughput screening of BBB drug permeability studies (Nielsen et al., 2011; Geldenhuys et al., 2012) It is this underlying premise of evolutionary conservation which provides confidence that understanding the BBB in rodent and other model organisms will be relevant to the human BBB.

Primate studies, on the other hand, can illuminate more recent evolutionary innovations relevant to the human BBB. Gene expression differences between neurons and BECs from human postmortem tissue isolated by LCM were compared with published data sets on chimpanzees and rhesus macaques for analysis of rates of transcriptome evolution in neuronal vs. endothelial cell types (Giger et al., 2010). The authors found that transcriptomes of neurons and endothelial cells evolve at different rates within brain tissue. This finding adds complexity to the challenge of translating BBB results from other species, even closely related species, into human models.

3.6. HUMAN BBB DATA SETS FOCUSED ON AGING, DISEASE, AND DYSFUNCTION

During normal aging, the blood brain barrier experiences functional changes, which can result in impairment and dysfunction of the barrier. Marques et al. (2013) provide a review of these changes in both the BBB and blood-CSF barriers. In the BBB, these changes include loosening of tight junctions, increases in pinocytotic vesicles, and decreases in mitochondrial density within ECs. The authors highlight the similarity between normal aging, and CNS disease related changes of the BBB. Since human BBB data from patients typically comes from those with obviously progressed symptoms, it is a challenge to determine if the changes in BBB function are causal or consequential to disease progression. Improvements in animal models of CNS diseases with BBB impairment may help answer such questions.

Nevertheless, several human studies in diverse disease paradigms have sought to understand vascular expression differences between healthy control and disease tissue. Microvascular endothelial cells from postmortem schizophrenia brains were isolated by LCM and their functional profile was compared to neurons and control tissue in a study by Harris et al. (2008). They found that the cerebral microvasculature of schizophrenic patients displayed a hypo-inflammatory status and this observation was reproducible on a separate microarray platform. This gene set could be useful in comparison studies with similar rodent models of cognitive dysfunction or with human BBB gene sets from patients with other cognitive or behavioral impairments. Likewise, the use of LCM to isolate vessels from glioblastoma multiforme brain tissue followed by microarray analysis and qPCR validation identified uniquely upregulated genes specific to tumor tissue and absent in nonmalignant human brain (Pen et al., 2007). Interestingly, a similar study from another group did not identify the same upregulated genes and describe a different expression signature (Dieterich et al., 2012). Another recent study also used LCM to query genes expressed at the BBB from multiple sclerosis lesions isolated from postmortem tissue (Cunnea et al., 2010).

Brain endothelial cell transcriptomes from human neurodegenerative diseases have been distinctly underrepresented. However, there is no shortage of studies reporting genome-wide data sets from Alzheimers disease brain or sub-regions such as hippocampus (Blalock et al., 2004; Dunckley et al., 2006; Webster et al., 2009; Blalock et al., 2011). To the best of our knowledge, the only published data set generated thus far representing the BBB in human neurodegeneration is from a study where brain microvessels from control and Alzheimers disease tissue were transcriptionally profiled to identify abnormal gene expression or differentially expressed genes (Wang et al., 2012a). A comparison of this data set with brain microvasculature gene expression data derived from mouse models of Alzheimer's disease may serve as a useful tool for model validation.

3.7. RODENT BBB DATA SETS IN MODELS OF NEURODEGENERATION AND DISEASE

Transgenic mouse models of Alzheimers disease have been instrumental to the study of amyloid-β accumulation and its role in neuronal impairment and cognitive dysfunction. Transcriptome analysis of whole brain, specific subregions, various disease time points, and in multiple Alzheimer's disease transgenic models or after experimental treatments has been performed (Dickey et al., 2003; Reddy et al., 2004; Lazarov et al., 2005; Gatta et al., 2014). Genomic studies specifically using mouse brain vasculature from Alzheimer's disease models, on the other hand, remain sparse. The most recent study used a proteomics approach from homozygous Tg-SwDI mice which harbor three familial, autosomal dominant mutations on APP, and demonstrate sustained increases in vascular amyloid-β accumulation over time (Searcy et al., 2014). The authors compared brain microvessel fractions from 3- and 9-month old wild type and transgenic mice for aging-related effects on the mouse vascular proteome as well as amyloid-β-induced effects. They found distinct sets of proteins changed in young and old wild type and transgenic mice, indicating a differential effect of age on the cerebrovasculature.

An experimental mouse model of multiple sclerosis, experimental autoimmune encephalomyelitis, is characterized primarily by dysfunction of the BBB. Functional studies have produced insights into the role of particular genes, such as the chemokine CXCL12, and the permeability of the BBB in experimental autoimmune encephalomyelitis (McCandless et al., 2006, 2009). However, to our knowledge, there does not yet exist a genome wide expression data set derived from the BBB in this important model of multiple sclerosis.

Metabolic diseases, with obesity a leading factor, may also have a multitude of effects on the BBB and as a result, CNS function. A recent study on diet-induced obesity using a mouse model profiled the proteomic changes in brain vasculature after 2 months of high fat diet chow administered starting at 2 months of age (Ouyang et al., 2014). The samples were compared directly with mice maintained on normal chow and the authors found 47 downregulated and 2 upregulated proteins, indicating that in general, diet-induced obesity suppressed metabolic activity in brain microvessels (Ouyang et al., 2014).

Rodent models exist for other neurological diseases associated with BBB dysfunction, including stroke, epilepsy, ALS, and neuromyelitis optica. However, to date, there is a void of genome wide expression data on brain endothelial cells from these important models. Future data sets derived from these models will be invaluable in bridging the knowledge gap between our understanding of healthy BBB maintenance and BBB dysfunction in disease.

Another genomic data set that is publicly available and could be used as a valuable cross-reference tool describes the transcriptional changes in four rat brain tissues/regions including striatum, and parietal cortex, choroid plexus, and the meninges and its associated vasculature (Bowyer et al., 2013). This study also included a time course analysis to profile the effects of amphetamines or environment-induced hypothermia on choroid plexus and the meninges.

4. SUMMARY OF INSIGHTS FROM BBB GENOMIC STUDIES

4.1. OVERVIEW

Genomic studies on the BBB have provided a number of large data sets identifying genes that are expressed by BECs, enriched in BECs compared to peripheral ECs, and also genes that change levels during development or disease context. The challenge now is to sort through these vast data sets and untangle which of these large numbers of genes are functionally important for the formation and function of the BBB, and which can be targeted to either modulate the BBB during neurological disease or to use as carriers for drug delivery across the BBB. Two positive outcomes have arisen from these data sets: (1) many of these analyses that use completely different methodologies have identified the same BBB genes, and (2) virtually all of the data sets have verified the expression and BBB-enrichment of commonly studied genes important for BBB function including tight junctions (claudin 5, occludin, Zo-1, Zo-2), efflux transport (P-glycoprotein, and ABCG2, also known as Bcrp), nutrient transport (Glut-1, Mct-1, Lat-1) and others (basigin, carbonic anhydrase 4). The strong reproducibility and ability to verify positive hits suggests that these data sets will indeed provide an extremely strong blueprint for identification of novel genes important for BBB function.

4.2. SIGNALING REGULATORS

Several important discoveries have already been generated from these data sets. For instance, the identification that a cluster of Wnt/β-catenin signaling components and downstream targets (Fzd6, Lef1, Axin2, Dixdc1, Apcdd1, Troy) are greatly enriched in BECs compared to peripheral ECs led to the hypothesis that Wnt may be an important regulator of the BBB. As discussed above, several groups have verified and identified that Wnt/β-catenin signaling is required for driving CNS-specific angiogenesis, BBB induction and maintenance (Liebner et al., 2008; Stenman et al., 2008; Daneman et al., 2009; Wang et al., 2012b). Beyond the morphogens Wnt and Shh, and the canonical VEGF and Notch signaling pathways, a further understanding of other growth factors and kinases involved in angiogenesis have also been possible from expression data. Moreover, gene cluster/pathway analysis can provide an important method to sift through large data sets to find groups of genes that are functionally important. Other clusters associated with BBB-enrichment are genes involved in retinoid signaling, amino acid metabolism and glycolysis, suggesting that these may be important for unique function of BECs.

4.3. MOLECULAR COMPONENTS OF THE BARRIER

Many groups have used these data sets to identify individual genes that are important for BBB function. Lipolysis stimulated receptor (Lsr) was identified as enriched in BECs compared to peripheral ECs (Daneman et al., 2010a), has recently been shown to recruit tricellulin/Marveld2 to tricellular tight junctions for the formation of epithelial barriers (Masuda et al., 2011), and could potentially have a similar function at the BBB. Like Lsr, Marveld2 was identified as enriched at the BBB along with other tight junction components such as Jam4, Mpp7 and Cgnl1 (Daneman et al., 2010a), suggesting that these may also be important for formation of BBB tight junctions. Interestingly, the genomic data sets have not added much clarity as to which claudins may be important for BBB function. While it is well established that claudin 5 is most critical in transmembrane adhesion for BEC tight junctions (Nitta et al., 2003), various studies have also implicated claudin 1, claudin 3, claudin 12 and other claudins as expressed by BECs (Liebner et al., 2000; Nitta et al., 2003; Wolburg et al., 2003; Krause et al., 2008; Pfeiffer et al., 2011). Several different genomic data sets have essentially come to different conclusions as to which claudins are expressed by BECs. Array studies on purified mouse BECs have suggested that in addition to claudin 5, claudin 12 is the other claudin expressed by BECs (Daneman et al., 2010a; Tam et al., 2012), while cultured cells have identified claudin 3 as a component of BEC tight junctions (Liebner et al., 2008), and proteomics on human passaged endothelial cells have identified a wider array of claudins present at these junctions (Ohtsuki et al., 2013). These differences may result from species differences, differences in acutely isolated vs. cultured cells, or different sensitivities of analyses, and further work needs to be done to determine which are the important molecules.

4.4. TRANSPORTERS AND DRUG DELIVERY TARGETS

The genomic data sets have also identified a huge number of molecular transporters highly expressed and enriched in BECs compared to peripheral ECs. In addition to widely studied BBB transporters (Glut-1, Lat-1, Mct-1), a number of other transporters have been identified and include molecules that transport neurotransmitters (Slc6a6, Slc6a17), thiamine (Slc19a3), nucleotides (Slc25a33), carnitine (Slc25a20), zinc (Slc20a1, Slc39a10) and riboflavin (Slc52a2/Gpr172b) (Lyck et al., 2009; Daneman et al., 2010a). Determining the expression and function of this wide array of transporters may be important to understand the nutrient requirements of the CNS. A recent study by Ben-Zvi et al. (2014) selectively profiled E15.5 embryos for transcripts enriched at the BBB vs. lung endothelium and identified Mfsd2a, a lipid transporter required for docosahexaenoic acid transport (Nguyen et al., 2014), further confirming its high expression levels. Analyzing the expression of transporters and signaling components may also identify novel molecules to target for drug delivery to the CNS. The most commonly utilized target for BBB-specific receptor-mediated drug delivery to the CNS is transferrin receptor, which has been identified as highly expressed and enriched in BECs by a number of data sets (Li et al., 2001; Enerson and Drewes, 2006), suggesting that other targets may also be identified. Interestingly, a peptide targeting Lrp1 has been shown to target molecules across the BBB, however, several genomic studies identified Lrp8, and not Lrp1, as highly expressed and enriched in BECs (Daneman et al., 2010a; Tam et al., 2012). For a detailed review on the expression of transporters at the blood-brain and blood-CSF interfaces in the developing and adult brain, see Saunders et al. (2013).

5. EMERGING FRONTIERS

5.1. PROTEOMICS

One major criticism of transcriptomic approaches is that transcript abundance does not necessarily correlate with protein levels and actual functional activity. To that end, proteomic approaches may nicely complement gene expression studies. For a detailed review of proteomic studies which describe how various cell culturing conditions can significantly affect protein profiles and also how protein expression is explored using *in vivo* models of ischemia, stroke, inflammation, and disease, see Pottiez et al. (2009). Additionally, global genomic approaches are often followed with validation by qPCR assays and new developments in microfluidic devices have enabled higher throughput of expression validation studies from the same profiled samples, as well as the inclusion of a multitude of other samples, with or without experimental treatments, or from disease models and patients.

However, a major consideration of current proteomics BBB data is again the purity of the cell population being queried. Many BBB proteomics data are largely obtained from brain microvessel preparations consisting of additional pericytic or astrocytic connections that are in direct contact with BECs which are known to contain concentrated levels of cell-type specific receptors or channel proteins (see **Table 2**). Detection of known proteins such as those expressed on astrocytic endfeet (Chun et al., 2011), can be easily separated, however, lesser known hits may not be readily segregated by cell type or fall within a general category. A recent effort to profile one specific branch of CNS vasculature, the arteries comprising the Circle of Willis, generated an extensive data set of 6630 proteins, of which a third are specific to the cerebral arterial landscape (Badhwar et al., 2014). Interestingly, because isolation of the sampled tissue was via manual dissection and performed under light microscopy, whole units of arterial mediators such as neuronal regulators of vasoactivity, presumably from nerve terminals, as well as regulators of smooth muscle relaxation and contractility were identified. The cerebral artery-specific proteome was compared to the mouse microvessel proteome which revealed that intracortical microvessels had more BBB-unique protein numbers and that Circle of Willis arteries were less developed and specialized compared to microvessels (Badhwar et al., 2014). Additional studies have also compared human brain microvessel proteomic signatures with mouse (Uchida et al., 2011).

Investigators have tried to circumvent these issues by coupling gene expression with proteomics in analyses of human brain vasculature isolated from resected glioma or epileptic lesions (Dauchy et al., 2008; Shawahna et al., 2011). Furthermore, a proteomics report of young and aged primate brain microvasculature provides a highly quantitative snapshot of membrane proteins expressed at the BBB at two stages of development (Ito et al., 2011). The data were compared to mouse BBB proteomic findings, which revealed significant differences. These comparisons may provide a cautionary note when translating findings between rodents and primates, likely impacting nervous system drug development studies focused on using mouse BBB models to understand transporter and receptor expression levels (Kamiie et al., 2008; Ito et al., 2011).

Overall, proteomic studies have been incredibly useful in identifying novel molecules. In particular, proteomic analysis of lipid rafts isolated from cultured cells has identified leukocyte adhesion molecules, ninjurin, Alcam, and Mcam, that are critical for trafficking of specific subsets of immune cells into the CNS during neuroinflammatory disease (Wosik et al., 2007; Cayrol et al.,

Table 2 | Recent proteomics data sets for the BBB.

Method of BBB isolation	Relevant study details	Species	*Dev study	Other tissues	Disease
LCM					
Lu et al., 2008	Microvessels from CD31+ immunostained brain	Mouse			
Haqqani et al., 2005	*In vivo* ischemia	Rat			+
FILTRATION/CENTRIFUGATION					
Badhwar et al., 2014	Surgical dissection of circle of Willis brain artery	Mouse			
Ouyang et al., 2014	Mouse model of diet-induced obesity and control	Mouse			+
Searcy et al., 2014	Effect of aging on BMVs from wild type and Tg-SwDI mice	Mouse	+		+
Agarwal et al., 2012	BMVs from wild type and P-gp/Bcrp knockout	Mouse			
Chun et al., 2011	Membrane fraction of BMVs	Mouse			
Ito et al., 2011	BMVs from neonate, child, and adult	Cyno monkey	+		
Shawahna et al., 2011	BMVs from epilepsy patients and glioma patients	Human			+
Uchida et al., 2011	Human and mouse BMVs	Human and mouse			
Kamiie et al., 2008	Membrane fraction of microvessels from brain, liver and kidney	Mouse		+	
CELL CULTURE					
Ohtsuki et al., 2013	hCMEC/D3 compared to isolated human BMVs and HUVECs	Human		+	
Pottiez et al., 2010	BCECs co-cultured with glial cells	Cow			
Pottiez et al., 2009	BMECs cultured with and without astrocytes	Cow			
Lu et al., 2007	MECs from brain and heart	Rat		+	
Haqqani et al., 2007	Immortalized BECs and *in vitro* ischemia	Rat			+

**Developmental stages. BCEC, brain capillary endothelial cell; BEC, brain endothelial cell; BMEC, brain microvessel endothelial cell; BMV, brain microvessel; hCMEC/D3, human cerebral microvascular endothelial cell line; HUVEC, human umbilical vein endothelial cell.*

2008; Ifergan et al., 2011). This suggests that the cultured cells may provide a model for "activated" endothelial cells and thus a good model to study their interaction with immune cells that might occur during neurological disease. In addition to these established functions of the BBB, these data sets may identify novel and unknown genes that could point to novel functions of the BBB. Although a daunting task, examining the function and regulation of each of these genes and pathways should provide incredible insight into how our brain interacts with the humoral space.

5.2. MicroRNA

MicroRNA (miRNA) arrays have also been used to identify and understand their role in regulating gene expression levels at the BBB in disease. Using hCMEC/D3 cells treated with TNFα and IFNγ, Reijerkerk et al. (2013) set out to profile the microRNAs that modulate BBB function under inflammatory conditions. With a panel of miRNAs identified to have differential expression induced by inflammatory mediators that also displayed opposing changes after barrier induction in the cell line, the authors further examined their expression in brain capillaries isolated via filtration from resected multiple sclerosis patient lesions. These samples showed decreased expression of miR-125a-5p (Reijerkerk et al., 2013). In another study using a miRNA array of 318 candidates, mouse brain endothelioma line bEND3 cells were profiled for altered miRNA expression in response to lupus serum or C5a (Eadon et al., 2014). Studies similar to these, for example evaluating freshly isolated BECs for miRNA expression at different developmental times or in diverse disease models, will further expand our knowledge of how gene expression is regulated at the BBB.

5.3. RNA-SEQUENCING

RNA sequencing is a high-throughput, quantitative transcriptomic approach that is rapidly gaining popularity (Lister et al., 2008; Mortazavi et al., 2008; Nagalakshmi et al., 2008; Wilhelm et al., 2008), especially as more genome annotations are completed for more and more species. RNA-seq data also allows for the relatively unbiased discovery of alternative splicing within transcripts. Where the bulk of our transcriptome based knowledge has been driven by methods that illuminate overall gene expression (including microarray and SAGE), we have until recently, been lacking much of the important resolution afforded by identification of alternative splicing events. Many of the genes encoding proteins that form tight junctions and ABC transporters, for example, have distinct isoforms resulting from alternative splicing events. Future additional RNA-seq experiments with BBB data will provide a foundation for our future understanding of the relevance of such splicing behavior with respect to barrier development, maintenance, and dysfunction.

The high-throughput sequencing of transcriptomes afforded by RNA-seq technologies also facilitates the study of RNA editing. The process of RNA editing, which is most prevalent in the brain, is a post-transcriptional modification that can influence splicing patterns, coding sequence, and a host of other gene regulatory functions. Indeed, some of the best-studied RNA-editing events that result in altered protein isoforms occur within neuronal glutamate receptors. Future RNA-seq experiments will be needed to explore the role of RNA-editing within brain endothelial cells specifically.

Currently, BBB RNA-seq data is limited to a single dataset from mouse (at the time this review was submitted), which is already providing an extensive view of the expression landscape of not only BECs, but also neurons, astrocytes, oligodendrocytes, and microglia (Zhang et al., 2014). The authors of this study primarily used FACs and immunopanning methods to purify specific cell types, thus minimizing cross contamination and enabling greater quantitative comparisons. In addition, this valuable dataset has been made available to the public via a searchable website which includes differential splicing data (Zhang et al., 2014).

To supplement the paucity of RNA-seq data derived from the BBB, a recent developmental study using RNA sequencing to understand brain-CSF barrier formation assembled a comprehensive list of transcripts differentially enriched between E15 embryo and P42 adult rat lateral ventricle choroid plexus (Liddelow et al., 2013). This served as a quantitative approach to update a prior microarray study (Liddelow et al., 2012). The authors performed immunohistochemistry to demonstrate embryonic and choroid plexus epithelium-specific expression of genes they found enriched via RNA-seq (Liddelow et al., 2013).

The RNA-seq approach has also been used to profile expression signatures of single cells. In a study where cultured cortical neuron transcriptomes of single cells were compared to individual layer 5 pyramidal neurons *in situ*, the authors found that gene expression levels correlated better amongst single cultured neurons compared to the single neurons sampled *in situ* (Qiu et al., 2012). This *in vivo* heterogeneity may also apply to cells of the BBB and thus future gene expression studies sampling single BECs or capillary fragments from distinct disease regions or developmental stages of individual vascular branches may reveal further complexity in expression of specific transporters or receptors.

5.4. FINAL REMARKS

Advancements in techniques for the isolation and purification of BECs and in the technologies to study the resulting transcriptomes and proteomes make for an exciting and promising future for the BBB research community. Transcriptome wide data for human diseases associated with BBB dysfunction, and corresponding animal models are under-represented in the current selection of BBB data sets. Future studies may also identify sexual dimorphisms to the BBB, how the BBB changes in response to neuronal activity, during normal aging, as well as following intake of different drugs. Furthermore, understanding heterogeneity of the BBB between different segments of the vascular tree as well as between different regions of the brain may be important in our understanding of how the BBB interacts with neural cells to regulate brain function and behavior. Filling these gaps with data that are as close to the *in vivo* setting as possible, and utilizing techniques such as FACS or LCM, will be of great benefit. Finally, the continued commitment to share newly generated data sets in publicly accessible repositories will undoubtedly propel forward our understanding of BBB biology at an unprecedented pace.

ACKNOWLEDGMENTS

We sincerely thank Allison Bruce for her graphics, Sabya Biswas for LCM imaging, and all the investigators who have shared their data sets publicly for the benefit of the research community.

REFERENCES

Abbott, N. J. (2005). Dynamics of CNS barriers: evolution, differentiation, and modulation. *Cell Mol. Neurobiol.* 25, 5–23. doi: 10.1007/s10571-004-1374-y

Adams, R. H., and Alitalo, K. (2007). Molecular regulation of angiogenesis and lymphangiogenesis. *Nat. Rev. Mol. Cell Biol.* 8, 464–478. doi: 10.1038/nrm2183

Agarwal, S., Uchida, Y., Mittapalli, R. K., Sane, R., Terasaki, T., and Elmquist, W. F. (2012). Quantitative proteomics of transporter expression in brain capillary endothelial cells isolated from Pglycoprotein (P-gp), breast cancer resistance protein (Bcrp), and P-gp/Bcrp knockout mice. *Drug Metab. Dispos.* 40, 1164–1169. doi: 10.1124/dmd.112.044719

Armulik, A., Genove, G., and Betsholtz, C. (2011). Pericytes: developmental, physiological, and pathological perspectives, problems, and promises. *Dev. Cell.* 21, 193–215. doi: 10.1016/j.devcel.2011.07.001

Armulik, A., Genove, G., Mae, M., Nisancioglu, M. H., Wallgard, E., Niaudet, C., et al. (2010). Pericytes regulate the blood-brain barrier. *Nature* 468, 557–561. doi: 10.1038/nature09522

Badhwar, A., Stanimirovic, D. B., Hamel, E., and Haqqani, A. S. (2014). The proteome of mouse cerebral arteries. *J. Cereb. Blood Flow. Metab.* 34, 1033–1046. doi: 10.1038/jcbfm.2014.52

Ball, H. J., McParland, B., Driussi, C., and Hunt, N. H. (2002). Isolating vessels from the mouse brain for gene expression analysis using laser capture microdissection. *Brain Res. Brain Res. Protoc.* 9, 206–213. doi: 10.1016/S1385-299X(02)00147-2

Banerjee, S., Sousa, A. D., and Bhat, M. A. (2006). Organization and function of septate junctions, an evolutionary perspective. *Cell Biochem. Biophys.* 46, 65–77. doi: 10.1385/CBB:46:1:65

Barbier, M., Faille, D., Loriod, B., Textoris, J., Camus, C., Puthier, D., et al. (2011). Platelets alter gene expression profile in human brain endothelial cells in an *in vitro* model of cerebral malaria. *PLoS One* 6:e19651. doi: 10.1371/journal.pone.0019651

Ben-Zvi, A., Lacoste, B., Kur, E., Andreone, B. J., Mayshar, Y., Yan, H., et al. (2014). Mfsd2a is critical for the formation and function of the blood-brain barrier. *Nature* 509, 507–511. doi: 10.1038/nature13324

Betz, A. L., Csejtey, J., and Goldstein, G. W. (1979). Hexose transport and phosphorylation by capillaries isolated from rat brain. *Am. J. Physiol.* 236, c96–c102.

Blalock, E. M., Buechel, H. M., Popovic, J., Geddes, J. W., and Landfield, P. W. (2011). Microarray analyses of laser-captured hippocampus reveal distinct gray and white matter signatures associated with incipient Alzheimer's disease. *J. Chem. Neuroanat.* 42, 118–126. doi: 10.1016/j.jchemneu.2011.06.007

Blalock, E. M., Geddes, J. W., Chen, K. C., Porter, N. M., Markesbery, W. R., and Landfield, P. W. (2004). Incipient Alzheimer's disease: microarray correlation analyses reveal major transcriptional and tumor suppressor responses. *Proc. Natl. Acad. Sci. U.S.A.* 101, 2173–2178. doi: 10.1073/pnas.0308512100

Boado, R. J., and Pardridge, M. M. (1991). A one-step procedure for isolation of poly(A)+ mRNA from isolated brain capillaries and endothelial cells in culture. *J. Neurochem.* 57, 2136–2139. doi: 10.1111/j.1471-4159.1991.tb06433.x

Bowman, P. D., Betz, A. L., Ar, D., Wolinsky, J. S., Penney, J. B., Shivers, R. R., et al. (1981). Primary culture of capillary endothelium from rat brain. *In Vitro* 17, 353–362. doi: 10.1007/BF02618147

Bowyer, J. F., Patterson, T. A., Saini, U. T., Hanig, J. P., Thomas, M., Camacho, L., et al. (2013). Comparison of the global gene expression of choroid plexus and meninges and associated vasculature under control conditions and after pronounced hyperthermia or amphetamine toxicity. *BMC Genom.* 14, 147–2164. doi: 10.1186/1471-2164-14-147

Calabria, A. R., and Shusta, E. V. (2008). A genomic comparison of *in vivo* and *in vitro* brain microvascular endothelial cells. *J. Cereb. Blood Flow Metab.* 28, 135–148. doi: 10.1038/sj.jcbfm.9600518

Cayrol, R., Wosik, K., Berard, J. L., Dodelet-Devillers, A., Ifergan, I., Kebir, H., et al. (2008). Activated leukocyte cell adhesion molecule promotes leukocyte trafficking into the central nervous system. *Nat. Immunol.* 9, 137–145. doi: 10.1038/ni1551

Chun, H. B., Scott, M., Niessen, S., Hoover, H., Baird, A., Yates, J., et al. (2011). The proteome of mouse brain microvessel membranes and basal lamina. *J. Cereb. Blood Flow Metab.* 31, 2267–2281. doi: 10.1038/jcbfm.2011.104

Cunnea, P., McMahon, J., O'Connell, E., Mashayekhi, K., Fitzgerald, U., and McQuaid, S. (2010). Gene expression analysis of the microvascular compartment in multiple sclerosis using laser microdissected blood vessels. *Acta Neuropathol.* 119, 601–615. doi: 10.1007/s00401-009-0618-9

Daneman, R., Agalliu, D., Zhou, L., Kuhnert, F., Kuo, C. J., and Barres, B. A. (2009). Wnt/beta-catenin signaling is required for CNS, but not non-CNS, angiogenesis. *Proc. Natl. Acad. Sci. U.S. A.* 106, 641–646. doi: 10.1073/pnas.0805165106

Daneman, R., Zhou, L., Agalliu, D., Cahoy, J. D., Kaushal, A., and Barres, B. A. (2010a). The mouse blood-brain barrier transcriptome: a new resource for understanding the development and function of brain endothelial cells. *PLoS ONE* 5:e13741. doi: 10.1371/journal.pone.0013741

Daneman, R., Zhou, L., Kebede, A. A., and Barres, B. A. (2010b). Pericytes are required for blood-brain barrier integrity during embryogenesis. *Nature* 468, 562–566. doi: 10.1038/nature09513

Dauchy, S., Dutheil, F., Weaver, R. J., Chassoux, F., Daumas-Duport, C., Couraud, P. O., et al. (2008). ABC transporters, cytochromes P450 and their main transcription factors: expression at the human blood-brain barrier. *J. Neurochem.* 107, 1518–1528. doi: 10.1111/j.1471-4159.2008.05720.x

Dickey, C. A., Loring, J. F., Montgomery, J., Gordon, M. N., Eastman, P. S., and Morgan, D. (2003). Selectively reduced expression of synaptic plasticity-related genes in amyloid precursor protein + presenilin-1 transgenic mice. *J. Neurosci.* 23, 5219–5226.

Dieterich, L. C., Mellberg, S., Langenkamp, E., Zhang, L., Zieba, A., Salomaki, H., et al. (2012). Transcriptional profiling of human glioblastoma vessels indicates a key role of VEGF-A and TGFbeta2 in vascular abnormalization. *J. Pathol.* 228, 378–390. doi: 10.1002/path.4072

Dorr, A., Sled, J. G., and Kabani, N. (2007). Three-dimensional cerebral vasculature of the CBA mouse brain: a magnetic resonance imaging and micro computed tomography study. *Neuroimage* 35, 1409–1423. doi: 10.1016/j.neuroimage.2006.12.040

Dunckley, T., Beach, T. G., Ramsey, K. E., Grover, A., Mastroeni, D., Walker, D. G., et al. (2006). Gene expression correlates of neurofibrillary tangles in Alzheimer's disease. *Neurobiol. Aging.* 27, 1359–1371. doi: 10.1016/j.neurobiolaging.2005.08.013

Eadon, M. T., Jacob, A., Cunningham, P. N., Quigg, R. J., Garcia, J. G., and Alexander, J. J. (2014). Transcriptional profiling reveals that C5a alters miRNA in brain endothelial cells. *Immunology.* 143, 363–373. doi: 10.1111/imm.12314

Enerson, B. E., and Drewes, L. R. (2006). The rat blood-brain barrier transcriptome. *J. Cereb. Blood Flow Metab.* 26, 959–973. doi: 10.1038/sj.jcbfm.9600249

Engelhardt, B., and Liebner, S. (2014). Novel insights into the development and maintenance of the blood-brain barrier. *Cell Tissue Res.* 355, 687–699. doi: 10.1007/s00441-014-1811-2

Falcon, S., and Gentleman, R. (2007). Using GOstats to test gene lists for GO term association. *Bioinformatics* 23, 257–258. doi: 10.1093/bioinformatics/btl567

Franzen, B., Duvefelt, K., Jonsson, C., Engelhardt, B., Ottervald, J., Wickman, M., et al. (2003). Gene and protein expression profiling of human cerebral endothelial cells activated with tumor necrosis factor-alpha. *Brain Res. Mol. Brain Res.* 115, 130–146. doi: 10.1016/S0169-328X(03)00185-2

Gatta, V., D'Aurora, M., Granzotto, A., Stuppia, L., and Sensi, S. L. (2014). Early and sustained altered expression of aging-related genes in young 3xTg-AD mice. *Cell Death Dis.* 5:e1054. doi: 10.1038/cddis.2014.11

Geldenhuys, W. J., Allen, D. D., and Bloomquist, J. R. (2012). Novel models for assessing blood-brain barrier drug permeation. *Expert Opin. Drug Metab Toxicol.* 8, 647–653. doi: 10.1517/17425255.2012.677433

Gentleman, R. C., Carey, V. J., Bates, D. M., Bolstad, B., Dettling, M., Dudoit, S., et al. (2004). Bioconductor: open software development for computational biology and bioinformatics. *Genome Biol.* 5:R80. doi: 10.1186/gb-2004-5-10-r80

Giger, T., Khaitovich, P., Somel, M., Lorenc, A., Lizano, E., Harris, L. W., et al. (2010). Evolution of neuronal and endothelial transcriptomes in primates. *Genome Biol. Evol.* 2, 284–292. doi: 10.1093/gbe/evq018

Goetz, I. E., Warren, J., Estrada, C., Roberts, E., and Krause, D. N. (1985). Long-term serial cultivation of arterial and capillary endothelium from adult bovine brain. *In Vitro Cell Dev. Biol.* 21, 172–180. doi: 10.1007/BF02621355

Harris, L. W., Wayland, M., Lan, M., Ryan, M., Giger, T., Lockstone, H., et al. (2008). The cerebral microvasculature in schizophrenia: a laser capture microdissection study. *PLoS ONE* 3:e3964. doi: 10.1371/journal.pone.0003964

Haqqani, A. S., Kelly, J., Baumann, E., Haseloff, R. F., Blasig, I. E., and Stanimirovic, D. B. (2007). Protein markers of ischemic insult in brain endothelial cells identified using 2D gel electrophoresis and ICAT-based quantitative proteomics. *J. Proteome Res.* 6, 226–239. doi: 10.1021/pr0603811

Haqqani, A. S., Nesic, M., Preston, E., Baumann, E., Kelly, J., and Stanimirovic, D. (2005). Characterization of vascular protein expression patterns in cerebral ischemia/reperfusion using laser capture microdissection and ICAT-nanoLC-MS/MS. *FASEB J.* 19, 1809–1821. doi: 10.1096/fj.05-3793com

Hawkins, B. T., and Egleton, R. D. (2008). Pathophysiology of the blood-brain barrier: animal models and methods. *Curr. Top Dev. Biol.* 80, 277–309. doi: 10.1016/S0070-2153(07)80007-X

He, Z., Cui, L., Patterson, T. A., and Paule, M. G. (2011). Defining the phosphodiesterase superfamily members in rat brain microvessels. *ACS Chem. Neurosci.* 2, 600–607. doi: 10.1021/cn2000487

Himburg, H. A., Muramoto, G. G., Daher, P., Meadows, S. K., Russell, J. L., Doan, P., et al. (2010). Pleiotrophin regulates the expansion and regeneration of hematopoietic stem cells. *Nat. Med.* 16, 475–482. doi: 10.1038/nm.2119

Hudson, L. C., Bragg, D. C., Tompkins, M. B., and Meeker, R. B. (2005). Astrocytes and microglia differentially regulate trafficking of lymphocyte subsets across brain endothelial cells. *Brain Res.* 1058, 148–160. doi: 10.1016/j.brainres.2005.07.071

Ifergan, I., Kebir, H., Terouz, S., Alvarez, J. I., Lecuyer, M. A., Gendron, S., et al. (2011). Role of Ninjurin-1 in the migration of myeloid cells to central nervous system inflammatory lesions. *Ann. Neurol.* 70, 751–763. doi: 10.1002/ana.22519

Irizarry, R. A., Hobbs, B., Collin, F., Beazer-Barclay, Y. D., Antonellis, K. J., Scherf, U., et al. (2003). Exploration, normalization, and summaries of high density oligonucleotide array probe level data. *Biostatistics* 4, 249–264. doi: 10.1093/biostatistics/4.2.249

Ito, K., Uchida, Y., Ohtsuki, S., Aizawa, S., Kawakami, H., Katsukura, Y., et al. (2011). Quantitative membrane protein expression at the blood-brain barrier of adult and younger cynomolgus monkeys. *J. Pharm. Sci.* 100, 3939–3950. doi: 10.1002/jps.22487

Kamiie, J., Ohtsuki, S., Iwase, R., Ohmine, K., Katsukura, Y., Yanai, K., et al. (2008). Quantitative atlas of membrane transporter proteins: development and application of a highly sensitive simultaneous LC/MS/MS method combined with novel in-silico peptide selection criteria. *Pharm. Res.* 25, 1469–1483. doi: 10.1007/s11095-008-9532-4

Kauffmann, A., Gentleman, R., and Huber, W. (2009). arrayQualityMetrics–a bioconductor package for quality assessment of microarray data. *Bioinformatics* 25, 415–416. doi: 10.1093/bioinformatics/btn647

Krause, G., Winkler, L., Mueller, S. L., Haseloff, R. F., Piontek, J., and Blasig, I. E. (2008). Structure and function of claudins. *Biochim. Biophys. Acta.* 1778, 631–645. doi: 10.1016/j.bbamem.2007.10.018

Lazarov, O., Robinson, J., Tang, Y. P., Hairston, I. S., Korade-Mirnics, Z., Lee, V. M., et al. (2005). Environmental enrichment reduces Abeta levels and amyloid deposition in transgenic mice. *Cell* 120, 701–713. doi: 10.1016/j.cell.2005.01.015

Li, J. Y., Boado, R. J., and Pardridge, W. M. (2001). Blood-brain barrier genomics. *J. Cereb. Blood Flow Metab.* 21, 61–68. doi: 10.1097/00004647-200101000-00008

Li, K., Dong, D., Yao, L., Dai, D., Gu, X., and Guo, L. (2008). Identification of STC1 as an beta-amyloid activated gene in human brain microvascular endothelial cells using cDNA microarray. *Biochem. Biophys. Res. Commun.* 376, 399–403. doi: 10.1016/j.bbrc.2008.08.158

Liddelow, S. A., Dziegielewska, K. M., Ek, C. J., Habgood, M. D., Bauer, H., Bauer, H. C., et al. (2013). Mechanisms that determine the internal environment of the developing brain: a transcriptomic, functional and ultrastructural approach. *PLoS ONE* 8:e65629. doi: 10.1371/journal.pone.0065629

Liddelow, S. A., Temple, S., Mollgard, K., Gehwolf, R., Wagner, A., Bauer, H., et al. (2012). Molecular characterisation of transport mechanisms at the developing mouse blood-CSF interface: a transcriptome approach. *PLoS ONE* 7:e33554. doi: 10.1371/journal.pone.0033554

Liebner, S., Corada, M., Bangsow, T., Babbage, J., Taddei, A., Czupalla, C. J., et al. (2008). Wnt/beta-catenin signaling controls development of the blood-brain barrier. *J. Cell Biol.* 183, 409–417. doi: 10.1083/jcb.200806024

Liebner, S., Fischmann, A., Rascher, G., Duffner, F., Grote, E. H., Kalbacher, H., et al. (2000). Claudin-1 and claudin-5 expression and tight junction morphology are altered in blood vessels of human glioblastoma multiforme. *Acta Neuropathol.* 100, 323–331. doi: 10.1007/s004010000180

Lindahl, P., Johansson, B. R., Leveen, P., and Betsholtz, C. (1997). Pericyte loss and microaneurysm formation in PDGF-B-deficient mice. *Science* 277, 242–245. doi: 10.1126/science.277.5323.242

Lister, R., O'Malley, R. C., Tonti-Filippini, J., Gregory, B. D., Berry, C. C., Millar, A. H., et al. (2008). Highly integrated single-base resolution maps of the epigenome in Arabidopsis. *Cell* 133, 523–536. doi: 10.1016/j.cell.2008.03.029

Lopez-Ramirez, M. A., Male, D. K., Wang, C., Sharrack, B., Wu, D., and Romero, I. A. (2013). Cytokine-induced changes in the gene expression profile of a human cerebral microvascular endothelial cell-line, hCMEC/D3. *Fluids Barriers CNS* 10, 27–8118. doi: 10.1186/2045-8118-10-27

Lyck, R., Ruderisch, N., Moll, A. G., Steiner, O., Cohen, C. D., Engelhardt, B., et al. (2009). Culture-induced changes in blood-brain barrier transcriptome: implications for amino-acid transporters *in vivo*. *J. Cereb. Blood Flow Metab.* 29, 1491–1502. doi: 10.1038/jcbfm.2009.72

Lu, L., Yang, P.-Y., Rui, Y.-Ch., Kang, H., Zhang, J., Zhang, J.-P., et al. (2007). Comparative proteome analysis of rat brain and coronary microvascular endothelial cells. *Physiol. Res.* 56, 159–168.

Lu, Q., Murugesan, N., Macdonald, J. A., Wu, S. L., Pachter, J. S., and Hancock, W. S. (2008). Analysis of mouse brain microvascular endothelium using immuno-laser capture microdissection coupled to a hybrid linear ion trap with Fourier transform-mass spectrometry proteomics platform. *Electrophoresis* 29, 2689–2695. doi: 10.1002/elps.200700936

Macdonald, J. A., Murugesan, N., and Pachter, J. S. (2008). Validation of immuno-laser capture microdissection coupled with quantitative RT-PCR to probe blood-brain barrier gene expression in situ. *J. Neurosci. Methods.* 174, 219–226. doi: 10.1016/j.jneumeth.2008.07.009

Macdonald, J. A., Murugesan, N., and Pachter, J. S. (2010). Endothelial cell heterogeneity of blood-brain barrier gene expression along the cerebral microvasculature. *J. Neurosci. Res.* 88, 1457–1474. doi: 10.1002/jnr.22316

Marques, F., Sousa, J. C., Sousa, N., and Palha, J. A. (2013). Blood-brain-barriers in aging and in Alzheimer's disease. *Mol. Neurodegener.* 8, 38–1326. doi: 10.1186/1750-1326-8-38

Marroni, M., Kight, K. M., Hossain, M., Cucullo, L., Desai, S. Y., and Janigro, D. (2003). Dynamic *in vitro* model of the blood-brain barrier. Gene profiling using cDNA microarray analysis. *Methods Mol. Med.* 89, 419–434. doi: 10.1385/1-59259-419-0:419

Masuda, S., Oda, Y., Sasaki, H., Ikenouchi, J., Higashi, T., Akashi, M., et al. (2011). LSR defines cell corners for tricellular tight junction formation in epithelial cells. *J. Cell Sci.* 124, 548–555. doi: 10.1242/jcs.072058

Mayer, F., Mayer, N., Chinn, L., Pinsonneault, R. L., Kroetz, D., and Bainton, R. J. (2009). Evolutionary conservation of vertebrate blood-brain barrier chemoprotective mechanisms in Drosophila. *J. Neurosci.* 29, 3538–3550. doi: 10.1523/JNEUROSCI.5564-08.2009

McCandless, E. E., Budde, M., Lees, J. R., Dorsey, D., Lyng, E., and Klein, R. S. (2009). IL-1R signaling within the central nervous system regulates CXCL12 expression at the blood-brain barrier and disease severity during experimental autoimmune encephalomyelitis. *J. Immunol.* 183, 613–620. doi: 10.4049/jimmunol.0802258

McCandless, E. E., Wang, Q., Woerner, B. M., Harper, J. M., and Klein, R. S. (2006). CXCL12 limits inflammation by localizing mononuclear infiltrates to the perivascular space during experimental autoimmune encephalomyelitis. *J. Immunol.* 177, 8053–8064. doi: 10.4049/jimmunol.177.11.8053

Mojsilovic-Petrovic, J., Nesic, M., Pen, A., Zhang, W., and Stanimirovic, D. (2004). Development of rapid staining protocols for laser-capture microdissection of brain vessels from human and rat coupled to gene expression analyses. *J. Neurosci. Methods.* 133, 39–48. doi: 10.1016/j.jneumeth.2003.09.026

Mortazavi, A., Williams, B. A., McCue, K., Schaeffer, L., and Wold, B. (2008). Mapping and quantifying mammalian transcriptomes by RNA-Seq. *Nat. Methods* 5, 621–628. doi: 10.1038/nmeth.1226

Murugesan, N., Macdonald, J. A., Lu, Q., Wu, S. L., Hancock, W. S., and Pachter, J. S. (2011). Analysis of mouse brain microvascular endothelium using laser capture microdissection coupled with proteomics. *Methods Mol. Biol.* 686, 297–311. doi: 10.1007/978-1-60761-938-3-14

Nagalakshmi, U., Wang, Z., Waern, K., Shou, C., Raha, D., Gerstein, M., et al. (2008). The transcriptional landscape of the yeast genome defined by RNA sequencing. *Science* 320, 1344–1349. doi: 10.1126/science.1158441

Navone, S. E., Marfia, G., Invernici, G., Cristini, S., Nava, S., Balbi, S., et al. (2013). Isolation and expansion of human and mouse brain microvascular endothelial cells. *Nat. Protoc.* 8, 1680–1693. doi: 10.1038/nprot.2013.107

Nguyen, L. N., Ma, D., Shui, G., Wong, P., Cazenave-Gassiot, A., Zhang, X., et al. (2014). Mfsd2a is a transporter for the essential omega-3 fatty acid docosahexaenoic acid. *Nature* 509, 503–506. doi: 10.1038/nature13241

Nielsen, P. A., Andersson, O., Hansen, S. H., Simonsen, K. B., and Andersson, G. (2011). Models for predicting blood-brain barrier permeation. *Drug Discov. Today.* 16, 472–475. doi: 10.1016/j.drudis.2011.04.004

Nitta, T., Hata, M., Gotoh, S., Seo, Y., Sasaki, H., Hashimoto, N., et al. (2003). Size-selective loosening of the blood-brain barrier in claudin-5-deficient mice. *J. Cell Biol.* 161, 653–660.

Obermeier, B., Daneman, R., and Ransohoff, R. M. (2013). Development, maintenance and disruption of the blood-brain barrier. *Nat. Med.* 19, 1584–1596. doi: 10.1038/nm.3407

Ohtsuki, S., Ikeda, C., Uchida, Y., Sakamoto, Y., Miller, F., Glacial, F., et al. (2013). Quantitative targeted absolute proteomic analysis of transporters, receptors and junction proteins for validation of human cerebral microvascular endothelial cell line hCMEC/D3 as a human blood-brain barrier model. *Mol. Pharm.* 10, 289–296. doi: 10.1021/mp3004308

Ouyang, S., Hsuchou, H., Kastin, A. J., Wang, Y., Yu, C., and Pan, W. (2014). Diet-induced obesity suppresses expression of many proteins at the blood-brain barrier. *J. Cereb. Blood Flow Metab.* 34, 43–51. doi: 10.1038/jcbfm.2013.166

Pen, A., Moreno, M. J., Martin, J., and Stanimirovic, D. B. (2007). Molecular markers of extracellular matrix remodeling in glioblastoma vessels: microarray study of laser-captured glioblastoma vessels. *Glia* 55, 559–572. doi: 10.1002/glia.20481

Pfeiffer, F., Schafer, J., Lyck, R., Makrides, V., Brunner, S., Schaeren-Wiemers, N., et al. (2011). Claudin-1 induced sealing of blood-brain barrier tight junctions ameliorates chronic experimental autoimmune encephalomyelitis. *Acta Neuropathol.* 122, 601–614. doi: 10.1007/s00401-011-0883-2

Pottiez, G., Deracinois, B., Duban-Deweer, S., Cecchelli, R., Fenart, L., Karamanos, Y., et al. (2010). A large-scale electrophoresis- and chromatography-based determination of gene expression profiles in bovine brain capillary endothelial cells after the re-induction of blood-brain barrier properties. *Proteome Sci.* 8:57. doi: 10.1186/1477-5956-8-57

Pottiez, G., Flahaut, C., Cecchelli, R., and Karamanos, Y. (2009). Understanding the blood-brain barrier using gene and protein expression profiling technologies. *Brain Res. Rev.* 62, 83–98. doi: 10.1016/j.brainresrev.2009.09.004

Qiu, S., Luo, S., Evgrafov, O., Li, R., Schroth, G. P., Levitt, P., et al. (2012). Single-neuron RNA-Seq: technical feasibility and reproducibility. *Front. Genet.* 3:124. doi: 10.3389/fgene.2012.00124

Reddy, P. H., McWeeney, S., Park, B. S., Manczak, M., Gutala, R. V., Partovi, D., et al. (2004). Gene expression profiles of transcripts in amyloid precursor protein transgenic mice: up-regulation of mitochondrial metabolism and apoptotic genes is an early cellular change in Alzheimer's disease. *Hum. Mol. Genet.* 13, 1225–1240. doi: 10.1093/hmg/ddh140

Reese, T. S., and Karnovsky, M. J. (1967). Fine structural localization of a blood-brain barrier to exogenous peroxidase. *J. Cell. Biol.* 34, 207–217. doi: 10.1083/jcb.34.1.207

Reijerkerk, A., Lopez-Ramirez, M. A., van Het Hof, B., Drexhage, J. A., Kamphuis, W. W., Kooij, G., et al. (2013). MicroRNAs regulate human brain endothelial cell-barrier function in inflammation: implications for multiple sclerosis. *J. Neurosci.* 33, 6857–6863. doi: 10.1523/JNEUROSCI.3965-12.2013

Risau, W., Hallmann, R., and Albrecht, U. (1986). Differentiation-dependent expression of proteins in brain endothelium during development of the blood-brain barrier. *Dev. Biol.* 117, 537–545. doi: 10.1016/0012-1606(86)90321-0

Saunders, N. R., Daneman, R., Dziegielewska, K. M., and Liddelow, S. A. (2013). Transporters of the blood-brain and blood-CSF interfaces in development and in the adult. *Mol. Aspects Med.* 34, 742–752. doi: 10.1016/j.mam.2012.11.006

Schwabe, T., Bainton, R. J., Fetter, R. D., Heberlein, U., and Gaul, U. (2005). GPCR signaling is required for blood-brain barrier formation in drosophila. *Cell* 123, 133–144. doi: 10.1016/j.cell.2005.08.037

Searcy, J. L., Le Bihan, T., Salvadores, N., McCulloch, J., and Horsburgh, K. (2014). Impact of age on the cerebrovascular proteomes of wild-type and Tg-SwDI mice. *PLoS ONE* 9:e89970. doi: 10.1371/journal.pone.0089970

Shawahna, R., Uchida, Y., Decleves, X., Ohtsuki, S., Yousif, S., Dauchy, S., et al. (2011). Transcriptomic and quantitative proteomic analysis of transporters and drug metabolizing enzymes in freshly isolated human brain microvessels. *Mol. Pharm.* 8, 1332–1341. doi: 10.1021/mp200129p

Shusta, E. V. (2005). Blood-brain barrier genomics, proteomics, and new transporter discovery. *NeuroRx* 2, 151–161. doi: 10.1602/neurorx.2.1.151

Shusta, E. V., Boado, R. J., Mathern, G. W., and Pardridge, W. M. (2002). Vascular genomics of the human brain. *J. Cereb. Blood Flow Metab.* 22, 245–252. doi: 10.1097/00004647-200203000-00001

Siegenthaler, J. A., Sohet, F., and Daneman, R. (2013). 'Sealing off the CNS': cellular and molecular regulation of blood-brain barriergenesis. *Curr. Opin. Neurobiol.* 23, 1057–1064. doi: 10.1016/j.conb.2013.06.006

Smyth, G. K. (2004). Linear models and empirical bayes methods for assessing differential expression in microarray experiments. *Stat. Appl. Genet. Mol. Biol.* 3:3. doi: 10.2202/1544-6115.1027

Stenman, J. M., Rajagopal, J., Carroll, T. J., Ishibashi, M., McMahon, J., and McMahon, A. P. (2008). Canonical Wnt signaling regulates organ-specific assembly and differentiation of CNS vasculature. *Science* 322, 1247–1250. doi: 10.1126/science.1164594

Stork, T., Engelen, D., Krudewig, A., Silies, M., Bainton, R. J., and Klambt, C. (2008). Organization and function of the blood-brain barrier in Drosophila. *J. Neurosci.* 28, 587–597. doi: 10.1523/JNEUROSCI.4367-07.2008

Tam, S. J., Richmond, D. L., Kaminker, J. S., Modrusan, Z., Martin-McNulty, B., Cao, T. C., et al. (2012). Death receptors DR6 and TROY regulate brain vascular development. *Dev. Cell* 22, 403–417. doi: 10.1016/j.devcel.2011.11.018

Tam, S. J., and Watts, R. J. (2010). Connecting vascular and nervous system development: angiogenesis and the blood-brain barrier. *Annu. Rev. Neurosci.* 33, 379–408. doi: 10.1146/annurev-neuro-060909-152829

Triguero, D., Buciak, J., and Pardridge, W. M. (1990). Capillary depletion method for quantification of blood-brain barrier transport of circulating peptides and plasma proteins. *J. Neurochem.* 54, 1882–1888. doi: 10.1111/j.1471-4159.1990.tb04886.x

Uchida, Y., Ohtsuki, S., Katsukura, Y., Ikeda, C., Suzuki, T., Kamiie, J., et al. (2011). Quantitative targeted absolute proteomics of human blood-brain barrier transporters and receptors. *J. Neurochem.* 117, 333–345. doi: 10.1111/j.1471-4159.2011.07208.x

Urich, E., Lazic, S. E., Molnos, J., Wells, I., and Freskgard, P. O. (2012). Transcriptional profiling of human brain endothelial cells reveals key properties crucial for predictive *in vitro* blood-brain barrier models. *PLoS ONE* 7:e38149. doi: 10.1371/journal.pone.0038149

Vinters, H. V., Reave, S., Costello, P., Girvin, J. P., and Moore, S. A. (1987). Isolation and culture of cells derived from human cerebral microvessels. *Cell Tissue Res.* 249, 657–667. doi: 10.1007/BF00217338

Wang, S., Qaisar, U., Yin, X., and Grammas, P. (2012a). Gene expression profiling in Alzheimer's disease brain microvessels. *J. Alzheimers Dis.* 31, 193–205. doi: 10.3233/JAD-2012-120454

Wang, Y., Rattner, A., Zhou, Y., Williams, J., Smallwood, P. M., and Nathans, J. (2012b). Norrin/Frizzled4 signaling in retinal vascular development and blood brain barrier plasticity. *Cell* 151, 1332–1344. doi: 10.1016/j.cell.2012.10.042

Webster, J. A., Gibbs, J. R., Clarke, J., Ray, M., Zhang, W., Holmans, P., et al. (2009). Genetic control of human brain transcript expression in Alzheimer disease. *Am. J. Hum. Genet.* 84, 445–458. doi: 10.1016/j.ajhg.2009.03.011

Wilhelm, B. T., Marguerat, S., Watt, S., Schubert, F., Wood, V., Goodhead, I., et al. (2008). Dynamic repertoire of a eukaryotic transcriptome surveyed at single-nucleotide resolution. *Nature* 453, 1239–1243. doi: 10.1038/nature07002

Wolburg, H., Wolburg-Buchholz, K., Kraus, J., Rascher-Eggstein, G., Liebner, S., Hamm, S., et al. (2003). Localization of claudin-3 in tight junctions of the blood-brain barrier is selectively lost during experimental autoimmune encephalomyelitis and human glioblastoma multiforme. *Acta Neuropathol.* 105, 586–592. doi: 10.1007/s00401-003-0688-z

Wosik, K., Cayrol, R., Dodelet-Devillers, A., Berthelet, F., Bernard, M., Moumdjian, R., et al. (2007). Angiotensin II controls occludin function and is required for blood brain barrier maintenance: relevance to multiple sclerosis. *J. Neurosci.* 27, 9032–9042. doi: 10.1523/JNEUROSCI.2088-07.2007

Wu, V. M., and Beitel, G. J. (2004). A junctional problem of apical proportions: epithelial tube-size control by septate junctions in the Drosophila tracheal system. *Curr. Opin. Cell Biol.* 16, 493–499. doi: 10.1016/j.ceb.2004.07.008

Yousif, S., Marie-Claire, C., Roux, F., Scherrmann, J. M., and Decleves, X. (2007). Expression of drug transporters at the blood-brain barrier using an optimized isolated rat brain microvessel strategy. *Brain Res.* 1134, 1–11. doi: 10.1016/j.brainres.2006.11.089

Yu, Y. J., and Watts, R. J. (2013). Developing therapeutic antibodies for neurodegenerative disease. *Neurotherapeutics* 10, 459–472. doi: 10.1007/s13311-013-0187-4

Zhang, Y., Chen, K., Sloan, S. A., Bennett, M. L., Scholze, A. R., O'Keeffe, S., et al. (2014). An RNA-Sequencing Transcriptome and Splicing Database of Glia, Neurons, and Vascular Cells of the Cerebral Cortex. *J. Neurosci.* 34, 11929–11947. doi: 10.1523/JNEUROSCI.1860-14.2014

Zhou, L., Sohet, F., and Daneman, R. (2014a). Purification and culture of central nervous system endothelial cells. *Cold Spring Harb. Protoc.* 2014, 44–46. doi: 10.1101/pdb.top070987

Zhou, Y., Wang, Y., Tischfield, M., Williams, J., Smallwood, P. M., Rattner, A., et al. (2014b). Canonical WNT signaling components in vascular development and barrier formation. *J. Clin. Invest.* 124, 3825–3846. doi: 10.1172/JCI76431

13

Barrier mechanisms in the *Drosophila* blood-brain barrier

Samantha J. Hindle* and Roland J. Bainton*

Department of Anesthesia and Perioperative Care, University of California, San Francisco, San Francisco, CA, USA

Correspondence:
Samantha J. Hindle and Roland J. Bainton, Department of Anesthesia and Perioperative Care, University of California, San Francisco, Genentech Hall, Room S312C 600 16th Street, San Francisco, CA 94158, USA
e-mail: hindles@anesthesia.ucsf.edu; baintonr@anesthesia.ucsf.edu

The invertebrate blood-brain barrier (BBB) field is growing at a rapid pace and, in recent years, studies have shown a physiologic and molecular complexity that has begun to rival its vertebrate counterpart. Novel mechanisms of paracellular barrier maintenance through G-protein coupled receptor signaling were the first demonstrations of the complex adaptive mechanisms of barrier physiology. Building upon this work, the integrity of the invertebrate BBB has recently been shown to require coordinated function of all layers of the compound barrier structure, analogous to signaling between the layers of the vertebrate neurovascular unit. These findings strengthen the notion that many BBB mechanisms are conserved between vertebrates and invertebrates, and suggest that novel findings in invertebrate model organisms will have a significant impact on the understanding of vertebrate BBB functions. In this vein, important roles in coordinating localized and systemic signaling to dictate organism development and growth are beginning to show how the BBB can govern whole animal physiologies. This includes novel functions of BBB gap junctions in orchestrating synchronized neuroblast proliferation, and of BBB secreted antagonists of insulin receptor signaling. These advancements and others are pushing the field forward in exciting new directions. In this review, we provide a synopsis of invertebrate BBB anatomy and physiology, with a focus on insights from the past 5 years, and highlight important areas for future study.

Keywords: invertebrates, blood-brain barrier, chemoprotection, drug delivery, conserved physiology

INTRODUCTION

In order for the nervous system to perform efficiently in coordinating sophisticated movements, behaviors and cognitive functions, it requires chemical isolation from the fluctuating, and potentially damaging, components in the blood. The blood-brain barrier (BBB) has evolved to provide this role, becoming more sophisticated with increasing complexity and demand of the nervous system (Abbott, 2005). Therefore, there are alternative cellular strategies for making BBB structures. In insects, crustacea, cephalopod molluscs and cartilaginous fish the BBB is formed by glial cells, whereas in higher order vertebrates the BBB is formed primarily by the brain vascular endothelium. The formation and functions of the vertebrate BBB are covered extensively by various reviews (e.g., Abbott, 2005; Abbott et al., 2010; Obermeier et al., 2013) and within this BBB series; the aim of this review is to describe the comparative compound structure and associated physiologies of the invertebrate BBB. In recent years, the invertebrate BBB field has flourished with interesting insights into the mechanisms of BBB maintenance, as well as discovering novel metabolic and signaling roles. In addition, both established and emerging invertebrate models are proving useful as drug screening tools to advance therapies for neurodegenerative diseases. These findings, and others, are providing many exciting avenues for future BBB investigations.

Abbreviations: BBB, blood-brain barrier; SPG, subperineurial glia; PG, perineurial glia; CNS, central nervous system; ABC, ATP-binding cassette; SLC, solute carrier; GPCR, G-protein coupled receptor; ARSs, actin-rich structures; IPCs, insulin producing cells; dILPs, *Drosophila* insulin-like peptides

ANATOMICAL OVERVIEW OF THE INVERTEBRATE BBB

Unlike in vertebrates, the blood (hemolymph) in insects does not circulate in a closed capillary network; instead, the hemolymph is freely flowing in the body cavity. As a result, protection of the insect nervous system from the high and often fluctuating concentrations of hemolymph potassium requires that the BBB entirely surrounds the nervous system. Therefore, at the gross anatomical level, the invertebrate BBB is quite different from that of the vascular endothelium in vertebrates. However, like its vertebrate counterpart, the invertebrate BBB is a compound structure (**Figure 1**), analogous to the vertebrate neurovascular unit (Stork et al., 2008; Mayer et al., 2009; DeSalvo et al., 2011, 2014). The invertebrate compound BBB is primarily composed of two surface glia cell types [the apical perineurial glia (PG) and the basal subperineurial glia (SPG)], and the exterior extracellular matrix layer known as the neural lamella (**Figures 1**, **2**). The absence of almost all glial cells in the *Drosophila glial cells missing* (*gcm*) mutant renders the nervous system permeable to a broad range of fluorescent dextran molecules ranging from 10 to 500 kDa (Stork et al., 2008), confirming the importance of glial cells for the invertebrate BBB.

The protective functions of the invertebrate BBB are apparent from embryonic stage 17 throughout development and into the adult stage (Bainton et al., 2005; Schwabe et al., 2005; Stork et al., 2008; Mayer et al., 2009). The PG, however, are not thought to contribute toward these BBB properties early in development as PG cells do not proliferate and completely surround the CNS until late larval stages (Stork et al., 2008). The roles of the BBB during early development are therefore attributed to the SPG, which entirely encapsulate the embryonic nervous system and maintain a tight barrier throughout development and into the adult stage (Stork et al., 2008). In order to maintain this tight diffusion barrier, the SPG cells do not proliferate as the nervous system grows; instead the SPG increase in size and become polyploid (Unhavaithaya and Orr-Weaver, 2012). The polyploid

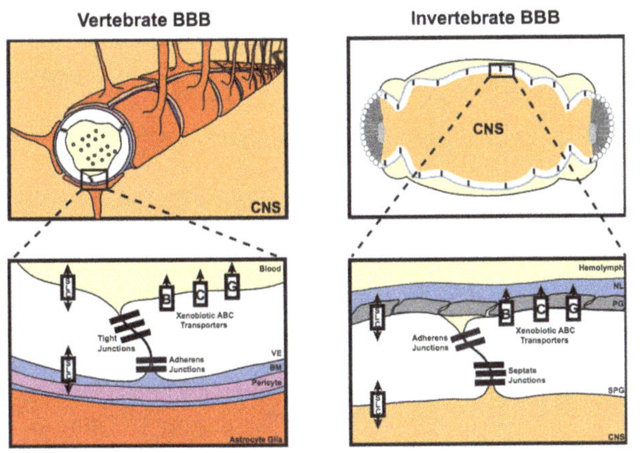

FIGURE 1 | Diagrammatical representation of the vertebrate and invertebrate blood-brain barrier (BBB). The vertebrate BBB is primarily formed by the vascular endothelial cells (VE) that form the capillaries in the brain; however, the surrounding pericytes within the basement membrane (BM), and the end feet of the astrocyte glia also contribute to vertebrate BBB functions. These cellular and non-cellular layers form a compound barrier structure known as the neurovascular unit (NVU). The invertebrate BBB is also a compound structure, consisting of the subperineurial glia (SPG), the perineurial glia (PG), and also a basement membrane known as the neural lamella (NL). Both the vertebrate and invertebrate barriers express tight/septate junction and adherens junction proteins, as well as various xenobiotic ATP-binding Cassette (ABC) and Solute Carrier (SLC) transporters required to maintain central nervous system (CNS) homeostasis.

nature of the SPG is essential to maintain the integrity of the septate junctions that are present between the SPG cells, as the nervous system grows. Inhibition of polyploidy in the SPG causes the septate junctions to rupture and diffusion barrier integrity to be lost (Unhavaithaya and Orr-Weaver, 2012). The formation of the invertebrate BBB has been covered extensively elsewhere (Stork et al., 2008; Edwards and Meinertzhagen, 2010; DeSalvo et al., 2011).

The majority of research on the invertebrate BBB has focused on the main BBB layer, the SPG. However, recent investigations have started to uncover additional roles for cellular and non-cellular layers external to the SPG cells. When the septate junction protein Neurexin IV was mutated in *Drosophila*, the brain penetration of 500 kDa dextran was delayed compared to in the *glial cells missing* mutant, which lacks almost all glial cells (Stork et al., 2008). This suggests that barriers other than the SPG septate junctions are present that can reduce the brain access of certain high molecular weight molecules. It is therefore possible that the PG and neural lamella layers act as non-specific, large molecular-weight filters. Moreover, DeSalvo et al. (2011, 2014) and Meyer et al. (2014) have recently suggested that the PG may have signaling and metabolic roles in BBB function, and in maintaining the neural lamella. Collagen IV, which forms a major part of the neural lamella, is secreted by hemocytes in the embryo and the fat body during post-embryonic development (Mirre et al., 1988; Pastor-Pareja and Xu, 2011); but Meyer et al. (2014) showed that, in addition to the fat body, the *Drosophila* BBB can also contribute to the integrity of the neural lamella. Mutations that affect the deposition of Collagen IV into the neural lamella, result in deformation of the central nervous system (CNS) and deficits in nervous system function (Olofsson and Page, 2005; Meyer et al., 2014). Knocking out matrix metalloproteinases specifically in the SPG or PG cells resulted in larval lethality or an extended ventral nerve cord phenotype, respectively (Meyer et al., 2014). This suggests that

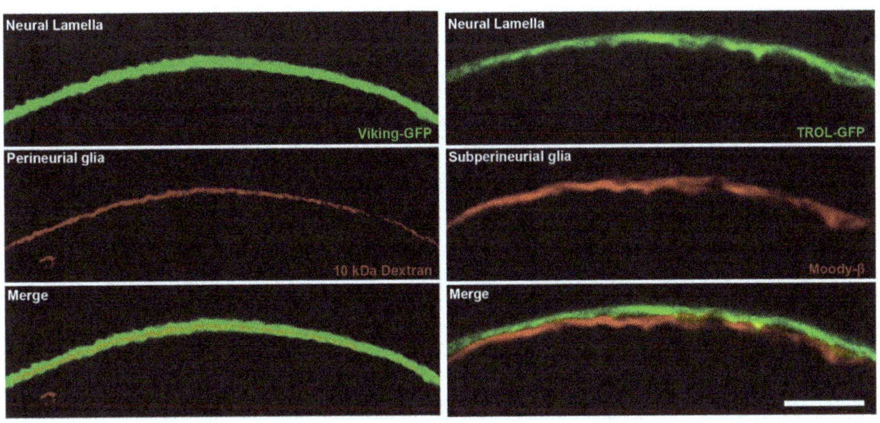

FIGURE 2 | The cellular and non-cellular layers of the *Drosophila* compound BBB. Confocal micrographs of cross sections of the adult *Drosophila* optic lobe showing the localization of the neural lamella (green, left and right panels), the perineurial glia (PG) layer (red, left panels) and the subperineurial glia (SPG) layer (red, right panels). The left panels show the positioning of the neural lamella (identified by the Collagen IV marker Viking-GFP) with respect to the PG (marked by 10 kDa Texas Red Dextran staining). The right panels show the closely apposed neural lamella (marked by the extracellular matrix proteoglycan TROL-GFP) and SPG layer (stained by Moody-β antibody). Scale bar, 20 μm.

the BBB glia are required to maintain the structural integrity of the lamella, which is necessary for correct CNS shape. It therefore appears that the glial cells of the BBB may coordinate with the fat body to maintain and restructure the neural lamella to respond to changing developmental and possibly metabolic demands.

In addition to coordination between the BBB and fat body for maintenance of BBB functions, evidence suggests that neurons also have a role to play. Rbp9, which is homologous to the RNA-binding proteins elav (invertebrates) and hu (vertebrates), has been shown to function in maintaining BBB integrity; loss of Rbp9 function leads to down-regulation of septate junction proteins (primarily Neurexin IV and Coracle), and a resultant porous BBB (Kim et al., 2010). Interestingly, Rbp9 is expressed in neurons, but not in glia, and is therefore not expressed in the BBB itself (Kim-Ha et al., 1999). As the *Rbp9* mutants initially form an intact BBB and only show a porous BBB phenotype upon adult eclosion (Kim et al., 2010), it appears that neuronal Rbp9 plays an important role in BBB maintenance in invertebrates, analogous to the involvement of neuronal signaling in vertebrate BBB integrity (Stewart and Wiley, 1981; Stenman et al., 2008; Daneman et al., 2009). In conclusion, it appears that, like the vertebrate neurovascular unit, there is an important involvement of all layers of the invertebrate compound BBB in the formation and maintenance of the BBB.

MOLECULAR OVERVIEW OF THE INVERTEBRATE BBB

As was mentioned above, the vertebrate vascular endothelium of the brain is specialized to provide an extremely tight barrier to transcellular and paracellular molecular transit. This is due to the following vascular endothelium properties: tight junction complexes between the vascular endothelium cells; enrichment of efflux ABC transporters, which are localized to the apical (luminal) face of the vascular endothelium; low rates of trancytosis due to reduced vesicular trafficking (Muir and Peters, 1962; Reese and Karnovsky, 1967; Brightman and Reese, 1969; Daneman et al., 2010; for reviews see Zlokovic, 2008; Abbott et al., 2010; Obermeier et al., 2013). Many of these molecular properties are also shared by the invertebrate BBB. As alluded to above, the SPG cells of the invertebrate BBB form a tight barrier to paracellular transit due to the presence of pleated septate junctions. These complexes are equivalent to the septate junctions that perform electrical and chemical insulation properties at the axo-glial paranodal junctions (Bhat et al., 2001; Bhat, 2003). SPG cells also express efflux ABC transporters, in particular the ABC B1 xenobiotic efflux transporter Mdr1/P-glycoprotein homolog (Mdr65) is both highly enriched and shows apical localization in the SPG cells (Mayer et al., 2009; DeSalvo et al., 2014). In addition to the chemoprotective properties, the BBB must also regulate the brain access of endogenous molecules, such as glucose and ions. For this, the BBB expresses various solute carrier proteins (SLCs). Recent evidence from *Drosophila* has also suggested interesting roles for the gap junctions that are expressed in both the vertebrate and invertebrate BBB. These findings are discussed in more detail below.

CHEMOPROTECTIVE ROLES OF THE INVERTEBRATE BBB

Septate junction formation and maintenance

The primary barrier of the invertebrate BBB is provided by the septate junctions, the functional equivalent of the vertebrate tight junctions and paranodal septate junctions. The formation and maintenance of a tight diffusion barrier protects the invertebrate nervous system from the high concentrations of potassium in the hemolymph; without this barrier, the embryos are unable to fire action potentials and cannot coordinate movements to hatch from the embryonic cuticle. Septate junction mutations therefore cause a porous BBB and embryonic lethality (e.g., Baumgartner et al., 1996; Schwabe et al., 2005; Stork et al., 2008). The 5 main components of the septate junctions are the membrane components Neurexin IV (Caspr in vertebrates), Neuroglian (vertebrate Neurofascin 155), ATPα and Nervana2 (Na^+/K^+ ATPase α and β subunits), and the intracellular component Coracle (protein 4.1 in vertebrates); however additional proteins are also thought to contribute toward the integrity and maintainance of the septate junctions, including Gliotactin (vertebrate Neuroligin-like), Contactin (vertebrate Contactin), Discs large (Dlg; vertebrate PSD-95-like), Fasciclin III, Moody, Sinuous, and Megatrachea (the latter 2 are vertebrate claudin-like proteins) (Fehon et al., 1994; Auld et al., 1995; Baumgartner et al., 1996; Behr et al., 2003; Genova and Fehon, 2003; Paul et al., 2003; Schulte et al., 2003; Faivre-Sarrailh et al., 2004; Bainton et al., 2005; Schwabe et al., 2005; Stork et al., 2008; Oshima and Fehon, 2011). The septate junction proteins interact with each other to form stable septae contacts between SPG cells that surround the CNS (**Figure 3**). Disruption of any septate junction component leads to a porous BBB phenotype, suggesting that they function interdependently to maintain BBB function. To further address the relationship between septate junction components, Oshima and Fehon (2011) investigated the dynamics of septate junction-associated proteins. Using fluorescence recovery after photobleaching (FRAP), they elegantly showed that the 5 main septate junction components form a very stable core unit, whereas other septate junction-associated proteins (e.g., Dlg) are more mobile. In addition, they discovered that mutating different septate junction-associated proteins had different mechanisms for causing a defective BBB. Loss of some septate junction-associated proteins (e.g., Dlg) caused delayed formation of the stable septate junction core; however, the dynamics of this stable core, once formed, was not affected by *Dlg* mutation. Furthermore, the loss of Gliotactin or endocytic proteins, such as clathrin heavy chain or the *Drosophila* dynamin homolog shibire, led to a mislocalisation of the core septate junction proteins, but had no effect on septate junction core formation (Oshima and Fehon, 2011).

Interestingly, a particular splice form of Neurexin IV (containing exon 3) was shown to be the septate junction-forming version of Neurexin IV and has been shown to be preferentially expressed in glia over neurons (Rodrigues et al., 2012). The mechanism of cell-specific splicing has recently been elucidated in *Drosophila* using elegantly designed genetic reagents that revealed the transcript pattern of the Neurexin IV isoform(s) present in neurons vs. glia (Rodrigues et al., 2012). The authors found that the cell-specific splicing of Neurexin IV involves the RNA-binding protein HOW (Held out wings). HOW is not expressed in neurons, but

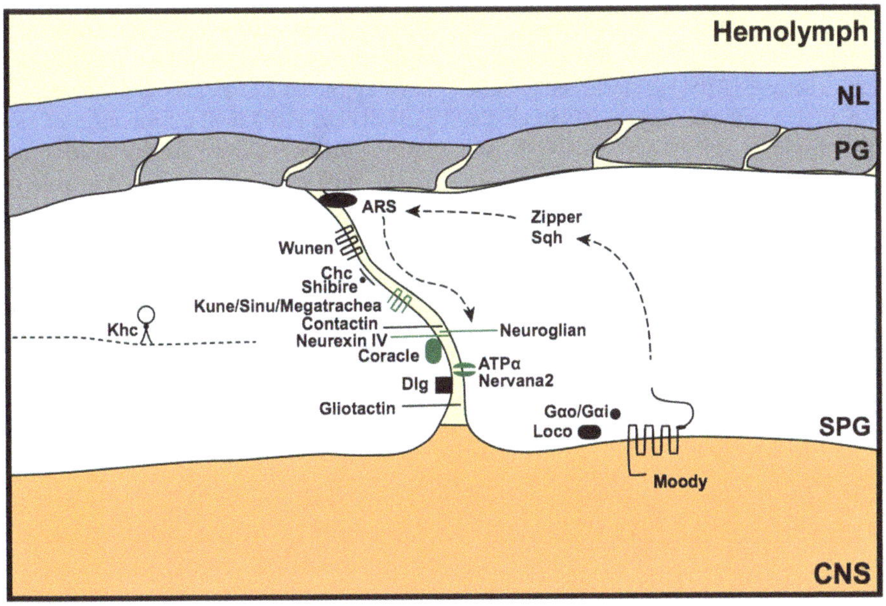

FIGURE 3 | Septate junction formation and maintenance in the invertebrate BBB. Components of the core septate junction (green) and the associated proteins that maintain BBB integrity (black) were identified from loss of function mutants that led to a porous BBB phenotype. *Discs large (Dlg)* mutants showed delayed assembly of the core septate junction components, whereas mutants of Gliotactin, and the endocytic proteins Clathrin-heavy chain (Chc) and Shibire, showed a mislocalization of the septate junction core. The Moody GPCR signaling pathway (Moody, $G_{\alpha o}/G_{\alpha i}$, loco) was shown to genetically interact with actin and non-muscle myosin components [actin-rich structures (ARS), Zipper, Spaghetti squash (Sqh)] to maintain septate junction integrity. Kinesin heavy chain (Khc) may regulate septate junction integrity by transporting Neurexin IV as a cargo protein. Loss of septate junction integrity by disrupting the function of wunen, the lipid phosphate phosphatase, suggests a role for bioactive lipids in paracellular barrier function. NL, neural lamella; PG, perineurial glia; SPG, subperineurial glia; CNS, central nervous system; kune (kune-kune).

ectopic neuronal expression of the constitutively nuclear form of HOW leads to a shift in Neurexin IV isoform expression to that of a glial pattern, leading to larval lethality. This showed that the expression and nuclear localization of HOW in glia predisposes glia to expression of the Neurexin IV (exon 3) form, promoting the formation of septate junctions. Rodrigues et al. (2012) showed the additional involvement of the kinase Cdk12 and the splicesomal component Prp40 in HOW function.

Recently, another claudin-like protein (Kune-kune) and a leukocyte antigen 6 family protein (Coiled) were identified in screens for disrupted BBB integrity (Nelson et al., 2010; Hijazi et al., 2011; Syed et al., 2011). The protein Kune-kune colocalizes with the septate junction component Coracle. Its localization is dependent on the presence of various septate junction components (e.g., Coracle, ATPα, Sinuous and Megatrachea) and, reciprocally, septate junction component localization is dependent on the presence of Kune-kune (Nelson et al., 2010). The authors discovered that Kune-kune regulates both septate junction localization and levels, whereas the other claudin-like proteins Sinuous and Megatrachea regulate septate junction component levels and localization, respectively. Analysis of septate junction levels and localization in single, double and triple mutants of these three claudin-like proteins showed that Kune-kune seems to have a more important role in coordinating septate junction components than Sinuous and Megatrachea (Nelson et al., 2010). The Ly6 family protein Coiled is required for septate junction formation in the embryo; *Coiled* mutations cause disrupted localization of septate junction proteins, including Neurexin IV, Coracle and Discs large, therefore abrogating BBB integrity (Hijazi et al., 2011; Syed et al., 2011).

The G protein-coupled receptors (GPCRs) encoded by the *moody* gene (Moody-α and Moody-β) are required to regulate BBB permeability (Bainton et al., 2005; Schwabe et al., 2005). In addition, the trimeric G proteins Gαi and Gαo, and the regulator of G protein signaling (RGS) loco are thought to signal in the same Moody pathway to regulate septate junction formation and maintenance (Schwabe et al., 2005). Mutations in any of these four components leads to a porous BBB and locomotor dysfunction; however, the *moody* null has a weaker BBB permeability to 10 kDa dextran compared to the *Gαi*, *Gαo*, and *loco* mutants, suggesting that these latter components of the GPCR signaling pathway may have additional upstream or downstream signaling partners involved in septate junction integrity. Interestingly, because loco is a negative regulator of GPCR signaling, this means that both loss and gain of GPCR signaling disrupts BBB integrity. This suggests that discreet, and localized control over this signaling pathway is required for correct septate junction formation and maintenance. That being said, the effect on septate junction integrity appears to be a secondary effect of disrupted GPCR signaling on the actin cytoskeleton and cell size/shape, which leads to reduced undulations of the SPG cells and a shortening of the septate junction length (Schwabe et al., 2005). As the length of the septate junction dictates the tightness of the BBB, this creates a more permeable septate junction barrier in *moody* mutants.

Additional evidence that BBB integrity requires the coordination of Moody signaling and actin dynamics was recently provided by Hatan et al. (2011). They discovered that highly dynamic actin-rich structures (ARSs) are localized in close proximity to, but not overlapping with, the septate junctions; the ARSs colocalized with the fusion proteins Neuroglian-GFP and Scribble-GFP, but not with Neurexin-IV. The regulation of ARS morphology and size was shown to require Moody signaling and also activation of non-muscle myosin components Zipper and Spaghetti squash, which are thought to be downstream of Moody signaling (Hatan et al., 2011). Disruption of ARSs by knocking down the actin nucleation components Arp2 and Arp3 led to dissociation of ARSs and Neuroglian, discontinuous Neuroglian labeling at the septate junction, and breakdown of BBB integrity. These findings suggest an interesting possibility that ARSs act as dynamic docking sites for septate junction components to allow their rapid incorporation into the septate junctions during development to maintain a tight BBB as the brain grows (**Figure 3**). Although the ARSs were only detectable during development, and not during adult stages (Hatan et al., 2011), it would be interesting to determine whether similar structures have a transitory role in the adult, perhaps during circumstances of BBB challenge (chemical, physical or pathological).

Another regulator of BBB integrity, the Kinesin heavy chain, was recently identified from a 5000 candidate-gene screen for locomotion defects (Schmidt et al., 2012). Kinesin heavy chain is classically known for its role in axonal transport. However, Schmidt et al. (2012) discovered an important role within SPG cells. Knocking down *Kinesin heavy chain* specifically in SPG cells led to disrupted axonal excitability resulting in spasticity in adult flies. They found that one of the cargoes of a Kinesin heavy chain-dependent Rab protein is Neurexin-IV, suggesting that Kinesin heavy chain may contribute toward the control of neuronal excitability by regulating Neurexin-IV incorporation into the septate junctions of the SPG cells. The vertebrate homologs of *Drosophila* Kinesin heavy chain are members of the KIF5 family. Both KIF5A and KIF5C are mainly expressed in neurons, but KIF5B shows some expression in glia (Kanai et al., 2000); however, no specific roles have been found for KIF5B in glia. Interestingly, the kinesin KIF13B has been shown to transport Discs large 1 (Dlg1) to sites of membrane remodeling during myelin formation in the Schwann glial cells that insulate the peripheral nervous system (Bolis et al., 2009). Therefore, homologous roles may exist for Kinesin heavy chain proteins in regulating tight junction integrity in the vertebrate BBB.

Wunen is a lipid phosphate phosphatase (LPP), an integral membrane enzyme that, in vertebrates, is required in the regulation of bioactive lipids (e.g., sphingosine-1-phosphate). In *Drosophila*, Wunen is known for its role in germ cell survival and migration (Zhang et al., 1997; Starz-Gaiano et al., 2001); however, it has recently been shown to also localize to septate junctions and to function in septate junction maintenance both in trachea and the BBB (Ile et al., 2012; **Figure 3**). *Wunen* mutant nerve cords show increased permeability to 10 kDa dextran, comparable to that of a Neurexin-IV mutant (Ile et al., 2012). A role for bioactive lipids in the maintenance of BBB integrity has previously been show in mammalian brain microvascular endothelial cells grown in culture (Lee et al., 2006). Treatment with sphingosine-1-phosphate caused relocalization of tight junction/cell-cell contact proteins (including ZO-1 and claudin-5) and increased the trans-epithelial electrical resistance. Also, an *in vivo* role for the mammalian LPP3 in the formation of vascular endothelial cell interactions was shown during development (Escalante-Alcalde et al., 2003). This shows that the role for bioactive lipids in BBB formation and maintenance is evolutionarily conserved, and supports the notion that the invertebrate septate junctions are functionally and mechanistically equivalent to the vertebrate tight junctions.

Xenobiotic efflux transporters

In the vertebrate vascular endothelium, the tight junctions provide chemoprotection to the brain by preventing the entry of molecules via the paracellular route. However, another mechanism is required to prevent transcellular access to the brain. This is provided by the xenobiotic efflux transporters (**Figure 4**). These transporters belong to the ATP-binding cassette (ABC) B, C, and G classes, and are localized to the apical membrane of the vascular endothelium. The xenobiotic efflux transporters are well-characterized for their role in removing lipophilic xenobiotics from the plasma membrane (Leslie et al., 2005), preventing access into the brain. Hence, these transporters are a major hindrance to the successful delivery of therapeutics into the brain (Abbott and Romero, 1996; Abbott, 2013). The main xenobiotic efflux transporters at the BBB are P-glycoprotein (P-gp/ABCB1/Mdr1) and Breast Cancer Resistance Protein (BCRP/ABCG2). In invertebrates a transcellular transport-barrier has been identified in the SPG cells, which is provided by the homolog of P-glycoprotein (Mdr65; Mayer et al., 2009). *Drosophila* Mdr65 shares 42% sequence identity with P-glycoprotein. In the *Drosophila* brain, Mdr65 expression is restricted to the SPG layer of the BBB and, like P-glycoprotein, localizes to the apical membrane. Mayer et al. (2009) identified Mdr65 in a screen for increased BBB permeability to the P-glycoprotein substrate Rhodamine B. Mdr65 is also required at the BBB to protect the brain from various P-glycoprotein xenobiotic substrates, and sensitivity of the *Mdr65* mutants to these xenobiotics can be rescued by expression of human P-glycoprotein specifically in the SPG cells, confirming that Mdr65 provides an evolutionarily conserved chemoprotective transport barrier at the invertebrate BBB. Interestingly, recent work in the migratory locust (*Locusta migratoria*) and the desert locust (*Schistocerca gregaria*) has shown that P-glycoprotein-like xenobiotic transporters also provide a transcellular barrier in the locust brain (Nielsen et al., 2011; Andersson et al., 2013). These findings advance the possibilities of using insect models to study the roles of xenobiotic efflux transporters at the BBB (see below).

In addition to Mdr65, other potential homologs of mammalian chemoprotective ABC transporters are expressed at the invertebrate BBB (DeSalvo et al., 2014). These candidates were identified based on their expression or enrichment in the adult *Drosophila* BBB; these include putative homologs for *ABCC-/MRP-1, 4, 5* and *6* (*CG5789, SUR, CG11897,* and *MRP*) and *ABCG2/BCRP* (*W, CG31689* and *CG3164*). Currently, there are no published reports showing whether these gene

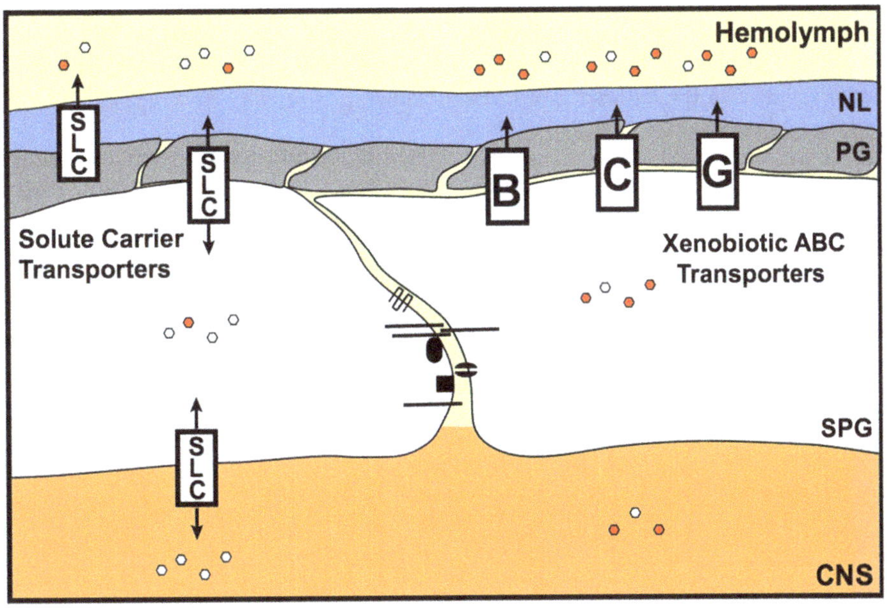

FIGURE 4 | Chemoprotective and endogenous molecule transporters of the invertebrate BBB. The transcellular chemoprotective barrier is primarily provided by the ATP-binding Cassette (ABC) transporters. These xenobiotic efflux transporters are localized to the apical surface of the subperineurial glia (SPG) and remove lipophilic molecules from the SPG membrane, preventing access to the brain. Members of the Solute Carrier (SLC) class of transporters also have some chemoprotective roles, but are mainly known as transporters of endogenous molecules. The SLCs control the entry of hydrophilic/charged molecules (e.g., glucose, amino acids and ions) into the brain, to support optimal brain function. SLCs are present both on the apical and basal surfaces of the SPG cells. Some SLC members, e.g., Oatp58Dc, are also expressed in the perineurial glia (PG). Red and white hexagons represent xenobiotics and endogenous molecules, respectively. NL, neural lamella; CNS, central nervous system.

products can perform chemoprotective functions at the invertebrate BBB.

The vertebrate organic anion transporters (Oats and Oatps) are primarily known for their roles in controlling the brain access of endogenous anions (Kusuhara and Sugiyama, 2005); however, they also have chemoprotective functions (Anderson and Thwaites, 2010). Potential homologs of vertebrate Oats and Oatps are also expressed at the *Drosophila* BBB (*CG6126, CG3168, CG6231, ORCT2, CG4630, ORCT, Oatp58Dc,* and *Oatp74D*; DeSalvo et al., 2014), providing candidates for determining whether Oat/Oatps can also contribute toward chemoprotection of the brain in invertebrates. The *Drosophila* genome encodes eight Oatp transporters, two of which have enriched transcript number in the *Drosophila* brain (*Oatp58Dc* and *Oatp74D*; http://flyatlas.org/). Seabrooke and O'Donnell (2013) have recently shown that Oatp58Dc is expressed in the PG, SPG and post-mitotic neurons, and is required specifically in PG cells for maintaining chemical protection of the brain from fluorescein. In the absence of Oatp58Dc, levels of hemolymph-injected fluorescein are higher in the brains of *Oatp58Dc Drosophila* brains. This shows that, at least for Oatp58Dc, invertebrate organic anion transporters can also provide chemoprotective functions to the BBB.

ENDOGENOUS MOLECULE REGULATION

Transcellular access to the brain is not only controlled by ATP-dependent xenobiotic efflux transporters; secondary/facilitated transporters and channel proteins are also expressed at the BBB in both vertebrates and invertebrates (**Figure 4**). The largest group of the facilitated transporters is the solute carrier (SLC) transporters. In vertebrates, the SLCs are grouped into 48 classes (SLC 1–48) based on sequence identity (Hediger et al., 2004). It was recently documented that *Drosophila* glia express SLCs from eight of these vertebrate SLC classes (*SLC1, SLC5, SLC6, SLC7, SLC24,* and *SLC29*), but it was not determined whether these SLCs were expressed or enriched in the BBB (Featherstone, 2011). Microarray analysis of the adult *Drosophila* BBB glia has recently identified which of these SLCs are expressed or enriched at the BBB, and also identified additional BBB SLC class candidates (DeSalvo et al., 2014). Of note, there are 18 SLC homologs that are both highly expressed and enriched at the *Drosophila* BBB (members from the SLCO, 2, 7, 16, 19, 22, and 39 classes) and would therefore be good candidates for further study.

A role for the SLC12 transporter Ncc69 (a cation chloride cotransporter) and its serine/threonine kinase regulator Fray has been shown in controlling extracellular volume in peripheral nerves (Leiserson et al., 2011). Mutants in either *Ncc69* or *Fray* lead to the accumulation of fluid between axons and glia, resulting in peripheral neuropathy. Both Ncc69 and Fray were also shown to function in the SPG cells of the blood-nerve barrier.

Eight potential SLC21 (Oatp) transporters have been identified in *Drosophila* (Seabrooke and O'Donnell, 2013). Of these eight, four are expressed in the *Drosophila* head or brain (*Oatp30B, Oatp33Ea, Oatp58Dc,* and *Oatp74D*; http://flyatlas.org/; Torrie et al., 2004; Seabrooke and O'Donnell, 2013). According to the data in DeSalvo et al. (2014), *Oatp30B* is primarily expressed in neurons, however, Meyer et al. (2014) suggested a glial role for Oatp30B in neural lamella integrity and CNS shape. *Oatp33Ea* shows very low expression in all cell types of the adult brain; as its expression was previously shown in the fly head, Oatp33Ea may therefore localize to the fat bodies of the head rather than the brain. As mentioned above, the organic anion transporter Oatp58Dc is expressed in the PG, SPG and post-mitotic neurons of the *Drosophila* CNS; however, its function was shown to be specifically required in the PG layer of the BBB (Seabrooke and O'Donnell, 2013). This suggests a novel role for the PG in regulating organic anion access to the brain. *Oatp74D* was also shown by DeSalvo et al. (2014) to be highly enriched in the BBB (21-fold and 64-fold enrichment compared to whole brain and neuron levels, respectively). It would be interesting to determine the function of this transporter, whether it is required in the SPG or PG, and whether there is any overlap or coordination in the BBB functions of Oatp58Dc and Oatp74D.

Although the BBB provides a paracellular barrier to the movement of inorganic ions between the hemolymph and the brain, transcellular transit does occur (Treherne, 1966). This involves both energy-dependent mechanisms (Na^+/K^+ ATPases) and also diffusion down the electrochemical gradient, which may be partially set up by V-type H^+-ATPases (Kocmarek and O'Donnell, 2011).

Another mode of transit across the BBB is provided by receptor-mediated transcytosis. In general, vesicular transcytosis is reduced in the vascular endothelial cells of the vertebrate BBB; however, small and large molecular weight molecules can transit the BBB by a specific, receptor-mediated route (see Xiao and Gan, 2013 for review). In *Drosophila*, the mechanism of receptor-mediated transcytosis of lipoprotein via the low-density lipoprotein receptor (LRP) has recently been investigated (Brankatschk and Eaton, 2010; Brankatschk et al., 2014). Lipophorin is the main lipoprotein present in *Drosophila*. The protein component of lipophorin (apolipophorin) can be cleaved into ApoLI and ApoLII, and this cleavage was shown to affect the localization of the lipoprotein once it had transited across the BBB. The full length ApoL localized to neurons, whereas ApoLII was found in the optic anlage. The authors further investigated the function of lipophorin in the brain and found that knocking down the production of lipophorin in its synthesis organ (the fat body) blocked neuroblast proliferation in the first/second instar larvae. They suggest that this may be due to the reduced BBB transit of GPI-linked proteins, which they show requires the presence of lipophorin. Brankatschk and Eaton (2010) also showed that lipophorin-associated, sterol-linked fluorescent proteins only have limited access to the brain and primarily accumulate at the BBB. From this, one might conclude that sterol-linked proteins don't play a role in neuroblast proliferation as they scarcely enter the brain; however, recent work in the Brand lab discovered a role for synchronized BBB calcium signaling in coordinated neuroblast proliferation (Speder and Brand, 2014; see below). Therefore, sterol-linked proteins may not need to enter the brain to induce neuroblast proliferation. Instead their accumulation in the BBB may trigger a signaling cascade that induces the underlying neuroblasts to proliferate. Brankatschk et al. (2014) have also shown that BBB calcium release is required for the BBB transit and normal brain localization of Lipid Transfer Particle. This was shown to be important for the insulin-dependent regulation of systemic growth (see below).

METABOLIC AND SIGNALING ROLES OF THE INVERTEBRATE BBB

The previous sections have primarily dealt with the anatomy and function of the invertebrate BBB in chemoprotection of the brain, regulation of endogenous molecule access to the brain, and the maintenance of these functions. However, the BBB acts as more than just a selective filter. Exciting new findings have revealed that the *Drosophila* BBB can also sense and respond to systemic metabolic signals (Chell and Brand, 2010; Speder and Brand, 2014). Thus, the BBB appears to be a dynamic and communicative layer between the brain and the body (**Figure 5**). The insulin signaling pathway has long been known to sense nutritional status and dictate organism growth, reproductive output and lifespan, and this is evolutionarily conserved (Partridge et al., 2011; Wigby et al., 2011; Mirth and Shingleton, 2012). This systemic signaling is coordinated by the secretion of *Drosophila* insulin-like peptides (dILPs), which are secreted by insulin producing cells (IPCs) in the brain. The secretion of dILPs is triggered by a factor produced by the fat body (the *Drosophila* liver and adipose tissue equivalent) in response to dietary amino acids [through the Slimfast and target of rapamycin (TOR) signaling pathways; Geminard et al., 2009], and fat and sugar (through the *Drosophila* cytokine Unpaired2; Rajan and Perrimon, 2012; reviewed in Nassel et al., 2013). In addition to the IPCs, the BBB glia have recently been shown to be a source of dILPs required for the reactivation of proliferation in the underlying neuroblasts (Chell and Brand, 2010; Speder and Brand, 2014; **Figure 5**). The BBB glia expression of dILP2 and dILP6 is nutrient-dependent, suggesting that a humoral signal from the fat body (possibly Unpaired2; Rajan and Perrimon, 2012) is sensed by the surface glia leading to dILP production and secretion to reactivate neuroblast proliferation in the larval brain (Chell and Brand, 2010). It would be interesting to determine whether this humoral signal is the same signal that depends upon lipophorin particles to induce neuroblast proliferation, as shown by Brankatschk and Eaton (2010).

Additional evidence for the role of BBB glia in coordinating neuroblast proliferation was provided by Speder and Brand (2014) who discovered that gap junctional proteins expressed in the SPG cells were required for synchronized calcium oscillations within the SPG, and for neuroblast proliferation. The synchronized calcium oscillations were nutrient-dependent, and were therefore suggested to be a bridge in the gap between the nutrition-dependent fat body-derived signal and the synchronous nutrient-dependent exit of neuroblasts from quiescence. Although this work suggests a direct role for the BBB glia in neuroblast proliferation, Sousa-Nunes et al. (2011) suggest that neuroblast proliferation requires dILP6 expression by the underlying cortex glia rather than the SPG cells. Therefore, the role of the BBB may be to coordinate a complex signaling network, bringing together systemic nutritional signals and relaying this information to the underlying cortex glia to regulate neuroblast proliferation (**Figure 5**).

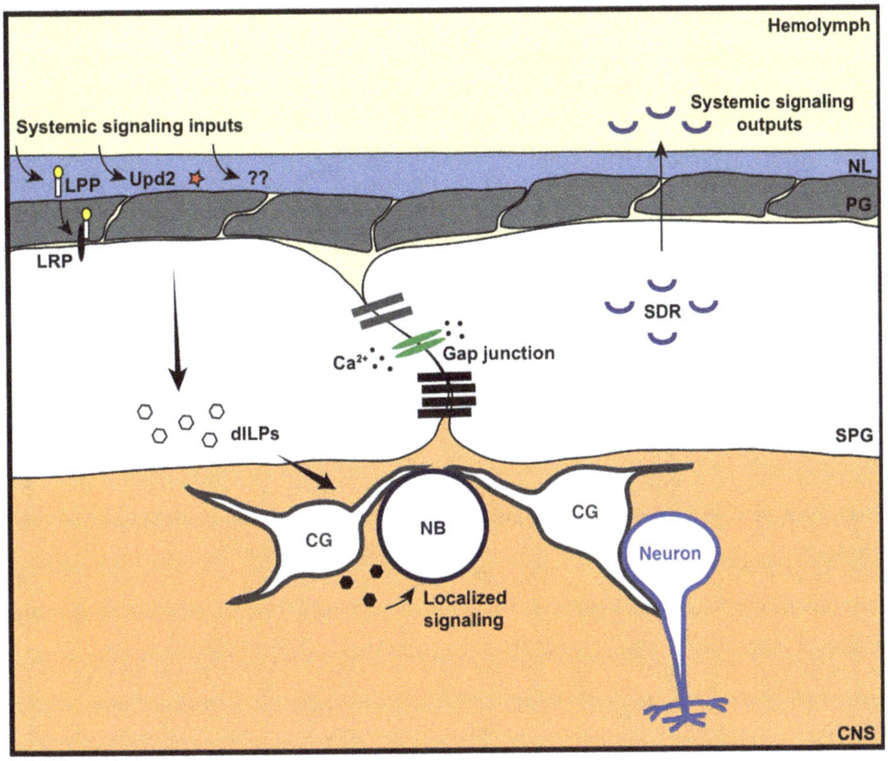

FIGURE 5 | Metabolic and signaling roles of the invertebrate BBB. The *Drosophila* BBB can sense and respond to various systemic signaling inputs. This includes the lipoprotein-like receptor (LRP) ligand lipophorin (LPP), the cytokine-like molecule Unpaired-2 (Upd2) and other unidentified signaling molecules (??) that are released in response to metabolic/nutritional triggers. This leads to localized secretion of *Drosophila* insulin-like peptide (dILP) by the subperineurial glia (SPG) and/or cortex glia (CG) to coordinate neuroblast (NB) proliferation. The coordinated response of the SPG is thought to occur through synchronous calcium (Ca^{2+}) oscillations via gap junction proteins. In addition to localized growth regulation, the *Drosophila* BBB can also regulate systemic growth (whole organism growth). The SPG cells both express and constitutively secrete a negative regulator of insulin signaling: the secreted decoy of insulin receptor (SDR); SDR mutants lead to excessive growth of the whole animal.

In extension of this work, Brankatschk et al. (2014) have shown that the BBB can also regulate growth systemically (whole organism growth) in addition to localized growth control (neuroblast proliferation). They found that the BBB controls Lipid Transfer Particle brain access and localization to Dilp2-recruiting neurons in the brain; this resulted in systemic secretion of Dilp2 from insulin producing cells in the brain, impacting on whole organism growth. This BBB function is nutrition-dependent and requires calcium signaling in the BBB. In fact, genetic manipulations that forced an increase in BBB calcium release resulted in normal systemic insulin signaling despite an inappropriate nutritional state. Together, these fascinating findings show that the BBB can have a master role in linking nutritional input to both local and systemic growth outputs.

A further role for the *Drosophila* BBB in growth control was shown by Okamoto et al. (2013). The authors discovered a negative regulator of insulin signaling, the secreted decoy of insulin receptor (SDR), in an RNAi screen for secreted regulators of body growth; *SDR* mutants had a larger body weight. SDR is expressed in the BBB glia of the CNS, the midgut muscles and imaginal discs of the larva; however, its function in body growth was shown to be dependent on its BBB glia expression (Okamoto et al., 2013). Although SDR expression and secretion was shown to be constitutive, and not dependent on nutritional status, it proved to be crucial for controlling body weight during adverse nutritional conditions; *SDR* mutants were lethal when grown in adverse nutritional conditions whereas wild type larvae survived. These results suggest a further role for the BBB in controlling body growth during development. The body size of the adult fly is predetermined during the larval and pupal stages (Mirth and Shingleton, 2012); however, DeSalvo et al. (2014) showed that *SDR* is highly expressed and enriched in the BBB glia of the adult brain. Therefore, this begs a number of questions. What is the role of SDR in the adult? Is its secretion regulated or constitutive in the adult? Does its expression level change with age? Does SDR have a role in regulating aging? These are exciting questions that can easily be addressed in the *Drosophila* model organism.

This additional role of the BBB in coordinating both localized and systemic insulin signaling to regulate localized and organism-wide growth is likely to be one in a number of ways that the BBB can communicate with various organs of the body.

THE INVERTEBRATE BBB AS A TOOL FOR ADVANCING THERAPEUTIC INTERVENTIONS

One of the major hindrances in neuropharmacology is the resistance of the BBB for drug delivery to the brain. This is primarily due to the efficient functioning of P-glycoprotein. Furthermore, the pre-clinical to clinical translation of CNS drug penetration following the use of P-glycoprotein inhibitors has proved unsuccessful due to incomplete P-glycoprotein inhibition (see Kalvass et al., 2013 for a detailed review). Therefore, being able to develop drugs that are not P-glycoprotein substrates would be a beneficial strategy. Drug screening largely depends upon *in vitro* tests using brain microvascular endothelial cell monolayers. However, studies have shown that brain microvascular endothelial cells grown in culture do not maintain their full BBB properties; of particular note, they show a down regulation of P-glycoprotein (Calabria and Shusta, 2008), suggesting that this methodology is not ideal. Early phase drug screening using rodents would be too costly; therefore, there is a need for a cost-effective *in vivo* approach to further the development of CNS drugs. With this in mind, DeSalvo et al. (2011) developed an approach to perform live screening of chemical fluor penetration into the *Drosophila* brain. This approach involved visualizing a change in the fluorescence intensity in the fly eye, due to a change in permeability of the blood-eye barrier. DeSalvo et al. (2011) showed this approach could be used to screen for genetic modifiers of BBB integrity and identified various interesting candidate genes that were expressed in different layers of the compound BBB, supporting the notion that all layers of the compound barrier are important for full BBB integrity. In addition to genetic modifiers, this live imaging approach can be used for large-scale drug screening to identify drugs that will penetrate the BBB and are therefore not likely P-glycoprotein (Mdr65) substrates.

Interestingly, other invertebrate BBB models have been developed to allow *in vivo* drug screening. Using the grasshopper system, Nielsen et al. (2011) showed that co-administration of a P-glycoprotein inhibitor with a test P-glycoprotein substrate rendered the BBB more permeable to the P-glycoprotein substrate. Furthermore, Andersson et al. (2013) were able to use this methodology to distinguish P-glycoprotein substrates from non-substrates using liquid chromatography-mass spectrometry to measure the drug content in the brain, either in the absence or presence of a P-glycoprotein inhibitor. This confirmed that P-glycoprotein substrates could be identified using this model system. These invertebrate BBB models provide a valuable bridge between endothelial cell culture models and vertebrate P-glycoprotein knock-out models for drug screening.

In addition to using invertebrate BBB models to assess BBB permeability of test drugs, these model systems can also be used to test new technologies for increasing drug delivery to the brain. The cost of performing these trials in invertebrates would be comparatively small and would therefore allow for a much broader scaled testing strategy than can be applied to vertebrate systems. The use of *Drosophila* to address the problem of brain drug delivery was shown by Sarantseva et al. (2011), where they tested the ability of dendrimers to cross the BBB. Dendrimers are nanopolymers that can encapsulate various cargo and therefore have been utilized in many biological (and non-biological) fields (see Kesharwani et al., 2014 for a review). The advantage of using these nanopolymers as a CNS drug delivery strategy is the ability to customize the dendrimer to very specific requirements. For example, the functional group on the polymer surface can be modified to allow tissue-specific targeting, and they are also able to "carry" various types of cargo, including nucleic acids, proteins and drugs across cell membranes (Kesharwani et al., 2014). The use of these biological vectors in drug delivery have been shown for epithelial barriers, such as the skin and intestine (e.g., Kaminskas et al., 2012). Moreover, the ability of the lysine-based dendrimer D5 to carry peptides across the *Drosophila* BBB has been shown (Sarantseva et al., 2011), suggesting that this nanotechnology could be a useful strategy for improving CNS drug delivery in vertebrates.

FUTURE QUESTIONS AND EMERGING AREAS OF BBB RESEARCH

We have highlighted that the invertebrate BBB is a compound structure, like the vertebrate neurovascular unit, and each of its cellular and non-cellular layers appears to have a coordinated role in maintaining BBB integrity and for signaling purposes. However, there is still much to learn about the nature of the communication between these layers, how this is regulated, and how the individual layers respond to physical, chemical or pathological perturbations. In particular, understanding the compensations that occur within these BBB layers during a disease state will likely be required to advance therapeutic design to combat these disorders. Expression changes of chemoprotective transporters, such as P-glycoprotein and Breast Cancer Resistance Protein, have already been shown to occur in disease states including Alzheimer's disease and epilepsy (Vogelgesang et al., 2002; Loscher and Potschka, 2005; Miller, 2010). These expression changes are thought to explain the multidrug resistance phenotypes seen in some neurological disorders. Therefore, investigations that show ways to counter these compensations would be valuable for treating these diseases. Furthermore, being able to parse the contribution of the PG and SPG toward CNS protection would be a valuable endeavor. This could involve a genetic approach, like used by DeSalvo et al. (2014), to produce separate PG and SPG transcriptomes in both the wild type and diseased states.

In addition to parsing the contributions of the SPG and PG toward BBB function, an important future question for the field is to determine whether there are regional specializations across the invertebrate compound BBB. We have seen evidence of coordinated BBB functions via gap junction signaling within the SPG cells, which impacted upon the synchrony of neuroblast proliferation (Speder and Brand, 2014); equally possible is the presence of regional BBB responses to localized signals, in terms of developmental and pathological signals, as well as localized immune cell transmigration. In extension of this, it is important to understand how the different layers of the compound BBB network can respond to localized signals and perturbations. For example, it would be interesting to determine whether there are different subsets of underlying cortex glia that can sense and respond to chemical perturbations of the BBB and other subsets that can respond to the metabolic status of the CNS, to provide both broad and localized "feedback circuitry" to relay information about CNS homeostasis to the BBB. Due to the powerful genetic strengths of the *Drosophila* system and the accessible architecture of the invertebrate BBB, this is an area where invertebrate model organisms can help to pave the way forward.

An exciting, emerging area of BBB research that deserves further attention is whether there are sex-specific traits of the BBB. It is already known that there are sex-specific differences in the CNS, a concept that is evolutionarily conserved (Cachero et al., 2010). However, very little is known about sex-specific components of the BBB and its impact on physiology. This is another research area where *Drosophila* can advance the field, as it is possible to specifically change the sex of the BBB using targeted genetics. This allows the separation of sex-specific BBB effects from sex-specific effects of the whole organism. This approach is possible because sex determination is cell autonomous in flies; therefore, one can express a master regulator of sex determination (e.g., *TraF*) in a specific cell type and alter the sex identity of that cell type. This has been shown for the *Drosophila* liver and adipose tissue equivalent (the fat body), showing that male courtship behavior can be altered by changing the sex identity of the fat body cells (Lazareva et al., 2007). This technique was recently applied to the BBB, showing a behavioral impact of sex-specificity in the BBB (Hoxha et al., 2013). BBB-specific, ectopic expression of a gene that feminizes cells (*TraF*) led to reduced courtship behavior in males. Hoxha et al. (2013) showed that this was not solely a developmental effect, as BBB-specific expression of TraF only during the adult stages of the fly still reduced courtship in males. The authors also showed that this reduction in courtship behavior required the GPCR Moody, which Bainton et al. (2005) previously showed to have separable roles in maintaining BBB integrity (a structural role) and behavioral drug responses (a signaling role). Interestingly, there are sex-specific enrichments of *Moody* isoforms in the BBB (Hoxha et al., 2013). Of the four *Moody* isoforms, there is an enrichment of one of the *Moody-α* isoforms in male heads and an enrichment of both *Moody-β* isoforms in female heads. Therefore, Hoxha et al. (2013) have already identified that sex-specific transcripts do exist in the BBB and that sex identity of the BBB can impact upon behavior. It would be interesting to determine whether sex-specific differences in the BBB can also impact upon pharmacokinetics, as this could have major implications for treatments of CNS disorders.

REFERENCES

Abbott, N. J. (2005). Dynamics of CNS barriers: evolution, differentiation, and modulation. *Cell. Mol. Neurobiol.* 25, 5–23. doi: 10.1007/s10571-004-1374-y

Abbott, N. J. (2013). Blood-brain barrier structure and function and the challenges for CNS drug delivery. *J. Inherit. Metab. Dis.* 36, 437–449. doi: 10.1007/s10545-013-9608-0

Abbott, N. J., Patabendige, A. A., Dolman, D. E., Yusof, S. R., and Begley, D. J. (2010). Structure and function of the blood-brain barrier. *Neurobiol. Dis.* 37, 13–25. doi: 10.1016/j.nbd.2009.07.030

Abbott, N. J., and Romero, I. A. (1996). Transporting therapeutics across the blood-brain barrier. *Mol. Med. Today* 2, 106–113. doi: 10.1016/1357-4310(96)88720-X

Anderson, C. M., and Thwaites, D. T. (2010). Hijacking solute carriers for proton-coupled drug transport. *Physiology (Bethesda)* 25, 364–377. doi: 10.1152/physiol.00027.2010

Andersson, O., Hansen, S. H., Hellman, K., Olsen, L. R., Andersson, G., Badolo, L., et al. (2013). The grasshopper: a novel model for assessing vertebrate brain uptake. *J. Pharmacol. Exp. Ther.* 346, 211–218. doi: 10.1124/jpet.113.205476

Auld, V. J., Fetter, R. D., Broadie, K., and Goodman, C. S. (1995). Gliotactin, a novel transmembrane protein on peripheral glia, is required to form the blood-nerve barrier in Drosophila. *Cell* 81, 757–767. doi: 10.1016/0092-8674(95)90537-5

Bainton, R. J., Tsai, L. T., Schwabe, T., DeSalvo, M., Gaul, U., and Heberlein, U. (2005). moody encodes two GPCRs that regulate cocaine behaviors and blood-brain barrier permeability in Drosophila. *Cell* 123, 145–156. doi: 10.1016/j.cell.2005.07.029

Baumgartner, S., Littleton, J. T., Broadie, K., Bhat, M. A., Harbecke, R., Lengyel, J. A., et al. (1996). A Drosophila neurexin is required for septate junction and blood-nerve barrier formation and function. *Cell* 87, 1059–1068. doi: 10.1016/S0092-8674(00)81800-0

Behr, M., Riedel, D., and Schuh, R. (2003). The claudin-like megatrachea is essential in septate junctions for the epithelial barrier function in Drosophila. *Dev. Cell* 5, 611–620. doi: 10.1016/S1534-5807(03)00275-2

Bhat, M. A. (2003). Molecular organization of axo-glial junctions. *Curr. Opin. Neurobiol.* 13, 552–559. doi: 10.1016/j.conb.2003.09.004

Bhat, M. A., Rios, J. C., Lu, Y., Garcia-Fresco, G. P., Ching, W., St Martin, M., et al. (2001). Axon-glia interactions and the domain organization of myelinated axons requires neurexin IV/Caspr/Paranodin. *Neuron* 30, 369–383. doi: 10.1016/S0896-6273(01)00294-X

Bolis, A., Coviello, S., Visigalli, I., Taveggia, C., Bachi, A., Chishti, A. H., et al. (2009). Dlg1, Sec8, and Mtmr2 regulate membrane homeostasis in Schwann cell myelination. *J. Neurosci.* 29, 8858–8870. doi: 10.1523/JNEUROSCI.1423-09.2009

Brankatschk, M., Dunst, S., Nemetschke, L., and Eaton, S. (2014). Delivery of circulating lipoproteins to specific neurons in the *Drosophila* brain regulates systemic insulin signaling. *Elife* 3:e02862. doi: 10.7554/eLife.02862

Brankatschk, M., and Eaton, S. (2010). Lipoprotein particles cross the blood-brain barrier in Drosophila. *J. Neurosci.* 30, 10441–10447. doi: 10.1523/JNEUROSCI.5943-09.2010

Brightman, M. W., and Reese, T. S. (1969). Junctions between intimately apposed cell membranes in the vertebrate brain. *J. Cell Biol.* 40, 648–677. doi: 10.1083/jcb.40.3.648

Cachero, S., Ostrovsky, A. D., Yu, J. Y., Dickson, B. J., and Jefferis, G. S. (2010). Sexual dimorphism in the fly brain. *Curr. Biol.* 20, 1589–1601. doi: 10.1016/j.cub.2010.07.045

Calabria, A. R., and Shusta, E. V. (2008). A genomic comparison of *in vivo* and *in vitro* brain microvascular endothelial cells. *J. Cereb. Blood Flow Metab.* 28, 135–148. doi: 10.1038/sj.jcbfm.9600518

Chell, J. M., and Brand, A. H. (2010). Nutrition-responsive glia control exit of neural stem cells from quiescence. *Cell* 143, 1161–1173. doi: 10.1016/j.cell.2010.12.007

Daneman, R., Agalliu, D., Zhou, L., Kuhnert, F., Kuo, C. J., and Barres, B. A. (2009). Wnt/beta-catenin signaling is required for CNS, but not non-CNS, angiogenesis. *Proc. Natl. Acad. Sci. U.S.A.* 106, 641–646. doi: 10.1073/pnas.0805165106

Daneman, R., Zhou, L., Agalliu, D., Cahoy, J. D., Kaushal, A., and Barres, B. A. (2010). The mouse blood-brain barrier transcriptome: a new resource for understanding the development and function of brain endothelial cells. *PLoS ONE* 5:e13741. doi: 10.1371/journal.pone.0013741

DeSalvo, M. K., Hindle, S. J., Rusan, Z. M., Orng, S., Eddison, M., Halliwell, K., et al. (2014). The Drosophila surface glia transcriptome: evolutionary conserved blood-brain barrier processes. *Front. Neurosci.* 8:346. doi: 10.3389/fnins.2014.00346

DeSalvo, M. K., Mayer, N., Mayer, F., and Bainton, R. J. (2011). Physiologic and anatomic characterization of the brain surface glia barrier of Drosophila. *Glia* 59, 1322–1340. doi: 10.1002/glia.21147

Edwards, T. N., and Meinertzhagen, I. A. (2010). The functional organisation of glia in the adult brain of Drosophila and other insects. *Prog. Neurobiol.* 90, 471–497. doi: 10.1016/j.pneurobio.2010.01.001

Escalante-Alcalde, D., Hernandez, L., Le Stunff, H., Maeda, R., Lee, H. S., Gang, C. Jr., et al. (2003). The lipid phosphatase LPP3 regulates extra-embryonic vasculogenesis and axis patterning. *Development* 130, 4623–4637. doi: 10.1242/dev.00635

Faivre-Sarrailh, C., Banerjee, S., Li, J., Hortsch, M., Laval, M., and Bhat, M. A. (2004). Drosophila contactin, a homolog of vertebrate contactin, is required for septate junction organization and paracellular barrier function. *Development* 131, 4931–4942. doi: 10.1242/dev.01372

Featherstone, D. E. (2011). Glial solute carrier transporters in Drosophila and mice. *Glia* 59, 1351–1363. doi: 10.1002/glia.21085

Fehon, R. G., Dawson, I. A., and Artavanis-Tsakonas, S. (1994). A Drosophila homologue of membrane-skeleton protein 4.1 is associated with septate junctions and is encoded by the coracle gene. *Development* 120, 545–557.

Geminard, C., Rulifson, E. J., and Leopold, P. (2009). Remote control of insulin secretion by fat cells in Drosophila. *Cell Metab.* 10, 199–207. doi: 10.1016/j.cmet.2009.08.002

Genova, J. L., and Fehon, R. G. (2003). Neuroglian, Gliotactin, and the Na+/K+ ATPase are essential for septate junction function in Drosophila. *J. Cell Biol.* 161, 979–989. doi: 10.1083/jcb.200212054

Hatan, M., Shinder, V., Israeli, D., Schnorrer, F., and Volk, T. (2011). The Drosophila blood brain barrier is maintained by GPCR-dependent dynamic actin structures. *J. Cell Biol.* 192, 307–319. doi: 10.1083/jcb.201007095

Hediger, M. A., Romero, M. F., Peng, J. B., Rolfs, A., Takanaga, H., and Bruford, E. A. (2004). The ABCs of solute carriers: physiological, pathological and therapeutic implications of human membrane transport proteinsIntroduction. *Pflugers Arch.* 447, 465–468. doi: 10.1007/s00424-003-1192-y

Hijazi, A., Haenlin, M., Waltzer, L., and Roch, F. (2011). The Ly6 protein coiled is required for septate junction and blood brain barrier organisation in Drosophila. *PLoS ONE* 6:e17763. doi: 10.1371/journal.pone.0017763

Hoxha, V., Lama, C., Chang, P. L., Saurabh, S., Patel, N., Olate, N., et al. (2013). Sex-specific signaling in the blood-brain barrier is required for male courtship in Drosophila. *PLoS Genet.* 9:e1003217. doi: 10.1371/journal.pgen.1003217

Ile, K. E., Tripathy, R., Goldfinger, V., and Renault, A. D. (2012). Wunen, a Drosophila lipid phosphate phosphatase, is required for septate junction-mediated barrier function. *Development* 139, 2535–2546. doi: 10.1242/dev.077289

Kalvass, J. C., Polli, J. W., Bourdet, D. L., Feng, B., Huang, S. M., Liu, X., et al. (2013). Why clinical modulation of efflux transport at the human blood-brain barrier is unlikely: the ITC evidence-based position. *Clin. Pharmacol. Ther.* 94, 80–94. doi: 10.1038/clpt.2013.34

Kaminskas, L. M., Boyd, B. J., and Porter, C. J. H. (2012). Dendrimer pharmacokinetics: the effect of size, structure and surface characteristics on ADME properties (vol 6, pg 1063, 2011). *Nanomedicine* 7, 167–168. doi: 10.2217/nnm.11.67

Kanai, Y., Okada, Y., Tanaka, Y., Harada, A., Terada, S., and Hirokawa, N. (2000). KIF5C, a novel neuronal kinesin enriched in motor neurons. *J. Neurosci.* 20, 6374–6384.

Kesharwani, P., Jain, K., and Jain, N. K. (2014). Dendrimer as nanocarrier for drug delivery. *Prog. Polymer Sci.* 39, 268–307. doi: 10.1016/j.progpolymsci.2013.07.005

Kim, J., Kim, Y. J., and Kim-Ha, J. (2010). Blood-brain barrier defects associated with Rbp9 mutation. *Mol Cells* 29, 93–98. doi: 10.1007/s10059-010-0040-0

Kim-Ha, J., Kim, J., and Kim, Y. J. (1999). Requirement of RBP9, a Drosophila Hu homolog, for regulation of cystocyte differentiation and oocyte determination during oogenesis. *Mol. Cell. Biol.* 19, 2505–2514.

Kocmarek, A. L., and O'Donnell, M. J. (2011). Potassium fluxes across the blood brain barrier of the cockroach, Periplaneta americana. *J. Insect Physiol.* 57, 127–135. doi: 10.1016/j.jinsphys.2010.09.011

Kusuhara, H., and Sugiyama, Y. (2005). Active efflux across the blood-brain barrier: role of the solute carrier family. *NeuroRx* 2, 73–85. doi: 10.1602/neurorx.2.1.73

Lazareva, A. A., Roman, G., Mattox, W., Hardin, P. E., and Dauwalder, B. (2007). A role for the adult fat body in Drosophila male courtship behavior. *PLoS Genet.* 3:e16. doi: 10.1371/journal.pgen.0030016

Lee, J. F., Zeng, Q., Ozaki, H., Wang, L., Hand, A. R., Hla, T., et al. (2006). Dual roles of tight junction-associated protein, zonula occludens-1, in sphingosine 1-phosphate-mediated endothelial chemotaxis and barrier integrity. *J. Biol. Chem.* 281, 29190–29200. doi: 10.1074/jbc.M604310200

Leiserson, W. M., Forbush, B., and Keshishian, H. (2011). Drosophila glia use a conserved cotransporter mechanism to regulate extracellular volume. *Glia* 59, 320–332. doi: 10.1002/glia.21103

Leslie, E. M., Deeley, R. G., and Cole, S. P. (2005). Multidrug resistance proteins: role of P-glycoprotein, MRP1, MRP2, and BCRP (ABCG2) in tissue defense. *Toxicol. Appl. Pharmacol.* 204, 216–237. doi: 10.1016/j.taap.2004.10.012

Loscher, W., and Potschka, H. (2005). Drug resistance in brain diseases and the role of drug efflux transporters. *Nat. Rev. Neurosci.* 6, 591–602. doi: 10.1038/nrn1728

Mayer, F., Mayer, N., Chinn, L., Pinsonneault, R. L., Kroetz, D., and Bainton, R. J. (2009). Evolutionary conservation of vertebrate blood-brain barrier chemoprotective mechanisms in Drosophila. *J. Neurosci.* 29, 3538–3550. doi: 10.1523/JNEUROSCI.5564-08.2009

Meyer, S., Schmidt, I., and Klambt, C. (2014). Glia ECM interactions are required to shape the Drosophila nervous system. *Mech. Dev.* 133C, 105–116. doi: 10.1016/j.mod.2014.05.003

Miller, D. S. (2010). Regulation of P-glycoprotein and other ABC drug transporters at the blood-brain barrier. *Trends Pharmacol. Sci.* 31, 246–254. doi: 10.1016/j.tips.2010.03.003

Mirre, C., Cecchini, J. P., Le Parco, Y., and Knibiehler, B. (1988). *De novo* expression of a type IV collagen gene in Drosophila embryos is restricted to mesodermal derivatives and occurs at germ band shortening. *Development* 102, 369–376.

Mirth, C. K., and Shingleton, A. W. (2012). Integrating body and organ size in Drosophila: recent advances and outstanding problems. *Front. Endocrinol. (Lausanne)* 3:49. doi: 10.3389/fendo.2012.00049

Muir, A. R., and Peters, A. (1962). Quintuple-layered membrane junctions at terminal bars between endothelial cells. *J. Cell Biol.* 12, 443–448. doi: 10.1083/jcb.12.2.443

Nassel, D. R., Kubrak, O. I., Liu, Y., Luo, J., and Lushchak, O. V. (2013). Factors that regulate insulin producing cells and their output in Drosophila. *Front. Physiol.* 4:252. doi: 10.3389/fphys.2013.00252

Nelson, K. S., Furuse, M., and Beitel, G. J. (2010). The Drosophila Claudin Kune-kune is required for septate junction organization and tracheal tube size control. *Genetics* 185, 831–839. doi: 10.1534/genetics.110.114959

Nielsen, P. A., Andersson, O., Hansen, S. H., Simonsen, K. B., and Andersson, G. (2011). Models for predicting blood-brain barrier permeation. *Drug Discov. Today* 16, 472–475. doi: 10.1016/j.drudis.2011.04.004

Obermeier, B., Daneman, R., and Ransohoff, R. M. (2013). Development, maintenance and disruption of the blood-brain barrier. *Nat. Med.* 19, 1584–1596. doi: 10.1038/nm.3407

Okamoto, N., Nakamori, R., Murai, T., Yamauchi, Y., Masuda, A., and Nishimura, T. (2013). A secreted decoy of InR antagonizes insulin/IGF signaling to restrict body growth in Drosophila. *Genes Dev.* 27, 87–97. doi: 10.1101/gad.204479.112

Olofsson, B., and Page, D. T. (2005). Condensation of the central nervous system in embryonic Drosophila is inhibited by blocking hemocyte migration or neural activity. *Dev. Biol.* 279, 233–243. doi: 10.1016/j.ydbio.2004.12.020

Oshima, K., and Fehon, R. G. (2011). Analysis of protein dynamics within the septate junction reveals a highly stable core protein complex that does not include the basolateral polarity protein Discs large. *J. Cell Sci.* 124, 2861–2871. doi: 10.1242/jcs.087700

Partridge, L., Alic, N., Bjedov, I., and Piper, M. D. (2011). Ageing in Drosophila: the role of the insulin/Igf and TOR signalling network. *Exp. Gerontol.* 46, 376–381. doi: 10.1016/j.exger.2010.09.003

Pastor-Pareja, J. C., and Xu, T. (2011). Shaping cells and organs in Drosophila by opposing roles of fat body-secreted Collagen IV and perlecan. *Dev. Cell* 21, 245–256. doi: 10.1016/j.devcel.2011.06.026

Paul, S. M., Ternet, M., Salvaterra, P. M., and Beitel, G. J. (2003). The Na+/K+ ATPase is required for septate junction function and epithelial tube-size control in the Drosophila tracheal system. *Development* 130, 4963–4974. doi: 10.1242/dev.00691

Rajan, A., and Perrimon, N. (2012). Drosophila cytokine unpaired 2 regulates physiological homeostasis by remotely controlling insulin secretion. *Cell* 151, 123–137. doi: 10.1016/j.cell.2012.08.019

Reese, T. S., and Karnovsky, M. J. (1967). Fine structural localization of a blood-brain barrier to exogenous peroxidase. *J. Cell Biol.* 34, 207–217. doi: 10.1083/jcb.34.1.207

Rodrigues, F., Thuma, L., and Klambt, C. (2012). The regulation of glial-specific splicing of Neurexin IV requires HOW and Cdk12 activity. *Development* 139, 1765–1776. doi: 10.1242/dev.074070

Sarantseva, S. V., Bolshakova, O. I., Timoshenko, S. I., Kolobov, A. A., and Schwarzman, A. L. (2011). Dendrimer D5 is a vector for peptide transport to brain cells. *Bull. Exp. Biol. Med.* 150, 429–431. doi: 10.1007/s10517-011-1160-z

Schmidt, I., Thomas, S., Kain, P., Risse, B., Naffin, E., and Klambt, C. (2012). Kinesin heavy chain function in Drosophila glial cells controls neuronal activity. *J. Neurosci.* 32, 7466–7476. doi: 10.1523/JNEUROSCI.0349-12.2012

Schulte, J., Tepass, U., and Auld, V. J. (2003). Gliotactin, a novel marker of tricellular junctions, is necessary for septate junction development in Drosophila. *J. Cell Biol.* 161, 991–1000. doi: 10.1083/jcb.200303192

Schwabe, T., Bainton, R. J., Fetter, R. D., Heberlein, U., and Gaul, U. (2005). GPCR signaling is required for blood-brain barrier formation in drosophila. *Cell* 123, 133–144. doi: 10.1016/j.cell.2005.08.037

Seabrooke, S., and O'Donnell, M. J. (2013). Oatp58Dc contributes to blood-brain barrier function by excluding organic anions from the Drosophila brain. *Am. J. Physiol. Cell Physiol.* 305, C558–C567. doi: 10.1152/ajpcell.00408.2012

Sousa-Nunes, R., Yee, L. L., and Gould, A. P. (2011). Fat cells reactivate quiescent neuroblasts via TOR and glial insulin relays in Drosophila. *Nature* 471, 508–512. doi: 10.1038/nature09867

Speder, P., and Brand, A. H. (2014). Gap junction proteins in the blood-brain barrier control nutrient-dependent reactivation of Drosophila neural stem cells. *Dev. Cell* 30, 309–321. doi: 10.1016/j.devcel.2014.05.021

Starz-Gaiano, M., Cho, N. K., Forbes, A., and Lehmann, R. (2001). Spatially restricted activity of a Drosophila lipid phosphatase guides migrating germ cells. *Development* 128, 983–991.

Stenman, J. M., Rajagopal, J., Carroll, T. J., Ishibashi, M., McMahon, J., and McMahon, A. P. (2008). Canonical wnt signaling regulates organ-specific assembly and differentiation of CNS vasculature. *Science* 322, 1247–1250. doi: 10.1126/science.1164594

Stewart, P. A., and Wiley, M. J. (1981). Developing nervous tissue induces formation of blood-brain barrier characteristics in invading endothelial cells: a study using quail–chick transplantation chimeras. *Dev. Biol.* 84, 183–192. doi: 10.1016/0012-1606(81)90382-1

Stork, T., Engelen, D., Krudewig, A., Silies, M., Bainton, R. J., and Klambt, C. (2008). Organization and function of the blood-brain barrier in Drosophila. *J. Neurosci.* 28, 587–597. doi: 10.1523/JNEUROSCI.4367-07.2008

Syed, M. H., Krudewig, A., Engelen, D., Stork, T., and Klambt, C. (2011). The CD59 family member Leaky/Coiled is required for the establishment of the blood-brain barrier in Drosophila. *J Neurosci* 31, 7876–7885. doi: 10.1523/JNEUROSCI.0766-11.2011

Torrie, L. S., Radford, J. C., Southall, T. D., Kean, L., Dinsmore, A. J., Davies, S. A., et al. (2004). Resolution of the insect ouabain paradox. *Proc. Natl. Acad. Sci. U.S.A.* 101, 13689–13693. doi: 10.1073/pnas.0403087101

Treherne, J. E. (1966). The effect of ouabain on the efflux of sodium ions in the nerve cords of two insect species (*Periplaneta americana* and *Carausius morosus*). *J. Exp. Biol.* 44, 355–362.

Unhavaithaya, Y., and Orr-Weaver, T. L. (2012). Polyploidization of glia in neural development links tissue growth to blood-brain barrier integrity. *Genes Dev.* 26, 31–36. doi: 10.1101/gad.177436.111

Vogelgesang, S., Cascorbi, I., Schroeder, E., Pahnke, J., Kroemer, H. K., Siegmund, W., et al. (2002). Deposition of Alzheimer's beta-amyloid is inversely correlated with P-glycoprotein expression in the brains of elderly non-demented humans. *Pharmacogenetics* 12, 535–541. doi: 10.1097/00008571-200210000-00005

Wigby, S., Slack, C., Gronke, S., Martinez, P., Calboli, F. C., Chapman, T., et al. (2011). Insulin signalling regulates remating in female Drosophila. *Proc. Biol. Sci.* 278, 424–431. doi: 10.1098/rspb.2010.1390

Xiao, G., and Gan, L. S. (2013). Receptor-mediated endocytosis and brain delivery of therapeutic biologics. *Int. J. Cell Biol.* 2013:703545. doi: 10.1155/2013/703545

Zhang, N., Zhang, J., Purcell, K. J., Cheng, Y., and Howard, K. (1997). The Drosophila protein Wunen repels migrating germ cells. *Nature* 385, 64–67. doi: 10.1038/385064a0

Zlokovic, B. V. (2008). The blood-brain barrier in health and chronic neurodegenerative disorders. *Neuron* 57, 178–201. doi: 10.1016/j.neuron.2008.01.003

14

Embryonic blood-cerebrospinal fluid barrier formation and function

David Bueno*, Maryam Parvas, Ismaïl Hermelo and Jordi Garcia-Fernàndez

Department of Genetics, Faculty of Biological Sciences, University of Barcelona, Barcelona, Spain

Correspondence:
David Bueno, Departament de Genètica, Facultat de Biologia, Universitat de Barcelona, Av. Diagonal 643, 08028 Barcelona, Spain
e-mail: dbueno@ub.edu

During embryonic development and adult life, brain cavities and ventricles are filled with cerebrospinal fluid (CSF). CSF has attracted interest as an active signaling medium that regulates brain development, homeostasis and disease. CSF is a complex protein-rich fluid containing growth factors and signaling molecules that regulate multiple cell functions in the central nervous system (CNS). The composition and substance concentrations of CSF are tightly controlled. In recent years, it has been demonstrated that embryonic CSF (eCSF) has a key function as a fluid pathway for delivering diffusible signals to the developing brain, thus contributing to the proliferation, differentiation and survival of neural progenitor cells, and to the expansion and patterning of the brain. From fetal stages through to adult life, CSF is primarily produced by the choroid plexus. The development and functional activities of the choroid plexus and other blood–brain barrier (BBB) systems in adults and fetuses have been extensively analyzed. However, eCSF production and control of its homeostasis in embryos, from the closure of the anterior neuropore when the brain cavities become physiologically sealed, to the formation of the functional fetal choroid plexus, has not been studied in as much depth and remains open to debate. This review brings together the existing literature, some of which is based on experiments conducted by our research group, concerning the formation and function of a temporary embryonic blood–CSF barrier in the context of the crucial roles played by the molecules in eCSF.

Keywords: embryonic cerebrospinal fluid, blood-eCSF barrier, primary neurogenesis, neural progenitor cells, brain development, cephalic vesicles

INTRODUCTION

Many civilizations have developed along riverbanks and seashores, in order to use the fluid medium to promote cohesion and transport, and to favor the survival of the people living at its edge. Surprisingly, the brain is also organized, from its embryonic beginnings and throughout adult life, around an extraordinarily dynamic and complex fluid, called cerebrospinal fluid (CSF), which the cells lining the brain and spinal cord bathe in. CSF is a subject that attracts growing interest in brain development research. In the last two decades, this has led to an understanding of normal adult brain function and disease, including migration of neuroblasts created in the subventricular zone of the adult brain from the lateral ventricles to the olfactory bulb (Sawamoto et al., 2006). CSF composition during embryogenesis and the fetal period is highly complex, as demonstrated by several proteomic analyses (Dziegielewska et al., 1980a, 1981; Fielitz et al., 1984; Gato et al., 2004; Parada et al., 2005a, 2006; Zappaterra et al., 2007). In addition, CSF composition and its biological properties change throughout development in a tightly regulated manner in parallel with its function, as demonstrated for some of the molecules contained within the embryonic CSF (eCSF), e.g., retinol binding protein (RBP), and fibroblast growth factor no. 2 (FGF2), with regard to the initiation of primary brain neurogenesis (Parvas et al., 2008a).

The development of the brain involves three main distinct phases: formation of the tube from the neural plate; polarization of the tube into a posterior spinal cord, and an anterior expanded brain, which is initially a hollow eCSF-filled vesicle surrounded by a pseudo-monostratified neuroepithelium; and histiogenesis of the neuroepithelium (**Figure 1**; for a general description of central nervous system (CNS) development, see Smith and Schoenwolf, 1997; Copp et al., 2003; Copp, 2005). During most of the last century, developmental neuroscience focused primarily on neuroepithelial events at the molecular, cellular, and tissue level. For example, it has been demonstrated that diffusible molecules such as growth factors and morphogens secreted locally by organizing centers regulate these processes by controlling neighboring cells in an autocrine/paracrine way (Bally-Cuif and Boncinelli, 1997), and that they regulate the expression of a number of transcription factors through which complex molecular, and genetic networks are established.

Only in the last two decades has the eCSF in the cavities of the brain primordium started to attract attention and be considered

Abbreviations: BBB, blood–brain barrier; CG, Carnegie Stage (for human embryo development); CNS, central nervous system; CSF, cerebrospinal fluid; E, embryonic developmental day; eCSF, embryonic cerebrospinal fluid; EGF, epidermal growth factor ESI-MS/MS: electrospray ionization coupled with tandem mass spectrometry; fCSF, fetal cerebrospinal fluid; FGF2, fibroblast growth factor no. 2; HRP, horse radish peroxidase; IsO, mesencephalic-rhombencephalic isthmus organizing center; RBP, retinol binding protein; SDS-PAGE, sodium dodecyl sulfate polyacrylamide gel electrophoresis.

an essential part of the developing brain which exerts a direct influence on basic neuroepithelial cell behavior, i.e., promoting cellular survival, replication, and neurogenic differentiation, and also contributing to the regulation of neuroepithelial gene expression, thus playing a key role in brain development (Gato et al., 2005; Martin et al., 2006, 2009; Parada et al., 2008a; Alonso et al., 2011; Feliciano et al., 2014). In fetuses and adults, these cavities become the brain's ventricular system, since eCSF is the precursor of fetal and adult CSF (reviewed by Miyan et al., 2003). It has also been demonstrated that fetal CSF (fCSF) contributes to cortical development (Miyan et al., 2006).

CSF composition and homeostasis in fetuses and the adult brain are tightly regulated by the choroid plexus, whose epithelial cells establish a blood–CSF barrier (**Figure 2**; Møllgård et al., 1979; Tauc et al., 1984). The choroid plexus is a vascular structure in the brain ventricles that manufactures CSF by promoting the transport of certain molecules from blood plasma and producing others that are delivered directly to the ventricles. Acting in parallel, CNS homeostasis in adult vertebrates is also controlled by the blood–brain barrier (BBB) vessels in

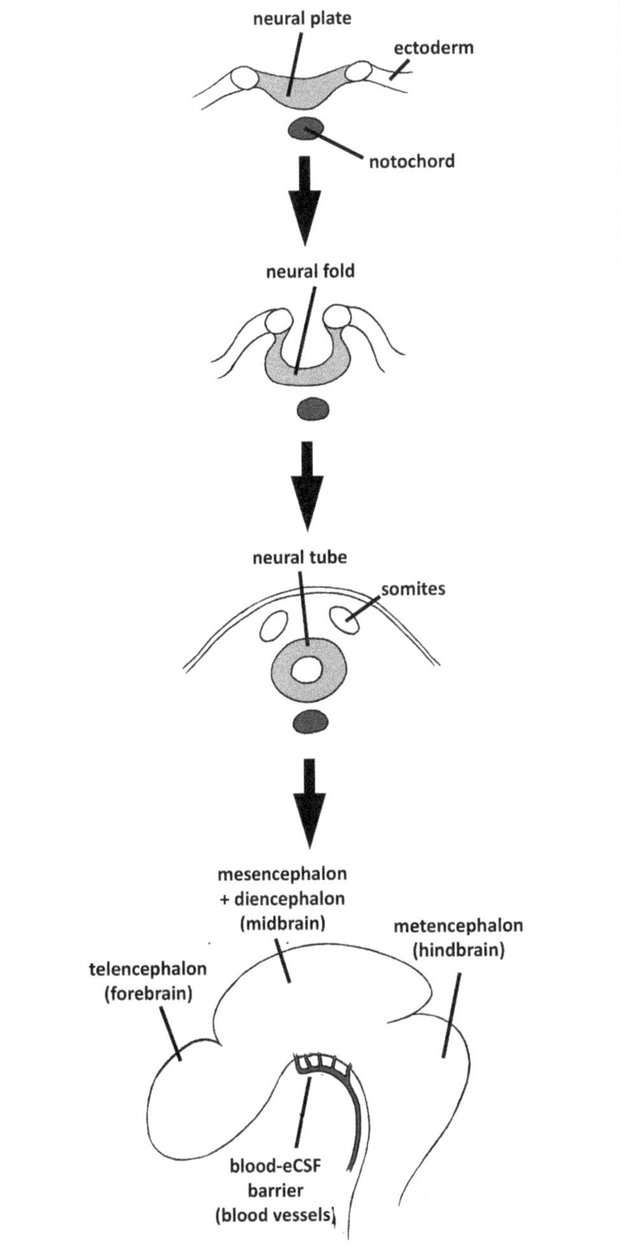

FIGURE 1 | Summary of CNS development and brain cavities formation from the differentiation of the neural plate to the initiation of brain primary neurogenesis (corresponding to embryonic stage E4 in chick embryos or E12.7 in rat embryos, according to the experiments reviewed in this paper). The embryonic blood–eCSF barrier is also indicated.

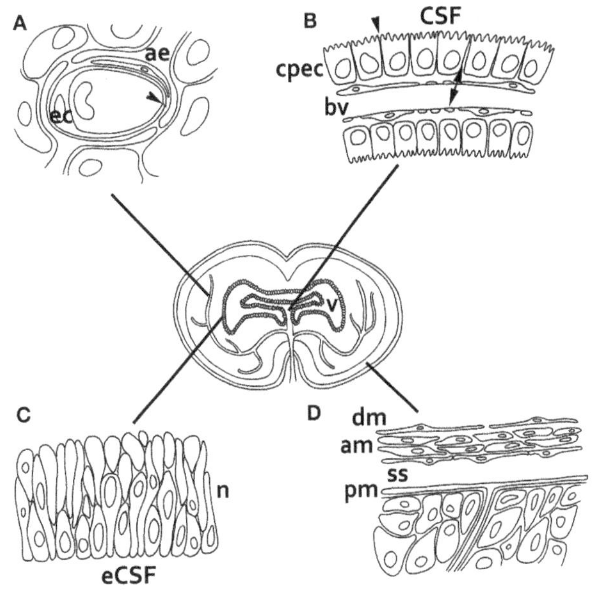

FIGURE 2 | Barriers of the developing and adult brain. (A) The blood–brain barrier between the lumen of cerebral blood vessels and the brain parenchyma. The endothelial cells have luminal tight junctions (arrowheads) that form a physical barrier, preventing the movement of molecules from the blood plasma, except those that are allowed to enter the brain via active and specific transport. In embryos, some blood vessels and the neuroectodermal cells adjacent to them also perform this function. **(B)** The blood–CSF barrier between choroid plexus blood vessels and the adult and fetal CSF. These blood vessels are fenestrated and form a non-restrictive barrier (arrows), but the choroid plexus epithelial cells are joined by tight junctions to stop the movement of molecules (arrowheads). **(C)** The inner CSF–brain barrier between the eCSF and the brain parenchyma, which is present only during early development. The neuroependymal cells lining the brain cavities do not allow the exchange of large molecules such as proteins between the eCSF and brain, but they do allow exchange of smaller molecules such as sucrose. This implies that the influence of eCSF on basic neuroepithelial cell behavior—e.g., promoting cellular survival, replication and neurogenic differentiation—has to be accounted for through specific receptors located at the apical pole of neural progenitor cells, which are in contact with the lumen of the cavities. There is no crossing restriction in the adult brain. **(D)** The outer CSF–brain barrier between the subarachnoid space and overlaying structures. The blood vessels are fenestrated, but the outer cells of the arachnoid membrane are connected by tight junctions. Abbreviations: ae, astrocitic endfoot; am, arachnoid membrane; bv, blood vessel; cpec, choroid plexus endothelial cell; dm, dura mater; ec, endothelial cell; n, neuroepithelium; pm, pia mater; ss, subarachnoid space; v, ventricle.

the brain; this significantly impedes entry from the blood to the brain of virtually all molecules, except those that are small and lipophilic. However, BBB vessels also allow sets of small and large hydrophilic molecules, e.g., gene products, to enter the brain via active transport (reviewed by Rubin and Staddon, 1999; see **Figure 2** for a more extensive summary of brain barriers).

In parallel with eCSF studies, control of eCSF production and homeostasis in vertebrate embryos from the closure of the anterior neuropore to the formation of the choroid plexus during fetal stages have not been analyzed until recently. However, this developmental stage is particularly interesting for brain formation, since it is mainly characterized by rapid brain anlagen growth and initiation of primary neurogenesis in the neural progenitor cells lining the cavities. This review brings together the existing literature on the formation and function of embryonic blood–CSF barriers, from the closure of the anterior neuropore to the formation of choroid plexuses in vertebrates, using avians (chicks), and mammals (mainly mice and rats) as model systems. We highlight the crucial role played by eCSF in neural development. As stated by Gato (2013) in a short but revealing commentary, "eCSF—and by extension the barriers and mechanisms controlling its formation, composition and homeostasis—constitute a rising subject in brain development."

PHYLOGENETIC ORIGIN OF THE CSF SYSTEM

It is thought that the CSF system evolved in the deuterostome lineage from the ancestor of echinoderms and chordates to maintain the chemical environment necessary for the functioning of the cells of the CNS, including the neuroendocrine pathways (Brocklehurst, 1979). For example, it is known that in starfish, the neurons of the radial nerves and "brain" are always in contact with seawater; this allows them to detect the composition of the seawater, as well as other physical parameters such as water temperature, and modulate the activity of the nervous system accordingly. However, its open nature means that this system does not respond to neuroendocrine or other signaling molecule pathways (**Figure 3**).

During the larval stages of morphologically and evolutionarily more complex lancelets, such as the chordate amphioxus *Branchiostoma lanceolatum*, seawater enters the ventricular lumen of the "brain" through the anterior neuropore, which remains open until adulthood. Seawater represents the first "internal" fluid environment of lancelet brain tissue and depends directly on the environment. However, when lancelets reach adulthood, the anterior neuropore closes and the ventricular lumen of the "brain" becomes a closed system (**Figure 3**). Thus, the composition of this fluid no longer depends directly on the environment, but on the activity and metabolism of the organism. Finally, the composition of eCSF in craniata, such as lampreys, and vertebrates depends exclusively on the surrounding tissue and the rest of the embryo from early embryonic stages, since the anterior neuropore closes very early in neural tube development, before brain primary neurogenesis starts. This suggests that this condition was first developed by the ancestor of these two phylogenetic groups (**Figure 3**; reviewed by Vígh et al., 2004).

eCSF PROTEIN CONTENT

In vertebrates, brain development depends on regional character specification, which in turn depends on a progressive series of precisely coordinated morphogenetic movements in combination with cell proliferation and differentiation. These processes are controlled by the sequential action of patterning molecules, which give neural progenitor cells specific characteristics, including transcription factors and diffusible molecules such as growth factors and morphogens (Martinez, 2001; Stern, 2001, 2002). During early stages of brain development, when the architecture of the brain anlagen is formed by a pseudo-monostratified neuroepithelium that develops around the cephalic cavities with its lining surface in close contact with the eCSF, these diffusible molecules may come from both the surrounding tissues, such as the mesencephalic-rhombencephalic isthmus (IsO) organizing center (Nakamura et al., 2005), and eCSF, which may be used as a fluid pathway for their delivery.

Classic studies performed on chick embryos at developmental stages E2.5 to E6.5 (E = embryonic developmental day) showed that eCSF has a higher concentration of total proteins than adult CSF (Birge et al., 1974; Gato et al., 2004). A similar situation has been observed in sheep at E35 (youngest fetus) as compared with E60 (sheep gestation, 145 days), and in rat from E12 to E22 (birth), and neonatal. Some phylogenetic differences in CSF maturation have been identified, however, when comparing these mammalian species, regarding, for example, the developmental stages at which the reduction in total CSF protein occurs (Dziegielewska et al., 1980a,b, 1981; Checiu et al., 1984; Fielitz et al., 1984).

The first published studies of the specific protein content of eCSF were based on crossed immunoelectrophoresis to identify individual proteins, and radial immunodiffusion to quantitate them. It was suggested that the protein fractions identified in sheep eCSF were albumin, fetuin, alpha-fetoprotein, transferrin, lipoproteins, alpha1-antitypsin, and prealbumin (Dziegielewska et al., 1980a, 1981). Rat eCSF exhibits a similar electrophoretic pattern, with the possible presence of IgGs (Dziegielewska et al., 1981). As regards chick eCSF, Gato et al. (2004) identified 21 protein fractions by SDS-PAGE protein separation and molecular mass inference, which coincide with previously reported proteins such as transferrin, alpha-fetoprotein, immunoglobulins, and transthyretin.

Proteomic analyses of avian and mammalian eCSF that confirm and significantly expand on most of the abovementioned findings have also been published. The first reports to use conventional proteomic techniques (2D-electrophoresis, in-gel digestion, and ESI-MS/MS mass spectrometry analysis) on chick and rat eCSF at E4 and E12.5, respectively, which correspond to the developmental stages in which brain development is characterized by maximum neuroepithelial progenitor cell proliferation and the beginning of neural differentiation, showed the presence of dozens of different specific proteins within this fluid, most of which may be involved in brain development (Parada et al., 2005a, 2006). These proteins were classified into several different groups according to their functional characteristics, as previously reported in systems other than eCSF (**Table 1**). The most remarkable dissimilarity between chick and rat eCSF proteomes is the

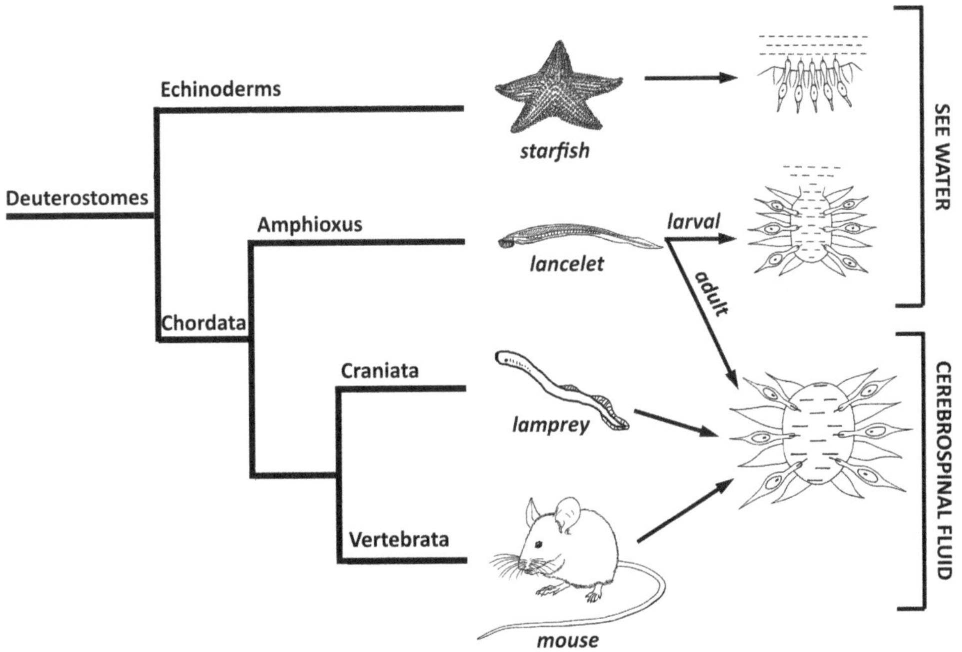

FIGURE 3 | Scheme of the evolution of the phylogenetic increase in the control that the chemical environment has over the cerebrospinal fluid.

presence of enzymes and enzyme regulators in rat eCSF, as well as an increased number of members of the apolipoprotein family, from two different apolipoproteins identified in chicks, AI and AIV, to at least five in rats, including AI and AIV, as well as B, E, and M. It has been suggested that this relates to the higher complexity of the CNS in mammals, although apolipoprotein B was later identified in chick eCSF by Western-blot analysis using specific antibodies (Parada et al., 2008a). These dissimilarities may also be due to differences in choroid plexus formation. E4.5 chick embryos correspond to a developmental stage 2.5 days before the first appearance of the choroid plexus; while in E12.5 rat embryos, transthyretin-positive choroid plexus primordium starts to be detected. However, rat choroid plexus primordium at this developmental stage is not fully functional and, as discussed below (see Sections Protein Traffic Occurs in Very Specific Blood Vessels and Includes Both Endothelial and Neuroepithelial Cells, and Traffic of Water, ions, And Glucose Occurs at the Same Transport Site as Proteins), these rat embryos still maintain a specific and temporary embryonic blood–eCSF barrier.

Zappaterra et al. (2007) also reported an extensive and thorough proteome analysis of rat eCSF from three different stages: E12.5, E14.5 from both the lateral and fourth ventricles, and E17.5 during cortical development. They identified 423, 318, 249, and 382 proteins, respectively, which were also classified into several groups according to their function (**Table 1**). The human eCSF proteome has been analyzed at Carnegie Stage (CG) 20 (Zappaterra et al., 2007), revealing the presence of 188 proteins; 130 of which are shared with rats. The categorization of these proteins based on their molecular function and the biological processes they are involved in are almost identical, which would suggest that they represent essential eCSF functions.

More recently, proteomic analysis performed on both eCSF from chick and rat embryos at E4 and E13 respectively, but using a more sensitive technique (a high-performance liquid chromatography ion-trap column coupled to an ESI MS/MS mass spectrometer), showed the presence of 121 (chick), and 100 (rat) different proteins within the fluid, although all of them may be classified in the same general groups (Bueno et al., unpublished results). All of these studies, whose overall results are relatively similar, have proved to be complementary and reinforce the putative capacity of eCSF to influence the behavior of neuroepithelial cells through the molecules it contains, as has been demonstrated in several studies (Gato et al., 2005; Martin et al., 2006, 2009; Parada et al., 2008a,b).

However, one of the limitations of this proteomic analysis is the almost complete lack of growth factors and cytokines within eCSF proteomes, since these molecules, which are crucial for controlling developmental processes, exert their actions at very low concentrations. They may therefore be masked by the more abundant proteins or may be below the detection threshold of the techniques used. Nevertheless, Western-blot analysis of both avian and mammalian eCSF using specific antibodies revealed the presence of some growth factors and cytokines within this fluid. These include fibroblast growth factor 2 (FGF2) (Martin et al., 2006), epidermal growth factor (EGF) (Birecree et al., 1991), and leukemia inhibitory factor (Hatta et al., 2006), which are known to be involved in the regulation of a number of developmental processes.

Although interpreting these different results is complex because of the different classifications used (see **Table 1**), and the fact that some gene products may correspond to different functional groups in different studies, it is evident that eCSF acts as

Table 1 | Summary of the classifications of proteins identified in chick, rat and human eCSF proteomes.

Chick eCSF	Rat eCSF	Human eCSF
Parada et al., 2006 Bueno et al., unpublished results 1. Extracellular matrix 2. Osmotic pressure and ion carriers 3. Cell death and quiescence 4. Apolipoproteins 5. Retinol and vitamin D carriers 6. Antioxidant and antimicrobial 7. Intracellular 8. Unknown	Parada et al., 2005a 1. Extracellular matrix 2. Osmotic pressure and ion carriers 3. Regulators of lipid metabolism 4. Retinol and corticosteroid carriers 5. Enzymes and enzyme regulators 6. Antioxidant and antimicrobial 7. Unknown function during embryonic development ——————— Zappaterra et al., 2007 Bueno et al., unpublished results <u>According to subcellular location</u> 1. Secreted 2. Secreted, extracellular matrix 3. Cell membrane 4. Cytoplasm 5. Nucleus 6. Intracellular 7. Golgi 8. Lysosome 9. ER <u>According to molecular function</u> 1. Cell adhesion 2. Chaperone 3. Cytoskeletal 4. Defense/immunity 5. Extracellular matrix 6. Hydrolase 7. Kinase 8. Ligase 9. Membrane traffic 10. Miscellanea 11. Unclassified 12. Nucleic acid binding 13. Oxidoreductase 14. Phosphatase 15. Protease 16. Receptor 17. Calcium binding 18. Regulatory molecule 19. Signaling molecule 20. Synthase and synthetase 21. Transcription factor 22. Transfer 23. Transferase 24. Transporter 25. Isomerase <u>According to biological process</u> 1. Neuronal activities 2. Signal transduction 3. Developmental processes 4. Cell proliferation and differentiation 5. Coenzyme and prosthetic group metabolism	Zappaterra et al., 2007 <u>According to subcellular location</u> 1. Secreted 2. Secreted, extracellular matrix 3. Cell membrane 4. Cytoplasm 5. Nucleus 6. Intracellular 7. Golgi 8. Lysosome <u>According to molecular function</u> 1. Cell adhesion 2. Chaperone 3. Cytoskeletal 4. Defense/immunity 5. Extracellular matrix 6. Hydrolase 7. Kinase 8. Ligase 9. Membrane traffic 10. Miscellanea 11. Unclassified 12. Nucleic acid binding 13. Oxidoreductase 14. Phosphatase 15. Protease 16. Receptor 17. Calcium binding 18. Regulatory molecule 19. Signaling molecule 20. Synthase and synthetase 21. Transcription factor 22. Transfer 23. Transferase 24. Transporter 25. Cell junction protein <u>According to biological process</u> 1. Neuronal activities 2. Signal transduction 3. Developmental processes 4. Cell proliferation and differentiation 5. Coenzyme and prosthetic group metabolism 6. Cell structure and motility 7. Immunity and defense 8. Apoptosis 9. Oncogenesis 10. Muscle contraction 11. Transport 12. Blood circulation and gas exchange 13. Carbohydrate metabolism 14. Nucleoside, nucleotide and nucleic acid metabolism 15. Homeostasis 16. Protein metabolism and modification 17. Cell cycle

(Continued)

Table 1 | Continued

Chick eCSF	Rat eCSF	Human eCSF
	6. Cell structure and motility 7. Immunity and defense 8. Apoptosis 9. Oncogenesis 10. Muscle contraction 11. Transport 12. Blood circulation and gas exchange 13. Carbohydrate metabolism 14. Nucleoside, nucleotide and nucleic acid metabolism 15. Homeostasis 16. Protein metabolism and modification 17. Cell cycle 18. Intracellular protein traffic 18. Cell adhesion 19. Lipid, fatty acid and steroid metabolism 20. Sensory perception 21. Electron transport 22. Amino acid metabolism 23. Biological process unclassified 24. Protein targeting and location 25. Miscellaneous	18. Intracellular protein traffic 18. Cell adhesion 19. Lipid, fatty acid and steroid metabolism 20. Sensory perception 21. Electron transport 22. Amino acid metabolism 23. Biological process unclassified 24. Protein targeting and location 25. Miscellaneous

References are shown in the table.

a fluid pathway to transfer proteins to and from the neuroepithelial cells. It thus influences neuroepithelial cell behavior and, hence, brain development (Gato et al., 2005; Parada et al., 2005a, 2008a,b; Martin et al., 2006, 2009; Alonso et al., 2011; Castells et al., 2012; see Gato and Desmond, 2009 for a review).

eCSF FUNCTION

Through the specific molecules it contains and certain of its mechanical properties, eCSF plays several crucial roles during the early stages of brain development: just after the closure of the anterior neuropore when the brain ventricles become physiologically sealed cavities, during initial brain anlagen growth, and during the initiation of the primary neurogenesis of the neural progenitor cells. Using several experimental approaches in chick and mouse embryos, it has been reported that the progressive increase in eCSF volume exerts positive pressure against the neuroepithelial walls and generates an expansive force, thus contributing to brain expansion. An experimentally inflicted decrease in eCSF pressure leads to severe dysmorphogenesis and brain collapse (Desmond and Jacobson, 1977; Desmond and Levitan, 2002). The rapid expansion, which accounts for 70% of brain enlargement in the early stages, occurs in parallel with occlusion of the spinal neurocoele (Desmond and Jacobson, 1977). This renders the cephalic cavities a physiologically sealed system, which would indicate the existence of mechanisms that control the influx of water and ions into the brain cavities. Moreover, as proteoglycans are the major components of the extracellular matrix in embryo brain cavities (Alonso et al., 1998, 1999), it has been suggested that the special osmotic properties of chondroitin sulfate proteoglycan and other proteoglycans in eCSF may cause water retention in the cavities. This would generate and regulate the inner cephalic hydrostatic pressure, although other proteins, e.g., major eCSF proteins, may also contribute to this function.

In addition to the mechanical properties of eCSF, it has also been shown to contribute to the regulation of some basic cellular functions, e.g., the survival, proliferation, and differentiation of neural progenitor cells. Through the use of *in vitro* cultures of mesencephalic neuroectodermal explants from both chick and rat embryos at E4 and E12.5, respectively, the diffusible molecules in eCSF have been shown to actively contribute to the regulation of the survival, proliferation, and neurogenesis of neuroepithelial progenitor cells, directly from this embryonic fluid (Gato et al., 2005; Martin et al., 2009). Mesencephalic explants cultured with only a chemically defined medium show a reduction in the number of proliferating cells, an increased rate of apoptotic cells, and a severe decrease in the number of cells engaged in the process of neural differentiation (i.e., primary neurogenesis) compared to control embryos. However, when the explants are cultured with a chemically defined medium supplemented with eCSF, the cellular parameters remain close to those of the control embryos.

Most of the proteins identified in eCSF in the abovementioned proteomic analysis have known physiological functions during embryonic development that are consistent with the overall roles reported for eCSF during CNS development. Functional *in vivo* and *in vitro* analysis of the particular role of some of these gene products at the beginning of primary neurogenesis, before the formation of functional choroid plexuses, has revealed their specific roles in the overall function of eCSF in neuroepithelial progenitor cell behavior. For example, it has been reported that the deglycosylation of eCSF proteoglycans with beta-d-xyloside alters brain enlargement in chick embryos (Alonso et al., 1998), and that immunoblocking of the FGF2 in eCSF severely disrupts neuroepithelial stem cell proliferation and differentiation (Martin et al., 2006). Similarly, it has been reported that the LDL lipid fraction, transported by apolipoprotein B in eCSF, is also involved in regulating neuroepithelial progenitor cell proliferation and differentiation (Parada et al., 2008a). Other reports have shown that retinol-binding protein (RBP) is responsible for transporting and transferring all-*trans*-retinol from the embryonic plasma to the eCSF, from where it reaches the neuroepithelium and is transformed into retinoic acid, the actual morphogen, by retinoic acid-synthesizing enzymes expressed in the neuroepithelium (Parada et al., 2008b; Alonso et al., 2011). Also that large glycoprotein SCO-spondin synthesized by the by the diencephalic roof plate contributes to the control of neuroepithelial cell proliferation via eCSF (Vera et al., 2013). As well as that eCSF nanovesicles carry evolutionarily conserved molecules that promote neural stem cell amplification (Feliciano et al., 2014); among other findings.

In addition to the effects of eCSF on neural progenitor cell behavior through some of the specific molecules it contains, its involvement in regulating the expression of genes known to be involved in brain patterning has also been established (Parada et al., 2005b). When dorsal mesencephalic neuroepithelial explants lacking IsO (a known organizing center for mesencephalon and brain development) or dorsal mesencephalic neuroepithelial explants including IsO are cultured in a chemically defined medium but in the absence of eCSF, the typical expression of dorsal mesencephalic, and IsO genes, i.e., *fgf8* and *otx2*, is disrupted. Conversely, when dorsal mesencephalic explants including IsO are cultured in an eCSF-supplemented medium, they do exhibit this expression. Interestingly, however, when dorsal mesencephalic explants lacking IsO are cultured with an eCSF-supplemented medium, they also show ectopic expression domains of *Shh* in the mesencephalic neuroectoderm; *Shh* is a gene that is typically expressed in the ventral but not dorsal neuroectoderm. Only the concurrence of eCSF within the culture medium and IsO in the dorsal mesencephalic explant makes this tissue mimic its typical pattern of gene expression, which would suggest that IsO and some molecules in eCSF exert a synergistic action.

MECHANISMS CONTROLLING eCSF FORMATION AND HOMEOSTASIS

The crucial roles played by eCSF during initial brain development together with the complexity of its composition (it includes proteins that may account for the overall function of this fluid in neuroepithelial development) raise some interesting questions about the origin of the gene products and other molecules within it. Further questions concern how the homeostasis of this fluid is controlled at the beginning of primary neurogenesis, just after the closure of the anterior neuropore when the cephalic cavities become physiologically sealed, since the development of a functional choroid plexus is known to occur a bit later in development.

THE NEED FOR A BLOOD–eCSF BARRIER FUNCTION: A HISTORICAL PERSPECTIVE

Developing choroid plexuses are first detected at E7 in chicks, at E12.5–E13 in rats and mice, and during the seventh week of gestation in humans (Bellairs and Osmond, 2005; Emerich et al., 2005). Despite the large amount of accurate information available on brain barriers encompassing fetal stages through to adulthood (Ferguson and Woodbury, 1969; Parada et al., 2007; Johanson et al., 2008, 2011; Gato and Desmond, 2009; Liddelow, 2011; Ek et al., 2012; Zappaterra and Lehtinen, 2012), the existence of an embryonic blood–eCSF barrier that controls eCSF composition and homeostasis during early embryonic development remains in doubt. This is partially due to a common belief that barriers in the developing brain are immature, although this implies neither the absence of mechanisms that control eCSF composition and homeostasis, nor that the embryonic brain does not require an environment of great chemical stability.

A further complicating factor is the way in which blood–CSF barrier permeability has traditionally been interpreted. Conventionally, the fact that the ratio of the concentration of particular molecules in CSF with respect to that in blood plasma is much higher in the developing brain than in the adult brain (Ferguson and Woodbury, 1969; Dziegielewska et al., 1979; Habgood et al., 1993; Ek et al., 2001) has been interpreted as evidence of greater barrier permeability (Spector and Johanson, 1989; Kniesel et al., 1996; Engelhardt, 2003; Lee et al., 2003). However, the morphological basis of these barriers formed by means of tight junctions is present from the earliest stages of development between endothelial blood vessel cells in BBB areas, as well as in the epithelial cells of the choroid plexuses in the blood–CSF barrier (Møllgård et al., 1979; Saunders and Møllgård, 1984; Tauc et al., 1984). To reconcile these two sets of evidence, it has been suggested that different transcellular mechanisms operate for protein and small molecule transfer across the embryonic blood–CSF interface (Johansson et al., 2006).

In the past 8 years, a number of studies have provided increasing evidence of the existence of a transient blood–eCSF barrier mechanism in both avian and mammal embryos between the closure of the anterior neuropore and the start of choroid plexus functionality (see below). It has also been demonstrated that at this developmental stage in avians, major eCSF protein fractions are not synthesized by the neuroectodermal cells, but are synthesized in other embryonic tissues or derived from the egg, and subsequently transported from the blood plasma to the cephalic cavities, most probably in a selective manner (Parvas et al., 2008b). These data suggest the need for a physiological blood–eCSF barrier to control the initial composition and homeostasis of the eCSF before the formation of a functional fetal choroid plexus.

THE CEPHALIC NEUROECTODERM BECOMES IMPERMEABLE JUST AFTER CLOSURE OF THE ANTERIOR NEUROPORE

The impermeability of the cephalic neuroectoderm is one of the key factors in the formation of a physiologically sealed system of brain cavities. Early experiments to test the integrity of the embryonic neuroectoderm relied on injected dyes such as trypan, or Evans blue, or enzymes such as horseradish peroxidase (HRP). They produced conflicting results, probably because of the fragility of embryos (Habgood et al., 1992). For example, Wakai and Hirokawa (1978) showed that blood–CSF interface permeability to HRP may follow a free diffusion pattern beginning to decrease at E12–E14 in chick embryos; although their results are probably an artifact due to the very high concentrations of HRP used in the work. However, much more recent experiments in which small concentrations of FGF2 conjugated to FITC or alternatively other proteins of a similar size not normally present in the eCSF are injected into the outflow of the embryo heart, show the existence of selective transport from the blood plasma to the eCSF from E4 onwards (Martin et al., 2006; Parvas et al., 2008a).

In a similar way, the microinjection of a small-sized tracer, biotin dextran amine of 3 kDa (BDA3000), into the outflow of the heart or the cephalic cavity of embryos at E3 and E4, showed that from E4 onwards its transport is restricted to a small subset of endothelial cells and cells adjacent to neuroepithelial cells, located in the ventral mesencephalon and the most anterior part of the ventral prosencephalon, lateral to the floor plate, via transcellular routes (Parvas et al., 2008a) (**Figure 4**). The existence of these specialist transport cells is a key factor in blood–eCSF barrier activity and in some respects may parallel the function of the fetal choroid plexus (Møllgård and Saunders, 1977; Balslev et al., 1997; Ek et al., 2001; Johansson et al., 2006).

PROTEIN TRAFFIC IS SPECIFIC AND HOMEOSTASIS TIGHTLY REGULATED

Initially, eCSF is derived from trapped amniotic fluid; a situation formally equivalent to that of lancelets with respect to seawater during the shift from larval to adult life (see Section Phylogenetic Origin of the CSF System Above; Vígh et al., 2004). After the closure of the anterior neuropore, however, the brain cavities

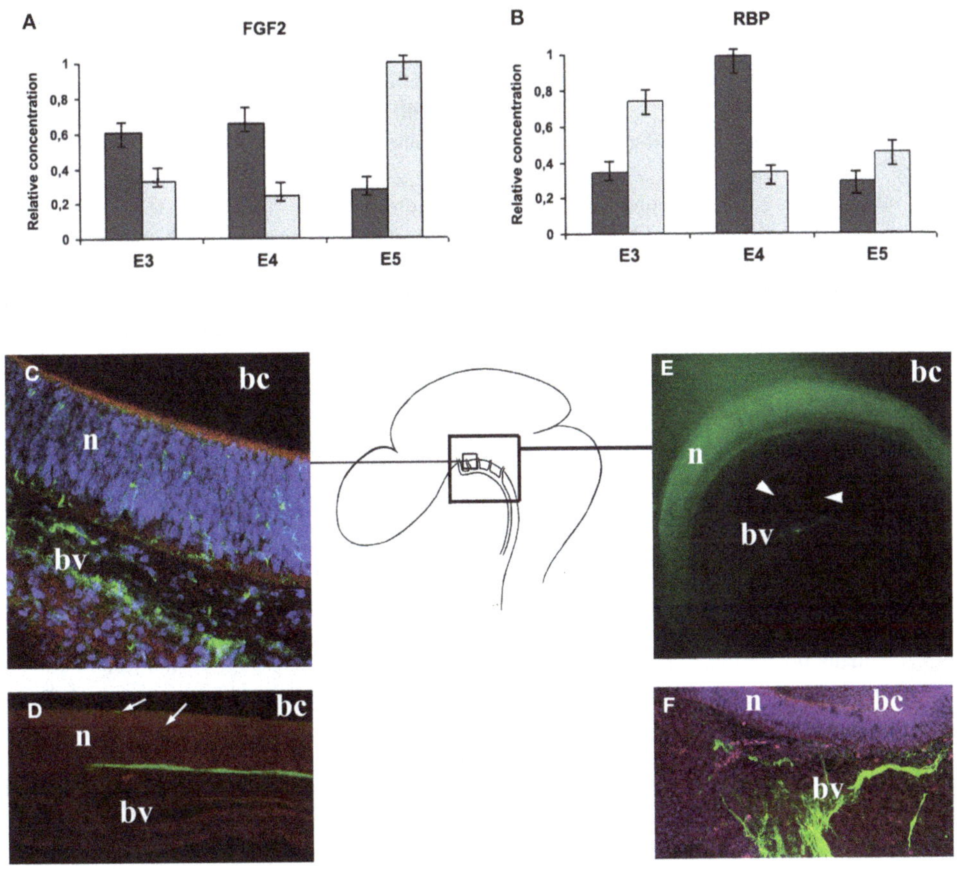

FIGURE 4 | Transport of molecules across the blood–eCSF barrier in chick embryos. (A-B) Relative concentrations of some endogenous proteins in the embryonic serum (light gray), and in the eCSF (dark gray), at E3, E4, and E5 developmental stages (Parvas et al., 2008a). **(C)** Vibratome section showing transport of BDA3000 injected into the cephalic cavities at the ventral mesencephalon, lateral to the floor plate, at E4 (Parvas et al., 2008a). Note the presence of fluorescent dextran in both blood vessels (bv) and across the neuroectoderm (n). **(D)** Vibratome section showing transport of BSA microinjected into the cephalic cavities from the eCSF to the embryonic serum, at E4 (Parvas et al., 2008a). Note the accumulation of BSA in the mesenchyme, at the interface between the neuroectoderm (n) and the blood vessels (bv). Also note the presence of BSA within neuroectodermal cells (arrows). **(E)** AQP1 immunostaining of half head, at E5. Note the immunostained blood vessels and capillary sprouts (arrowheads) (Parvas and Bueno, 2010b). **(F)** Magnification of a blood vessel immunostained with an anti-AQP1 antibody, at E6. Abbreviations: bc, brain cavity; bv, brain vesicles; n, neuroectoderm.

become a physiologically sealed system, hence its composition becomes tightly regulated. Interestingly, most of the molecules identified in chick eCSF are not produced by the neuroectoderm itself. They are stored in the yolk or white of the egg and taken up by the chorioallantoic membrane, or produced by other embryonic structures. This would suggest that they are transported from the production or storage site to the eCSF, most probably via the blood plasma (Martin et al., 2006; Parvas et al., 2008a,b).

In this way, the quantification of the relative concentration of endogenous chick proteins normally present in both blood plasma and the eCSF, e.g., ovalbumin, pRBP, and FGF2, at different developmental stages, demonstrated that their physiological ratio is developmentally regulated. They vary from E3 to E5 in a way which is consistent with their known activities in brain development (Parvas et al., 2008a; **Figure 4**). For example, the eCSF/blood plasma ratio for FGF2 is higher at E5 than at E3 or E4, the developmental period at which this growth factor acts from the eCSF to influence neuroepithelial progenitor cell proliferation (Martin et al., 2006). While for pRBP, the eCSF/blood plasma ratio is much higher at E4 than at E3 or E5, coinciding exactly with its reported period of activity in retinol transport from blood plasma to the eCSF (Parada et al., 2008b).

It has also been demonstrated that the transfer of microinjected proteins across the blood–eCSF interface is protein-specific (Parvas et al., 2008a). Thus, proteins from non-chick sources are never transported from the blood plasma to the eCSF when experimentally microinjected into the outflow of the heart; with the notable exception of HRP, as discussed above. In the same way, neither were proteins which are not normally present in eCSF but are in the blood plasma transported from the blood plasma to this fluid, even when their concentration was experimentally increased 10- to 100-fold by microinjection (Parvas et al., 2008a).

Conversely, when chick proteins such as ovalbumin, FGF2 and pRBP, which are transported between these two embryonic compartments under normal physiological conditions, were bound to FITC to distinguish them from their endogenously produced counterparts and experimentally microinjected into the outflow of the heart, they were actively transported across the blood–eCSF interface (Parvas et al., 2008a; **Figure 4**). However, the transfer ratio of these proteins was maintained in its normal range, indicating that eCSF homeostasis is strongly controlled by the barrier system. For example, when ovalbumin, FGF2 or pRBP bound to FITC were microinjected into the outflow of the heart of chick embryos at E4, they were effectively transferred from the blood plasma to the eCSF, but the total concentration of each of these molecules did not increase in eCSF: it remained stable despite their 10- to 100-fold increase in the blood plasma (Parvas et al., 2008a). In other words, the rate of traffic does not depend on the relative concentrations between the blood plasma and the eCSF, but on some kind of "sensor" that controls eCSF homeostasis, paralleling those identified in the choroid plexus for several sets of molecules.

Moreover, the experimental microinjection of these chick endogenous proteins into the cephalic cavities to directly raise their concentration in the eCSF was rapidly compensated by the eCSF–blood plasma transport system (Parvas et al., 2008a). Similarly, when the microinjected proteins came from non-chick sources, they were rapidly eliminated from the eCSF (**Figure 4**). All of these data strongly suggest blood–eCSF barrier activity in both directions (from blood plasma to eCSF and vice versa) to control eCSF composition before the formation of the functional fetal choroid plexus, thereby ensuring that the eCSF activity is maximally efficient during neural development (Parvas and Bueno, 2011; Castells et al., 2012).

The importance of the blood–eCSF barrier in the control of eCSF composition and homeostasis, and thus, indirectly, in early brain development, has been tested by disrupting it with 6-aminonicotinamide gliotoxin (6-AN); a known antimetabolite of nicotinamide that blocks protein transport across the BBB by halting transcellular caveolae transport (Bertossi et al., 2003; Parvas and Bueno, 2011). Chick embryos treated with 6-AN showed caveolae transport disruption and a lack of protein transport across the blood–eCSF barrier; and this had a clear effect on neuroepithelial cell survival, proliferation and neurogenesis. This blockage also disrupted water influx to the eCSF, leading to an alteration in brain anlagen growth.

PROTEIN TRAFFIC OCCURS IN VERY SPECIFIC BLOOD VESSELS AND INCLUDES BOTH ENDOTHELIAL AND NEUROEPITHELIAL CELLS

Histological analysis was carried out on embryos when transporting endogenous proteins linked to FITC microinjected into the outflow of the heart from the blood plasma to the eCSF, or when microinjected into the cephalic cavities from the eCSF to the blood plasma, as well as proteins from non-chick sources in the same direction. The results demonstrated that, within the developmental period analyzed, transfer from blood plasma to the eCSF, and vice versa occurs only in a specific area of the embryo: in the brain stem lateral to the floor plate, in the ventral mesencephalon and the most anterior part of the ventral prosencephalon (**Figure 4**). Interestingly, this location does not correspond to the area in which fetal choroid plexus development starts, i.e., from an invagination of the dorsal roof plate along the midline of the neural tube. This would seem to indicate that barrier properties are controlled by different independent systems at different stages of development. Moreover, the histological analysis showed that this blood–eCSF barrier function includes endothelial cells of specific perineural blood vessels and some vascular sprouts located within the neuroectoderm cells and adjacent neuroepithelial cells, as well as their adjacent neuroectodermal cells (Parvas et al., 2008a).

Similarly, immunohistological analysis revealed the presence of caveolin 1 in the endothelial cells of blood vessels involved in the blood–eCSF barrier function and in the adjacent neuroectodermal cells, which would indicate that proteins are transported via transcellular routes (Parvas and Bueno, 2010a). Caveolin 1 is the main structural component of caveolae, which are 50 to 100 nm vesicular invaginations of the plasma membrane that are involved in transcellular molecular transport, cell adhesion and signal transduction. Endothelial cells usually show the highest expression of caveolin 1, which is also found in the human BBB vessels (Dermeitzel and Krause, 1991; Laterra and Goldstein, 1993).

Interestingly, caveolin 1 has also been detected in the same embryonic area in rat embryos, including endothelial cells of blood vessels and the adjacent neuroectodermal cells, at an equivalent developmental stage (E12.7) (Parvas and Bueno, 2010a). Although few data are available on protein transport from blood plasma to eCSF in mammals at this developmental stage, the presence of caveolin 1 in the same region that involves both endothelial and neuroepithelial cells has led to the suggestion that there is a barrier function in mammals that acts in the same way as the function that has been demonstrated in chick embryos (Parvas and Bueno, 2010a).

TRAFFIC OF WATER, IONS AND GLUCOSE OCCURS AT THE SAME TRANSPORT SITE AS PROTEINS

During the initial stages of brain development, the control of water flux and regulation of solute transport is critical, since the increase in brain cavity volume is accompanied by a parallel increase in eCSF volume (reviewed by Gato and Desmond, 2009). Aquaporins (AQPs), a family of transmembrane proteins that form molecular water channels that mediate rapid membrane water transport, have been identified in epithelial and endothelial cells at numerous locations in higher vertebrates (Nielsen and Agre, 1995; Verkman et al., 1996; Agre et al., 1998, 2002). Of the 12 AQPs described to date (AQP0 to AQP11), AQP1 and AQP4 appear to play a role in water transport across brain barriers. AQP1 is expressed at very early stages of choroid plexus development in a range of mammalian species (Johansson et al., 2005), and AQP4 is present in adult brain endothelial cells (Amiry-Moghaddam et al., 2004). Findings from several studies suggest that choroid plexus apical expression of AQP1 is closely related to the rate of CSF formation. For example, AQP1-null mice have lowered CSF formation and pressure (Oshio et al., 2005).

Similarly, ion transfer appears to be critical for eCSF production and brain anlagen growth. Ions can move through cell membranes, both actively via ion pumps and passively via ion channels. In the adult, AQP4 co-localizes with the inwardly rectifying K^+ channel Kir4.1 (Nagelhus et al., 2004), and it has been suggested that together, these two proteins play a key role in K^+ and water balance. A study using PCR analysis and immunohistochemical procedures revealed that Kir4.1, AQP1, and AQP4 are present in both chick and rat embryos in the same blood vessels where specific protein transport has also been detected (Parvas and Bueno, 2010b; **Figure 4**). In chick embryos, AQP1 is present from E4, and AQP4, and Kir4.1 from E5; and in rat embryos AQP1 is detected from E12.7 and AQP4, and Kir4.1 from E13.7, i.e., at the equivalent developmental stages. These results may explain the control of the rapid expansion of brain anlagen at this developmental stage by means of water and ion influx, as previously suggested by Desmond and Jacobson (1977).

In addition to water and ion influx, the transfer of energy molecules such as glucose is crucial for the developing neuroepithelium. Glucose is an important energy source for the brain, and although few data are available on embryos, it has been recently shown that several glucose transporters are expressed at a much higher level in the rat embryonic choroid plexus than in the adult (Liddelow et al., 2014). Glucose is transported across cell membranes mainly by the GLUT family of solute carriers. In adults, GLUT1 is located in the brain barriers and also in the choroid plexus epithelial cells (Saunders et al., 2013). Similarly, a study using PCR analysis and immunohistochemical procedures demonstrated that in chick and rat embryos, GLUT1 is also present in the same blood vessels where protein transport and the presence of AQP1, AQP4, and Kir4.1 have been detected (Parvas and Bueno, 2010b).

CONCLUSION

Taken together, all of these findings seem to confirm that a blood–eCSF barrier function controls eCSF composition and homeostasis from early stages of brain development in chick embryos. That control includes protein, glucose, water, and ion influx, and thus regulates eCSF osmolarity. It has been proposed that a similar blood–eCSF barrier is also present in mammals at the equivalent brain development stages (Parvas and Bueno, 2010a,b). The roles ascribed to this transient barrier confirm the crucial importance of the eCSF milieu for brain development at the beginning of primary neurogenesis; after the closure of the anterior neuropore and before the fetal choroid plexus is fully functional, which occurs shortly afterwards. Thus, the blood–eCSF barrier function should be considered as an actual barrier system that operates in early embryos in a transcellular way, and which includes specific transporters for particular molecules and sensors to monitor eCSF homeostasis. Just as most civilizations develop along riverbanks and seashores, using the fluid medium that is immediately available to them to promote cohesion and transport, and to enhance the chances of survival of the people who live at the edge of the liquid medium, so the brain is also organized, from its embryonic beginnings and throughout adult life, around an extraordinarily dynamic, and complex fluid: the CSF. Continuing this simile, as civilizations build harbors from which to ship goods and control transport that becomes ever more complex as they develop, so the brain has evolved barrier mechanisms, which start to form very early in brain development and change their morphology and physiology in accordance with the changing developmental stages.

ACKNOWLEDGMENTS

Financial support from the Spanish Ministerio de Educación y Ciencia, via grant BFU2011-23921 is gratefully acknowledged. We also thank the reviewers and editors for comments and suggestions that have made the paper more comprehensive and sounder.

REFERENCES

Agre, P., Bonhivers, M., and Borgnia, M. J. (1998). The aquaporins, blueprints for cellular plumbing systems. *J. Biol. Chem.* 273, 14659–14662.

Agre, P., King, L. S., Yasui, M., Guggino, W. B., Ottersen, O. P., Fujiyoshi, Y., et al. (2002). Aquaporin water channels–from atomic structure to clinical medicine. *J. Physiol.* 542, 3–16. doi: 10.1113/jphysiol.2002.020818

Alonso, M. I., Gato, A., Moro, J. A., and Barbosa, E. (1998). Disruption of proteoglycans in neural tube fluid by beta-D-xyloside alters brain enlargement in chick embryos. *Anat. Rec.* 252, 499–508.

Alonso, M. I., Gato, A., Moro, J. A., Martin, P., and Barbosa, E. (1999). Involvement of sulfated proteoglycans in embryonic brain expansion at earliest stages of development in rat embryos. *Cells Tissues Organs* 165, 1–9. doi: 10.1159/000016667

Alonso, M. I., Martín, C., Carnicero, E., Bueno, D., and Gato, A. (2011). Cerebrospinal fluid control of neurogenesis induced by retinoic acid during early brain development. *Dev. Dyn.* 240, 1650–1659. doi: 10.1002/dvdy.22657

Amiry-Moghaddam, M., Frydenlund, D. S., and Ottersen, O. P. (2004). Anchoring of aquaporin-4 in brain: molecular mechanisms and implications for the physiology and pathophysiology of water transport. *Neuroscience* 129, 999–1010. doi: 10.1016/j.neuroscience.2004.08.049

Bally-Cuif, L., and Boncinelli, E. (1997). Transcription factors and head formation in vertebrates. *Bioessays* 19, 127–135. doi: 10.1002/bies.950190207

Balslev, Y., Dziegielewska, K. M., Møllgard, K., and Saunders, N. R. (1997). Intercellular barriers to and transcellular transfer of albumin in the fetal sheep brain. *Anat. Embryol. (Berl.)* 195, 229–236. doi: 10.1007/s004290050042

Bellairs, R., and Osmond, M. (2005). *Atlas of Chick Development*. London: Elsevier Academy Press.

Bertossi, M., Girolamo, F., Errede, M., Virgintino, D., and Roncali, L. (2003). Effects of 6-aminonicotinamide gliotoxin on blood-brain barrier differentiation in the chick embryo cerebellum. *Anat. Embryol. (Berl.)* 207, 209–219. doi: 10.1007/s00429-003-0335-4

Birecree, E., King, L. E. J., and Nanney, L. B. (1991). Epidermal growth factor and its receptor in the developing human nervous system. *Brain Res. Dev. Brain Res.* 60, 145–154. doi: 10.1016/0165-3806(91)90043-I

Birge, W. J., Rose, A. D., Haywood, J. R., and Doolin, P. F. (1974). Development of the blood-cerebrospinal fluid barrier to proteins and differentiation of cerebrospinal fluid in the chick embryo. *Dev. Biol.* 41, 245–254.

Brocklehurst, G. (1979). The significance of the evolution of the cerebrospinal fluid system. *Ann. Rev. Coll. Surg. Engl.* 61, 349–356.

Castells, A., Parvas, M., and Bueno, D. (2012). Homeostasis of cerebrospinal fluid has a role in early brain development. *Neuroreport* 23, 917–921. doi: 10.1097/WNR.0b013e3283582067

Checiu, I., Prelipceanu, O., and Popescu, O. (1984). The role of cerebrospinal fluid during embryonic development. A biochemical study. *Morphol. Embryol.* 30, 243–250.

Copp, A. J. (2005). Neurulation in the cranial region-normal and abnormal. *J. Anat.* 207, 623–635. doi: 10.1111/j.1469-7580.2005.00476.x

Copp, A. J., Greene, N. D., and Murdoch, J. N. (2003). The genetic basis of mammalian neurulation. *Nat. Rev. Genet.* 4, 784–793. doi: 10.1038/nrg1181

Dermeitzel, R., and Krause, D. (1991). "Molecular anatomy of the blood brain barrier as defined by immunocyto-chemistry," in *International Review of Cytology*, eds K. W. Jeon and M. Friedlander (New York, NY: Academic Press), 57–109.

Desmond, M. E., and Jacobson, A. G. (1977). Embryonic brain enlargement requires cerebrospinal fluid pressure. *Dev. Biol.* 57, 188–198. doi: 10.1016/0012-1606(77)90364-5

Desmond, M. E., and Levitan, M. L. (2002). Brain expansion in the chick embryo initiated by experimentally produced occlusion of the spinal neurocoel. *Anat. Rec.* 268, 147–159. doi: 10.1002/ar.10146

Dziegielewska, K. M., Evans, C. A., and Fossan, G. (1980a). Proteins in cerebrospinal fluid and plasma of fetal sheep during development. *J. Physiol.* 300, 441–455.

Dziegielewska, K. M., Evans, C. A., and Lai, P. C. (1981). Proteins in cerebrospinal fluid and plasma of fetal rats during development. *Dev. Biol.* 83, 193–200. doi: 10.1016/S0012-1606(81)80024-3

Dziegielewska, K. M., Evans, C. A., Malinowska, D. H., Møllgård, K., Reynolds, J. M., Reynolds, M. L., et al. (1979). Studies of the development of brain barrier systems to lipid insoluble molecules in fetal sheep. *J. Physiol.* 292, 207–231.

Dziegielewska, K. M., Evans, C. A., Malinowska, D. H., Møllgård, K., Reynolds, M. L., and Saunders, N. R. (1980b). Blood-cerebrospinal fluid transfer of plasma proteins during fetal development in the sheep. *J. Physiol.* 300, 457–465.

Ek, C. J., Dziegielewska, K. M., Habgood, M. D., and Saunders, N. R. (2012). Barriers in the developing brain and Neurotoxicology. *Neurotoxicology* 33, 586–604. doi: 10.1016/j.neuro.2011.12.009

Ek, C. J., Habgood, M. D., Dziegielewska, K. M., Potter, A., and Saunders, N. R. (2001). Permeability and route of entry for lipid-insoluble molecules across brain barriers in developing *Monodelphis domes*tica. *J. Physiol.* 536, 841–853. doi: 10.1111/j.1469-7793.2001.00841

Emerich, D. F., Skinner, S. J. M., Borlongan, C. V., Vasconcellos, A. V., and Thanos, C. G. (2005). The choroid plexus in the rise, fall and repair of the brain. *Bioessays* 27, 262–274. doi: 10.1002/bies.20193

Engelhardt, B. (2003). Development of the blood-brain barrier. *Cell Tissue Res.* 314, 119–129. doi: 10.1387/ijdb.103224sl

Feliciano, D. M., Zhang, S., Nasrallah, C. M., Lisgo, S. N., and Bordey, A. (2014). Embryonic cerebrospinal fluid nanovesicles carry evolutionarily conserved molecules that promote neural stem cell amplification. *PLoS ONE* 9:e88810. doi: 10.1371/journal.pone.0088810

Ferguson, R. K., and Woodbury, D. M. (1969). Penetration of 14C-inulin and 14C-sucrose into brain, cerebrospinal fluid, and skeletal muscle of developing rats. *Exp. Brain Res.* 7, 181–194.

Fielitz, W., Esteves, A., and Moro, R. (1984). Protein composition of cerebrospinal fluid in the developing chick embryo. *Brain Res.* 315, 111–115. doi: 10.1016/0165-3806(84)90082-8

Gato, A. (2013). Cerebrospinal fluid: a rising subject in brain development. *Front. Mol. Neurosci.* 6, 1. doi: 10.3389/fnmol.2013.00030

Gato, A., and Desmond, M. E. (2009). Why the embryo still matters: CSF and the neuroepithelium as interdependent regulators of embryonic brain growth, morphogenesis and histiogenesis. *Dev. Biol.* 327, 263–272. doi: 10.1016/j.ydbio.2008.12.029

Gato, A., Martín, P., Alonso, M. I., Martín, C., Pulgar, M. A., and Moro, J. A. (2004). Analysis of cerebro-spinal fluid protein composition in early developmental stages in chick embryos. *J. Exp. Zool. A Comp. Exp. Biol.* 301, 280–289. doi: 10.1002/jez.a.20035

Gato, A., Moro, J. A., Alonso, M. I., Bueno, D., De La Mano, A., and Martín, C. (2005). Embryonic cerebrospinal fluid regulates neuroepithelial survival, proliferation, and neurogenesis in chick embryos. *Anat. Rec. A Discov. Mol. Cell Evol. Biol.* 284, 475–484. doi: 10.1002/ar.a.20185

Habgood, M. D., Knott, G. W., Dziegielewska, K. M., and Saunders, N. R. (1993). The nature of the decrease in blood-cerebrospinal fluid barrier exchange during postnatal brain development in the rat. *J. Physiol.* 468, 73–83.

Habgood, M. D., Sedgwick, J. E., Dziegielewska, K. M., and Saunders, N. R. (1992). A developmentally regulated blood-cerebrospinal fluid transfer mechanism for albumin in immature rats. *J. Physiol.* 456, 181–192.

Hatta, T., Matsumoto, A., Ono, A., Udagawa, J., Nimura, M., Hashimoto, R., et al. (2006). Quantitative analyses of leukemia inhibitory factor in the cerebrospinal fluid in mouse embryos. *Neuroreport* 17, 1863–1866. doi: 10.1097/WNR.0b013e3280113962

Johanson, C. E., Duncan, J. A., Klinge, P. M., Brinker, T., Stopa, E. G., and Silverberg, G. D. (2008). Multiplicity of cerebrospinal fluid functions: new challenges in health and disease. *Cerebrospinal Fluid Res.* 5, 10. doi: 10.1186/1743-8454-5-10

Johanson, C. E., Stopa, E. G., and McMillan, P. N. (2011). The blood-cerebrospinal fluid barrier: structure and functional significance. *Methods Mol. Biol.* 686, 101–131. doi: 10.1007/978-1-60761-938-3_4

Johansson, P. A., Dziegielewska, K. M., Ek, C. J., Habgood, M. D., Liddelow, S. A., Potter, A. M., et al. (2006). Blood-CSF barrier function in the rat embryo. *Eur. J. Neurosci.* 24, 65–76. doi: 10.1111/j.1460-9568.2006.04904.x

Johansson, P. A., Dziegielewska, K. M., Ek, C. J., Habgood, M. D., Møllgård, K., Potter, A., et al. (2005). Aquaporin-1 in the choroid plexuses of developing mammalian brain. *Cell Tissue Res.* 322, 353–364. doi: 10.1007/s00441-005-1120-x

Kniesel, U., Risau, W., and Wolburg, H. (1996). Development of blood-brain barrier tight junctions in the rat cortex. *Brain Res. Dev. Brain Res.* 96, 229–240.

Laterra, J., and Goldstein, G. W. (1993). "Brain microves-sels and microvascular cells *in vitro*," in *The Blood-Brain Barrier Pardridge*, ed W. M. Pardridge (New York, NY: Raven Press), 1–24.

Lee, S. W., Kim, W. J., Choi, Y. K., Song, H. S., Son, M. J., Gelman, I. H., et al. (2003). SSeCKS regulates angiogenesis and tight junction formation in blood-brain barrier. *Nat. Med.* 9, 900–906. doi: 10.1038/nm889

Liddelow, S. A. (2011). Fluids and barriers of the CNS: a historical viewpoint. *Fluids Barriers CNS* 8:2. doi: 10.1186/2045-8118-8-2

Liddelow, S. H., Dziegielewska, K. M., Møllgård, K., Habgood, M. D., Wakefield, M. J., Lyndsay, H., et al. (2014). Influx mechanisms in the embryonic and adult rat choroid plexus: a transcriptome study. *Front. Neurosci.*

Martin, C., Alonso, M. I., Santiago, C., Moro, J. A., De la Mano, A., Carretero, R., et al. (2009). Early embryonic brain development in rats requires the trophic influence of cerebrospinal fluid. *Int. J. Dev. Neurosci.* 27, 733–740. doi: 10.1016/j.ijdevneu.2009.06.002

Martin, C., Bueno, D., Alonso, M. I., Moro, J. A., Callejo, S., Parada, C., et al. (2006). FGF2 plays a key role in embryonic cerebrospinal fluid trophic properties over chick embryo neuroepithelial stem cells. *Dev. Biol.* 297, 402–416 doi: 10.1016/j.ydbio.2006.05.010

Martinez, S. (2001). The isthmic organizer and brain regionalization. *Int. J. Dev. Biol.* 44, 367–371. Available online at: http://www.ijdb.ehu.es/web/paper.php?doi=11291867

Miyan, J. A., Nabiyouni, M., and Zendah, M. (2003). Development of the brain: a vital role for cerebrospinal fluid. *Can. J. Physiol. Pharmacol.* 81, 317–328. doi: 10.1139/y03-027

Miyan, J. A., Zendah, M., Mashayekhi, F., and Owen-Lynch, P. J. (2006). Cerebrospinal fluid supports viability and proliferation of cortical cells *in vitro*, mirroring *in vivo* development. *Cerebrospinal Fluid Res.* 3:2. doi: 10.1186/1743-8454-3-2

Møllgård, K., Lauritzen, B., and Saunders, N. R. (1979). Double replica technique applied to choroid plexus from early foetal sheep: completeness and complexity of tight junctions. *J. Neurocytol.* 8, 139–149. doi: 10.1007/BF01175557

Møllgård, K., and Saunders, N. R. (1977). A possible transepithelial pathway via endoplasmic reticulum in foetal sheep choroid plexus. *Proc. R. Soc. Lond. B Biol. Sci.* 199, 321–326. doi: 10.1098/rspb.1977.0142

Nagelhus, E. A., Mathiisen, T. M., and Ottersen, O. P. (2004). Aquaporin-4 in the central nervous system: cellular and subcellular distribution and coexpression with KIR4.1. *Neuroscience* 129, 905–913. doi: 10.1016/j.neuroscience.2004.08.053

Nakamura, H., Katahira, T., Matsunaga, E., and Sato, T. (2005). Isthmus organizer for midbrain and hindbrain development. *Brain Res. Brain Res. Rev.* 49, 120–126. doi: 10.1016/j.brainresrev.2004.10.005

Nielsen, S., and Agre, P. (1995). The aquaporin family of water channels in kidney. *Kidney Int.* 48, 1057–1068.

Oshio, K., Watanabe, H., Song, Y., Verkman, A. S., and Manley, G. T. (2005). Reduced cerebrospinal fluid production and intracranial pressure in mice lacking choroid plexus water channel Aquaporin-1. *FASEB J.* 19, 76–78. doi: 10.1096/fj.04-1711fje

Parada, C., Gato, A., Aparicio, M., and Bueno, D. (2006). Proteome analysis of chick embryonic cerebrospinal fluid. *Proteomics* 6, 312–320. doi: 10.1002/pmic.200500085

Parada, C., Escolà-Gil, J. C., and Bueno, D. (2008a). Low-density lipoproteins from embryonic cerebrospinal fluid are required for neural differentiation. *J. Neurosci. Res.* 86, 2674–2684. doi: 10.1002/jnr.21724

Parada, C., Gato, A., and Bueno, D. (2005a). Mammalian embryonic cerebrospinal fluid proteome has greater apolipoprotein and enzyme pattern complexity than the avian proteome. *J. Proteome Res.* 4, 2420–2428. doi: 10.1021/pr050213t

Parada, C., Gato, A., and Bueno, D. (2008b). All-trans retinol and retinol-binding protein from embryonic cerebrospinal fluid exhibit dynamic behavior during early central nervous system development. *Neuroreport* 19, 945–950. doi: 10.1097/WNR.0b013e3283021c94

Parada, C., Martín, C., Alonso, M. I., Moro, J. A., Bueno, D., and Gato, A. (2005b). Embryonic cerebrospinal fluid collaborates with the isthmic organizer to regulate mesencephalic gene expression. *J. Neurosci. Res.* 82, 333–345. doi: 10.1002/jnr.20618

Parada, C., Parvas, M., and Bueno, D. (2007). Cerebrospinal fluid proteomes: from neural development to neurodegenerative diseases. *Curr. Proteomics* 4, 89–106. doi: 10.2174/157016407782194611

Parvas, M., and Bueno, D. (2010a). The embryonic blood-CSF barrier has molecular elements for specific glucose transport and for the general transport of molecules via transcellular routes. *Adv. Biosci. Biotechnol.* 1, 315–321. doi: 10.4236/abb.2010.14041

Parvas, M., and Bueno, D. (2010b). The embryonic blood-CSF barrier has molecular elements to control E-CSF osmolarity during early CNS development. *J. Neurosci. Res.* 88, 1205–1212. doi: 10.1002/jnr.22293

Parvas, M., and Bueno, D. (2011). Disruption of embryonic blood-CSF barrier in chick embryos reveals the actual importance of this barrier to control E-CSF composition and homeostasis in early brain development. *Open J. Neurosci.* 1, 1–11. Available online at: http://rossscience.org/ojns/articles/2075-9088-1-3.pdf

Parvas, M., Parada, C., and Bueno, D. (2008a). A blood-CSF barrier function controls embryonic CSF protein composition and homeostasis during early CNS development. *Dev. Biol.* 321, 51–63. doi: 10.1016/j.ydbio.2008.05.552

Parvas, M., Rius, M., and Bueno, D. (2008b). Most of the abundant protein fractions of embryonic cerebrospinal fluid are produced out of the brain anlagen. *Open Proteomics J.* 1, 1–4. doi: 10.2174/1875039700801010001

Rubin, L. L., and Staddon, J. M. (1999). The cell biology of the blood-brain barrier. *Annu. Rev. Neurosci.* 22, 11–28. doi: 10.1146/annurev.neuro.22.1.11

Saunders, N. R., Daneman, R., Dziegielewska, K. M., and Liddelow, S. A. (2013). Transporters of the blood-brain and blood-CSF interfaces in development and in the adult. *Mol. Aspects Med.* 34, 742–752. doi: 10.1016/j.mam.2012.11.006

Saunders, N. R., and Møllgård, K. (1984). Development of the blood-brain barrier. *J. Dev. Physiol.* 6, 45–57.

Sawamoto, K., Wichterle, H., Gonzalez-Perez, O., Cholfin, J. A., Yamada, M., Spassky, N., et al. (2006). New neurons follow the flow of cerebrospinal fluid in the adult brain. *Science* 311, 629–632 doi: 10.1126/science.1119133

Smith, J. L., and Schoenwolf, G. C. (1997). Neurulation: coming to closure. *Trends Neurosci.* 20, 510–517.

Spector, R., and Johanson, C. E. (1989). The mammalian choroid plexus. *Sci. Am.* 261, 68–74.

Stern, C. D. (2001). Initial patterning of the central nervous system: how many organizers? *Nat. Rev. Neurosci.* 2, 92–98. doi: 10.1038/35053563

Stern, C. D. (2002). Induction and initial patterning of the nervous system–the chick embryo enters the scene. *Curr. Opin. Genet. Dev.* 12, 447–451. doi: 10.1016/S0959-437X(02)00324-6

Tauc, M., Vignon, X., and Bouchaud, C. (1984). Evidence for the effectiveness of the blood–CSF barrier in the fetal rat choroid plexus. A freeze-fracture and peroxidase diffusion study. *Tissue Cell* 16, 65–74.

Vera, A., Stanic, K., Montecinos, H., Torrejón, M., Marcellini, S., and Caprile, T. (2013). SCO-spondin from embryonic cerebrospinal fluid is required for neurogenesis during early brain development. *Front. Cell Neurosci.* 7:80. doi: 10.3389/fncel.2013.00080

Verkman, A. S., van Hoek, A. N., Ma, T., Frigeri, A., Skach, W. R., Mitra, A., et al. (1996). Water transport across mammalian cell membranes. *Am. J. Physiol.* 270, C12–30.

Vígh, B., Manzano e Silva, M. J., Frank, C. L., Vincze, C., Czirok, S. J., Szabo, A., et al. (2004). The system of cerebrospinal fluid-contacting neurons. Its supposed role in the nonsynaptic signal transmission of the brain. *Histol. Histopathol.* 19, 607–628. Available online at: http://www.hh.um.es/pdf/Vol_19/19_2/Vigh-19-607-628-2004.pdf

Wakai, S., and Hirokawa, N. (1978). Development of the blood-brain barrier to horseradish peroxidase in the chick embryo. *Cell Tissue Res.* 195, 195–203. doi: 10.1007/BF00236719

Zappaterra, M. D., and Lehtinen, M. K. (2012). The cerebrospinal fluid: regulator of neurogenesis, behavior, and beyond. *Cell Mol. Life Sci.* 69, 2863–2878. doi: 10.1007/s00018-012-0957-x

Zappaterra, M. D., Lisgo, S. N., Lindsay, S., Gygi, S. P., Walsh, C. A., and Ballif, B. A. (2007). A comparative proteomic analysis of human and rat embryonic cerebrospinal fluid. *J. Proteome Res.* 6, 3537–3548. doi: 10.1021/pr070247w

15

"You Shall Not Pass"—tight junctions of the blood brain barrier

Hans-Christian Bauer[1,2,3], István A. Krizbai[4,5], Hannelore Bauer[6] and Andreas Traweger[1,3]*

[1] Institute of Tendon and Bone Regeneration, Paracelsus Medical University - Spinal Cord Injury and Tissue Regeneration Center Salzburg, Salzburg, Austria
[2] Department of Traumatology and Sports Injuries, Paracelsus Medical University, Salzburg, Austria
[3] Austrian Cluster for Tissue Regeneration, Vienna, Austria
[4] Biological Research Centre, Institute of Biophysics, Hungarian Academy of Sciences, Szeged, Hungary
[5] Institute of Life Sciences, Vasile Goldis Western University of Arad, Arad, Romania
[6] Department of Organismic Biology, University of Salzburg, Salzburg, Austria

***Correspondence:**
Andreas Traweger, Institute of Tendon and Bone Regeneration, Paracelsus Medical University - Spinal Cord Injury and Tissue Regeneration Center Salzburg, Strubergasse 22, A-5020 Salzburg, Austria
e-mail: andreas.traweger@pmu.ac.at

The structure and function of the barrier layers restricting the free diffusion of substances between the central nervous system (brain and spinal cord) and the systemic circulation is of great medical interest as various pathological conditions often lead to their impairment. Excessive leakage of blood-borne molecules into the parenchyma and the concomitant fluctuations in the microenvironment following a transient breakdown of the blood-brain barrier (BBB) during ischemic/hypoxic conditions or because of an autoimmune disease are detrimental to the physiological functioning of nervous tissue. On the other hand, the treatment of neurological disorders is often hampered as only minimal amounts of therapeutic agents are able to penetrate a fully functional BBB or blood cerebrospinal fluid barrier. An in-depth understanding of the molecular machinery governing the establishment and maintenance of these barriers is necessary to develop rational strategies allowing a controlled delivery of appropriate drugs to the CNS. At the basis of such tissue barriers are intimate cell-cell contacts (*zonulae occludentes*, tight junctions) which are present in all polarized epithelia and endothelia. By creating a paracellular diffusion constraint TJs enable the vectorial transport across cell monolayers. More recent findings indicate that functional barriers are already established during development, protecting the fetal brain. As an understanding of the biogenesis of TJs might reveal the underlying mechanisms of barrier formation during ontogenic development numerous *in vitro* systems have been developed to study the assembly and disassembly of TJs. In addition, monitoring the stage-specific expression of TJ-associated proteins during development has brought much insight into the "developmental tightening" of tissue barriers. Over the last two decades a detailed molecular map of transmembrane and cytoplasmic TJ-proteins has been identified. These proteins not only form a cell-cell adhesion structure, but integrate various signaling pathways, thereby directly or indirectly impacting upon processes such as cell-cell adhesion, cytoskeletal rearrangement, and transcriptional control. This review will provide a brief overview on the establishment of the BBB during embryonic development in mammals and a detailed description of the ultrastructure, biogenesis, and molecular composition of epithelial and endothelial TJs will be given.

Keywords: blood-brain barrier, tight junctions, PDZ scaffolds, MAGUK proteins, cell polarity, brain capillary endothelial cells, vascular permeability

ESTABLISHMENT OF THE BBB DURING MAMMALIAN EMBRYOGENESIS

During evolution organisms with a complex nervous system have developed mechanisms to selectively restrict the blood-to-brain traffic of compounds allowing a tight regulation of the neuroparenchymal microenvironment. Such cerebral

Abbreviations: CD31/34, cluster of differentiation 31/34; Cdc42, cell division control protein 42; CD2AP, CD2-associated protein; CDK4, cyclin-dependent kinase 4/cell division protein kinase 4; C/EBP, CCAAT/enhancer-binding-protein; cECs, capillary endothelial cells; CNS, central nervous system; ECM, extracellular matrix; ES cells, embryonic stem cells; GAP, GTPase activating protein; GDNF, glial-derived neurotrophic factor; GEF-H1, guanine nucleotide exchange factor-H1; Glut-1, glucose transporter-1; GUK, guanylate kinase; hCMEC/D3, human cerebral microvascular endothelial cell line/D3; hnRNP, heterogeneous nuclear ribonucleoprotein; MAGI, membrane-associated guanylate kinase inverted; MAGUK, membrane-associated guanylate kinase; MARVEL, MAL (myelin and lymphocyte) and related proteins for vesicle trafficking and membrane link; NVU, neurovascular unit; PDZ, PSD-95, discs large, ZO-1; SMAD, SMA (small)/ MAD: Mothers against decapentaplegic; TAMPs, TJ-associated MARVEL proteins; TEER, transepithelial electrical resistance; Unc-5, uncoordinated locomotion-5; VEGF, vascular endothelial growth factor; WD40, tryptophan-aspartic acid (WD) repeat; Wnt, wingless/Int-1.

homeostasis is fundamental for proper function of synapses and neural networks. However, despite the burgeoning literature on when the BBB is established in the course of mammalian development, the topic is still heavily debated. This is largely the result of inconsistent and partially contradictive results stemming from different animal models used and due to misinterpretation of experiments (*for review see Saunders et al. in this volume*). In addition, not a single barrier, but the sum of several cellular and molecular barriers ensures the stable environment needed for the proper function of the central nervous system, further complicating the analysis. Of the three main CNS barriers the brain endothelium constituting the blood-brain barrier (BBB) represents the major interface between the blood and the brain interstitial fluid with an estimated total surface area of 20 m^2 (Begley and Brightman, 2003). The endothelial cells are fitted with specialized structures, such as cell-cell adhesion complexes obliterating the paracellular space (tight junctions) and an array of transport and shuttle proteins controlling the flux of ions and solutes. The term BBB has been coined nearly 100 years ago by Stern et al. (Stern and Rothlin, 1918; Stern and Gauthier, 1921), implying a structure completely preventing an exchange between blood and nervous tissue. However, since then it has become increasingly clear that the BBB is a complex and dynamic structure allowing a controlled passage of blood-borne substances. In addition, the functional BBB, at least in the adult, is not only composed of the endothelial cells (ECs) lining the microvasculature but also requires the contact and/or input of other cell types, including astrocytes, neurons, and pericytes separated only by a basement membrane. All these contributing building blocks of the BBB are commonly being referred to as "neurovascular unit," a term which has been introduced for the first time by members of the Stroke Progress Review Group in 2002 at the NIH, USA. During embryonic development however, the composition of the NVU and the nature of the cerebral capillary endothelial cells (cECs) most likely is very different from those seen in the adult. At an even more fundamental level, at which developmental stage can we speak of a structure exerting barrier functions and does BBB formation in cEC coincide with the early vascularization of the growing CNS?

In mice angiogenesis in the brain begins at day E9 of development, when pial vessels encircle the telencephalon (Vasudevan et al., 2008). By E10 pial vessels sprout and start forming a primitive vascular plexus within the telencephalon. The newly formed vessels have a premature appearance (see **Figures 1A,B**) but allow already erythrocyte traffic (Bauer et al., 1993, 1995). In parallel, periventricular vessels migrate into the dorsal telencephalon resulting in a ventrolateral to dorsomedial angiogenesis gradient (Vasudevan et al., 2008). It is proposed that the pial vessels develop into venous sinuses and the periventricular vessels into arteries. The assumption that the plexus of the CNS likely arises from two different endothelial cell populations is further supported by the demonstration of different expression patterns of homeobox transcription factors, namely Dlx1/2, Nkx2.1 in periventricular ventral vessels and Pax6 in pial vessels. Intriguingly, these transcription factors also regulate neuroepithelial cell proliferation and neuronal migration (Sussel et al., 1999; Nery et al., 2003). Therefore, it is tempting to speculate that angiogenesis in due course influences and regulates neuronal proliferation and differentiation.

Several proteins, morphogenetic molecules and their receptors are involved in both, angiogenesis of the brain and in the formation of the BBB: VEGF has been identified as one of the first of these effectors. This morphogenetic molecule is secreted by neuronal precursor cells and promotes via binding to endothelial tyrosine kinase receptors (FLT-1/VEGFR-1; FLK-1/VEGFR-2) vessel sprouting during the early phases of CNS development (Breier et al., 1992; Raab et al., 2004). VEGF is also secreted by brain endothelial cells and exerts its influence on the cortical cytoarchitecture during later stages of embryonic development allowing the establishment of a functional neuronal architecture in the CNS (Li et al., 2013). Other effector molecules include members of the Wnt family (Wnt7a/b, Wnt3a) together with the action of ß-catenin, Tie-2 (an endothelial cell-specific receptor tyrosine kinase) and its ligands angiopoietin-1 and angiopoietin-2 (Ang-1, Ang-2), as well as sonic hedgehog and Norrin (Engelhardt and Liebner, 2014). The important role of Ang-1 during BBB formation is additionally strengthened by the identification of SSeCKS, a soluble protein which induces the expression of Ang-1 in cEC of the BBB (Lee et al., 2003). Next to these effectors which exert their action throughout the entire CNS, others are restricted to specific areas. For example GPR124 (orphan G protein-coupled receptor 124) is specifically expressed in endothelial cells regulating sprouting in the forebrain and in spinal cord but not in other regions of the CNS (Kuhnert et al., 2010). GPR124 also modulates TGF-ß signaling, thereby influencing pericyte and astrocyte differentiation and further impacts upon glucose transport by regulating the expression of Glut-1 in cECs. Taken together, the factors described above are intimately related to the induction of a functional BBB as they promote differentiation of the cECs, ultimately resulting in the formation of occluding cell adhesion structures and the expression of specific transporter receptors and shuttling molecules such as the multidrug resistance molecule.

The early transplantation experiments by Stewart and Wiley and Ikeda et al. demonstrated the induction of BBB features of invading endothelial cells by ectopic transplantation of embryonic brain tissue, indicating that the acquisition of BBB function is not merely an intrinsic property of cerebral endothelial cells (Stewart and Wiley, 1981; Ikeda et al., 1996) but requires the direct and indirect communication with neighboring neuronal cells. In the early brain these are the neuroepithelial cells and neuroblasts and later in embryonic development and postnatally, neurons, pericytes and glial cells (Bauer and Bauer, 2000). However, the underlying molecular machinery and ramifications of this interaction are not fully understood mainly due to its complex nature and its constant modulation during embryonic and postnatal development. Lindahl et al. showed that platelet derived growth factor–B (PDGF-B) secreted from migrating cECs led to the recruitment of pericytes and their attachment to the newly formed vessels (Lindahl et al., 1997). In the following years *in vivo* and *in vitro* studies demonstrated that pericytes are imperative for BBB formation (Deli et al., 2005; Armulik et al., 2010; Daneman et al., 2010b). Recently, another effector was described by Ben-Zvi et al. (2014) named Mfsd2a, a transmembrane protein

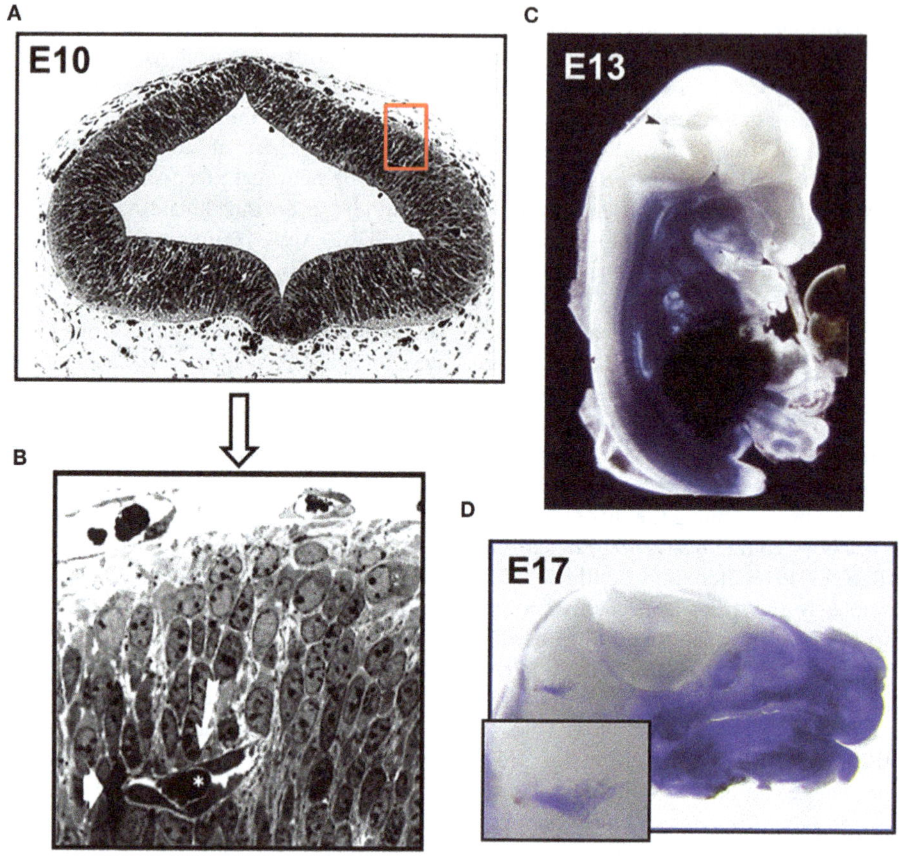

FIGURE 1 | Establishment of the intraneural vascular plexus and a functional BBB during mouse embryogenesis. (A) Semithin section of embryonic mouse neocortex at E10 showing the intraneural and parts of the surrounding perineural domain **(B)** neuroepithelial cells surround a primitive capillary (white arrow) containing a red blood cell (asterisk). Murine E13 **(C)** and E17 **(D)** embryos microperfused with 0.5% Trypan blue solution. After fixation specimens were cut medially and photographed. Arrowhead indicates and enlarged area depicts stained choroid plexus (Bauer et al., 1993, 1995).

exclusively expressed in cerebral endothelial cells. Mfsd2a suppresses transcytosis in endothelial cells and thus the transport of plasma proteins. Interestingly, the protein is expressed in mice at embryonic day 13.5 and its expression depends on the presence of pericytes. In Mfsd2a-knockout mice the BBB is impaired from embryonic day 15.5 to adulthood what led the authors to the conclusion that vascularization and the establishment of a functional BBB are not coinciding. In earlier findings however it has been shown that the BBB becomes functional even before E15 (Bauer et al., 1993, 1995). Microperfusion of E12–E13 mouse embryos with Trypan Blue revealed that the CNS remained void of staining except for the choroid plexus anlage, indicating that at least certain plasma proteins have been excluded (see **Figures 1C,D**). Further, the number of pinocytotic vesicles in endothelial cells of intraneural capillaries decreased from E12 onwards, whereas the number of vesicles in endothelial cells of the perineural domain in the CNS increased (see **Table 1**).

In summary, the formation of a functional BBB, or more precisely, of a neurovascular unit with specific barrier structures and transport functions is a complex, multifactorial process requiring the concerted action and interaction of various cell types including cECs, astrocytes, neuronal and glial cells, as well as pericytes. Finally, although the developmental stage at which a functional BBB is present is still under debate, there is good evidence that a barrier toward large molecules exists very early in embryonic brain development, which then fully matures postnatally.

TIGHT JUNCTION MORPHOLOGY AND FUNCTION

Next to an extensive transport machinery, tight junctions sealing the microvascular endothelium represent the core structure of the BBB. The tight junction (TJ) is the most apical cell-cell junction complex in polarized epithelia and endothelia and can be visualized by ultrathin-section electron microscopy as focal points or "kissing points" where membranes of adjacent cells come into close apposition, completely obliterating the intercellular cleft (Farquhar and Palade, 1963). The application of freeze-fracture electron microscopy provided a more detailed description of TJs. TJs of epithelial cells appear as a complex network of anastomosing and continuous cylindrical strands on the protoplasmic leaflet (P-face) of the plasma membrane, with complementary grooves on the exoplasmic leaflet (E-face), completely encircling the apical aspect of the cell (Chalcroft and Bullivant, 1970; Staehelin, 1973, 1974; Van Deurs and Koehler, 1979). In contrast, depending

Table 1 | Frequency of endothelial fenestrations (f), junctional complexes (j.c.) and pinocytotic vesicles (p.v.) in intraneural and perineural capillaries during murine embryonic development.

Day of embryonic development	Intraneural capillaries			Perineural capillaries		
	f	j.c.	p.v.	f	j.c.	p.v.
E9	No capillaries present			0.9	3.2	2.0
E10	nd	1.7	2.9	0.13	2.9	1.9
E12	nd	2.58	2.33	nd	3.25	3.0
E14	nd	2.29	1.57	nd	2.43	3.29
E17	nd	2.25	1.63	nd	2.75	4.13

Values were determined as follows: number of f, j.c., or p.v. divided by the number of capillaries examined (7–17 capillaries; mean values are shown). n.d., not detected (Bauer et al., 1993).

on the vascular bed investigated, TJ strands of endothelial cells generally display a significantly lower level of P-face association. Whereas endothelial cells of the peripheral vasculature show predominantly E-face associated strands (Simionescu et al., 1976; Muhleisen et al., 1989), freeze fracture replicas of TJs located at the BBB reveal a high degree of P-face association and are among the most complex found in the entire vasculature (Nagy et al., 1984; Liebner et al., 2000b). It seems that not only the complexity of the strand network but also the association of the TJ-strands with the P- or E-face reflects the functional quality (i.e., permeability and electrical resistance) of the barrier (Lippoldt et al., 2000). The varying P-face/E-face ratios possibly are a consequence of altered attachment of the TJ strands to the epithelial or endothelial cytoskeleton, but much detail is still missing.

Next to the establishment and maintenance of a size and charge selective paracellular barrier (Gumbiner, 1987, 1993; Cereijido et al., 1993), TJs also serve to create an intramembrane diffusion barrier ("fence") restricting the intermixing of apical and basolateral components within the exoplasmic leaflet of plasma membranes (Van Meer et al., 1986). In addition, they guide a selective distribution and clustering of membrane components to distinct cell-surfaces (Fanning and Anderson, 1999) and assemble large protein complexes around scaffolding proteins at their cytoplasmic aspect. The modular nature of these adaptor proteins allows the spatial and temporal assembly of multi-protein complexes not only ensuring the structural integrity of the TJ, but also integrating various regulatory pathways which are pivotal for TJ physiology, i.e., establishment of apico-basal polarity, gene expression, and cell proliferation (Gonzalez-Mariscal et al., 2008; Guillemot et al., 2008; Balda and Matter, 2009; McCrea et al., 2009). Finally, the junctional cytoplasmic plaque provides a direct and indirect link to the cytoskeleton.

Generally, much of our understanding of TJ biology stems from studying polarized epithelial cells. However, several aspects of the core structure of endothelial and epithelial TJs are similar and many of the reported findings apply most likely for both cell types. The identification of an ever increasing number of TJ-associated proteins (Gonzalez-Mariscal and Nava, 2005; Wang and Margolis, 2007; Ebnet, 2008; Gonzalez-Mariscal et al., 2008; Giepmans and Van Ijzendoorn, 2009; Steed et al., 2010; Bauer et al., 2011) has led to a wide acceptance of the "protein model", proposing that linear arrays of polymerized transmembrane adhesion molecules form TJ-strands and adhere with strands from apposing plasma membranes (Staehelin, 1973; Tsukita et al., 2001; Furuse, 2010). However, it remains to be unequivocally proven that the high transcellular electrical resistance of epithelia and endothelia can solely be attributed to the molecular interaction of TJ-strands. The involvement of lipid components ("lipid model") cannot be fully ruled out and a "lipid-protein hybrid model" might explain the complexity of TJ physiology (Kan, 1993; Yamagata et al., 2003; Lee et al., 2008; Chen-Quay et al., 2009). But information on the functional and structural relationship of proteins and lipids in the junctional complex remain scarce.

THE BIOGENESIS OF TIGHT JUNCTIONS

Functional TJs not only seal the paracellular space between epithelial and endothelial cells, they are also imperative for the establishment of a polarized, transporting epithelial and endothelial phenotype. The cellular constituents of tissue barriers are polarized, displaying apico-basal polarity through the selective distribution of specific lipid- and protein complexes to distinct sites at the cell surface. Generally, the cells are oriented with their apical aspect of the plasma membrane toward the lumen ("free surface"), whereas the lateral domains are in close contact with neighboring cells and basally adhere to other solid tissues (or parenchyme), only separated by a basement membrane. Epithelial and endothelial cells grown in suspension, or loss of matrix anchorage results in programmed cell death (anoikis), whereas grown on a surface, even single cells polarize. Therefore, the contact to the extracellular matrix, mainly conferred by the family of integrin transmembrane proteins, is crucial to ensure robust cell polarization and morphogenesis *in vivo* (Lee and Streuli, 2014). As soon as an appropriate vectorial transport machinery is in place, epithelia and endothelia are considered fully differentiated, separating tissue and organ compartments and allowing the establishment and maintenance of distinct internal and external milieus.

However, in spite of considerable structural similarities the functional properties of epithelial and endothelial barriers in various tissues and organs can significantly vary. This is largely due to the expression of different transmembrane (i.e., claudins; see further below) and accessory TJ proteins. However, also parameters other than mere structural features need to be taken into account when comparing barriers of various origin and organs. For example, environmental factors (i.e., soluble factors or contacting cells) can influence the barrier properties in developing and mature organs. A beautiful example is the intimate association of cerebral endothelial cells with neuroectoderm-derived accessory cells (astroglia, neurons, and neural precursor cells), which is a unique feature of the BBB and imperative for its physiological functioning. These cells not only contribute physically to the barrier but also induce barrier properties in differentiating cerebral endothelial cells (Bauer and Bauer, 2000; Abbott, 2002; Haseloff et al., 2005; Abbott et al., 2006; Weidenfeller et al., 2007).

Most of our knowledge about tissue barrier formation stems from studies on epithelial and endothelial cells *in vitro* (Gonzalez-Mariscal et al., 1985; Stevenson et al., 1988; Bauer et al., 2011; Watson et al., 2013; Czupalla et al., 2014; Wilhelm and Krizbai, 2014). In this respect, particularly the re-establishment of TJs following calcium depletion and the concomitant breakdown of cell-cell contacts has been investigated (Gonzalez-Mariscal et al., 1990; Contreras et al., 1992; Stuart et al., 1994). Much of our understanding of TJ formation in primary (and secondary) epithelia also comes from studying embryogenesis of *D. melanogaster* (cellularization) and *C. elegans* (Knust and Bossinger, 2002; St Johnston and Ahringer, 2010). Mammalian TJ biogenesis has mainly been described in cultured preimplantation mouse embryos, which serve as a valuable model to determine the expression of junctional proteins during the earliest steps of cell lineage differentiation. Cultured preimplantation mouse embryos can easily be manipulated to precisely determine the role of junction-related proteins at early developmental stages such as compaction and cavitation (formation of the blastocoel) (Dard et al., 2008; Eckert and Fleming, 2008). Early signs of junction establishment appear during formation of tubular structures or cavities, a process which is fundamental to organ development in both vertebrates and invertebrates. From a range of investigations describing the epithelial and endothelial tubular biogenesis, three major morphologic mechanisms are being proposed, commonly referred to as *cell hollowing*, *cord hollowing*, and *cavitation*. In all of them, tubes or cavities arise from lumenless, unpolarized cell aggregates or single unpolarized cells. While cell and cord hollowing are common in vascular structures, cavitation is rather attributed to epithelial tubulogenesis and is only scarcely observed in endothelial vessel formation (Lubarsky and Krasnow, 2003). Cavitation has extensively been described in the preimplantation mouse embryo and coincides with the first occurrence of a differentiated epithelium in the mammalian embryo (Eckert and Fleming, 2008). The undifferentiated mammalian blastomeres are subjected to three rounds of cleavage, resulting in the formation of the eight-cell embryo, also referred to as the "early morula" stage. Subsequently, compaction of the embryo is initiated, representing the moment of establishment of an epithelial phenotype and the generation of an apical-basal axis. This asymmetric cellular organization is then coupled with a specific orientation of the mitotic spindle during cell division, resulting in asymmetric division of the blastomeres giving rise to two different cell populations. The inner, non-polarized blastomeres form the inner cell mass (ICM) of the blastocyst, and the outer polarized blastomeres giving rise to the first polarized epithelium, the trophectoderm (TE) which develops into the chorioallantoic placenta later during development. The ICM then develops into the epiblast, the origin of all tissues of the embryo proper, and the primitive endoderm which gives rise to the extra-embryonic membranes. A more detailed description on embryonic axis establishment and blastocyst lineage formation is beyond the scope of this review and the reader is referred to a series of excellent reviews (Larue et al., 1994; Arnold and Robertson, 2009; Rossant and Tam, 2009; Morris and Zernicka-Goetz, 2012; Takaoka and Hamada, 2012).

Overall, premature intercellular contacts serve as an initial spatial cue for the establishment of polarity not only in blastomeres but also in cells in general. Early studies then identified E-cadherin as the prime epithelial signature marker. During compaction of the early mouse embryo, diffusely localized E-cadherin becomes redistributed to long filopodia protruding from the blastomeres which facilitate the attachment of two neighboring cells via homophilic binding of opposing E-cadherin clusters (Fierro-Gonzalez et al., 2013). Interestingly, mouse embryos deficient in E-cadherin fail to form a proper trophectoderm and die around the time of implantation, compaction not being affected. This late phenotype is explained by the presence of a residual maternal E-cadherin pool, which is sufficient to drive compaction (Larue et al., 1994). Next to E-cadherin, the homophilic binding of nectin family members at developing adhesive structures takes place very early during the establishment of the polarized epithelial phenotype (Sato et al., 2006; Takai et al., 2008b). Nectins constitute a family of single-pass, calcium-independent transmembrane adhesive molecules which, together with clusters of cadherins form mature adherens junctions (Indra et al., 2013). During the early phases of polarization it is believed that nectin controls the initiation of cadherin clustering by preventing the endocytotic removal of cadherin (Takai et al., 2008a). The majority of nectin function is conferred via its association with the cytoplasmic protein afadin, which allows cross-talk with other junctional complexes. Afadin not only functionally couples the E-cadherin and nectin complex (Tachibana et al., 2000), but also directly interacts with the TJ-associated protein JAM-A, thereby influencing tight junction assembly during further progression of the polarity program (Fukuhara et al., 2002). JAM-A assembles at the cell membranes of the early 8-cell mouse embryo prior to compaction and unlike any other TJ constituent its recruitment to the cell-cell contact initiation sites is independent of cadherin-mediated adhesion (Thomas et al., 2004). Therefore, JAM-A recruitment occurs substantially ahead of other TJ transmembrane proteins, with occludin and claudin assembly taking place from the late morula stage onwards (Thomas et al., 2004; Eckert and Fleming, 2008). Importantly, only compact embryos treated with an E-cadherin neutralizing antibody disassemble rapidly, whereas inactivation of JAM-A does not perturb compaction and only results in a delayed cavitation of the embryo (Thomas et al., 2004). This result underscores the importance of cadherin-based cell-cell adhesion during compaction and indicates that JAM-A cell surface expression does not contribute to the initiation of cell adhesion *per se* within the embryo.

CELL POLARIZATION—A KEY STEP TOWARD BARRIER FORMATION

The establishment of mutually exclusive cortical domains in epithelia and endothelia in part relies on the asymmetric distribution of a set of evolutionary conserved biochemical factors controlling cell polarity. Genetic studies in *C. elegans* and *D. melanogaster* have identified three polarity groups, the Crb, Par, and Scrib groups, with the members of each group having interdependent and partly antagonistic functions. Although the majority of our understanding of the complex polarity signaling pathways in mammals is based on studies carried out in 2D and 3D cultured epithelial cells more recent studies indicate that the same set of proteins is critical for endothelial polarity (Lizama and Zovein, 2013). The Par complex is located sub-apically in epithelial cells and assembles around Par-6 isoforms (Macara, 2004). Par6 binds atypical protein kinase C (aPKC) λ/ι or ξ and selectively engages GTP-bound Cdc42 (Joberty et al., 2000; Johansson et al., 2000; Lin et al., 2000), which stimulates the activity of Par6-associated aPKC several-fold, potentially through a conformational rearrangement of the complex. The Par6/aPKC complex appears to be a general determinant of polarity, which undergoes cell-specific interactions with other polarity proteins. Members of the Par-complex act in synergy with the Crumbs/Pals/Patj group of proteins to define the apical cell surface (Hurd et al., 2003; Ebnet et al., 2008). As Jam-A (and all other isoforms; see further below) directly interacts with Par3, it most likely serves as a spatial landmark to tether the Par3/Par6/aPKC polarity complex to the primordial junction. The expression of the Par6/aPKC complex has been confirmed in brain endothelial cells (Daneman et al., 2010a) and it has also been shown to be important for the establishment of endothelial polarity and lumen formation in general (Zovein et al., 2010). Genetic deletion of β1-integrin results in decreased Par3 expression, leading to a loss of endothelial polarity (Osada et al., 2011). More recently, it has been shown that the non-canonical Wnt/planar cell polarity (PCP) pathway contributes to TJ integrity of hCMEC/D3 cell *in vitro*, suggesting that this pathway might act as a key regulator of the BBB *in vivo* (Artus et al., 2014). However, similarly to what has been reported for epithelial cells (Chen and Macara, 2005; Qin et al., 2005) the knock-down of Par3 only delays but does not fully inhibit TJ formation in brain endothelial cells.

The Crumbs group (Crb) localizes apically or at apical junctions and consists of the transmembrane Crb proteins and the large scaffolding proteins Pals1 and Patj through which the complex physically is connected to the Par group via Par6 (Bilder et al., 2003; Hurd et al., 2003; Assemat et al., 2008; Tepass, 2012). In ECs tight junction integrity is also maintained by angiomotin and angiomotin-like proteins (Amot, AmotL1), in part through the action of the associated RhoGEF Syx and loss of any of these proteins results in increased vascular permeability and/or reduced sprouting angiogenesis (Garnaas et al., 2008; Zheng et al., 2009; Ngok et al., 2012).

The basolateral region of epithelial cells is specified by a group of tumor suppressor genes, the Scrib complex. These include Scribble, which encodes a LAP protein (with leucine-rich repeats and four PDZ domains), Dlg, a MAGUK protein, and Lgl, comprised of WD40 repeats (Yamanaka and Ohno, 2008). Scrib, Dlg and Lgl are membrane-associated adaptors implicated in cytoskeletal organization and protein trafficking and potentially in coupling tissue architecture to withdrawal from the cell cycle. Although little is known about Scribble in endothelial cells, a recent study provides evidence that loss of Scrib does exhibit vascular hemorrhaging suggestive of defective permeability barriers and a likely role in endothelial cell tube formation and angiogenesis (Michaelis et al., 2013). In breast cancer epithelia Scribble has been demonstrated to interact with TAZ, a member of the Hippo signaling pathway (Cordenonsi et al., 2011). Interestingly, knock-down of angiomotin-like 2 (amotL2), another member of the hippo cascade with ties to the Crb-polarity complex, results in decreased tubulogenesis *in vitro* (Wang et al., 2011). Therefore, it is tempting to speculate that the opposing functions of Crumbs/Amot and Scribble polarity complexes also antagonistically impact upon the Hippo pathway to regulate endothelial polarity and lumen formation.

One of the essential polarity regulators from yeast to man is the RhoGTPase Cdc42. In epithelial cells PTEN-mediated segregation of phosphoinositides has been shown to initiate polarization by recruiting Cdc42 to apical domains (Martin-Belmonte et al., 2007). Further, the small GTPase Rac1 has been shown to play an important role downstream of the Par complex (Iden and Collard, 2008). Independent of their polarity actions the best studied function of Rho GTPases is their role als molecular organizers of the actin cytoskeleton. These two processes are interconnected as cell polarization and the establishment of a functional TJ also entails a complex rearrangement of the actin cytoskeleton, microtubule organizing centers, and the establishment of a vesicle trafficking machinery, all together facilitating vectorial transport functions (Rodriguez-Boulan and Macara, 2014).

After establishment of cell polarity additional junctional proteins are being sequentially delivered to the site of the adhesion structure resulting in the maturation of the adherens junction (AJ) and TJ (Eckert and Fleming, 2008). Initially, during compaction an immature junction, containing AJ and TJ constituents, is formed serving as an initial landmark which is required for proper cell polarization. Next to cadherin-catenin components, the TJ-related proteins ZO-1 (the shorter ZO-1α-isoform) and JAM-A localize to the immature junction. In addition, the rab GTPase rab13 relocates early to the apico-lateral contact site (Sheth et al., 2000). During the following 16-cell stage the TJ proteins ZO-2 (Sheth et al., 2008) and cingulin (Javed et al., 1993) enter the stage of junctional biogenesis and subsequently the transmembrane proteins occludin and claudin-1 and -3 are targeted to the junction. Concomitantly the segregation into an apical tight junction and an adherens junction located more basally takes place (Rajasekaran et al., 1996; Sheth et al., 2000). Interestingly, although the formation of tight junctions and cell polarity are intimately related, *in vitro* the Par protein- and Scribble-complex have minor effects on TJ establishment in epithelial cells. The knock-down of either protein only delays but does not inhibit TJ formation (Chen and Macara, 2005; Qin et al., 2005). In contrast, perturbation of the Crbs/Pals1/Patj complex results in persistent TJ defects (Fogg et al., 2005; Shin et al., 2005; Wang et al., 2007). As the junction further matures, together with a complex rearrangement of the cytoskeleton and the establishment of a vectorial transport system, a permeability seal is formed which is the prerequisite for the formation of the nascent blastocoel cavity.

Similar to epithelial differentiation, blood vessel formation relies on cell-cell contact and apical-basal polarization of endothelial cells prior to lumen formation and junctional maturation. As already mentioned above, various models have been proposed to explain vascular lumenization, including the intracellular vacuole coalescence model (*cell hollowing*), or extracellular vacuole exocytosis and lumenal repulsion model (*cord hollowing*) (Iruela-Arispe and Davis, 2009; Zeeb et al., 2010; Axnick and Lammert, 2012). While cell hollowing involves the generation and fusion of intracellular vacuoles of individual cells, cord hollowing is based on lumen formation between two or more ECs (or an EC cord) (Lubarsky and Krasnow, 2003; Blum et al., 2008; Chung and Andrew, 2008; Lee and Bautch, 2011). Both types of lumen formation make use of a similar set of proteins and pathways and distinguishing them from each other *in vivo* is a difficult task. Generally, lumina of small capillaries (maximum diameter of a single cell) are formed by cell hollowing while lumenization of larger vessels follows the process of cord hollowing. However, using a computational model of lumen formation it was recently suggested that cell hollowing and cord hollowing may operate in parallel (Boas and Merks, 2014).

The initial phase of cord hollowing is characterized by cell-cell adhesion, exocytosis and apical membrane repulsion (see **Figure 2**). Initial intercellular contacts are established by homotypic interaction of VE-cadherin and Pecam-1/CD31 which are distributed along the entire contacting plasma membrane. Additionally, the uniform distribution of the polarity proteins Par3 in contacting ECs is indicative of a yet unpolarized state of the cells. Besides VE-cadherin also N-cadherin was found at EC contact sites, which is believed to increase the amount of VE-cadherin at cell-cell contacts (Luo and Radice, 2005). Subsequently, de-adhesive glycoproteins (CD34-sialomucins) are delivered from cytoplasmic vesicles to the contacting plasma membrane delineating the future apical surface. The specific targeting of CD34-sialomucins to EC contact sites depends on VE-cadherin and involves PTEN signaling together with PIP2/PIP3 conversion (Zeeb et al., 2010). It is believed that the negatively

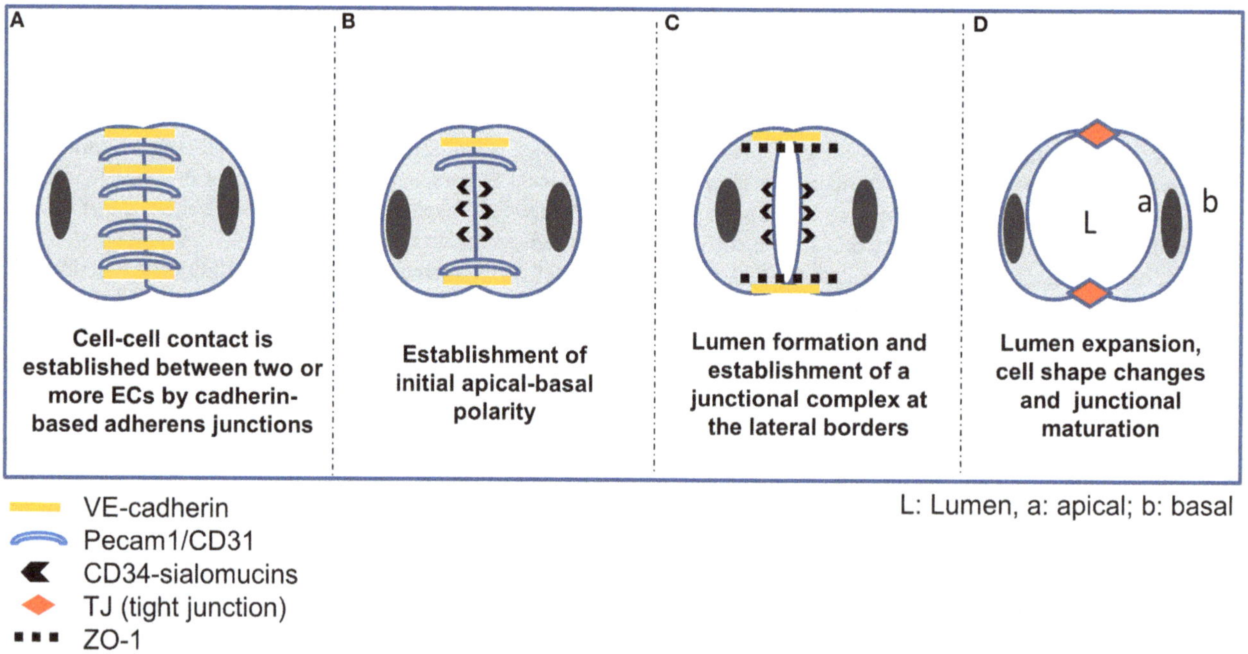

FIGURE 2 | Vascular lumen formation by cord hollowing. (A) Intercellular adhesion of two or more ECs is accomplished by homophilic interaction of VE-cadherin and Pecam-1. **(B)** Following establishment of Par3-mediated apicobasal polarity via ß-1 integrin matrix interaction and the adaptor protein RASIP1, CD34-sialomucins (CD34 and podocalyxin; PODXL) are recruited to cell-cell contacts delineating the future apical border. VE-cadherin is required for specifically targeting CD34-sialomucins to contact sites, and the delivery depends on PTEN-mediated transformation of PIP3 to PIP2. Rasip1 localizes at inter-endothelial junctions and acts downstream of Rap1 (Ras-related protein1), mediating EC-ECM adhesion and stabilizing junctional integrity by actin bundling. In cooperation with Radil (ras-association and dilute domain-containing protein), Rasip1 further inhibits Rho-mediated stress fiber formation, thereby increasing endothelial barrier function. Further, CCM1 mediates the stabilization of β-catenin-containing endothelial cell-cell junctions downstream of the Rap1 GTPase. **(C)** Due to the negatively charged CD34-sialomucins, electrostatic repulsion leads to separation of the contacting plasma membranes thereby creating a free (non-contacting) surface and a small lumen between ECs. Concomitantly, cadherin-based AJs are redistributed to lateral borders, indicating the establishment of a lateral junctional complex. Following phosphorylation by protein kinase C, pMoesin, the major ERM protein in endothelial cells, is recruited to the future apical membrane and links CD34-sialomucins to F-actin, supporting cytoskeletal rearrangements in ECs during lumen expansion. Further, non-muscle myosin assembles at the apical plasma membrane and interacts with F-actin in response to VEGF signaling to support lumen expansion and cell shape changes. **(D)** Further maturation of the endothelial TJs is then mediated by claudin-5, occludin, members of the junctional adhesion molecule (JAM) family, or by EC-selective adhesion molecule (ESAM).

charged extracellular domains of CD34 sialomucins initiate the repulsion of opposing leaflets creating a narrow space between the cells, commonly referred to as "slit formation" (Robbins and Beitel, 2010; Strilic et al., 2010). One of the CD34-related sialomucins is podocalyxin (PODXL). Originally, PODXL has been described as the major sialoprotein in the glycocalyx of glomerular podocytes (Kerjaschki et al., 1986). However, it has been recognized early that PODXL is a widespread component of vascular endothelial cells (Born and Palinski, 1985; Horvat et al., 1986). It localizes to the luminal domain of endothelial plasma membranes in a patchy distribution and is absent from the abluminal aspect (Horvat et al., 1986). Although the function of endothelial sialoproteins has long remained elusive, a role in regulating the thrombogenic properties of the endothelial surface was proposed (Gorog et al., 1982; Born and Palinski, 1985). More recently it has been shown that PODXL (syn. gp135) is a key regulator of apical domain structure establishment in epithelial cells (Meder et al., 2005) and it recruits filamentous actin and ezrin to the plasma membrane, inducing microvillus formation (Nielsen et al., 2007). Interestingly, embryoid bodies lacking ZO-1 or ZO-1/ZO-2 (but not ZO-2 alone) exhibit reduced expression of PODXL at the apical plasma membrane and lack TJs in the extraembryonic endoderm (Phua et al., 2014). Further, quantitative PCR profiling of RNA samples from laser capture microdissected microvessels revealed that PODXL is preferably expressed in brain microvessels (Agarwal et al., 2010) suggesting a role in BBB establishment and/or function.

CD34-sialomucins are further linked to the actin cytoskeleton via protein kinase C- (PKC) phosphorylated moesin, thereby contributing to cell shape changes during lumenization (Strilic et al., 2009). Lumen extension then depends on cytoskeletal rearrangements involving non-muscle myosin and recruitment thereof to the apical F-actin is accomplished by activation of the Rho-associated protein kinase (ROCK) and VEGF-A signaling (reviewed in Lee and Bautch, 2011). Finally, the assembly of CD34-sialomucins at the future apical membrane triggers the redistribution of junctional proteins to the lateral border, constituting the initial step in the formation of a lateral junctional complex.

Disturbance of endothelial polarization is observed in cerebral cavernous malformations (CCM), the most common vascular dysplasia in the brain, which is characterized by hemorrhagic stroke, focal neurological deficits and seizures (reviewed in Draheim et al., 2014). CCM1 binds to and is regulated by the small GTPase Rap1, enhancing the adhesive properties of VE-cadherin (Glading et al., 2007). The CCM1 FERM domain is unmasked by the activated Rap1, targeting CCM1 to the junction and promoting endothelial polarization in a Par-dependent manner (Lampugnani et al., 2010) (see **Figure 3**). In the absence of CCM1, endothelial lumenization is severely disturbed, as evidenced by grossly dilated capillaries and multicavernous structures (Clatterbuck et al., 2001). Endothelial-specific disruption of the CCM1 gene in mice induces endothelial to mesenchymal transition due to increased BMP6–SMAD signaling, a process which is characterized by the loss of cell polarity, increased cell proliferation and migratory capacity (Maddaluno et al., 2013). Although CCM genes are inactivated in all types of endothelial cells under pathological conditions, CCM lesions are mostly apparent in the brain vasculature. Therefore, the loss of endothelial polarity and the concomitant impaired astroglia-endothelial interaction, which is imperative for BBB function, seems to be the underlying cause of frequent vascular lesions in the brain (Maddaluno et al., 2013). This and other studies elegantly demonstrate that cell-cell adhesion and apical-basal polarization appears to be a universal event preceding epithelial and endothelial tubulogenesis, a mechanism imperative for organ development and vascularization.

Results from numerous studies on various developmental models converge on a crucial role for apical membrane specialization prior to junctional maturation. The establishment of a cadherin-based primordial junctional complex prior to segregation of a more apically located TJ appears to be a conserved step in epithelial and endothelial differentiation. Besides the indispensability of cadherin-based cell-cell contacts, the early and bi-phasic role of ZO-1 isoforms appears to be crucial for endothelial and epithelial barrier formation. Following *de novo* establishment of tight junctions, a dizzying number of proteins localize to the cytoplasmic aspect of TJ not only ensuring the integrity of the barrier but also allowing a remodeling and change in permeability properties in response to physiological and pathological stimuli. Of the known TJ constituents, the *zonula occludens* (ZO) proteins lie at the heart of the TJ cytoplasmic plaque. Below, the major tight junction proteins are being discussed, focusing on proteins that have been shown to localize to endothelial TJs.

TIGHT JUNCTION PROTEINS

MEMBRANE-SPANNING TJ CONSTITUENTS

Overall, 3 distinct TJ-associated transmembrane protein groups can be distinguished (see **Figure 4B**): (1) claudins, a family of proteins comprising at least 27 different members in mammals (Mineta et al., 2011); (2) TAMPs (TJ-associated MARVEL proteins)—a group of proteins containing the structural tetraspanning MARVEL motif, including occludin (Furuse et al., 1993), tricellulin (Ikenouchi et al., 2005), and MarvelD3 (Steed et al., 2009); (3) Immunoglobulin superfamily membrane proteins JAM-A/-B/-C (Martin-Padura et al., 1998; Aurrand-Lions et al., 2000; Palmeri et al., 2000; Ebnet et al., 2003), coxsackie adenovirus receptor (CAR) (Carson et al., 1999; Cohen et al., 2001), and endothelial cell-selective adhesion molecule (ESAM) (Nasdala et al., 2002).

Occludin was the first integral membrane protein shown to localize to TJs (Furuse et al., 1993) and is characterized by four transmembrane domains, a short intracellular turn, two extracellular loops, and a long carboxy- and a short amino-terminal cytoplasmic domain. Cis-oligomerization of occludin seems to be mediated by the MARVEL motif (Blasig et al., 2006; Yaffe et al., 2012), whereas the extracellular loops are believed to contribute to the gate-keeping function of TJs. The last 150 aa of the carboxyl terminus of occludin interact directly with F-actin (Wittchen et al., 1999) and the scaffold proteins ZO-1 (Furuse et al., 1994), ZO-2 (Itoh et al., 1999b), and ZO-3 (Haskins et al., 1998). Information regarding the physiological relevance of the N-terminal domain remains scarce. Using a yeast-based two-hybrid screen the E3 ubiquitin protein ligase Itch was found to directly

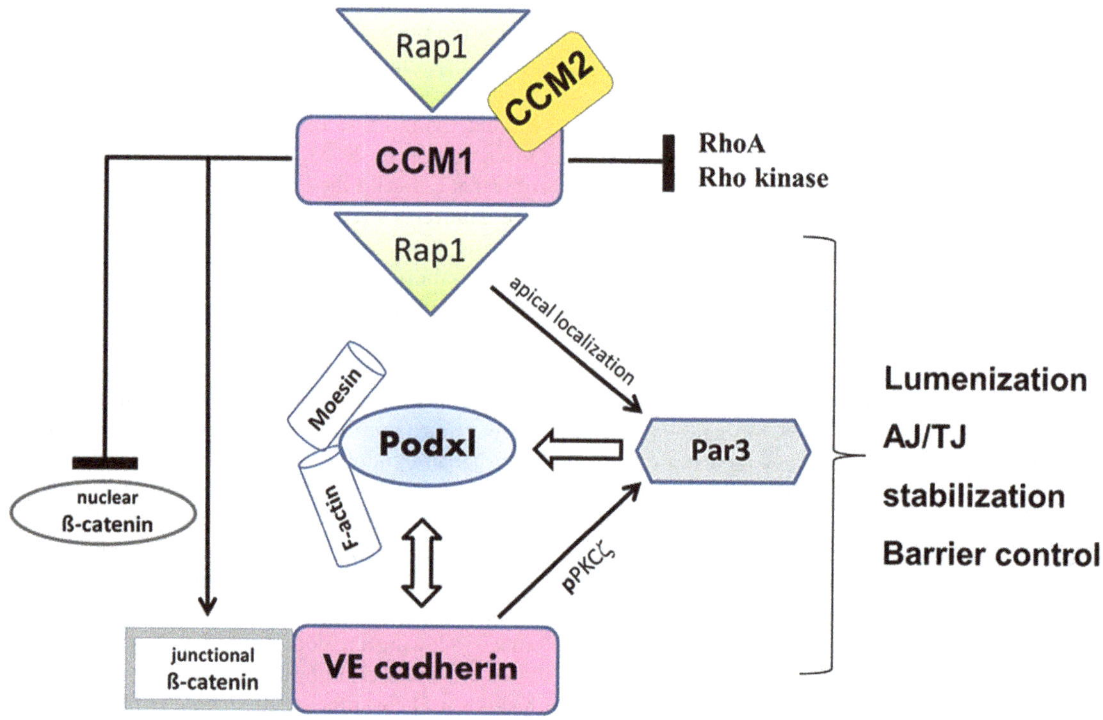

FIGURE 3 | VE-cadherin and CCM1 act in concert to establish endothelial polarization and lumen formation. Rap1 regulates the junctional localization of CCM1 and mediates CCM1 activity in endothelial polarization and lumen formation. CCM1 stabilizes VE-cadherin at AJs, by associating with ß-catenin and inhibiting dissociation of ß-catenin from AJs. Thereby, nuclear accumulation of ß-catenin and ß-catenin transcriptional signaling is impaired. VE-cadherin promotes the apical localization and activation of the Par3 polarity complex. While VE-cadherin is needed for phosphorylation of PKCξ, CCM1/Rap1 is responsible for the junctional recruitment of the polarity complex. The accumulation of podocalyxin (PODXL) at the presumptive apical membrane is controlled by VE-cadherin and ß1 integrin. PODXL in turn recruits moesin and filamentous actin (F-actin) to the apical domain initiating endothelial lumen formation.

interact with the outermost NH_2-terminal domain of occludin (Traweger et al., 2002). Indeed, following VEGF-induced phosphorylation occludin is targeted for proteasomal degradation via Itch, resulting in increased endothelial permeability (Murakami et al., 2009). Occludin is targeted by several kinases and is phosphorylated on serine, threonine (Sakakibara et al., 1997; Wong, 1997), and tyrosine residues (Tsukamoto and Nigam, 1999; Chen et al., 2002) and reversible phosphorylation is an important regulatory mechanism to control TJ assembly and maintenance. For example, endothelial cells subjected to shear stress showed a significantly reduced, but tyrosine-phosphorylated pool of occludin (DeMaio et al., 2001). However, controversial results on the role of occludin phosphorylation in epithelial and endothelial cells exist.

Early investigations led to the assumption that occludin is the core transmembrane protein of TJs (Furuse et al., 1996; McCarthy et al., 1996). However, the TJ scientific community was stunned to learn that occludin is dispensable for the formation of tight junction strands. Occludin-deficient ES cells were found to be morphologically indistinguishable from their wild type counterparts (Saitou et al., 1998) and occludin-deficient mouse embryos were viable and did not show any gross morphological alterations of TJs (Saitou et al., 2000). However, phenotypically *ocln-/-* animals displayed multiple histological abnormalities, including chronic inflammation and hyperplasia of the gastric epithelium, calcification of the brain, cortical bone thinning, and testicular atrophy. Subsequent analysis of the knockout animals suggested occludin may play a role in epithelial differentiation and proliferation (Schulzke et al., 2005). In man, mutations of the occludin gene cause band-like calcification with simplified gyration and polymicrogyria (BLC-PMG), a rare neurological disorder resulting in malformations of cortical development, implicating a role of occludin for TJs at the BBB (O'Driscoll et al., 2010). Most likely, other proteins of the TAMP family (i.e., tricellulin or MarvelD3) act redundantly partially masking the function of occludin. In summary, although occludin clearly is not of fundamental importance for the core TJ structure the findings outlined above suggest that it has a regulatory and accessory function in TJ formation and physiology.

After having realized that occludin is not the major TJ-strand protein, the search for a new protein began. Furuse and Tsukita identified small proteins that co-fractionated with occludin in a junction-enriched chicken liver fraction (Furuse et al., 1998). Since the initial discovery of these small proteins, termed claudin-1 and claudin-2, a total of 27 different *claudin* family members have been identified in man and mouse (Mineta et al., 2011). Although the predicted protein folding topology of claudins (21–28 kD) is very similar to that of occludin, they do

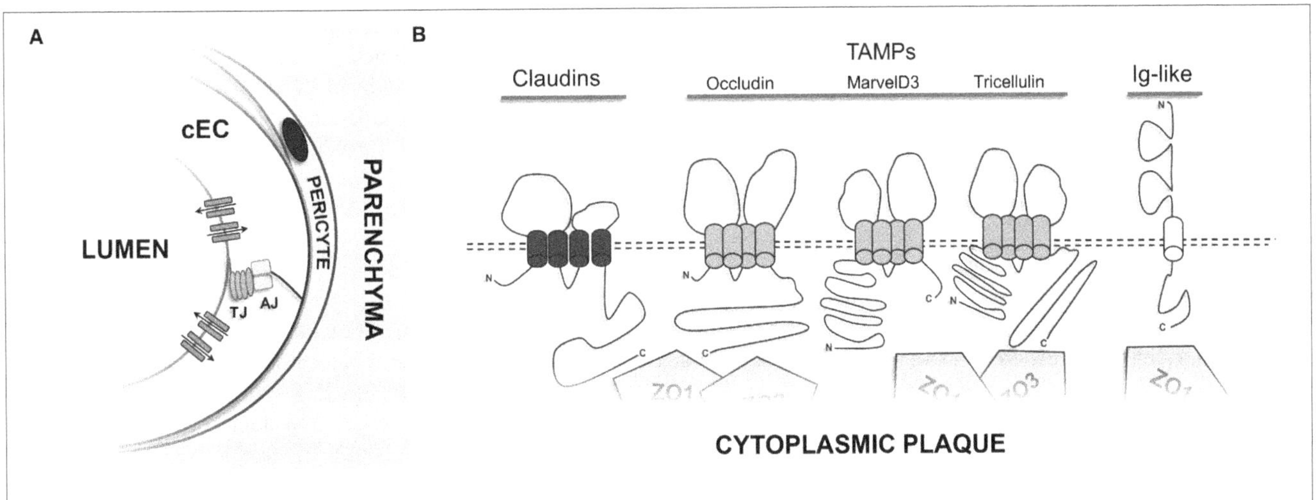

FIGURE 4 | Transmembrane proteins of the TJ. (A) Cerebral endothelial cells constitute the cellular building block of the BBB and control the para- and transcellular routes via elaborate influx and efflux transporters and cell-cell adhesion structures. Astroglial endfeet, neurons, and microglia which are present at the neurovascular unit have been omitted for clarity. **(B)** Schematic membrane-spanning models of the transmembrane components present at TJs.

not share any sequence homology (Furuse et al., 1998). Several gain-of-function and loss-of-function studies have led to the current model that claudins are the prime transmembrane proteins responsible for the formation of higher-order tight junction strands. For example, claudin-1 deficient mice die shortly after birth due to excessive transepidermal water loss (Furuse et al., 2002) and claudin-11 knockout animals show a complete loss of TJs in Sertoli cells, oligodendrocytes, and the marginal cells of the inner ear (Gow et al., 1999, 2004; Mazaud-Guittot et al., 2010).

It is believed that claudins and TAMPs oligomerize in a homo- and heterophilic fashion and TJ-strands are formed by mosaics of different claudin-family members and the combination and stoichiometry of various isoforms determines the charge- and size-selective properties of the barrier (Sonoda et al., 1999; Anderson and Van Itallie, 2009). Further, claudins show a tissue-specific expression pattern, contributing to tissue specific barrier properties. Therefore, for each tissue a unique combination of claudins which oligomerize with other TAMPS most likely determines the paracellular tightness of the junction toward different solutes.

Overall, claudins-1, -3, -5, -11, -14, -19 appear to be sealing components of tight junctions and for several of them human mutations have been characterized. Mutations in claudin-1 cause the neonatal ichtyosis and sclerosing cholangitis (NISCH) syndrome. Claudin-14 mutations are the underlying cause of autosomal recessive deafness 29 and 49 and mutations in claudin-19 cause renal hypomagnesemia with ocular involvement. Next to acting as "sealants" claudins have been proposed to form paracellular ion-selective channels (Amasheh et al., 2002) and so far claudin-2, -10a, -10b, -15, and -17 have been shown to have channel-forming properties. Whereas claudins-2, 10b, and 15 display cation selectivity, -10a and 17 have been described as anion-selective channels (reviewed in Gunzel and Fromm, 2012).

At the BBB, mainly claudin-3 (Wolburg et al., 2003) and claudin-5 (Morita et al., 1999) are being expressed, claudin-12 likely also being part of the BBB-TJ (Ohtsuki et al., 2007; Schrade et al., 2012). Early studies also have demonstrated the presence of claudin-1 at brain capillary endothelial cells (Liebner et al., 2000a), however this was a false report due to antibody cross-reactivity with claudin-3. Subsequent studies using claudin-1 specific antibodies failed to detect any claudin-1 in CNS parenchymal microvessels and/or in primary mouse or human brain endothelial cells (Wolburg et al., 2003; Hamm et al., 2004; Coisne et al., 2005; Weksler et al., 2005).

Of those having been described so far, claudin-5 is the most abundant isoform at the BBB as also shown by a SAGE analysis of rat brain microvasculature (Enerson and Drewes, 2006). It is crucial for the "tightness" of TJs at the mammalian BBB as its deletion resulted in a size-selective opening of the BBB *in vivo*, allowing the diffusion of molecules smaller than 800 Da (Nitta et al., 2003). Interestingly, the TJs of the BBB were morphologically normal, nevertheless the knockout of claudin-5 resulted in early neonatal death. This study also shows that the increase in paracellular flux is tolerated during embryogenesis, potentially due to the presence of the placental barrier. This indicates that the BBB in the mouse embryo is "immature," even though it already restricts the flux of blood-borne products into the neuroparenchyma (see **Figures 1C,D**).

Additional data establishes the key role of claudin-5 and claudin-3 in TJ integrity at the BBB. For example, overexpression of claudin-5 increases the paracellular tightness in cultured brain microvascular endothelial cells (Ohtsuki et al., 2007) and the selective loss of claudin-3 in experimental autoimmune encephalomyelitis or human glioblastoma multiforme is associated with BBB breakdown, suggesting that it also contributes to BBB integrity and function (Wolburg et al., 2003). Interestingly, a specific role of claudin-3 at the BBB is also underscored by the observation that its expression correlates with the maturation of the BBB in response to Wnt/β-catenin signaling during development (Liebner et al., 2008). However, the exact role of claudin-3 at the BBB remains to be seen.

The greatest sequence diversity of claudins is located in the C-terminal domain, suggesting that their diverse functions are in part conferred by their association with cytoplasmic proteins.

Generally, the last C-terminal amino acids constitute a PDZ binding motif resulting in the recruitment of the TJ-plaque proteins ZO-1, ZO-2, ZO-3 (Itoh et al., 1999a), which seem to instruct claudins to form functional TJ strands (Umeda et al., 2006). Similarly to occludin, claudins are also phosphorylated on serine or threonine residues, regulating their function and intracellular localization (Ishizaki et al., 2003; D'Souza et al., 2005; Ikari et al., 2006; Aono and Hirai, 2008).

Next to bicellular contacts, the formation of specialized tricellular contacts is required to maintain the integrity of cellular sheets. At these contacts a specialized TJ structure (tTJs) is formed where three sealing elements are in close apposition and form a narrow tube in the intercellular cleft (Friend and Gilula, 1972; Staehelin, 1973; Ikenouchi et al., 2005). Specialized transmembrane proteins, tricellulin and proteins of the angulin family are located at these contacts and recently have been identified in endothelial cells of the brain and retina (Mariano et al., 2013; Iwamoto et al., 2014). Tricellulin shares some sequence similarity with occludin and depending on the cell type can also be found at bicellular contacts where it possibly acts as a substitute for occludin (Ikenouchi et al., 2005; Krug et al., 2009). Taken together, TJ-associated MARVEL proteins are able to partially exert redundant functions, but also show tissue-specific expression and are involved in distinct aspects of tight junction assembly, maintenance, and regulation (Raleigh et al., 2010).

So far, the last class of transmembrane proteins found to localize to the TJ are members of the immunoglobulin superfamily. *Junction adhesion molecules* or more precisely the first isoform JAM-A was identified by using monoclonal antibodies raised against endothelial antigens (Martin-Padura et al., 1998). They form homotypic cell-cell contacts between endothelial and epithelial cells and are highly enriched at TJs (Bazzoni et al., 2000a; Liu et al., 2000). JAMs are generally glycosilated and encompass two extracellular variable type Ig domains and a single transmembrane domain. Through a classical type II PDZ binding motif located in its outermost C-terminus JAM-A interacts with several cytoplasmic proteins, aiding in the establishment of the cytoplasmic plaque of TJs (Bazzoni et al., 2000b; Ebnet et al., 2000; Martinez-Estrada et al., 2001; Hamazaki et al., 2002). Interestingly, JAM-/- mice show little alterations of the overall epithelial architecture in the intestinal tract, but display increased colonic inflammation and paracellular permeability (Laukoetter et al., 2007). Next to JAM-A, the closely related proteins JAM-B (JAM2) and JAM-C (JAM3) have been cloned and characterized (Aurrand-Lions et al., 2000; Cunningham et al., 2000; Palmeri et al., 2000; Arrate et al., 2001; Aurrand-Lions et al., 2001). In contrast to JAM-A, JAM-B/-C seem restricted to endothelial cells and have been demonstrated to form heterodimers in cell-cell contacts, thereby counteracting the interaction with the leukocyte receptor alpha(M)beta2 integrin (Cunningham et al., 2002; Lamagna et al., 2005). In humans, homozygous mutations of JAM-C result in intracerebral hemorrhages, subependymal calcification, and congenital cataracts (Mochida et al., 2010). However, overall little is known about their exact role at the BBB.

Strikingly, among all TJ-associated transmembrane proteins only JAM-A/-B/-C interact directly with the cell polarity protein Par3 (Ebnet et al., 2001, 2003; Itoh et al., 2001). JAMs localize to sites of early cell-cell contact formation, so called puncta or primordial spot-like junctions, where they most likely "flag" this region for the recruitment of the Par3/Par6/aPKC polarity complex during early junctional biogenesis in epithelial and endothelial cells (see also further above). Next to their involvement in cell-cell adhesion JAMs also mediate the transendothelial migration of leukocytes which is of particular importance for BBB function (Fraemohs et al., 2004; Aurrand-Lions et al., 2005).

Four additional Ig-superfamily protein members have been found to localize to TJs: CAR—coxsackie- and adenovirus receptor (Cohen et al., 2001; Raschperger et al., 2006), CLMP-coxsackie- and adenovirus receptor-like membrane protein (Raschperger et al., 2004), JAM 4 (Hirabayashi et al., 2003), and ESAM—endothelial cell-selective adhesion molecule (Hirata et al., 2001; Nasdala et al., 2002). Of these, ESAM seems to be the only endothelial-specific transmembrane protein. ESAM-/- mice did not show any major vascular defects, however endothelial tube formation was impaired suggesting a role of ESAM in cell-cell contact formation (Ishida et al., 2003). More recently, ESAM was also suggested to support the extravasation of neutrophils during the early phase of an inflammatory response (Wegmann et al., 2006).

Taken together, transmembrane proteins of the TJ not only facilitate cell-cell adhesion and impede paracellular flux, they also target cytoplasmic protein assemblies to distinct cell membrane domains, endowing endothelial and epithelial cells with their critical biological properties.

TJ CYTOPLASMIC PLAQUE PROTEINS

The most prominent subgroup of scaffolding proteins localizing to tight junctions is represented by the MAGUK (membrane-associated guanylate kinase) proteins (Dimitratos et al., 1999; Gonzalez-Mariscal et al., 2000; Funke et al., 2005). The modular nature of MAGUK proteins was early recognized as they all share a common structural core consisting of one or several PDZ domains and an SH3 domain followed by a catalytically inactive guanylate kinase (GUK) domain (see **Figure 5A**). Originally, MAGUKs only referred to a group of proteins including the mammalian synaptic scaffold protein Psd-95, the Drosophila tumor suppressor Dlg, and the tight junction protein ZO-1. Since then a large number of scaffold proteins belonging to this family have been identified. Generally, at junctions they serve as molecular hubs coordinating large protein assemblies which transduce the signals impinging on and emanating from the apical plasma membrane, thereby influencing diverse cellular processes, including the establishment and maintenance of cell polarity and cell-cell adhesion complexes, synaptic plasticity, and cell survival (Funke et al., 2005; Te Velthuis et al., 2007; De Mendoza et al., 2010).

Stevenson and Goodenough identified the first TJ-associated MAGUK ZO-1 (zonula occludens-1) by generating monoclonal antibodies against a TJ-enriched plasma membrane fraction from rodent liver (Stevenson et al., 1986). Subsequently, ZO-2 (Gumbiner et al., 1991) and ZO-3 (Balda et al., 1993; Haskins et al., 1998) were discovered by co-immunoprecipitation studies. The ZO proteins are at the core of large protein networks which are anchored to the TJ through their association with the

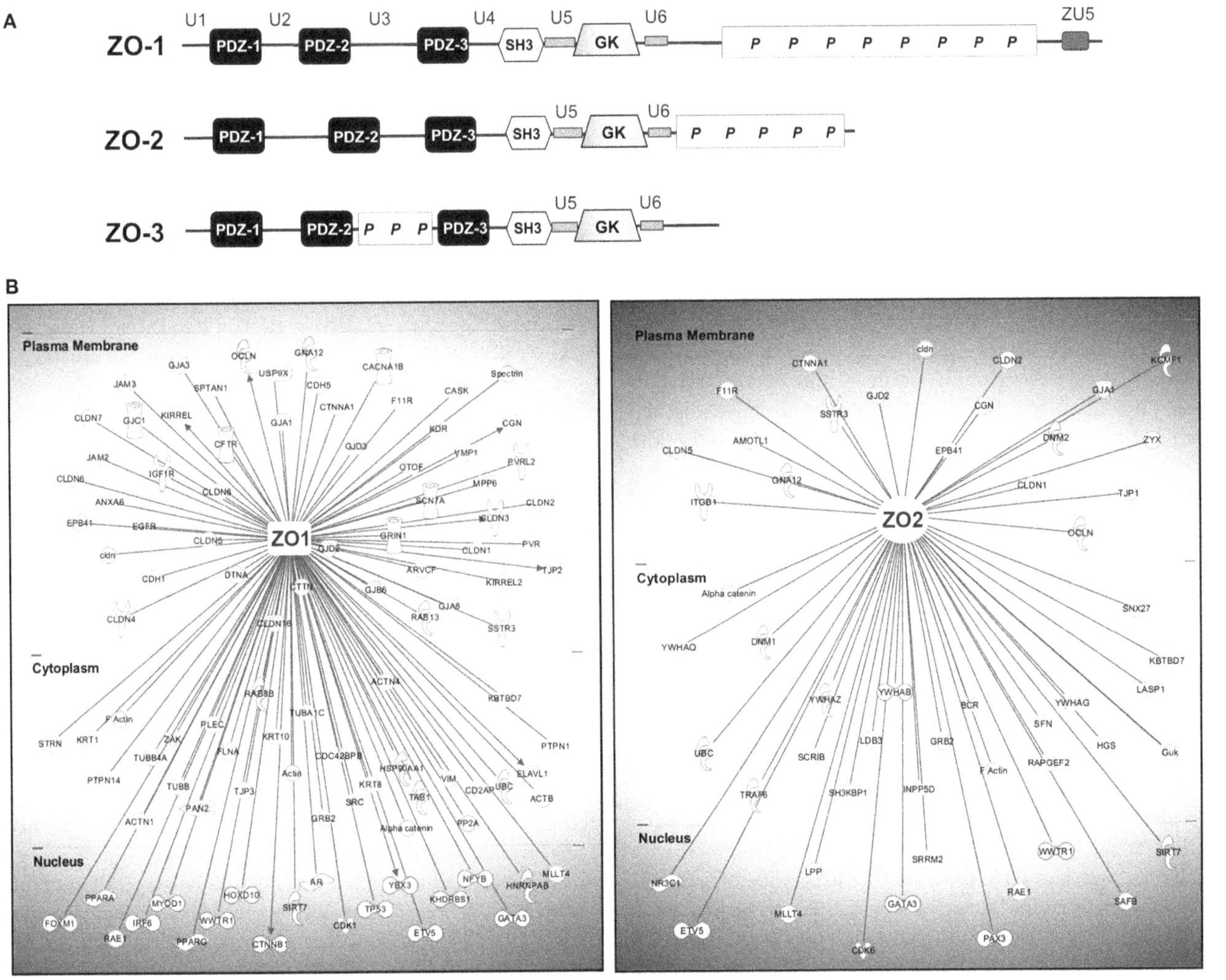

FIGURE 5 | TJ-MAGUKS are membrane-associated adaptor proteins assembling the tight junction plaque. (A) ZO-1, ZO-2, and ZO-3 are multi-domain proteins composed of three PDZ domains, one SH3 and a catalytically inactive GUK domain. Next to these MAGUK-related domains, ZO proteins also contain various ZO-specific unique (U) and proline-rich (*P*) regions. ZU5 is a region found in ZO-1 and Unc5-like netrin receptors. **(B)** ZO-1 and ZO-2 are at the basis of large protein assemblies containing structural and signaling molecules. Shown are proteins that have been demonstrated to interact with ZO-1 or ZO-2 in epithelial and endothelial cells. Gene symbols according to the H.G.N.C. nomenclature are indicated.

C-terminal domains of JAM-A (Bazzoni et al., 2000b; Ebnet et al., 2000; Itoh et al., 2001), occludin (Furuse et al., 1994; Fanning et al., 1998), and most claudins (Itoh et al., 1999a). They further interact physically or functionally with a multitude of cytoplasmic proteins forming the TJ-plaque and they provide a direct link to the actin cytoskeleton via a direct interaction with actin filaments (Itoh et al., 1997; Fanning et al., 1998; Wittchen et al., 1999; Fanning et al., 2002) or the actin binding proteins fodrin/spectrin, cortactin, and protein 4.1R (Katsube et al., 1998; Mattagajasingh et al., 2000). This association to intact cytoskeletal arrays is critical for the physiology of cell–cell junctions.

ZO-1 and ZO-2 are expressed in both epithelial and endothelial cells and have been shown to be indispensable for TJ- strand formation (Umeda et al., 2006; Katsuno et al., 2008). ZO-3 seems to be confined to epithelial cells (Inoko et al., 2003) and is less critical for TJ function (Adachi et al., 2006; Xu et al., 2008). Structurally, ZO proteins share a high degree of sequence similarity across their protein-binding modules, however display significant variability within their C-terminus suggesting that these regions are functionally distinct. Next to the core MAGUK domains of the ZO proteins, several unique (U) regions have been identified (see **Figure 5A**). In the case of ZO-1 these regions influence its intracellular localization and its scaffolding properties (Fanning et al., 2007; Fanning and Anderson, 2009), but little is known about their relevance for ZO-2 and ZO-3. Although the high sequence similarity also suggests a fair degree of functional redundancy, specific roles have been described for the different ZO proteins. Deficiency of ZO-1 results in mislocalization of endothelial junctional adhesion complexes and defects in angiogenesis were evident, resulting in early embryonic lethality (Katsuno et al., 2008). Deletion of ZO-2 in mice is embryonic lethal shortly after implantation due to an arrest in early gastrulation, embryos showing a decreased proliferation rate and an increase in apoptotic cells (Xu et al., 2008).

In brain cECs a decrease in the expression of ZO-1 and occludin after cerebral embolism has been reported (Kago et al., 2006) and *in vitro* under hypoxic conditions the localization of ZO-1 and ZO-2 was altered with a concurrent decrease in TEER (Mark and Davis, 2002; Fischer et al., 2004). Further, disruption of the TJs at the BBB occurs in many neurological disorders (Rosenberg, 2012). However, in most cases the changes in TJ structure and function are most likely the result of indirect downstream signaling events triggered secondary to an inflammatory or traumatic event and are not directly exerted by the junctional proteins themselves. Generally, the reduced expression of ZO-1 correlates with increased proliferation of cells and/or transformation. For example, in highly proliferative brain microvascular endothelial cells from human brain tumors ZO-1 levels are low. Apart from reduced expression, ZO proteins may also regulate proliferation by nuclear translocation. A large body of evidence demonstrates that ZO-1 and ZO-2 are not only present at cell-cell junctions but also target the cell nucleus. Even though the majority of these findings relate to epithelial cells, it is likely that many of these processes also take place in endothelial cells. All ZO proteins harbor conserved nuclear localization and nuclear export sequences (Lopez-Bayghen et al., 2006) and in sparse cultures, ZO-1 and ZO-2 are present in cell nuclei but become re-distributed to the plasma membrane as soon as cells reach confluence (Gottardi et al., 1996; Islas et al., 2002; Traweger et al., 2003; Jaramillo et al., 2004; Gonzalez-Mariscal et al., 2006). ZO-1 further perturbs gene expression by sequestering the Y-box transcription factor ZONAB to the cytoplasm. ZONAB interacts with the cell cycle regulator CDK4 and controls expression of cell cycle regulators such as cyclin D1 and PCNA (for review see Balda and Matter, 2009). ZO-2 has been shown to inhibit the transcription of G1 cyclin after translocating to the nucleus (Gonzalez-Mariscal et al., 2009). In addition, several proteins interact with ZO-2 during nuclear shuttling or within the nucleus itself. For example, the interaction of the armadillo-repeat protein ARVCF (armadillo repeat gene deleted in velocardiofacial syndrome) depends on an N-terminal PDZ domain of ZO-2 (Kausalya et al., 2004), a region which is also targeted by the non-receptor tyrosine kinase JAK1. Also, the transcription factors Jun, Fos, and C/EBP were shown to associate with ZO-2 within the nucleus and at TJs in epithelial cells (Betanzos et al., 2004). Next to directly associating with and/or influencing transcription factors, ZO-2 possibly impacts upon the transcription machinery via its association with the hnRNP SAF-B/HET (Traweger et al., 2003), a molecular platform which assembles a transcription complex in the vicinity of actively transcribed genes (Renz and Fackelmayer, 1996). Taken together, ZO proteins potentially act as direct or indirect regulators of cell proliferation through nuclear translocation and/or their ability to sequester transcription factors and signaling molecules to the cytoplasm. However, our understanding of the signaling pathways and their biochemical properties through which ZO proteins exert their effects beyond cell-cell adhesion remains fragmentary.

Next to the TJ-MAGUKs members of the so called MAGI protein family (membrane-associated guanylate kinase with inverted orientation) localize to TJs. They are large adaptor proteins containing 6 PDZ domains and a module of a GuK domain and two WW domains C-terminal to the first PDZ domain. Of the identified MAGI proteins, only MAGI-1 has been shown to localize to TJs of brain endothelial cells where it interacts with ESAM and promotes maturation of TJs in a Rho-dependent manner (Wegmann et al., 2004; Kimura et al., 2010). In vascular endothelial cells MAGI-1 physically interacts with β-catenin and localizes to VE-cadherin-based AJs (Sakurai et al., 2006), however much detail about the role of MAGI-1 at AJs and TJs is still missing.

Several other regulatory cytoplasmic plaque proteins have been demonstrated to localize to the TJ-plaque, including heterotrimeric G-proteins (Denker et al., 1996; Fabian et al., 1998; Saha et al., 1998). In brain capillary endothelial cells $G_{\alpha i2}$ is found in a complex together with claudin-5 and its depletion results in increased paracellular permeability and delayed TJ-formation after a hyperosmotic shock of cultured cECs (Luissint et al., 2012). Another class of proteins influencing TJ physiology are Rho family GTPases. In rat brain endothelial cells C3 transferase, a toxin which specifically inactivates RhoA-C, abrogated lymphocyte transmigration, suggesting that Rho is required for junction intergrity (Adamson et al., 1999). In addition, expression of mutant Rho GTPases in epithelial and endothelial cells affected barrier properties (Nusrat et al., 1995; Jou et al., 1998; Wojciak-Stothard et al., 2001; Bruewer et al., 2004) and the paracellular flux of sucrose was increased in cerebral endothelial cells treated with lysophoshatidic acid (Schulze et al., 1997). So far, 3 TJ-associated Rho-specific regulators have been identified. (1) The Rho-activator GEF-H1 has been shown to regulate paracellular permeability in epithelial and endothelial cells (Benais-Pont et al., 2003; Birukova et al., 2006). (2) Tuba, an activator for Cdc42, which is recruited to epithelial TJs in a ZO-1-dependent manner (Otani et al., 2006). (3) The GAP protein SH3BP1 which restricts the activity of Cdc42 and Rac when complexed with the scaffold protein CD2AP, parcingulin, and the actin filament capping protein CapZ (Elbediwy et al., 2012).

Cingulin and the closely related protein paracingulin (JACOP) have also been shown to concentrate at TJs of epithelial and endothelial cells, providing a direct link to the cytoskeleton and to regulate the activity of Rho family GTPases at junctions by recruiting guanidine exchange factors of RhoA and Rac1 (Paschoud et al., 2011). Overall, little is known about how the activities of RhoGTPases are regulated and how they feed into the signaling networks that control tight junction formation and integrity. Most likely a Rho-dependent regulation of the actinomyosin cytoskeleton perturbs TJ integrity.

Taken together, the modular structure of a set of adaptor proteins allows the spatio-temporal assembly of multi-protein complexes (see **Figure 5B**) at discrete regions of epithelial and endothelial cells through their interaction with clustered transmembrane TJ proteins, not only ensuring the structural integrity of the TJ, but also integrating various regulatory pathways at the cytoplasmic plaque which are pivotal for TJ physiology.

THE NVU—COUPLING BBB INTEGRITY AND NEURONAL ACTIVITY

The endothelial cells forming the lining of the microvasculature of the brain are set up to actively provide the brain with oxygen and essential nutrients, allowing not only a timely response to local demands but also buffering, which is crucial to physiological neuronal function (Abbott et al., 2006; Abbott, 2013). Brain cECs are wrapped by pericytes, both sharing a common basement membrane onto which astrocytes project their endfeet, ensheathing over 95% of the abluminal microvascular surface (see **Figure 4A**). In addition, cECs receive input from neurons.

Early *in vivo* grafting studies and experiments using astrocyte-conditioned media highlighted the role of astrocyte-derived secreted factors to influence the BBB properties of brain cECs by inducing junction formation (Arthur et al., 1987; Janzer and Raff, 1987; Tao-Cheng et al., 1987; Haseloff et al., 2005). Glial-derived neurotrophic factor (GDNF) has been demonstrated to enhance the barrier properties of brain cECs *in vitro* (Igarashi et al., 1999) and FGF was found to decrease BBB permeability (El Hafny et al., 1996), which is in line with the BBB integrity loss seen in FGF-$2^{-/-}$/FGF-$5^{-/-}$ double mutant mice (Reuss et al., 2003). Recently, sonic hedgehog (Shh) has been shown to be secreted by perivascular astrocytes and endothelial-specific deletion of Smoothened (Smo), a downstream target of Shh, resulted in incomplete BBB maturation early during mouse embryonic development (Alvarez et al., 2011). Further, Shh knockout mice displayed a decrease in TJ proteins in brain cECs.

Next to astrocytes, pericytes have been shown to directly influence the BBB (Hori et al., 2004; Daneman et al., 2010b). The canonical Wnt/β-catenin has also been shown to influence TJ integrity and BBB formation, increasing the expression of several genes, including the TJ protein claudin-3 (Liebner et al., 2008; Daneman et al., 2009). *In vitro*, activation of Wnt pathway controls the expression several TJ proteins (Paolinelli et al., 2013). Further, genetic ablation of Wnt7a/b results in the breakdown of the BBB and a severe CNS-specific hemorrhaging phenotype early in embryonic development (Stenman et al., 2008).

Next to astrocytes and pericytes, noradrenergic, serotonergic, cholinergic, and GABA-ergic neurons have been found to directly contact brain cECs (Cohen et al., 1996, 1997; Tong and Hamel, 1999; Vaucher et al., 2000). It is believed that neurons innervating the brain cECs and astrocytes of the NVU regulate BBB permeability; however the mechanism of action remains unknown.

Taken together, the BBB is a dynamic structure receiving continuous input from the CNS. It is this intimate association of cerebral endothelial cells with neuroectoderm-derived accessory cells that influences barrier function (i.e., tightness) in a spatio-temporal manner in the developing and mature brain.

CONCLUDING REMARKS

The basic structure of the BBB has been described more than 100 years ago. Much progress has been made on elucidating the molecular programs that govern tight junction biogenesis and many of the core molecular components of the endothelial TJ complex which constitutes the main physical paracellular barrier at the BBB have been identified. TJs are now appreciated as dynamic structures where multiple signaling pathways converge, fitting the BBB of the cerebral vascular bed with a high degree of plasticity in response to physiological and pathological stimuli. Next to cell-cell adhesion, processes such as cellular polarization, cytoskeletal rearrangements, integrin-mediated attachment to the ECM, and polarized trafficking are pivotal to the physiological functioning of the BBB. These mechanisms have so far mainly been described in epithelial cells and although most of the key players are present in endothelial cells, their actions may vary markedly in different physiological contexts. Therefore, it will be central to gain a better understanding of the spatio-temporal establishment of functional TJs at the BBB during early vascularization of the embryonic brain. Clearly, further insights have largely been hampered by the lack of suitable *in vitro* culture systems appropriately replicating the vascular properties of the brain microcapillaries. As for many neurological diseases it remains problematic to deliver appropriate drugs to the CNS, a transient modulation of the TJs or transcytosis at the BBB may constitute an alternative approach. Undoubtedly, a more detailed understanding of the complex structure and physiology of endothelial TJs will aid in developing practical solutions for the future.

ACKNOWLEDGMENTS

We apologize to those authors whose work we were unable to cite because of space limitations. Hans-Christian Bauer, Hannelore Bauer, and Andreas Traweger gratefully acknowledge funding by the Paracelsus Medical University Research Fund (PMU-FFF), the European Community' s 7th framework program NEUROBID, and the Lorenz Böhler Fund. The authors have no potential conflicts of interest.

REFERENCES

Abbott, N. J. (2002). Astrocyte-endothelial interactions and blood-brain barrier permeability. *J. Anat.* 200, 629–638. doi: 10.1046/j.1469-7580.2002.00064.x

Abbott, N. J. (2013). Blood-brain barrier structure and function and the challenges for CNS drug delivery. *J. Inherit. Metab. Dis.* 36, 437–449. doi: 10.1007/s10545-013-9608-0

Abbott, N. J., Ronnback, L., and Hansson, E. (2006). Astrocyte-endothelial interactions at the blood-brain barrier. *Nat. Rev. Neurosci.* 7, 41–53. doi: 10.1038/nrn1824

Adachi, M., Inoko, A., Hata, M., Furuse, K., Umeda, K., Itoh, M., et al. (2006). Normal establishment of epithelial tight junctions in mice and cultured cells lacking expression of ZO-3, a tight-junction MAGUK protein. *Mol. Cell. Biol.* 26, 9003–9015. doi: 10.1128/MCB.01811-05

Adamson, P., Etienne, S., Couraud, P. O., Calder, V., and Greenwood, J. (1999). Lymphocyte migration through brain endothelial cell monolayers involves signaling through endothelial ICAM-1 via a rho-dependent pathway. *J. Immunol.* 162, 2964–2973.

Agarwal, N., Lippmann, E. S., and Shusta, E. V. (2010). Identification and expression profiling of blood-brain barrier membrane proteins. *J. Neurochem.* 112, 625–635. doi: 10.1111/j.1471-4159.2009.06481.x

Alvarez, J. I., Dodelet-Devillers, A., Kebir, H., Ifergan, I., Fabre, P. J., Terouz, S., et al. (2011). The Hedgehog pathway promotes blood-brain barrier integrity and CNS immune quiescence. *Science* 334, 1727–1731. doi: 10.1126/science.1206936

Amasheh, S., Meiri, N., Gitter, A. H., Schoneberg, T., Mankertz, J., Schulzke, J. D., et al. (2002). Claudin-2 expression induces cation-selective channels in tight junctions of epithelial cells. *J. Cell Sci.* 115, 4969–4976. doi: 10.1242/jcs.00165

Anderson, J. M., and Van Itallie, C. M. (2009). Physiology and function of the tight junction. *Cold Spring Harb. Perspect. Biol.* 1:a002584. doi: 10.1101/cshperspect.a002584

Aono, S., and Hirai, Y. (2008). Phosphorylation of claudin-4 is required for tight junction formation in a human keratinocyte cell line. *Exp. Cell Res.* 314, 3326–3339. doi: 10.1016/j.yexcr.2008.08.012

Armulik, A., Genove, G., Mae, M., Nisancioglu, M. H., Wallgard, E., Niaudet, C., et al. (2010). Pericytes regulate the blood-brain barrier. *Nature* 468, 557–561. doi: 10.1038/nature09522

Arnold, S. J., and Robertson, E. J. (2009). Making a commitment: cell lineage allocation and axis patterning in the early mouse embryo. *Nat. Rev. Mol. Cell Biol.* 10, 91–103. doi: 10.1038/nrm2618

Arrate, M. P., Rodriguez, J. M., Tran, T. M., Brock, T. A., and Cunningham, S. A. (2001). Cloning of human junctional adhesion molecule 3 (JAM3) and its identification as the JAM2 counter-receptor. *J. Biol. Chem.* 276, 45826–45832. doi: 10.1074/jbc.M105972200

Arthur, F. E., Shivers, R. R., and Bowman, P. D. (1987). Astrocyte-mediated induction of tight junctions in brain capillary endothelium: an efficient *in vitro* model. *Brain Res.* 433, 155–159. doi: 10.1016/0165-3806(87)90075-7

Artus, C., Glacial, F., Ganeshamoorthy, K., Ziegler, N., Godet, M., Guilbert, T., et al. (2014). The Wnt/planar cell polarity signaling pathway contributes to the integrity of tight junctions in brain endothelial cells. *J. Cereb. Blood Flow Metab.* 34, 433–440. doi: 10.1038/jcbfm.2013.213

Assemat, E., Bazellieres, E., Pallesi-Pocachard, E., Le Bivic, A., and Massey-Harroche, D. (2008). Polarity complex proteins. *Biochim. Biophys. Acta* 1778, 614–630. doi: 10.1016/j.bbamem.2007.08.029

Aurrand-Lions, M., Duncan, L., Ballestrem, C., and Imhof, B. A. (2001). JAM-2, a novel immunoglobulin superfamily molecule, expressed by endothelial and lymphatic cells. *J. Biol. Chem.* 276, 2733–2741. doi: 10.1074/jbc.M005458200

Aurrand-Lions, M., Lamagna, C., Dangerfield, J. P., Wang, S., Herrera, P., Nourshargh, S., et al. (2005). Junctional adhesion molecule-C regulates the early influx of leukocytes into tissues during inflammation. *J. Immunol.* 174, 6406–6415. doi: 10.4049/jimmunol.174.10.6406

Aurrand-Lions, M. A., Duncan, L., Du Pasquier, L., and Imhof, B. A. (2000). Cloning of JAM-2 and JAM-3: an emerging junctional adhesion molecular family? *Curr. Top. Microbiol. Immunol.* 251, 91–98. doi: 10.1007/978-3-642-57276-0_12

Axnick, J., and Lammert, E. (2012). Vascular lumen formation. *Curr. Opin. Hematol.* 19, 192–198. doi: 10.1097/MOH.0b013e3283523ebc

Balda, M. S., Gonzalez-Mariscal, L., Matter, K., Cereijido, M., and Anderson, J. M. (1993). Assembly of the tight junction: the role of diacylglycerol. *J. Cell Biol.* 123, 293–302. doi: 10.1083/jcb.123.2.293

Balda, M. S., and Matter, K. (2009). Tight junctions and the regulation of gene expression. *Biochim. Biophys. Acta* 1788, 761–767. doi: 10.1016/j.bbamem.2008.11.024

Bauer, H., Sonnleitner, U., Lametschwandtner, A., Steiner, M., Adam, H., and Bauer, H. C. (1995). Ontogenic expression of the erythroid-type glucose transporter (Glut 1) in the telencephalon of the mouse: correlation to the tightening of the blood-brain barrier. *Brain Res. Dev. Brain Res.* 86, 317–325. doi: 10.1016/0165-3806(95)00044-E

Bauer, H. C., and Bauer, H. (2000). Neural induction of the blood-brain barrier: still an enigma. *Cell. Mol. Neurobiol.* 20, 13–28. doi: 10.1023/A:1006939825857

Bauer, H. C., Bauer, H., Lametschwandtner, A., Amberger, A., Ruiz, P., and Steiner, M. (1993). Neovascularization and the appearance of morphological characteristics of the blood-brain barrier in the embryonic mouse central nervous system. *Brain Res. Dev. Brain Res.* 75, 269–278. doi: 10.1016/0165-3806(93)90031-5

Bauer, H. C., Traweger, A., Zweimueller-Mayer, J., Lehner, C., Tempfer, H., Krizbai, I., et al. (2011). New aspects of the molecular constituents of tissue barriers. *J. Neural Transm.* 118, 7–21. doi: 10.1007/s00702-010-0484-6

Bazzoni, G., Martinez-Estrada, O. M., Mueller, F., Nelboeck, P., Schmid, G., Bartfai, T., et al. (2000a). Homophilic interaction of junctional adhesion molecule. *J. Biol. Chem.* 275, 30970–30976. doi: 10.1074/jbc.M003946200

Bazzoni, G., Martinez-Estrada, O. M., Orsenigo, F., Cordenonsi, M., Citi, S., and Dejana, E. (2000b). Interaction of junctional adhesion molecule with the tight junction components ZO-1, cingulin, and occludin. *J. Biol. Chem.* 275, 20520–20526. doi: 10.1074/jbc.M905251199

Begley, D. J., and Brightman, M. W. (2003). Structural and functional aspects of the blood-brain barrier. *Prog. Drug Res.* 61, 39–78.

Benais-Pont, G., Punn, A., Flores-Maldonado, C., Eckert, J., Raposo, G., Fleming, T. P., et al. (2003). Identification of a tight junction-associated guanine nucleotide exchange factor that activates Rho and regulates paracellular permeability. *J. Cell Biol.* 160, 729–740. doi: 10.1083/jcb.200211047

Ben-Zvi, A., Lacoste, B., Kur, E., Andreone, B. J., Mayshar, Y., Yan, H., et al. (2014). Mfsd2a is critical for the formation and function of the blood-brain barrier. *Nature* 509, 507–511. doi: 10.1038/nature13324

Betanzos, A., Huerta, M., Lopez-Bayghen, E., Azuara, E., Amerena, J., and Gonzalez-Mariscal, L. (2004). The tight junction protein ZO-2 associates with Jun, Fos and C/EBP transcription factors in epithelial cells. *Exp. Cell Res.* 292, 51–66. doi: 10.1016/j.yexcr.2003.08.007

Bilder, D., Schober, M., and Perrimon, N. (2003). Integrated activity of PDZ protein complexes regulates epithelial polarity. *Nat. Cell Biol.* 5, 53–58. doi: 10.1038/ncb897

Birukova, A. A., Adyshev, D., Gorshkov, B., Bokoch, G. M., Birukov, K. G., and Verin, A. D. (2006). GEF-H1 is involved in agonist-induced human pulmonary endothelial barrier dysfunction. *Am. J. Physiol. Lung Cell. Mol. Physiol.* 290, L540–L548. doi: 10.1152/ajplung.00259.2005

Blasig, I. E., Winkler, L., Lassowski, B., Mueller, S. L., Zuleger, N., Krause, E., et al. (2006). On the self-association potential of transmembrane tight junction proteins. *Cell. Mol. Life Sci.* 63, 505–514. doi: 10.1007/s00018-005-5472-x

Blum, Y., Belting, H. G., Ellertsdottir, E., Herwig, L., Luders, F., and Affolter, M. (2008). Complex cell rearrangements during intersegmental vessel sprouting and vessel fusion in the zebrafish embryo. *Dev. Biol.* 316, 312–322. doi: 10.1016/j.ydbio.2008.01.038

Boas, S. E., and Merks, R. M. (2014). Synergy of cell-cell repulsion and vacuolation in a computational model of lumen formation. *J. R. Soc. Interface* 11:20131049. doi: 10.1098/rsif.2013.1049

Born, G. V., and Palinski, W. (1985). Unusually high concentrations of sialic acids on the surface of vascular endothelia. *Br. J. Exp. Pathol.* 66, 543–549.

Breier, G., Albrecht, U., Sterrer, S., and Risau, W. (1992). Expression of vascular endothelial growth factor during embryonic angiogenesis and endothelial cell differentiation. *Development* 114, 521–532.

Bruewer, M., Hopkins, A. M., Hobert, M. E., Nusrat, A., and Madara, J. L. (2004). RhoA, Rac1, and Cdc42 exert distinct effects on epithelial barrier via selective structural and biochemical modulation of junctional proteins and F-actin. *Am. J. Physiol. Cell Physiol.* 287, C327–C335. doi: 10.1152/ajpcell.00087.2004

Carson, S. D., Hobbs, J. T., Tracy, S. M., and Chapman, N. M. (1999). Expression of the coxsackievirus and adenovirus receptor in cultured human umbilical vein endothelial cells: regulation in response to cell density. *J. Virol.* 73, 7077–7079.

Cereijido, M., Gonzalez-Mariscal, L., Contreras, R. G., Gallardo, J. M., Garcia-Villegas, R., and Valdes, J. (1993). The making of a tight junction. *J. Cell Sci. Suppl.* 17, 127–132. doi: 10.1242/jcs.1993.Supplement_17.18

Chalcroft, J. P., and Bullivant, S. (1970). An interpretation of liver cell membrane and junction structure based on observation of freeze-fracture replicas of both sides of the fracture. *J. Cell Biol.* 47, 49–60.

Chen, X., and Macara, I. G. (2005). Par-3 controls tight junction assembly through the Rac exchange factor Tiam1. *Nat. Cell Biol.* 7, 262–269. doi: 10.1038/ncb1226

Chen, Y. H., Lu, Q., Goodenough, D. A., and Jeansonne, B. (2002). Nonreceptor tyrosine kinase c-Yes interacts with occludin during tight junction formation in canine kidney epithelial cells. *Mol. Biol. Cell* 13, 1227–1237. doi: 10.1091/mbc.01-08-0423

Chen-Quay, S. C., Eiting, K. T., Li, A. W., Lamharzi, N., and Quay, S. C. (2009). Identification of tight junction modulating lipids. *J. Pharm. Sci.* 98, 606–619. doi: 10.1002/jps.21462

Chung, S., and Andrew, D. J. (2008). The formation of epithelial tubes. *J. Cell Sci.* 121, 3501–3504. doi: 10.1242/jcs.037887

Clatterbuck, R. E., Eberhart, C. G., Crain, B. J., and Rigamonti, D. (2001). Ultrastructural and immunocytochemical evidence that an incompetent blood-brain barrier is related to the pathophysiology of cavernous malformations. *J. Neurol. Neurosurg. Psychiatr.* 71, 188–192. doi: 10.1136/jnnp.71.2.188

Cohen, C. J., Shieh, J. T., Pickles, R. J., Okegawa, T., Hsieh, J. T., and Bergelson, J. M. (2001). The coxsackievirus and adenovirus receptor is a transmembrane component of the tight junction. *Proc. Natl. Acad. Sci. U.S.A.* 98, 15191–15196. doi: 10.1073/pnas.261452898

Cohen, Z., Bonvento, G., Lacombe, P., and Hamel, E. (1996). Serotonin in the regulation of brain microcirculation. *Prog. Neurobiol.* 50, 335–362. doi: 10.1016/S0301-0082(96)00033-0

Cohen, Z., Molinatti, G., and Hamel, E. (1997). Astroglial and vascular interactions of noradrenaline terminals in the rat cerebral cortex. *J. Cereb. Blood Flow Metab.* 17, 894–904. doi: 10.1097/00004647-199708000-00008

Coisne, C., Dehouck, L., Faveeuw, C., Delplace, Y., Miller, F., Landry, C., et al. (2005). Mouse syngenic *in vitro* blood-brain barrier model: a new tool to examine inflammatory events in cerebral endothelium. *Lab. Invest.* 85, 734–746. doi: 10.1038/labinvest.3700281

Contreras, R. G., Miller, J. H., Zamora, M., Gonzalez-Mariscal, L., and Cereijido, M. (1992). Interaction of calcium with plasma membrane of epithelial (MDCK) cells during junction formation. *Am. J. Physiol.* 263, C313–C318.

Cordenonsi, M., Zanconato, F., Azzolin, L., Forcato, M., Rosato, A., Frasson, C., et al. (2011). The Hippo transducer TAZ confers cancer stem cell-related traits on breast cancer cells. *Cell* 147, 759–772. doi: 10.1016/j.cell.2011.09.048

Cunningham, S. A., Arrate, M. P., Rodriguez, J. M., Bjercke, R. J., Vanderslice, P., Morris, A. P., et al. (2000). A novel protein with homology to the junctional adhesion molecule. Characterization of leukocyte interactions. *J. Biol. Chem.* 275, 34750–34756. doi: 10.1074/jbc.M002718200

Cunningham, S. A., Rodriguez, J. M., Arrate, M. P., Tran, T. M., and Brock, T. A. (2002). JAM2 interacts with alpha4beta1. Facilitation by JAM3. *J. Biol. Chem.* 277, 27589–27592. doi: 10.1074/jbc.C200331200

Czupalla, C. J., Liebner, S., and Devraj, K. (2014). *In vitro* models of the blood-brain barrier. *Methods Mol. Biol.* 1135, 415–437. doi: 10.1007/978-1-4939-0320-7_34

Daneman, R., Agalliu, D., Zhou, L., Kuhnert, F., Kuo, C. J., and Barres, B. A. (2009). Wnt/beta-catenin signaling is required for CNS, but not non-CNS, angiogenesis. *Proc. Natl. Acad. Sci. U.S.A.* 106, 641–646. doi: 10.1073/pnas.0805165106

Daneman, R., Zhou, L., Agalliu, D., Cahoy, J. D., Kaushal, A., and Barres, B. A. (2010a). The mouse blood-brain barrier transcriptome: a new resource for understanding the development and function of brain endothelial cells. *PLoS ONE* 5:e13741. doi: 10.1371/journal.pone.0013741

Daneman, R., Zhou, L., Kebede, A. A., and Barres, B. A. (2010b). Pericytes are required for blood-brain barrier integrity during embryogenesis. *Nature* 468, 562–566. doi: 10.1038/nature09513

Dard, N., Breuer, M., Maro, B., and Louvet-Vallee, S. (2008). Morphogenesis of the mammalian blastocyst. *Mol. Cell. Endocrinol.* 282, 70–77. doi: 10.1016/j.mce.2007.11.004

De Mendoza, A., Suga, H., and Ruiz-Trillo, I. (2010). Evolution of the MAGUK protein gene family in premetazoan lineages. *BMC Evol. Biol.* 10:93. doi: 10.1186/1471-2148-10-93

Deli, M. A., Abraham, C. S., Kataoka, Y., and Niwa, M. (2005). Permeability studies on *in vitro* blood-brain barrier models: physiology, pathology, and pharmacology. *Cell. Mol. Neurobiol.* 25, 59–127. doi: 10.1007/s10571-004-1377-8

DeMaio, L., Chang, Y. S., Gardner, T. W., Tarbell, J. M., and Antonetti, D. A. (2001). Shear stress regulates occludin content and phosphorylation. *Am. J. Physiol. Heart Circ. Physiol.* 281, H105–H113.

Denker, B. M., Saha, C., Khawaja, S., and Nigam, S. K. (1996). Involvement of a heterotrimeric G protein alpha subunit in tight junction biogenesis. *J. Biol. Chem.* 271, 25750–25753. doi: 10.1074/jbc.271.42.25750

Dimitratos, S. D., Woods, D. F., Stathakis, D. G., and Bryant, P. J. (1999). Signaling pathways are focused at specialized regions of the plasma membrane by scaffolding proteins of the MAGUK family. *Bioessays* 21, 912–921.

Draheim, K. M., Fisher, O. S., Boggon, T. J., and Calderwood, D. A. (2014). Cerebral cavernous malformation proteins at a glance. *J. Cell Sci.* 127, 701–707. doi: 10.1242/jcs.138388

D'Souza, T., Agarwal, R., and Morin, P. J. (2005). Phosphorylation of claudin-3 at threonine 192 by cAMP-dependent protein kinase regulates tight junction barrier function in ovarian cancer cells. *J. Biol. Chem.* 280, 26233–26240. doi: 10.1074/jbc.M502003200

Ebnet, K. (2008). Organization of multiprotein complexes at cell-cell junctions. *Histochem. Cell Biol.* 130, 1–20. doi: 10.1007/s00418-008-0418-7

Ebnet, K., Aurrand-Lions, M., Kuhn, A., Kiefer, F., Butz, S., Zander, K., et al. (2003). The junctional adhesion molecule (JAM) family members JAM-2 and JAM-3 associate with the cell polarity protein PAR-3: a possible role for JAMs in endothelial cell polarity. *J. Cell Sci.* 116, 3879–3891. doi: 10.1242/jcs.00704

Ebnet, K., Iden, S., Gerke, V., and Suzuki, A. (2008). Regulation of epithelial and endothelial junctions by PAR proteins. *Front. Biosci.* 13, 6520–6536. doi: 10.2741/3172

Ebnet, K., Schulz, C. U., Meyer Zu Brickwedde, M. K., Pendl, G. G., and Vestweber, D. (2000). Junctional adhesion molecule interacts with the PDZ domain-containing proteins AF-6 and ZO-1. *J. Biol. Chem.* 275, 27979–27988. doi: 10.1074/jbc.M002363200

Ebnet, K., Suzuki, A., Horikoshi, Y., Hirose, T., Meyer Zu Brickwedde, M. K., Ohno, S., et al. (2001). The cell polarity protein ASIP/PAR-3 directly associates with junctional adhesion molecule (JAM). *EMBO J.* 20, 3738–3748. doi: 10.1093/emboj/20.14.3738

Eckert, J. J., and Fleming, T. P. (2008). Tight junction biogenesis during early development. *Biochim. Biophys. Acta* 1778, 717–728. doi: 10.1016/j.bbamem.2007.09.031

Elbediwy, A., Zihni, C., Terry, S. J., Clark, P., Matter, K., and Balda, M. S. (2012). Epithelial junction formation requires confinement of Cdc42 activity by a novel SH3BP1 complex. *J. Cell Biol.* 198, 677–693. doi: 10.1083/jcb.201202094

El Hafny, B., Bourre, J. M., and Roux, F. (1996). Synergistic stimulation of gamma-glutamyl transpeptidase and alkaline phosphatase activities by retinoic acid and astroglial factors in immortalized rat brain microvessel endothelial cells. *J. Cell. Physiol.* 167, 451–460.

Enerson, B. E., and Drewes, L. R. (2006). The rat blood-brain barrier transcriptome. *J. Cereb. Blood Flow Metab.* 26, 959–973. doi: 10.1038/sj.jcbfm.9600249

Engelhardt, B., and Liebner, S. (2014). Novel insights into the development and maintenance of the blood-brain barrier. *Cell Tissue Res.* 355, 687–699. doi: 10.1007/s00441-014-1811-2

Fabian, G., Szabo, C. A., Bozo, B., Greenwood, J., Adamson, P., Deli, M. A., et al. (1998). Expression of G-protein subtypes in cultured cerebral endothelial cells. *Neurochem. Int.* 33, 179–185. doi: 10.1016/S0197-0186(98)00008-4

Fanning, A. S., and Anderson, J. M. (1999). Protein modules as organizers of membrane structure. *Curr. Opin. Cell Biol.* 11, 432–439. doi: 10.1016/S0955-0674(99)80062-3

Fanning, A. S., and Anderson, J. M. (2009). Zonula occludens-1 and -2 are cytosolic scaffolds that regulate the assembly of cellular junctions. *Ann. N.Y. Acad. Sci.* 1165, 113–120. doi: 10.1111/j.1749-6632.2009.04440.x

Fanning, A. S., Jameson, B. J., Jesaitis, L. A., and Anderson, J. M. (1998). The tight junction protein ZO-1 establishes a link between the transmembrane protein occludin and the actin cytoskeleton. *J. Biol. Chem.* 273, 29745–29753. doi: 10.1074/jbc.273.45.29745

Fanning, A. S., Little, B. P., Rahner, C., Utepbergenov, D., Walther, Z., and Anderson, J. M. (2007). The unique-5 and -6 motifs of ZO-1 regulate tight junction strand localization and scaffolding properties. *Mol. Biol. Cell* 18, 721–731. doi: 10.1091/mbc.E06-08-0764

Fanning, A. S., Ma, T. Y., and Anderson, J. M. (2002). Isolation and functional characterization of the actin binding region in the tight junction protein ZO-1. *FASEB J.* 16, 1835–1837. doi: 10.1096/fj.02-0121fje

Farquhar, M. G., and Palade, G. E. (1963). Junctional complexes in various epithelia. *J. Cell Biol.* 17, 375–412. doi: 10.1083/jcb.17.2.375

Fierro-Gonzalez, J. C., White, M. D., Silva, J. C., and Plachta, N. (2013). Cadherin-dependent filopodia control preimplantation embryo compaction. *Nat. Cell Biol.* 15, 1424–1433. doi: 10.1038/ncb2875

Fischer, S., Wiesnet, M., Marti, H. H., Renz, D., and Schaper, W. (2004). Simultaneous activation of several second messengers in hypoxia-induced hyperpermeability of brain derived endothelial cells. *J. Cell. Physiol.* 198, 359–369. doi: 10.1002/jcp.10417

Fogg, V. C., Liu, C. J., and Margolis, B. (2005). Multiple regions of Crumbs3 are required for tight junction formation in MCF10A cells. *J. Cell Sci.* 118, 2859–2869. doi: 10.1242/jcs.02412

Fraemohs, L., Koenen, R. R., Ostermann, G., Heinemann, B., and Weber, C. (2004). The functional interaction of the beta 2 integrin lymphocyte function-associated antigen-1 with junctional adhesion molecule-A is mediated by the I domain. *J. Immunol.* 173, 6259–6264. doi: 10.4049/jimmunol.173.10.6259

Friend, D. S., and Gilula, N. B. (1972). Variations in tight and gap junctions in mammalian tissues. *J. Cell Biol.* 53, 758–776. doi: 10.1083/jcb.53.3.758

Fukuhara, A., Irie, K., Nakanishi, H., Takekuni, K., Kawakatsu, T., Ikeda, W., et al. (2002). Involvement of nectin in the localization of junctional adhesion molecule at tight junctions. *Oncogene* 21, 7642–7655. doi: 10.1038/sj.onc.1205875

Funke, L., Dakoji, S., and Bredt, D. S. (2005). Membrane-associated guanylate kinases regulate adhesion and plasticity at cell junctions. *Annu. Rev. Biochem.* 74, 219–245. doi: 10.1146/annurev.biochem.74.082803.133339

Furuse, M. (2010). Molecular basis of the core structure of tight junctions. *Cold Spring Harb. Perspect. Biol.* 2:a002907. doi: 10.1101/cshperspect.a002907

Furuse, M., Fujimoto, K., Sato, N., Hirase, T., and Tsukita, S. (1996). Overexpression of occludin, a tight junction-associated integral membrane protein, induces the formation of intracellular multilamellar bodies bearing tight junction-like structures. *J. Cell Sci.* 109(Pt 2), 429–435.

Furuse, M., Fujita, K., Hiragi, T., Fujimoto, K., and Tsukita, S. (1998). Claudin-1 and -2: novel integral membrane proteins localizing at tight junctions with no sequence similarity to occludin. *J. Cell Biol.* 141, 1539–1550. doi: 10.1083/jcb.141.7.1539

Furuse, M., Hata, M., Furuse, K., Yoshida, Y., Haratake, A., Sugitani, Y., et al. (2002). Claudin-based tight junctions are crucial for the mammalian epidermal barrier: a lesson from claudin-1-deficient mice. *J. Cell Biol.* 156, 1099–1111. doi: 10.1083/jcb.200110122

Furuse, M., Hirase, T., Itoh, M., Nagafuchi, A., Yonemura, S., and Tsukita, S. (1993). Occludin: a novel integral membrane protein localizing at tight junctions [see comments]. *J. Cell Biol.* 123, 1777–1788. doi: 10.1083/jcb.123.6.1777

Furuse, M., Itoh, M., Hirase, T., Nagafuchi, A., Yonemura, S., Tsukita, S., et al. (1994). Direct association of occludin with ZO-1 and its possible involvement in the localization of occludin at tight junctions. *J. Cell Biol.* 127, 1617–1626. doi: 10.1083/jcb.127.6.1617

Garnaas, M. K., Moodie, K. L., Liu, M. L., Samant, G. V., Li, K., Marx, R., et al. (2008). Syx, a RhoA guanine exchange factor, is essential for angiogenesis *in vivo*. *Circ. Res.* 103, 710–716. doi: 10.1161/CIRCRESAHA.108.181388

Giepmans, B. N., and Van Ijzendoorn, S. C. (2009). Epithelial cell-cell junctions and plasma membrane domains. *Biochim. Biophys. Acta* 1788, 820–831. doi: 10.1016/j.bbamem.2008.07.015

Glading, A., Han, J., Stockton, R. A., and Ginsberg, M. H. (2007). KRIT-1/CCM1 is a Rap1 effector that regulates endothelial cell cell junctions. *J. Cell Biol.* 179, 247–254. doi: 10.1083/jcb.200705175

Gonzalez-Mariscal, L., Betanzos, A., and Avila-Flores, A. (2000). MAGUK proteins: structure and role in the tight junction. *Semin. Cell Dev. Biol.* 11, 315–324. doi: 10.1006/scdb.2000.0178

Gonzalez-Mariscal, L., Chavez De Ramirez, B., and Cereijido, M. (1985). Tight junction formation in cultured epithelial cells (MDCK). *J. Membr. Biol.* 86, 113–125. doi: 10.1007/BF01870778

Gonzalez-Mariscal, L., Contreras, R. G., Bolivar, J. J., Ponce, A., Chavez De Ramirez, B., and Cereijido, M. (1990). Role of calcium in tight junction formation between epithelial cells. *Am. J. Physiol.* 259, C978–C986.

Gonzalez-Mariscal, L., and Nava, P. (2005). Tight junctions, from tight intercellular seals to sophisticated protein complexes involved in drug delivery, pathogens interaction and cell proliferation. *Adv. Drug Deliv. Rev.* 57, 811–814. doi: 10.1016/j.addr.2005.01.004

Gonzalez-Mariscal, L., Ponce, A., Alarcon, L., and Jaramillo, B. E. (2006). The tight junction protein ZO-2 has several functional nuclear export signals. *Exp. Cell Res.* 312, 3323–3335. doi: 10.1016/j.yexcr.2006.07.006

Gonzalez-Mariscal, L., Tapia, R., and Chamorro, D. (2008). Crosstalk of tight junction components with signaling pathways. *Biochim. Biophys. Acta* 1778, 729–756. doi: 10.1016/j.bbamem.2007.08.018

Gonzalez-Mariscal, L., Tapia, R., Huerta, M., and Lopez-Bayghen, E. (2009). The tight junction protein ZO-2 blocks cell cycle progression and inhibits cyclin D1 expression. *Ann. N.Y. Acad. Sci.* 1165, 121–125. doi: 10.1111/j.1749-6632.2009.04024.x

Gorog, P., Schraufstatter, I., and Born, G. V. (1982). Effect of removing sialic acids from endothelium on the adherence of circulating platelets in arteries *in vivo*. *Proc. R. Soc. Lond. B Biol. Sci.* 214, 471–480. doi: 10.1098/rspb.1982.0022

Gottardi, C. J., Arpin, M., Fanning, A. S., and Louvard, D. (1996). The junction-associated protein, zonula occludens-1, localizes to the nucleus before the maturation and during the remodeling of cell-cell contacts. *Proc. Natl. Acad. Sci. U.S.A.* 93, 10779–10784. doi: 10.1073/pnas.93.20.10779

Gow, A., Davies, C., Southwood, C. M., Frolenkov, G., Chrustowski, M., Ng, L., et al. (2004). Deafness in Claudin 11-null mice reveals the critical contribution of basal cell tight junctions to stria vascularis function. *J. Neurosci.* 24, 7051–7062. doi: 10.1523/JNEUROSCI.1640-04.2004

Gow, A., Southwood, C. M., Li, J. S., Pariali, M., Riordan, G. P., Brodie, S. E., et al. (1999). CNS myelin and sertoli cell tight junction strands are absent in Osp/claudin-11 null mice. *Cell* 99, 649–659. doi: 10.1016/S0092-8674(00)81553-6

Guillemot, L., Paschoud, S., Pulimeno, P., Foglia, A., and Citi, S. (2008). The cytoplasmic plaque of tight junctions: a scaffolding and signalling center. *Biochim. Biophys. Acta* 1778, 601–613. doi: 10.1016/j.bbamem.2007.09.032

Gumbiner, B. (1987). Structure, biochemistry, and assembly of epithelial tight junctions. *Am. J. Physiol.* 253, C749–C758.

Gumbiner, B., Lowenkopf, T., and Apatira, D. (1991). Identification of a 160-kDa polypeptide that binds to the tight junction protein ZO-1. *Proc. Natl. Acad. Sci. U.S.A.* 88, 3460–3464. doi: 10.1073/pnas.88.8.3460

Gumbiner, B. M. (1993). Breaking through the tight junction barrier [comment]. *J. Cell Biol.* 123, 1631–1633. doi: 10.1083/jcb.123.6.1631

Gunzel, D., and Fromm, M. (2012). Claudins and other tight junction proteins. *Compr. Physiol.* 2, 1819–1852. doi: 10.1002/cphy.c110045

Hamazaki, Y., Itoh, M., Sasaki, H., Furuse, M., and Tsukita, S. (2002). Multi-PDZ domain protein 1 (MUPP1) is concentrated at tight junctions through its possible interaction with claudin-1 and junctional adhesion molecule. *J. Biol. Chem.* 277, 455–461. doi: 10.1074/jbc.M109005200

Hamm, S., Dehouck, B., Kraus, J., Wolburg-Buchholz, K., Wolburg, H., Risau, W., et al. (2004). Astrocyte mediated modulation of blood-brain barrier permeability does not correlate with a loss of tight junction proteins from the cellular contacts. *Cell Tissue Res.* 315, 157–166. doi: 10.1007/s00441-003-0825-y

Haseloff, R. F., Blasig, I. E., Bauer, H. C., and Bauer, H. (2005). In search of the astrocytic factor(s) modulating blood-brain barrier functions in brain capillary endothelial cells *in vitro*. *Cell. Mol. Neurobiol.* 25, 25–39. doi: 10.1007/s10571-004-1375-x

Haskins, J., Gu, L., Wittchen, E. S., Hibbard, J., and Stevenson, B. R. (1998). ZO-3, a novel member of the MAGUK protein family found at the tight junction, interacts with ZO-1 and occludin. *J. Cell Biol.* 141, 199–208. doi: 10.1083/jcb.141.1.199

Hirabayashi, S., Tajima, M., Yao, I., Nishimura, W., Mori, H., and Hata, Y. (2003). JAM4, a junctional cell adhesion molecule interacting with a tight junction protein, MAGI-1. *Mol. Cell. Biol.* 23, 4267–4282. doi: 10.1128/MCB.23.12.4267-4282.2003

Hirata, K., Ishida, T., Penta, K., Rezaee, M., Yang, E., Wohlgemuth, J., et al. (2001). Cloning of an immunoglobulin family adhesion molecule selectively expressed by endothelial cells. *J. Biol. Chem.* 276, 16223–16231. doi: 10.1074/jbc.M100630200

Hori, S., Ohtsuki, S., Hosoya, K., Nakashima, E., and Terasaki, T. (2004). A pericyte-derived angiopoietin-1 multimeric complex induces occludin gene expression in brain capillary endothelial cells through Tie-2 activation *in vitro*. *J. Neurochem.* 89, 503–513. doi: 10.1111/j.1471-4159.2004.02343.x

Horvat, R., Hovorka, A., Dekan, G., Poczewski, H., and Kerjaschki, D. (1986). Endothelial cell membranes contain podocalyxin—the major sialoprotein of visceral glomerular epithelial cells. *J. Cell Biol.* 102, 484–491. doi: 10.1083/jcb.102.2.484

Hurd, T. W., Gao, L., Roh, M. H., Macara, I. G., and Margolis, B. (2003). Direct interaction of two polarity complexes implicated in epithelial tight junction assembly. *Nat. Cell Biol.* 5, 137–142. doi: 10.1038/ncb923

Iden, S., and Collard, J. G. (2008). Crosstalk between small GTPases and polarity proteins in cell polarization. *Nat. Rev. Mol. Cell Biol.* 9, 846–859. doi: 10.1038/nrm2521

Igarashi, Y., Utsumi, H., Chiba, H., Yamada-Sasamori, Y., Tobioka, H., Kamimura, Y., et al. (1999). Glial cell line-derived neurotrophic factor induces barrier function of endothelial cells forming the blood-brain barrier. *Biochem. Biophys. Res. Commun.* 261, 108–112. doi: 10.1006/bbrc.1999.0992

Ikari, A., Matsumoto, S., Harada, H., Takagi, K., Hayashi, H., Suzuki, Y., et al. (2006). Phosphorylation of paracellin-1 at Ser217 by protein kinase A is essential for localization in tight junctions. *J. Cell Sci.* 119, 1781–1789. doi: 10.1242/jcs.02901

Ikeda, E., Flamme, I., and Risau, W. (1996). Developing brain cells produce factors capable of inducing the HT7 antigen, a blood-brain barrier-specific molecule, in chick endothelial cells. *Neurosci. Lett.* 209, 149–152. doi: 10.1016/0304-3940(96)12625-2

Ikenouchi, J., Furuse, M., Furuse, K., Sasaki, H., and Tsukita, S. (2005). Tricellulin constitutes a novel barrier at tricellular contacts of epithelial cells. *J. Cell Biol.* 171, 939–945. doi: 10.1083/jcb.200510043

Indra, I., Hong, S., Troyanovsky, R., Kormos, B., and Troyanovsky, S. (2013). The adherens junction: a mosaic of cadherin and nectin clusters bundled by actin filaments. *J. Invest. Dermatol.* 133, 2546–2554. doi: 10.1038/jid.2013.200

Inoko, A., Itoh, M., Tamura, A., Matsuda, M., Furuse, M., and Tsukita, S. (2003). Expression and distribution of ZO-3, a tight junction MAGUK protein, in mouse tissues. *Genes cells* 8, 837–845. doi: 10.1046/j.1365-2443.2003.00681.x

Iruela-Arispe, M. L., and Davis, G. E. (2009). Cellular and molecular mechanisms of vascular lumen formation. *Dev. Cell* 16, 222–231. doi: 10.1016/j.devcel.2009.01.013

Ishida, T., Kundu, R. K., Yang, E., Hirata, K., Ho, Y. D., and Quertermous, T. (2003). Targeted disruption of endothelial cell-selective adhesion molecule inhibits angiogenic processes *in vitro* and *in vivo*. *J. Biol. Chem.* 278, 34598–34604. doi: 10.1074/jbc.M304890200

Ishizaki, T., Chiba, H., Kojima, T., Fujibe, M., Soma, T., Miyajima, H., et al. (2003). Cyclic AMP induces phosphorylation of claudin-5 immunoprecipitates and expression of claudin-5 gene in blood-brain-barrier endothelial cells via protein kinase A-dependent and -independent pathways. *Exp. Cell Res.* 290, 275–288. doi: 10.1016/S0014-4827(03)00354-9

Islas, S., Vega, J., Ponce, L., and Gonzalez-Mariscal, L. (2002). Nuclear localization of the tight junction protein ZO-2 in epithelial cells. *Exp. Cell Res.* 274, 138–148. doi: 10.1006/excr.2001.5457

Itoh, M., Furuse, M., Morita, K., Kubota, K., Saitou, M., and Tsukita, S. (1999a). Direct binding of three tight junction-associated MAGUKs, ZO-1, ZO-2, and ZO-3, with the COOH termini of claudins. *J. Cell Biol.* 147, 1351–1363. doi: 10.1083/jcb.147.6.1351

Itoh, M., Morita, K., and Tsukita, S. (1999b). Characterization of ZO-2 as a MAGUK family member associated with tight as well as adherens junctions with a binding affinity to occludin and alpha catenin. *J. Biol. Chem.* 274, 5981–5986. doi: 10.1074/jbc.274.9.5981

Itoh, M., Nagafuchi, A., Moroi, S., and Tsukita, S. (1997). Involvement of ZO-1 in cadherin-based cell adhesion through its direct binding to alpha catenin and actin filaments. *J. Cell Biol.* 138, 181–192. doi: 10.1083/jcb.138.1.181

Itoh, M., Sasaki, H., Furuse, M., Ozaki, H., Kita, T., and Tsukita, S. (2001). Junctional adhesion molecule (JAM) binds to PAR-3: a possible mechanism for the recruitment of PAR-3 to tight junctions. *J. Cell Biol.* 154, 491–497. doi: 10.1083/jcb.200103047

Iwamoto, N., Higashi, T., and Furuse, M. (2014). Localization of Angulin-1/LSR and Tricellulin at Tricellular Contacts of Brain and Retinal Endothelial Cells *in vivo*. *Cell Struct. Funct.* 39, 1–8. doi: 10.1247/csf.13015

Janzer, R. C., and Raff, M. C. (1987). Astrocytes induce blood-brain barrier properties in endothelial cells. *Nature* 325, 253–257. doi: 10.1038/325253a0

Jaramillo, B. E., Ponce, A., Moreno, J., Betanzos, A., Huerta, M., Lopez-Bayghen, E., et al. (2004). Characterization of the tight junction protein ZO-2 localized at the nucleus of epithelial cells. *Exp. Cell Res.* 297, 247–258. doi: 10.1016/j.yexcr.2004.03.021

Javed, Q., Fleming, T. P., Hay, M., and Citi, S. (1993). Tight junction protein cingulin is expressed by maternal and embryonic genomes during early mouse development. *Development* 117, 1145–1151.

Joberty, G., Petersen, C., Gao, L., and Macara, I. G. (2000). The cell-polarity protein Par6 links Par3 and atypical protein kinase C to Cdc42. *Nat. Cell Biol.* 2, 531–539. doi: 10.1038/35019573

Johansson, A., Driessens, M., and Aspenstrom, P. (2000). The mammalian homologue of the Caenorhabditis elegans polarity protein PAR-6 is a binding partner for the Rho GTPases Cdc42 and Rac1. *J. Cell Sci.* 113(Pt 18), 3267–3275.

Jou, T. S., Schneeberger, E. E., and Nelson, W. J. (1998). Structural and functional regulation of tight junctions by RhoA and Rac1 small GTPases. *J. Cell Biol.* 142, 101–115. doi: 10.1083/jcb.142.1.101

Kago, T., Takagi, N., Date, I., Takenaga, Y., Takagi, K., and Takeo, S. (2006). Cerebral ischemia enhances tyrosine phosphorylation of occludin in brain capillaries. *Biochem. Biophys. Res. Commun.* 339, 1197–1203. doi: 10.1016/j.bbrc.2005.11.133

Kan, F. W. (1993). Cytochemical evidence for the presence of phospholipids in epithelial tight junction strands. *J. Histochem. Cytochem.* 41, 649–656. doi: 10.1177/41.5.8468446

Katsube, T., Takahisa, M., Ueda, R., Hashimoto, N., Kobayashi, M., and Togashi, S. (1998). Cortactin associates with the cell-cell junction protein ZO-1 in both Drosophila and mouse. *J. Biol. Chem.* 273, 29672–29677. doi: 10.1074/jbc.273.45.29672

Katsuno, T., Umeda, K., Matsui, T., Hata, M., Tamura, A., Itoh, M., et al. (2008). Deficiency of zonula occludens-1 causes embryonic lethal phenotype associated with defected yolk sac angiogenesis and apoptosis of embryonic cells. *Mol. Biol. Cell* 19, 2465–2475. doi: 10.1091/mbc.E07-12-1215

Kausalya, P. J., Phua, D. C., and Hunziker, W. (2004). Association of ARVCF with zonula occludens (ZO)-1 and ZO-2: binding to PDZ-domain proteins and cell-cell adhesion regulate plasma membrane and nuclear localization of ARVCF. *Mol. Biol. Cell* 15, 5503–5515. doi: 10.1091/mbc.E04-04-0350

Kerjaschki, D., Poczewski, H., Dekan, G., Horvat, R., Balzar, E., Kraft, N., et al. (1986). Identification of a major sialoprotein in the glycocalyx of human visceral glomerular epithelial cells. *J. Clin. Invest.* 78, 1142–1149. doi: 10.1172/JCI112694

Kimura, R., Ishida, T., Kuriyama, M., Hirata, K., and Hayashi, Y. (2010). Interaction of endothelial cell-selective adhesion molecule and MAGI-1 promotes mature cell-cell adhesion via activation of RhoA. *Genes Cells* 15, 385–396. doi: 10.1111/j.1365-2443.2010.01387.x

Knust, E., and Bossinger, O. (2002). Composition and formation of intercellular junctions in epithelial cells. *Science* 298, 1955–1959. doi: 10.1126/science.1072161

Krug, S. M., Amasheh, S., Richter, J. F., Milatz, S., Gunzel, D., Westphal, J. K., et al. (2009). Tricellulin forms a barrier to macromolecules in tricellular tight junctions without affecting ion permeability. *Mol. Biol. Cell* 20, 3713–3724. doi: 10.1091/mbc.E09-01-0080

Kuhnert, F., Mancuso, M. R., Shamloo, A., Wang, H. T., Choksi, V., Florek, M., et al. (2010). Essential regulation of CNS angiogenesis by the orphan G protein-coupled receptor GPR124. *Science* 330, 985–989. doi: 10.1126/science.1196554

Lamagna, C., Meda, P., Mandicourt, G., Brown, J., Gilbert, R. J., Jones, E. Y., et al. (2005). Dual interaction of JAM-C with JAM-B and alpha(M)beta2 integrin: function in junctional complexes and leukocyte adhesion. *Mol. Biol. Cell* 16, 4992–5003. doi: 10.1091/mbc.E05-04-0310

Lampugnani, M. G., Orsenigo, F., Rudini, N., Maddaluno, L., Boulday, G., Chapon, F., et al. (2010). CCM1 regulates vascular-lumen organization by inducing endothelial polarity. *J. Cell Sci.* 123, 1073–1080. doi: 10.1242/jcs.059329

Larue, L., Ohsugi, M., Hirchenhain, J., and Kemler, R. (1994). E-cadherin null mutant embryos fail to form a trophectoderm epithelium. *Proc. Natl. Acad. Sci. U.S.A.* 91, 8263–8267. doi: 10.1073/pnas.91.17.8263

Laukoetter, M. G., Nava, P., Lee, W. Y., Severson, E. A., Capaldo, C. T., Babbin, B. A., et al. (2007). JAM-A regulates permeability and inflammation in the intestine *in vivo*. *J. Exp. Med.* 204, 3067–3076. doi: 10.1084/jem.20071416

Lee, C. Y., and Bautch, V. L. (2011). Ups and downs of guided vessel sprouting: the role of polarity. *Physiology (Bethesda).* 26, 326–333. doi: 10.1152/physiol.00018.2011

Lee, D. B., Jamgotchian, N., Allen, S. G., Abeles, M. B., and Ward, H. J. (2008). A lipid-protein hybrid model for tight junction. *Am. J. Physiolo. Renal Physiol.* 295, F1601–F1612. doi: 10.1152/ajprenal.00097.2008

Lee, J. L., and Streuli, C. H. (2014). Integrins and epithelial cell polarity. *J. Cell Sci.* 127, 3217–3225. doi: 10.1242/jcs.146142

Lee, S. W., Kim, W. J., Choi, Y. K., Song, H. S., Son, M. J., Gelman, I. H., et al. (2003). SSeCKS regulates angiogenesis and tight junction formation in blood-brain barrier. *Nat. Med.* 9, 900–906. doi: 10.1038/nm889

Li, S., Haigh, K., Haigh, J. J., and Vasudevan, A. (2013). Endothelial VEGF sculpts cortical cytoarchitecture. *J. Neurosci.* 33, 14809–14815. doi: 10.1523/JNEUROSCI.1368-13.2013

Liebner, S., Corada, M., Bangsow, T., Babbage, J., Taddei, A., Czupalla, C. J., et al. (2008). Wnt/beta-catenin signaling controls development of the blood-brain barrier. *J. Cell Biol.* 183, 409–417. doi: 10.1083/jcb.200806024

Liebner, S., Fischmann, A., Rascher, G., Duffner, F., Grote, E. H., Kalbacher, H., et al. (2000a). Claudin-1 and claudin-5 expression and tight junction morphology are altered in blood vessels of human glioblastoma multiforme. *Acta Neuropathol. (Berl.)* 100, 323–331. doi: 10.1007/s004010000180

Liebner, S., Kniesel, U., Kalbacher, H., and Wolburg, H. (2000b). Correlation of tight junction morphology with the expression of tight junction proteins in blood-brain barrier endothelial cells. *Eur. J. Cell Biol.* 79, 707–717. doi: 10.1078/0171-9335-00101

Lin, D., Edwards, A. S., Fawcett, J. P., Mbamalu, G., Scott, J. D., and Pawson, T. (2000). A mammalian PAR-3-PAR-6 complex implicated in Cdc42/Rac1 and aPKC signalling and cell polarity. *Nat. Cell Biol.* 2, 540–547. doi: 10.1038/35019592

Lindahl, P., Johansson, B. R., Leveen, P., and Betsholtz, C. (1997). Pericyte loss and microaneurysm formation in PDGF-B-deficient mice. *Science* 277, 242–245. doi: 10.1126/science.277.5323.242

Lippoldt, A., Kniesel, U., Liebner, S., Kalbacher, H., Kirsch, T., Wolburg, H., et al. (2000). Structural alterations of tight junctions are associated with loss of polarity in stroke-prone spontaneously hypertensive rat blood-brain barrier endothelial cells. *Brain Res.* 885, 251–261. doi: 10.1016/S0006-8993(00)02954-1

Liu, Y., Nusrat, A., Schnell, F. J., Reaves, T. A., Walsh, S., Pochet, M., et al. (2000). Human junction adhesion molecule regulates tight junction resealing in epithelia [In Process Citation]. *J. Cell Sci.* 113, 2363–2374.

Lizama, C. O., and Zovein, A. C. (2013). Polarizing pathways: balancing endothelial polarity, permeability, and lumen formation. *Exp. Cell Res.* 319, 1247–1254. doi: 10.1016/j.yexcr.2013.03.028

Lopez-Bayghen, E., Jaramillo, B., Huerta, M., Betanzos, A., and Gonzalez-Mariscal, L. (2006). "TJ proteins that make round trips to the nucleus," in *Tight Junctions*, ed L. Gonzalez-Mariscal (Georgetown, TX: Landes Bioscience, Springer), 76–100.

Lubarsky, B., and Krasnow, M. A. (2003). Tube morphogenesis: making and shaping biological tubes. *Cell* 112, 19–28. doi: 10.1016/S0092-8674(02)01283-7

Luissint, A. C., Federici, C., Guillonneau, F., Chretien, F., Camoin, L., Glacial, F., et al. (2012). Guanine nucleotide-binding protein Galphai2: a new partner of claudin-5 that regulates tight junction integrity in human brain endothelial cells. *J. Cereb. Blood Flow Metab.* 32, 860–873. doi: 10.1038/jcbfm.2011.202

Luo, Y., and Radice, G. L. (2005). N-cadherin acts upstream of VE-cadherin in controlling vascular morphogenesis. *J. Cell Biol.* 169, 29–34. doi: 10.1083/jcb.200411127

Macara, I. G. (2004). Parsing the polarity code. *Nat. Rev. Mol. Cell Biol.* 5, 220–231. doi: 10.1038/nrm1332

Maddaluno, L., Rudini, N., Cuttano, R., Bravi, L., Giampietro, C., Corada, M., et al. (2013). EndMT contributes to the onset and progression of cerebral cavernous malformations. *Nature* 498, 492–496. doi: 10.1038/nature12207

Mariano, C., Palmela, I., Pereira, P., Fernandes, A., Falcao, A. S., Cardoso, F. L., et al. (2013). Tricellulin expression in brain endothelial and neural cells. *Cell Tissue Res.* 351, 397–407. doi: 10.1007/s00441-012-1529-y

Mark, K. S., and Davis, T. P. (2002). Cerebral microvascular changes in permeability and tight junctions induced by hypoxia-reoxygenation. *Am. J. Physiol. Heart Circ. Physiol.* 282, H1485–H1494. doi: 10.1152/ajpheart.00645.2001

Martin-Belmonte, F., Gassama, A., Datta, A., Yu, W., Rescher, U., Gerke, V., et al. (2007). PTEN-mediated apical segregation of phosphoinositides controls epithelial morphogenesis through Cdc42. *Cell* 128, 383–397. doi: 10.1016/j.cell.2006.11.051

Martin-Padura, I., Lostaglio, S., Schneemann, M., Williams, L., Romano, M., Fruscella, P., et al. (1998). Junctional adhesion molecule, a novel member of the immunoglobulin superfamily that distributes at intercellular junctions and modulates monocyte transmigration. *J. Cell Biol.* 142, 117–127. doi: 10.1083/jcb.142.1.117

Martinez-Estrada, O. M., Villa, A., Breviario, F., Orsenigo, F., Dejana, E., and Bazzoni, G. (2001). Association of junctional adhesion molecule with calcium/calmodulin-dependent serine protein kinase (CASK/LIN-2) in human epithelial caco-2 cells. *J. Biol. Chem.* 276, 9291–9296. doi: 10.1074/jbc.M006991200

Mattagajasingh, S. N., Huang, S. C., Hartenstein, J. S., and Benz, E. J. Jr. (2000). Characterization of the interaction between protein 4.1R and ZO-2: a possible link between the tight junction and the actin cytoskeleton. *J. Biol. Chem.* 275, 30573–30585. doi: 10.1074/jbc.M004578200

Mazaud-Guittot, S., Meugnier, E., Pesenti, S., Wu, X., Vidal, H., Gow, A., et al. (2010). Claudin 11 deficiency in mice results in loss of the Sertoli cell epithelial phenotype in the testis. *Biol. Reprod.* 82, 202–213. doi: 10.1095/biolreprod.109.078907

McCarthy, K. M., Skare, I. B., Stankewich, M. C., Furuse, M., Tsukita, S., Rogers, R. A., et al. (1996). Occludin is a functional component of the tight junction. *J. Cell Sci.* 109, 2287–2298.

McCrea, P. D., Gu, D., and Balda, M. S. (2009). Junctional music that the nucleus hears: cell-cell contact signaling and the modulation of gene activity. *Cold Spring Harb. Perspect. Biol.* 1:a002923. doi: 10.1101/cshperspect.a002923

Meder, D., Shevchenko, A., Simons, K., and Fullekrug, J. (2005). Gp135/podocalyxin and NHERF-2 participate in the formation of a preapical domain during polarization of MDCK cells. *J. Cell Biol.* 168, 303–313. doi: 10.1083/jcb.200407072

Michaelis, U. R., Chavakis, E., Kruse, C., Jungblut, B., Kaluza, D., Wandzioch, K., et al. (2013). The polarity protein Scrib is essential for directed endothelial cell migration. *Circ. Res.* 112, 924–934. doi: 10.1161/CIRCRESAHA.112.300592

Mineta, K., Yamamoto, Y., Yamazaki, Y., Tanaka, H., Tada, Y., Saito, K., et al. (2011). Predicted expansion of the claudin multigene family. *FEBS Lett.* 585, 606–612. doi: 10.1016/j.febslet.2011.01.028

Mochida, G. H., Ganesh, V. S., Felie, J. M., Gleason, D., Hill, R. S., Clapham, K. R., et al. (2010). A homozygous mutation in the tight-junction protein JAM3 causes hemorrhagic destruction of the brain, subependymal calcification, and congenital cataracts. *Am. J. Hum. Genet.* 87, 882–889. doi: 10.1016/j.ajhg.2010.10.026

Morita, K., Sasaki, H., Furuse, M., and Tsukita, S. (1999). Endothelial claudin: claudin-5/TMVCF constitutes tight junction strands in endothelial cells. *J. Cell Biol.* 147, 185–194. doi: 10.1083/jcb.147.1.185

Morris, S. A., and Zernicka-Goetz, M. (2012). Formation of distinct cell types in the mouse blastocyst. *Results Probl. Cell Differ.* 55, 203–217. doi: 10.1007/978-3-642-30406-4_11

Muhleisen, H., Wolburg, H., and Betz, E. (1989). Freeze-fracture analysis of endothelial cell membranes in rabbit carotid arteries subjected to short-term atherogenic stimuli. *Virchows Arch. B Cell Pathol. Incl. Mol. Pathol.* 56, 413–417. doi: 10.1007/BF02890045

Murakami, T., Felinski, E. A., and Antonetti, D. A. (2009). Occludin phosphorylation and ubiquitination regulate tight junction trafficking and vascular endothelial growth factor-induced permeability. *J. Biol. Chem.* 284, 21036–21046. doi: 10.1074/jbc.M109.016766

Nagy, Z., Peters, H., and Huttner, I. (1984). Fracture faces of cell junctions in cerebral endothelium during normal and hyperosmotic conditions. *Lab. Invest.* 50, 313–322.

Nasdala, I., Wolburg-Buchholz, K., Wolburg, H., Kuhn, A., Ebnet, K., Brachtendorf, G., et al. (2002). A transmembrane tight junction protein selectively expressed on endothelial cells and platelets. *J. Biol. Chem.* 277, 16294–16303. doi: 10.1074/jbc.M111999200

Nery, S., Corbin, J. G., and Fishell, G. (2003). Dlx2 progenitor migration in wild type and Nkx2.1 mutant telencephalon. *Cereb. Cortex* 13, 895–903. doi: 10.1093/cercor/13.9.895

Ngok, S. P., Geyer, R., Liu, M., Kourtidis, A., Agrawal, S., Wu, C., et al. (2012). VEGF and Angiopoietin-1 exert opposing effects on cell junctions by regulating the Rho GEF Syx. *J. Cell Biol.* 199, 1103–1115. doi: 10.1083/jcb.201207009

Nielsen, J. S., Graves, M. L., Chelliah, S., Vogl, A. W., Roskelley, C. D., and McNagny, K. M. (2007). The CD34-related molecule podocalyxin is a potent inducer of microvillus formation. *PLoS ONE* 2:e237. doi: 10.1371/journal.pone.0000237

Nitta, T., Hata, M., Gotoh, S., Seo, Y., Sasaki, H., Hashimoto, N., et al. (2003). Size-selective loosening of the blood-brain barrier in claudin-5-deficient mice. *J. Cell Biol.* 161, 653–660. doi: 10.1083/jcb.200302070

Nusrat, A., Giry, M., Turner, J. R., Colgan, S. P., Parkos, C. A., Carnes, D., et al. (1995). Rho protein regulates tight junctions and perijunctional actin organization in polarized epithelia. *Proc. Natl. Acad. Sci. U.S.A.* 92, 10629–10633. doi: 10.1073/pnas.92.23.10629

O'Driscoll, M. C., Daly, S. B., Urquhart, J. E., Black, G. C., Pilz, D. T., Brockmann, K., et al. (2010). Recessive mutations in the gene encoding the tight junction protein occludin cause band-like calcification with simplified gyration and polymicrogyria. *Am. J. Hum. Genet.* 87, 354–364. doi: 10.1016/j.ajhg.2010.07.012

Ohtsuki, S., Sato, S., Yamaguchi, H., Kamoi, M., Asashima, T., and Terasaki, T. (2007). Exogenous expression of claudin-5 induces barrier properties in cultured rat brain capillary endothelial cells. *J. Cell. Physiol.* 210, 81–86. doi: 10.1002/jcp.20823

Osada, T., Gu, Y. H., Kanazawa, M., Tsubota, Y., Hawkins, B. T., Spatz, M., et al. (2011). Interendothelial claudin-5 expression depends on cerebral endothelial cell-matrix adhesion by beta(1)-integrins. *J. Cerebral Blood Flow Metab.* 31, 1972–1985. doi: 10.1038/jcbfm.2011.99

Otani, T., Ichii, T., Aono, S., and Takeichi, M. (2006). Cdc42 GEF Tuba regulates the junctional configuration of simple epithelial cells. *J. Cell Biol.* 175, 135–146. doi: 10.1083/jcb.200605012

Palmeri, D., Van Zante, A., Huang, C. C., Hemmerich, S., and Rosen, S. D. (2000). Vascular endothelial junction-associated molecule, a novel member of the immunoglobulin superfamily, is localized to intercellular boundaries of endothelial cells. *J. Biol. Chem.* 275, 19139–19145. doi: 10.1074/jbc.M003189200

Paolinelli, R., Corada, M., Ferrarini, L., Devraj, K., Artus, C., Czupalla, C. J., et al. (2013). Wnt activation of immortalized brain endothelial cells as a tool for generating a standardized model of the blood brain barrier *in vitro*. *PLoS ONE* 8:e70233. doi: 10.1371/journal.pone.0070233

Paschoud, S., Yu, D., Pulimeno, P., Jond, L., Turner, J. R., and Citi, S. (2011). Cingulin and paracingulin show similar dynamic behaviour, but are recruited independently to junctions. *Mol. Membr. Biol.* 28, 123–135. doi: 10.3109/09687688.2010.538937

Phua, D. C., Xu, J., Ali, S. M., Boey, A., Gounko, N. V., and Hunziker, W. (2014). ZO-1 and ZO-2 are required for extra-embryonic endoderm integrity, primitive ectoderm survival and normal cavitation in embryoid bodies derived from mouse embryonic stem cells. *PLoS ONE* 9:e99532. doi: 10.1371/journal.pone.0099532

Qin, Y., Capaldo, C., Gumbiner, B. M., and Macara, I. G. (2005). The mammalian Scribble polarity protein regulates epithelial cell adhesion and migration through E-cadherin. *J. Cell Biol.* 171, 1061–1071. doi: 10.1083/jcb.200506094

Raab, S., Beck, H., Gaumann, A., Yuce, A., Gerber, H. P., Plate, K., et al. (2004). Impaired brain angiogenesis and neuronal apoptosis induced by conditional homozygous inactivation of vascular endothelial growth factor. *Thromb. Haemost.* 91, 595–605. doi: 10.1160/TH03-09-0582

Rajasekaran, A. K., Hojo, M., Huima, T., and Rodriguez-Boulan, E. (1996). Catenins and zonula occludens-1 form a complex during early stages in the assembly of tight junctions. *J. Cell Biol.* 132, 451–463. doi: 10.1083/jcb.132.3.451

Raleigh, D. R., Marchiando, A. M., Zhang, Y., Shen, L., Sasaki, H., Wang, Y., et al. (2010). Tight junction-associated MARVEL proteins marveld3, tricellulin, and occludin have distinct but overlapping functions. *Mol. Biol. Cell* 21, 1200–1213. doi: 10.1091/mbc.E09-08-0734

Raschperger, E., Engstrom, U., Pettersson, R. F., and Fuxe, J. (2004). CLMP, a novel member of the CTX family and a new component of epithelial tight junctions. *J. Biol. Chem.* 279, 796–804. doi: 10.1074/jbc.M308249200

Raschperger, E., Thyberg, J., Pettersson, S., Philipson, L., Fuxe, J., and Pettersson, R. F. (2006). The coxsackie- and adenovirus receptor (CAR) is an *in vivo* marker for epithelial tight junctions, with a potential role in regulating permeability and tissue homeostasis. *Exp. Cell Res.* 312, 1566–1580. doi: 10.1016/j.yexcr.2006.01.025

Renz, A., and Fackelmayer, F. O. (1996). Purification and molecular cloning of the scaffold attachment factor B (SAF-B), a novel human nuclear protein that specifically binds to S/MAR-DNA. *Nucleic Acids Res.* 24, 843–849. doi: 10.1093/nar/24.5.843

Reuss, B., Dono, R., and Unsicker, K. (2003). Functions of fibroblast growth factor (FGF)-2 and FGF-5 in astroglial differentiation and blood-brain barrier permeability: evidence from mouse mutants. *J. Neurosci.* 23, 6404–6412.

Robbins, R. M., and Beitel, G. J. (2010). Vascular lumen formation: negativity will tear us apart. *Curr. Biol.* 20, R973–R975. doi: 10.1016/j.cub.2010.10.032

Rodriguez-Boulan, E., and Macara, I. G. (2014). Organization and execution of the epithelial polarity programme. *Nat. Rev. Mol. Cell Biol.* 15, 225–242. doi: 10.1038/nrm3775

Rosenberg, G. A. (2012). Neurological diseases in relation to the blood-brain barrier. *J. Cereb. Blood Flow Metab.* 32, 1139–1151. doi: 10.1038/jcbfm.2011.197

Rossant, J., and Tam, P. P. (2009). Blastocyst lineage formation, early embryonic asymmetries and axis patterning in the mouse. *Development* 136, 701–713. doi: 10.1242/dev.017178

Saha, C., Nigam, S. K., and Denker, B. M. (1998). Involvement of Galphai2 in the maintenance and biogenesis of epithelial cell tight junctions. *J. Biol. Chem.* 273, 21629–21633. doi: 10.1074/jbc.273.34.21629

Saitou, M., Fujimoto, K., Doi, Y., Itoh, M., Fujimoto, T., Furuse, M., et al. (1998). Occludin-deficient embryonic stem cells can differentiate into polarized epithelial cells bearing tight junctions. *J. Cell Biol.* 141, 397–408. doi: 10.1083/jcb.141.2.397

Saitou, M., Furuse, M., Sasaki, H., Schulzke, J. D., Fromm, M., Takano, H., et al. (2000). Complex phenotype of mice lacking occludin, a component of tight junction strands. *Mol. Biol. Cell* 11, 4131–4142. doi: 10.1091/mbc.11.12.4131

Sakakibara, A., Furuse, M., Saitou, M., Ando-Akatsuka, Y., and Tsukita, S. (1997). Possible involvement of phosphorylation of occludin in tight junction formation. *J. Cell Biol.* 137, 1393–1401. doi: 10.1083/jcb.137.6.1393

Sakurai, A., Fukuhara, S., Yamagishi, A., Sako, K., Kamioka, Y., Masuda, M., et al. (2006). MAGI-1 is required for Rap1 activation upon cell-cell contact and for enhancement of vascular endothelial cadherin-mediated cell adhesion. *Mol. Biol. Cell* 17, 966–976. doi: 10.1091/mbc.E05-07-0647

Sato, T., Fujita, N., Yamada, A., Ooshio, T., Okamoto, R., Irie, K., et al. (2006). Regulation of the assembly and adhesion activity of E-cadherin by nectin and afadin for the formation of adherens junctions in Madin-Darby canine kidney cells. *J. Biol. Chem.* 281, 5288–5299. doi: 10.1074/jbc.M510070200

Schrade, A., Sade, H., Couraud, P. O., Romero, I. A., Weksler, B. B., and Niewoehner, J. (2012). Expression and localization of claudins-3 and -12 in transformed human brain endothelium. *Fluids Barriers CNS* 9:6. doi: 10.1186/2045-8118-9-6

Schulze, C., Smales, C., Rubin, L. L., and Staddon, J. M. (1997). Lysophosphatidic acid increases tight junction permeability in cultured brain endothelial cells. *J. Neurochem.* 68, 991–1000. doi: 10.1046/j.1471-4159.1997.68030991.x

Schulzke, J. D., Gitter, A. H., Mankertz, J., Spiegel, S., Seidler, U., Amasheh, S., et al. (2005). Epithelial transport and barrier function in occludin-deficient mice. *Biochim. Biophys. Acta* 1669, 34–42. doi: 10.1016/j.bbamem.2005.01.008

Sheth, B., Fontaine, J. J., Ponza, E., McCallum, A., Page, A., Citi, S., et al. (2000). Differentiation of the epithelial apical junctional complex during mouse preimplantation development: a role for rab13 in the early maturation of the tight junction. *Mech. Dev.* 97, 93–104. doi: 10.1016/S0925-4773(00)00416-0

Sheth, B., Nowak, R. L., Anderson, R., Kwong, W. Y., Papenbrock, T., and Fleming, T. P. (2008). Tight junction protein ZO-2 expression and relative function of ZO-1 and ZO-2 during mouse blastocyst formation. *Exp. Cell Res.* 314, 3356–3368. doi: 10.1016/j.yexcr.2008.08.021

Shin, K., Straight, S., and Margolis, B. (2005). PATJ regulates tight junction formation and polarity in mammalian epithelial cells. *J. Cell Biol.* 168, 705–711. doi: 10.1083/jcb.200408064

Simionescu, M., Simionescu, N., and Palade, G. E. (1976). Segmental differentiations of cell junctions in the vascular endothelium. Arteries and veins. *J. Cell Biol.* 68, 705–723. doi: 10.1083/jcb.68.3.705

Sonoda, N., Furuse, M., Sasaki, H., Yonemura, S., Katahira, J., Horiguchi, Y., et al. (1999). Clostridium perfringens enterotoxin fragment removes specific claudins from tight junction strands: evidence for direct involvement of claudins in tight junction barrier. *J. Cell Biol.* 147, 195–204. doi: 10.1083/jcb.147.1.195

St Johnston, D., and Ahringer, J. (2010). Cell polarity in eggs and epithelia: parallels and diversity. *Cell* 141, 757–774. doi: 10.1016/j.cell.2010.05.011

Staehelin, L. A. (1973). Further observations on the fine structure of freeze-cleaved tight junctions. *J. Cell Sci.* 13, 763–786.

Staehelin, L. A. (1974). Structure and function of intercellular junctions. *Int. Rev. Cytol.* 39, 191–283. doi: 10.1016/S0074-7696(08)60940-7

Steed, E., Balda, M. S., and Matter, K. (2010). Dynamics and functions of tight junctions. *Trends Cell Biol.* 20, 142–149. doi: 10.1016/j.tcb.2009.12.002

Steed, E., Rodrigues, N. T., Balda, M. S., and Matter, K. (2009). Identification of MarvelD3 as a tight junction-associated transmembrane protein of the occludin family. *BMC Cell Biol.* 10:95. doi: 10.1186/1471-2121-10-95

Stenman, J. M., Rajagopal, J., Carroll, T. J., Ishibashi, M., McMahon, J., and McMahon, A. P. (2008). Canonical Wnt signaling regulates organ-specific assembly and differentiation of CNS vasculature. *Science* 322, 1247–1250. doi: 10.1126/science.1164594

Stern, L., and Gauthier, R. (1921). Recherches sur le liquid cephalo-rachidien. 1. Les rapports entre le liquide cephalo-rachidien et la circulatioon sanguine. *Arch. Int. Physiol.* 17, 138–192. doi: 10.3109/13813452109146211

Stern, L., and Rothlin, E. (1918). Effets de l'action directe du curare sur les différentes parties du cervelet. *Schweiz Arch. Neurol. Psychiatry* 3, 234–254.

Stevenson, B. R., Anderson, J. M., and Bullivant, S. (1988). The epithelial tight junction: structure, function and preliminary biochemical characterization. *Mol. Cell. Biochem.* 83, 129–145. doi: 10.1007/BF00226141

Stevenson, B. R., Siliciano, J. D., Mooseker, M. S., and Goodenough, D. A. (1986). Identification of ZO-1: a high molecular weight polypeptide associated with the tight junction (zonula occludens) in a variety of epithelia. *J. Cell Biol.* 103, 755–766. doi: 10.1083/jcb.103.3.755

Stewart, P. A., and Wiley, M. J. (1981). Developing nervous tissue induces formation of blood-brain barrier characteristics in invading endothelial cells: a study using quail–chick transplantation chimeras. *Dev. Biol.* 84, 183–192. doi: 10.1016/0012-1606(81)90382-1

Strilic, B., Eglinger, J., Krieg, M., Zeeb, M., Axnick, J., Babal, P., et al. (2010). Electrostatic cell-surface repulsion initiates lumen formation in developing blood vessels. *Curr. Biol.* 20, 2003–2009. doi: 10.1016/j.cub.2010.09.061

Strilic, B., Kucera, T., Eglinger, J., Hughes, M. R., McNagny, K. M., Tsukita, S., et al. (2009). The molecular basis of vascular lumen formation in the developing mouse aorta. *Dev. Cell* 17, 505–515. doi: 10.1016/j.devcel.2009.08.011

Stuart, R. O., Sun, A., Panichas, M., Hebert, S. C., Brenner, B. M., and Nigam, S. K. (1994). Critical role for intracellular calcium in tight junction biogenesis. *J. Cell. Physiol.* 159, 423–433. doi: 10.1002/jcp.1041590306

Sussel, L., Marin, O., Kimura, S., and Rubenstein, J. L. (1999). Loss of Nkx2.1 homeobox gene function results in a ventral to dorsal molecular respecification within the basal telencephalon: evidence for a transformation of the pallidum into the striatum. *Development* 126, 3359–3370.

Tachibana, K., Nakanishi, H., Mandai, K., Ozaki, K., Ikeda, W., Yamamoto, Y., et al. (2000). Two cell adhesion molecules, nectin and cadherin, interact through their cytoplasmic domain-associated proteins. *J. Cell Biol.* 150, 1161–1176. doi: 10.1083/jcb.150.5.1161

Takai, Y., Ikeda, W., Ogita, H., and Rikitake, Y. (2008a). The immunoglobulin-like cell adhesion molecule nectin and its associated protein afadin. *Annu. Rev. Cell Dev. Biol.* 24, 309–342. doi: 10.1146/annurev.cellbio.24.110707.175339

Takai, Y., Miyoshi, J., Ikeda, W., and Ogita, H. (2008b). Nectins and nectin-like molecules: roles in contact inhibition of cell movement and proliferation. *Nat. Rev. Mol. Cell Biol.* 9, 603–615. doi: 10.1038/nrm2457

Takaoka, K., and Hamada, H. (2012). Cell fate decisions and axis determination in the early mouse embryo. *Development* 139, 3–14. doi: 10.1242/dev.060095

Tao-Cheng, J. H., Nagy, Z., and Brightman, M. W. (1987). Tight junctions of brain endothelium *in vitro* are enhanced by astroglia. *J. Neurosci.* 7, 3293–3299.

Te Velthuis, A. J., Admiraal, J. F., and Bagowski, C. P. (2007). Molecular evolution of the MAGUK family in metazoan genomes. *BMC Evol. Biol.* 7:129. doi: 10.1186/1471-2148-7-129

Tepass, U. (2012). The apical polarity protein network in Drosophila epithelial cells: regulation of polarity, junctions, morphogenesis, cell growth, and survival. *Annu. Rev. Cell Dev. Biol.* 28, 655–685. doi: 10.1146/annurev-cellbio-092910-154033

Thomas, F. C., Sheth, B., Eckert, J. J., Bazzoni, G., Dejana, E., and Fleming, T. P. (2004). Contribution of JAM-1 to epithelial differentiation and tight-junction biogenesis in the mouse preimplantation embryo. *J. Cell Sci.* 117, 5599–5608. doi: 10.1242/jcs.01424

Tong, X. K., and Hamel, E. (1999). Regional cholinergic denervation of cortical microvessels and nitric oxide synthase-containing neurons in Alzheimer's disease. *Neuroscience* 92, 163–175. doi: 10.1016/S0306-4522(98)00750-7

Traweger, A., Fang, D., Liu, Y. C., Stelzhammer, W., Krizbai, I. A., Fresser, F., et al. (2002). The Tight Junction-specific Protein Occludin Is a Functional Target of the E3 Ubiquitin-protein Ligase Itch. *J. Biol. Chem.* 277, 10201–10208. doi: 10.1074/jbc.M111384200

Traweger, A., Fuchs, R., Krizbai, I. A., Weiger, T. M., Bauer, H. C., and Bauer, H. (2003). The tight junction protein ZO-2 localizes to the nucleus and interacts with the heterogeneous nuclear ribonucleoprotein scaffold attachment factor-B. *J. Biol. Chem.* 278, 2692–2700. doi: 10.1074/jbc.M206821200

Tsukamoto, T., and Nigam, S. K. (1999). Role of tyrosine phosphorylation in the reassembly of occludin and other tight junction proteins. *Am. J. Physiol.* 276, F737–F750.

Tsukita, S., Furuse, M., and Itoh, M. (2001). Multifunctional strands in tight junctions. *Nat. Rev. Mol. Cell Biol.* 2, 285–293. doi: 10.1038/35067088

Umeda, K., Ikenouchi, J., Katahira-Tayama, S., Furuse, K., Sasaki, H., Nakayama, M., et al. (2006). ZO-1 and ZO-2 independently determine where claudins are polymerized in tight-junction strand formation. *Cell* 126, 741–754. doi: 10.1016/j.cell.2006.06.043

Van Deurs, B., and Koehler, J. K. (1979). Tight junctions in the choroid plexus epithelium. A freeze-fracture study including complementary replicas. *J. Cell Biol.* 80, 662–673. doi: 10.1083/jcb.80.3.662

Van Meer, G., Gumbiner, B., and Simons, K. (1986). The tight junction does not allow lipid molecules to diffuse from one epithelial cell to the next. *Nature* 322, 639–641. doi: 10.1038/322639a0

Vasudevan, A., Long, J. E., Crandall, J. E., Rubenstein, J. L., and Bhide, P. G. (2008). Compartment-specific transcription factors orchestrate angiogenesis gradients in the embryonic brain. *Nat. Neurosci.* 11, 429–439. doi: 10.1038/nn2074

Vaucher, E., Tong, X. K., Cholet, N., Lantin, S., and Hamel, E. (2000). GABA neurons provide a rich input to microvessels but not nitric oxide neurons in the rat cerebral cortex: a means for direct regulation of local cerebral blood flow. *J. Comp. Neurol.* 421, 161–171. doi: 10.1002/(SICI)1096-9861(20000529)421:2<161::AID-CNE3>3.0.CO;2-F

Wang, Q., Chen, X. W., and Margolis, B. (2007). PALS1 regulates E-cadherin trafficking in mammalian epithelial cells. *Mol. Biol. Cell* 18, 874–885. doi: 10.1091/mbc.E06-07-0651

Wang, Q., and Margolis, B. (2007). Apical junctional complexes and cell polarity. *Kidney Int.* 72, 1448–1458. doi: 10.1038/sj.ki.5002579

Wang, Y., Li, Z., Xu, P., Huang, L., Tong, J., Huang, H., et al. (2011). Angiomotin-like2 gene (amotl2) is required for migration and proliferation of endothelial cells during angiogenesis. *J. Biol. Chem.* 286, 41095–41104. doi: 10.1074/jbc.M111.296806

Watson, P. M., Paterson, J. C., Thom, G., Ginman, U., Lundquist, S., and Webster, C. I. (2013). Modelling the endothelial blood-CNS barriers: a method for the production of robust *in vitro* models of the rat blood-brain barrier and blood-spinal cord barrier. *BMC Neurosci.* 14:59. doi: 10.1186/1471-2202-14-59

Wegmann, F., Ebnet, K., Du Pasquier, L., Vestweber, D., and Butz, S. (2004). Endothelial adhesion molecule ESAM binds directly to the multidomain adaptor MAGI-1 and recruits it to cell contacts. *Exp. Cell Res.* 300, 121–133. doi: 10.1016/j.yexcr.2004.07.010

Wegmann, F., Petri, B., Khandoga, A. G., Moser, C., Khandoga, A., Volkery, S., et al. (2006). ESAM supports neutrophil extravasation, activation of Rho, and VEGF-induced vascular permeability. *J. Exp. Med.* 203, 1671–1677. doi: 10.1084/jem.20060565

Weidenfeller, C., Svendsen, C. N., and Shusta, E. V. (2007). Differentiating embryonic neural progenitor cells induce blood-brain barrier properties. *J. Neurochem.* 101, 555–565. doi: 10.1111/j.1471-4159.2006.04394.x

Weksler, B. B., Subileau, E. A., Perriere, N., Charneau, P., Holloway, K., Leveque, M., et al. (2005). Blood-brain barrier-specific properties of a human adult brain endothelial cell line. *FASEB J.* 19, 1872–1874. doi: 10.1096/fj.04-3458fje

Wilhelm, I., and Krizbai, I. A. (2014). *In vitro* models of the blood-brain barrier for the study of drug delivery to the brain. *Mol. Pharm.* 11, 1949–1963. doi: 10.1021/mp500046f

Wittchen, E. S., Haskins, J., and Stevenson, B. R. (1999). Protein interactions at the tight junction. Actin has multiple binding partners, and ZO-1 forms independent complexes with ZO-2 and ZO-3. *J. Biol. Chem.* 274, 35179–35185. doi: 10.1074/jbc.274.49.35179

Wojciak-Stothard, B., Potempa, S., Eichholtz, T., and Ridley, A. J. (2001). Rho and Rac but not Cdc42 regulate endothelial cell permeability. *J. Cell Sci.* 114, 1343–1355.

Wolburg, H., Wolburg-Buchholz, K., Kraus, J., Rascher-Eggstein, G., Liebner, S., Hamm, S., et al. (2003). Localization of claudin-3 in tight junctions of the blood-brain barrier is selectively lost during experimental autoimmune encephalomyelitis and human glioblastoma multiforme. *Acta Neuropathol.* 105, 586–592. doi: 10.1007/s00401-003-0688-z

Wong, V. (1997). Phosphorylation of occludin correlates with occludin localization and function at the tight junction. *Am. J. Physiol.* 273, C1859–C1867.

Xu, J., Kausalya, P. J., Phua, D. C., Ali, S. M., Hossain, Z., and Hunziker, W. (2008). Early embryonic lethality of mice lacking ZO-2, but Not ZO-3, reveals critical and nonredundant roles for individual zonula occludens proteins in mammalian development. *Mol. Cell. Biol.* 28, 1669–1678. doi: 10.1128/MCB.00891-07

Yaffe, Y., Shepshelovitch, J., Nevo-Yassaf, I., Yeheskel, A., Shmerling, H., Kwiatek, J. M., et al. (2012). The MARVEL transmembrane motif of occludin mediates oligomerization and targeting to the basolateral surface in epithelia. *J. Cell Sci.* 125, 3545–3556. doi: 10.1242/jcs.100289

Yamagata, K., Tagami, M., Takenaga, F., Yamori, Y., Nara, Y., and Itoh, S. (2003). Polyunsaturated fatty acids induce tight junctions to form in brain capillary endothelial cells. *Neuroscience* 116, 649–656. doi: 10.1016/S0306-4522(02)00715-7

Yamanaka, T., and Ohno, S. (2008). Role of Lgl/Dlg/Scribble in the regulation of epithelial junction, polarity and growth. *Front. Biosci.* 13, 6693–6707. doi: 10.2741/3182

Zeeb, M., Strilic, B., and Lammert, E. (2010). Resolving cell-cell junctions: lumen formation in blood vessels. *Curr. Opin. Cell Biol.* 22, 626–632. doi: 10.1016/j.ceb.2010.07.003

Zheng, Y., Vertuani, S., Nystrom, S., Audebert, S., Meijer, I., Tegnebratt, T., et al. (2009). Angiomotin-like protein 1 controls endothelial polarity and junction stability during sprouting angiogenesis. *Circ. Res.* 105, 260–270. doi: 10.1161/CIRCRESAHA.109.195156

Zovein, A. C., Luque, A., Turlo, K. A., Hofmann, J. J., Yee, K. M., Becker, M. S., et al. (2010). Beta1 integrin establishes endothelial cell polarity and arteriolar lumen formation via a Par3-dependent mechanism. *Dev. Cell* 18, 39–51. doi: 10.1016/j.devcel.2009.12.006

16

The choroid plexuses and their impact on developmental neurogenesis

Pia A. Johansson*

Institute for Stem Cell Research, Helmholtz Center Munich, German Research Center for Environmental Health, Munich, Germany

***Correspondence:**
Pia A. Johansson, Institute for Stem Cell Research, Helmholtz Center Munich, German Research Center for Environmental Health, Ingolstädterlandstr. 1, 85764 Neuherberg/Munich, Germany
e-mail: pia.johansson@helmholtz-muenchen.de

During brain development the neural stem cells are regulated by both intrinsic and extrinsic sources. One site of origin of extrinsic regulation is the developing choroid plexuses, primely situated inside the cerebral ventricles. The choroid plexuses are very active in terms of both secretion and barrier function as soon as they appear during development and control the production and contents of cerebrospinal fluid (CSF). This suggests that regulated secretion of signaling molecules from the choroid plexuses into CSF can regulate neural stem cell behavior (as they are in direct contact with CSF) and thereby neurogenesis and brain development. Here, choroid plexus development, particularly with regards to molecular regulation and specification, is reviewed. This is followed by a review and discussion of the role of the developing choroid plexuses in brain development. In particular, recent evidence suggests a region-specific reciprocal regulation between choroid plexuses and the neural stem cells. This is accomplished by site-specific secretion of signaling molecules from the different choroid plexuses into CSF, as well as brain region specific competence of the neural stem cells to respond to the signaling molecules present in CSF. In conclusion, although in its infancy, the field of choroid plexus regulation of neurogenesis has already and will likely continue to shed new light on our understanding of the control and fine-tuning of overall brain development.

Keywords: choroid plexus, cerebrospinal fluid, neurogenesis, neural stem cells, cerebral cortex, development

INTRODUCTION

Neurogenesis, both in the adult and during development, occurs in a specialized environment established by both the neurogenic (the neural stem cells) and non-neurogenic cells within the neurogenic area, and from cells and compartments in direct contact with the niche (Johansson et al., 2010; Braun and Jessberger, 2014, **Figure 1**). One of these compartments is cerebrospinal fluid (CSF). During development the neural stem cells are located at the apical (ventricle facing) surface of the developing brain tissue (as exemplified in **Figure 1** and **Box 1**). Thus, any molecule present in CSF has the potential to influence the behavior of the cells located at the ventricular surface (i.e., the neural stem cells) and thereby neurogenesis. The possible role of CSF itself in regulating neurogenesis has recently received more attention, however, there has been less focus on the tissue that produces the CSF; namely the choroid plexuses.

The most abundant proteins in CSF (albumin, transferrin, alpha-phetoprotein, fetuin) are derived from plasma and are transferred across the choroid plexus epithelium by a subset of choroid plexus epithelial cells in a highly specific and regulated manner (Johansson et al., 2006; Liddelow et al., 2009, 2011a,b). Over the last decade it has also been shown that in addition to the more classical plasma proteins, CSF contains a variety of comparatively less abundant signaling molecules (e.g., Shh, Igf1, Wnt4, Tgm2, Fgf2, see **Table 1**). Recent data from transcriptome analysis of the choroid plexus, in both the adult and during development (Marques et al., 2011; Johansson et al., 2013), has revealed the expression of a plethora of molecules previously not associated with the choroid plexus which can either intrinsically affect the function of the choroid plexus or be secreted into CSF. Indeed, a recent comparison of human adult CSF showed that of 1050 identified proteins in plasma 877 of these were also found in CSF whereas an astonishing 2204 proteins were found only in CSF (Guldbrandsen et al., 2014). As CSF is in direct contact with the neural stem cells in both the developing and the adult brain and as CSF is mostly regulated via the choroid plexuses, it is not far-fetched to assume that the choroid plexuses could be significant regulators of neurogenesis.

So far, only two papers have described a direct link between altered choroid plexus secretion (i.e., via direct choroid plexus manipulation) and alterations in developmental neurogenesis (Huang et al., 2010; Johansson et al., 2013). Hopefully, the recent increased focus on this signaling axis will lead to further contributions to this field over the coming years. Regulation of neurogenesis via molecules secreted (or transferred) from the choroid plexus into CSF could have potentially far-reaching ramifications for the understanding and treatment of both developmental disorders and pathological situations in the adult brain where modulation of neurogenesis might be beneficial. The role of the choroid plexus-CSF signaling axis in adult neurogenesis is beyond the scope of this review but the interested reader is referred to some recent articles and reviews which highlight this interaction (Falcao et al., 2012; Silva-Vargas et al., 2013; Baruch et al., 2014).

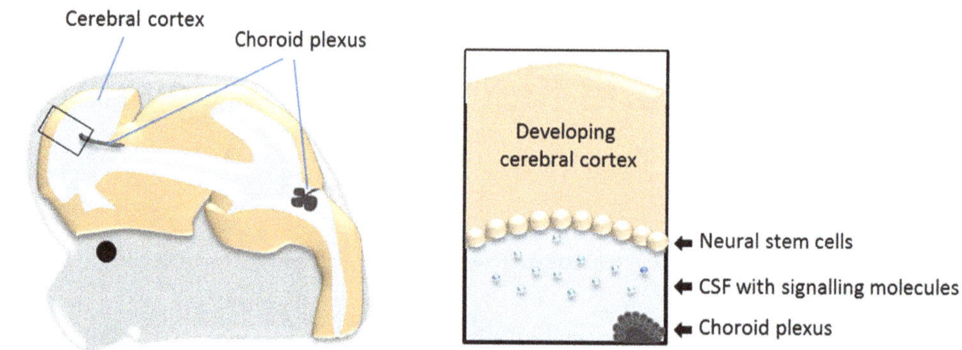

FIGURE 1 | The choroid plexuses, CSF and the neural stem cells during development. Schematic drawing showing the prime location of the choroid plexuses inside the cerebral ventricles and the bathing of the neural stem cells with CSF and molecules within it. CSF, cerebrospinal fluid.

STRUCTURE AND FUNCTION OF THE CHOROID PLEXUSES

The choroid plexuses are four modified epithelial structures suspended inside the cerebral ventricles. There are two lateral ventricular choroid plexuses, the third ventricular choroid plexus and the fourth ventricular (hindbrain) choroid plexus (**Figure 2**). The choroid plexuses consist of a central stroma covered by a single epithelial layer; the polarized choroid plexus epithelium (CPE). The stroma is highly vascularized, consisting of blood vessels, connective tissue and pericytes. The blood vessels are fenestrated and leaky, making them different from blood vessels in the brain parenchyma which are connected by tight junctions and form the blood-brain barrier. Thus, instead of having a barrier at the level of the blood vessels it is the cells of the CPE that are connected by continuous tight-junctional strands, restricting the entry of lipid-insoluble molecules into the CSF (the blood-CSF barrier, **Figure 2**, Brightman and Reese, 1969; Ek et al., 2003; Johansson et al., 2006).

In the adult, the choroid plexuses and CSF have several know functions such as: (i) protecting and regulating the internal environment of the brain via the blood-CSF barrier; (ii) secretion and modulation of CSF through the activity of the choroid plexus epithelial cells; and (iii) waste and metabolite removal, via the "CSF sink," through the continuous production and then removal of CSF into peripheral circulation. During development two out of these three functions are already performed by the choroid plexuses; protection of the brain via the blood-CSF barrier and regulation of CSF composition via specific and regulated transfer and secretion (see more below). However, due to the lack of CSF reabsorption during embryogenesis, the removal of waste and metabolites does not occur (Johansson et al., 2008a). There have also long been suggestions for additional roles for the choroid plexuses during development, such as the generation of an expansive pressure through CSF secretion (Desmond and Jacobson, 1977).

CHOROID PLEXUS DEVELOPMENT

The choroid plexuses are of dual embryonic origin, with the choroid plexus epithelium originating from the ectoderm and the central stroma from the mesoderm (Catala, 1998). The fourth ventricular choroid plexus develops first followed by the two lateral and then the third ventricular choroid plexuses (Dziegielewska et al., 2001). In the mouse the dorsal midline starts to invaginate (from dorsal to ventral) around E10, giving rise to the choroid plexus and, in the forebrain, the adjacent cortical hem (**Figure 3**). The choroid plexus and the hem both express *Lmhx1*, the hem expresses *Wnt* at high levels and the choroid plexus specifically expresses *transthyretin (Ttr)*. *Ttr* is known as *the* choroid plexus marker and is expressed in the mouse lateral ventricular choroid plexus from E11 (**Figure 3**). However, it should be noted that *Ttr* identifies choroid plexus tissue rather than determining the fate of the cells, as in the Ttr knock-out mice the choroid plexuses form normally.

Other molecules and signaling pathways have been shown to be involved in the specification and formation of the choroid plexus. The inhibition of BMP signaling via Foxg1Cre mediated deletion of Bmp1a receptors led to the absence of the lateral ventricular choroid plexuses (Hebert et al., 2002), however in this study the impact on brain development was not further investigated. A similar result was seen in the developing chick when the transcription factors Emx1 and 2 were mis-expressed in the roof plate region, which lead to the absence of *Bmp7* expression and a failure of the dorsal midline to invaginate (Von Frowein et al., 2006). Interestingly, what was also apparent during the latter experiments was that the transcription factor Otx2 was reciprocally inhibited by Emx1/2, suggesting a role of Otx2 in choroid plexus development. Further investigations into the role of Otx2 in choroid plexus development, this time in mice, revealed that it is indeed vital for choroid plexus specification and development (Johansson et al., 2013). Removal of Otx2 from all the choroid plexus anlage (tamoxifen mediated Cre-induction at E9) resulted in an almost complete absence of choroid plexus tissue. Both the Otx2 and Bmp1a deletion show specific roles for these molecules in choroid plexus development as the nearby cortical hem was unaffected in both mutants.

Another group of molecules involved in choroid plexus differentiation are members of the Notch signaling pathway. When the levels of Ngn2 or Hes5 were altered in the telencephalic midline (over-expressed and down-regulated respectively) the choroid plexus was reduced in size but Cajal-Retzius cells were increased in number (Imayoshi et al., 2008), suggesting a reciprocal

Box 1 | Schematic representation of neurogenesis in the developing cerebral cortex.

Neurogenesis in the cerebral cortex goes through a differentiation cascade starting with the neural stem cells (NSCs) lining the ventricle (a.k.a radial glial cells, blue cells). The processes of the NSCs span the entire thickness of the cortical wall and their nuclei move up and down in the ventricular zone (VZ) during the cell cycle (mitosis occurs at the ventricle and S-phase at the basal end of the VZ) but they stay in contact with the ventricle via the apical process and the cilium responsive to elements present in CSF through-out the cell cycle. The NSCs divide and give rise to the next cells in the differentiation cascade, the transient amplifying cells, TAPs (yellow cells) or neurons (green cells). The TAPs are a heterogeneous population and vary in their morphology, location and abundance (see Taverna et al., 2014) but in the mouse cerebral cortex the majority of the TAPs are what is known as basal (or intermediate) progenitors which migrated away from the VZ into the subventricular zone (SVZ). The TAPs then divide again and give rise to the neurons which migrate through the intermediate zone (IZ) into the cortical plate (CP) in an inside-out manner (i.e., the newly-born neurons migrate passed the older neurons and settle in a layer above the previous-born neurons, as illustrated by different shades of green). For a recent comprehensive review see Taverna et al., 2014.

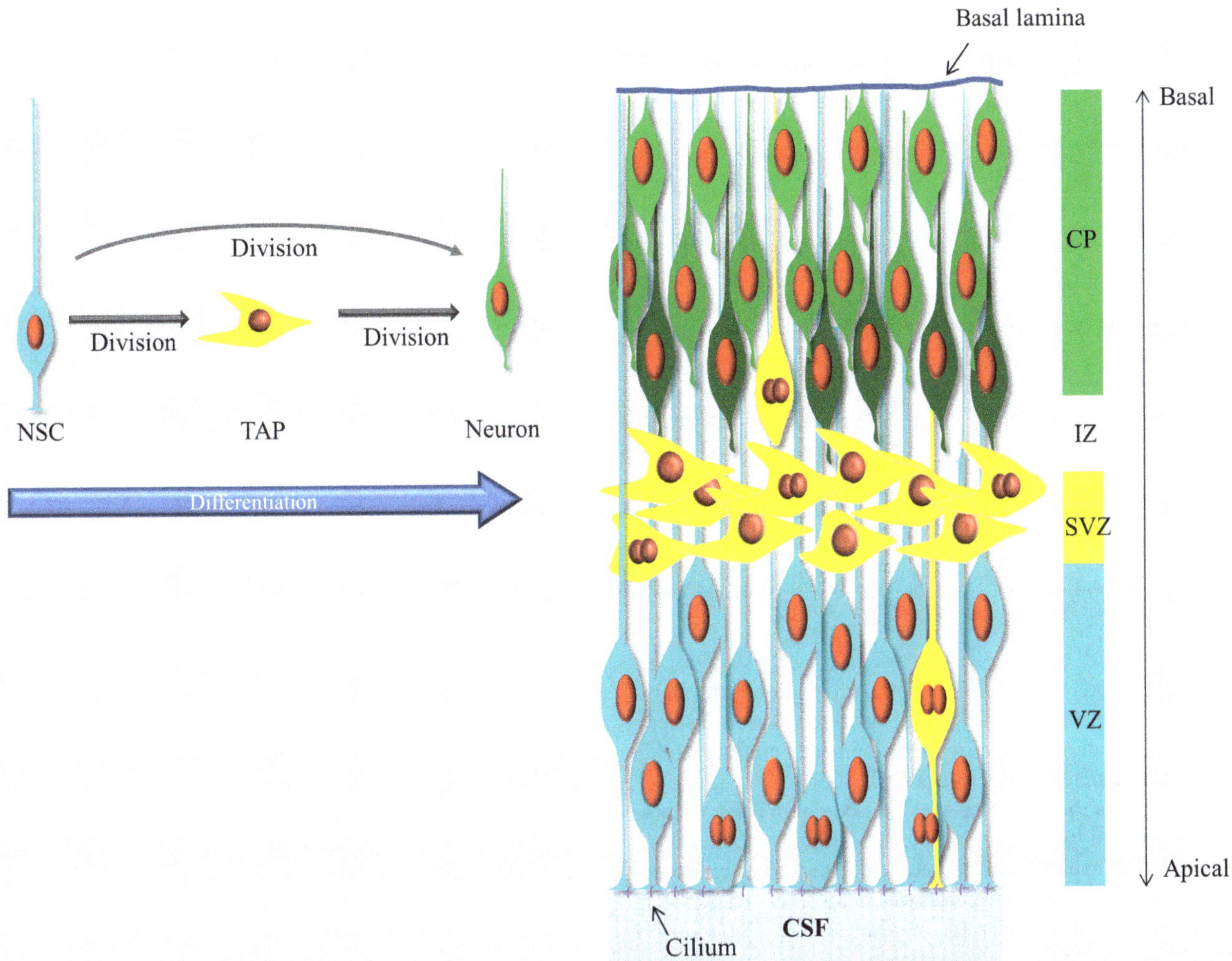

regulation of these cell types. An involvement of Notch signaling in the development of the Zebrafish (*Danio rerio*) choroid plexus has also been described (Bill et al., 2008). Overexpression of Notch1, on the other hand (activated Notch1 in the Gdf7-lineage), massively increased the size of the mouse hindbrain choroid plexus (Hunter and Dymecki, 2007). Further evidence for the involvement of Notch in choroid plexus development includes the formation of choroid plexus tumors after E9 injection of a virus encoding constitutively active Notch3 (Dang et al., 2006). Additionally, alterations in Notch-receptor localization and expression have been found in human choroid plexus tumors when compared to normal choroid plexus tissue (Beschorner et al., 2013).

After choroid plexus specification, the choroid plexus anlage go through a characteristic thinning of the epithelium, going from pseudostratified to a proper single layer epithelium as it starts to invaginate into the ventricles (Dziegielewska et al., 2001). The majority of the choroid plexus epithelial cells are post-mitotic and the plexus grows into the ventricle through addition of cells from the proliferative zone at "the root" (**Figure 3**, Liddelow et al.,

Table 1 | Selected list of secreted signaling molecules expressed in the choroid plexuses.

Gene symbol	Entrez	Gene title	Functional annotations/ Signaling pathways
(A) SECRETED MOLECULES WITH CONFIRMED PRESENCE IN EMBRYONIC CSF AND ABILITY TO INFLUENCE NEUROGENESIS			
Igf2	16002	Insulin-like growth factor 2	Growth factor activity
Shh	20423	Sonic hedgehog	Shh-signaling
Fgf2	14173	Fibroblast growth factor 2	Growth factor activity
Tgm2	21817	Transglutaminase 2, C polypeptide	Wnt-signaling
Wnt4	22417	Wingless-related MMTV integration site 4	Wnt-signaling
(B) SECRETED MOLECULES WITH THE POTENTIAL OF INFLUENCING NEUROGENESIS			
Cthrc1	68588	Collagen triple helix repeat containing 1	Wnt-signaling
Cxcl12	20315	Chemokine (C-X-C motif) ligand 12	Chemokine/growth factor activity
Reln	19699	Reelin	Nervous system development
Dkk2	56811	Dickkopf homolog 2 (Xenopus laevis)	Wnt-signaling
Fgf15	14170	Fibroblast growth factor 15	Growth factor activity
Fgf18	14172	Fibroblast growth factor 18	Growth factor activity
Gdf5	14563	Growth differentiation factor 5	Tgfβ /Hippo-signaling
Pmch	110312	Pro-melanin-concentrating hormone	Neuropeptide signaling
Sema3c	20348	Sema domain, immunoglobulin domain (Ig), short basic domain, secreted, (semaphorin) 3C	Nervous system development
Sfrp2	20319	Secreted frizzled-related protein 2	Wnt/BMP-signaling
Sostdc1	66042	Sclerostin domain containing 1	Wnt/BMP-signaling
Spp1	20750	Secreted phosphoprotein 1	BMP-signaling
Sulf1	240725	Sulfatase 1	Wnt/BMP/FGFreceptor signaling pathway
Tgfb1	21803	Transforming growth factor, beta 1	Tgfβ-signaling
Tgfb2	21808	Transforming growth factor, beta 2	Tgfβ-signaling
Tgfb3	21809	Transforming growth factor, beta 3	Tgfβ-signaling
Wfikkn2	278507	WAP, follistatin/kazal, immunoglobulin, kunitz and netrin domain containing 2	Tgfβ-signaling
Wnt1	22408	Wingless-type MMTV integration site 1	Wnt/BMP-signaling

Molecules in B from Johansson et al. (2013).

2010), which adds to the size of the choroid plexus throughout development. The choroid plexuses go through several stages of morphologically characterized development before reaching maturity postnatally (Dziegielewska et al., 2001).

The stroma of the choroid plexus (mesoderm derived, Catala, 1998), is induced by the choroid plexus anlage. Using chimeric transplantation experiments between chick and quail embryos, it was shown that the choroid plexus anlage (i.e., yet without stroma) from quail transplanted into the gut of a chick embryo induced the formation of a morphologically normal choroid plexus with organotypic fenestrated blood-vessels (Wilting and Christ, 1989). The blood vessels and the stroma were found to be of chick (host) origin demonstrating that the choroid plexus anlage induces the formation of the stroma and the blood vessels therein. In a different experiment they also showed that transplanting a non-choroid plexus forming neural epithelium to the normal site of choroid plexus development, in contact with the prospective stroma, did not induce choroid plexus characteristics (Wilting and Christ, 1989). However, even though neither the stroma nor the blood vessels induce choroid plexus formation, signaling from the stroma to the epithelial cells after stromal formation has been observed. This was seen recently when Shh was deleted from the choroid plexus epithelial cells, which lead to a decrease in Shh-signaling in the Shh responsive cells (choroid plexus progenitor cells and pericytes), which in turn resulted in a much smaller choroid plexus deficient in both vasculature and CPE cells (Huang et al., 2009; Nielsen and Dymecki, 2010).

Interestingly, this also leads us to one of the very few described regional differences between the choroid plexuses; *Shh* is not expressed in the forebrain choroid plexuses, suggesting that other molecules might be responsible for this regulation in the forebrain. Conversely, it appears that Otx2, which is expressed in and has an effect on the initial development of all the choroid plexuses, may have alternative functions in the different choroid plexuses after their specification and initial development, as deletion at E15 only affected survival in the hindbrain choroid plexus (Johansson et al., 2013). Further comparisons between the different choroid plexuses are currently under investigation.

REGULATION OF CSF SECRETION AND COMPOSITION DURING DEVELOPMENT

Three main components are required for fluid transport/secretion across an epithelium: (i) free passage of water and solutes between the cells has to be inhibited via the presence of tight-junctions

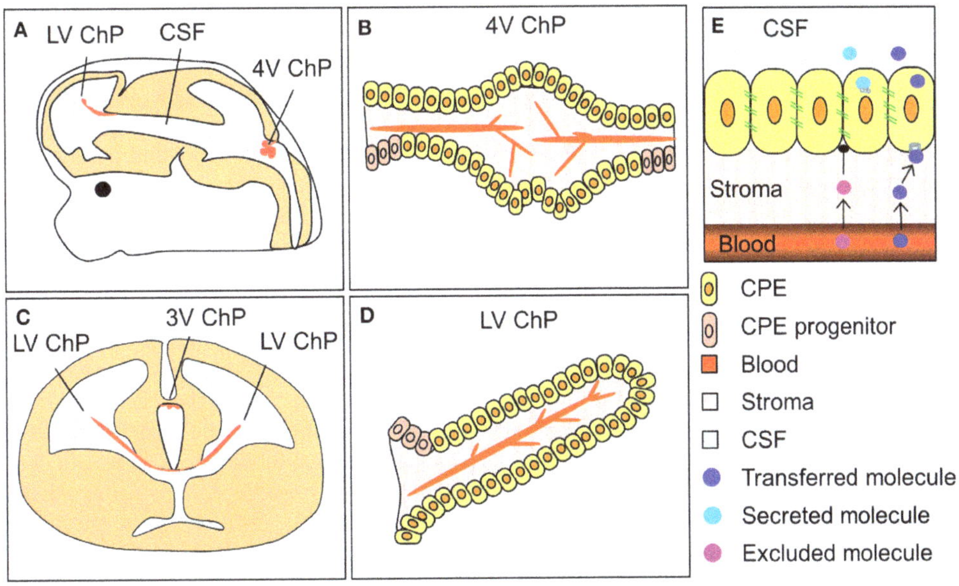

FIGURE 2 | The location and structure of the choroid plexuses and the blood-CSF barrier. (A,C) Schematic drawings of an embryonic brain in sagittal **(A)** and coronal **(C)** orientation depicting the location of the lateral, third and fourth ventricular choroid plexuses (LV ChP, 3V ChP and 4V ChP). **(B,D)** schematic drawing of the lateral and fourth ventricular choroid plexuses. **(E)** Simplified schematic depiction of the blood-CSF barrier and the transfer and secretion of molecules into CSF. ChP, choroid plexus.

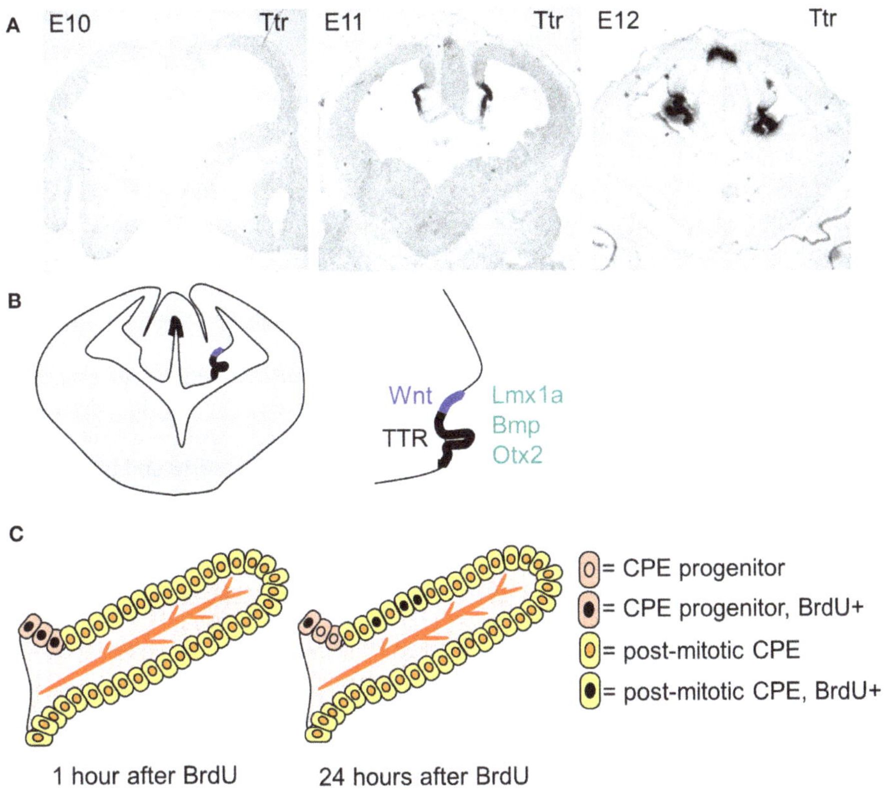

FIGURE 3 | The specification, differentiation and growth of the lateral ventricular choroid plexuses. (A) Photographs of *transthyretin (Ttr) in situ* hybridization sections, showing the choroid plexus anlage at E19, E11 and E12. **(B)** Schematic drawing showing the localization of the lateral ventricular choroid plexus and the cortical hem within the invaginated dorsal midline. **(C)** Schematic drawing (modified from Liddelow et al., 2010) showing the localization of the progenitor cells and the mode of growth of the choroid plexus.

(i.e., a barrier), (ii) the capacity of water transport across the cells (i.e., the presence of water channels), and (iii) the presence of transporters and exchangers that can create an ionic or osmotic gradient that drives water across the epithelium. These criteria are of course all met in the adult choroid plexus via the presence of the blood-CSF barrier, the presence of the water channel AQP1 and the creation of ion gradients between blood and CSF via a multitude of ion transporters and exchangers (see e.g., Wolburg and Paulus, 2010). In development the barrier criterion is met by the presence of continuous tight junctional strands as soon as the choroid plexus invaginates into the ventricles (Møllgård and Saunders, 1975; Møllgård et al., 1976; Ek et al., 2003; Johansson et al., 2006). Aquaporin-1, the only confirmed and consistently identified water channel in the choroid plexus, is present in the choroid plexus epithelial cells as soon as they start to differentiate (Johansson et al., 2005), making water transport possible from very early stages in choroid plexus development. The gradient, however, that drives the water transport, does not appear to be regulated in the same manner as in the adult (Johansson et al., 2008a,b; Liddelow et al., 2013). For example, two of the main components in creating the ion gradients in the adult (NaK-ATPase alpha subunit and carbonic anhydrase II) are not present in the early developing choroid plexus (Johansson et al., 2008b). Instead it has been suggested that the there is a colloid-osmotic gradient, created by the high protein concentration in CSF during development, that drives the water from blood (or more accurately from interstitial fluid) into CSF (see Johansson et al., 2008a). Experimental evidence for this suggestion was recently described, where the total protein concentration in CSF was artificially increased via systemic protein injections in early development (P9 *Monodelphis Domestica*), resulting in a transient doubling of the size of the lateral ventricles (Liddelow et al., 2011a).

In both development and in the adult little is known about the transcriptional regulation of CSF secretion. One transcription factor that appears to have a role in regulating CSF secretion is E2F5, which is expressed in the developing choroid plexus from E12.5 (Swetloff and Ferretti, 2005). Its deletion (homozygous full knock-out mice) resulted in post-natal non-obstructive hydrocephalus (Lindeman et al., 1998), suggesting that it normally suppresses secretion. However, as E2F5 protein levels appear to decrease in the choroid plexus as they mature (and its localization is shifted from nuclear to cytoplasmic), it was suggested that E2F5 plays a role in the maturation process of CPE cells (Lindeman et al., 1998). It was also found that E2F5 is one of the target genes of choroid plexus specific micro-RNA mir449, which is expressed through-out choroid plexus development (Redshaw et al., 2009), suggesting a yet unexplored role of microRNAs in choroid plexus function, CSF secretion and potentially in the regulation of neurogenesis.

THE IMPACT OF CSF PRESSURE AND COMPOSITION ON NEUROGENESIS

The continuous CSF production (originating mostly from the choroid plexuses) creates a pressure inside the cerebral ventricles. The requirement of this pressure for normal brain development was shown by a study in chick embryos (Stage18), where the intraventricular pressure was removed via insertion of hollow tubes into the ventricular system (Desmond and Jacobson, 1977). After 24 h the nervous tissue had folded into the ventricles. The ventricles themselves were smaller (only 20% of their normal size) and the surrounding brain tissue was not only disorganized but also reduced in size (Desmond and Jacobson, 1977).

However, the choroid plexuses not only regulate the level of CSF production but also modify its composition. CSF composition can be regulated in two main ways; either via changes in the transfer of molecules from blood into CSF across the epithelium (receptor or carrier mediated transfer as well as exclusion of molecules via efflux pumps) or via changes in the secretion of molecules produced by the choroid plexuses themselves (**Figure 2**). In the developing choroid plexuses both of these mechanisms are in play. The subset of epithelial cells that transport proteins from blood into CSF are not only present in development but their proportion is larger and they appear to be more specialized as they selectively transport certain plasma proteins and not others across the barrier, a mechanism that appears to not be present in the adult (for example see Johansson et al., 2008a; Liddelow et al., 2011b, 2013). In regards to other proteins capable of modifying CSF composition in the adult (efflux pumps, amino acid transporters, solute transporters), the majority are already present in the developing (e.g., E15 rat) choroid plexus but are often expressed at different levels (both higher and lower) compared to the adult (Ek et al., 2010; Kratzer et al., 2013; Liddelow et al., 2013) again suggesting a dynamic and regulated mechanisms of CSF composition control. In addition, recent choroid plexus transcriptome analyses have shown that the developing choroid plexuses also express a large amount of signaling type of molecules that can be secreted into the ventricles and affect the behavior of the neural stem cells lining the ventricles (e.g., Johansson et al., 2013, **Table 1**).

That CSF can modulate brain development has been shown in *in vitro* experiments. Here it was shown that isolated cortical cells can be maintained on embryonic CSF alone (Miyan et al., 2006). Neuroepithelial explants from chick were shown to survive and proliferate just as well in CSF serum free media as in serum supplemented media (Gato et al., 2005). Further, CSF from different ages affects the CSF differently, as seen in rat cortical cultures where E19 cells proliferated more in CSF from E19 and E20 compared to CSF from E18 and E21 (Miyan et al., 2006). Similar results were shown with E14 rat neurospheres, which, when cultured with E17 CSF, generated more spheres than when grown in CSF from E14, P6 or adult CSF (Lehtinen et al., 2011). This is consistent with the age-dependent changes in CSF composition previously observed using both proteomics (Zappaterra et al., 2007), total protein measurements (see Johansson et al., 2008a) and individual protein measurements (Dziegielewska et al., 1981; Huang et al., 2010; Lehtinen et al., 2011). The proteome study compared embryonic mouse CSF from three different ages and reported 423 proteins in E12.5 CSF, 318 in E14.5 and 382 in E17.5 CSF (all sampled from the lateral ventricle). Only 137 proteins were common to all three ages, suggesting a highly dynamic regulation of CSF composition (Zappaterra et al., 2007). In studies investigating particular molecules, the levels of different plasma derived proteins was found to vary between different embryonic stages and although the individual proteins were following the same pattern (increase, peak, and decrease) the peak was reached at different ages (Dziegielewska et al., 1981). Igf2 was found in CSF from embryonic rat at all ages investigated but showed a significant increase late in embryogenesis and a decrease again perinatally (Lehtinen et al., 2011). However, in a study measuring Shh levels, the concentration of this particular molecule did not change in mouse CSF between E12.5 and E15.5 (Huang et al., 2009). Together these studies show a highly regulated control of CSF composition during development and during the period of neurogenesis.

In support of the regulation of CSF content having a physiological function, direct manipulation of CSF composition has been shown to alter the behavior of the stem cells in direct contact with the CSF. Here, both loss and gain of function experiments have been performed *in vivo* using either neutralizing antibodies or recombinant proteins injected into the embryonic ventricles. For example, the removal of Fgf2 from chick CSF caused a loss of proliferation and increased neural differentiation (Martin et al., 2006). Similar experiments with another type of growth factor Igf1, in embryonic mice and rats, showed an increase in proliferation after intraventricular injections of recombinant proteins and a decrease after IGF-neutralizing antibodies were injected (Mairet-Coello et al., 2009). Thus, the link between CSF composition and alteration in neural stem cell behavior has been experimentally shown but the link between choroid plexus development and brain development remains less clear.

THE SPECIFIC IMPACT OF THE CHOROID PLEXUSES ON DEVELOPMENTAL NEUROGENESIS

The choroid plexuses appear whilst neurogenesis is occurring through-out the nervous system. This gives the potential for the choroid plexuses (via their modulation of CSF) to alter the behavior of the neural stem cells along the neuroaxis (**Figure 1**, **Box 1**). As described above, the capability of the CSF to alter both proliferation and survival in different brains regions *in vitro* has long been known, likely due to the signaling molecules present in CSF. However, to what extent these molecules are regulated or even secreted by the choroid plexuses has not been sufficiently investigated (perhaps in part due to the technical difficulties such an approach poses).

With the advancement of region and time specific deletion techniques new strategies to isolate choroid plexuses involvement in neurogenesis are available. Along these lines, some recent work has demonstrated, via choroid plexus specific deletions, that molecules expressed in the choroid plexus have the capability to influence brain development at other sites. This was first achieved by deletion of Shh from the hindbrain choroid plexus (using the Wnt1-Cre), resulting in a more than 50% decrease in the proliferation of the neural stem cells in the nearby cerebellum and impaired GABAergic progenitor expansion (Huang et al., 2010).

Recently, in work done by the author and colleagues, it has also been shown that when the transcription factor Otx2 was deleted from the hindbrain choroid plexus using the Gd7-Cre (only very sparse recombination in other regions) it not only significantly altered the size of the choroid plexus but also the relative expression of many secreted signaling molecules (Johansson et al., 2013). To our surprise, this deletion led to a region-specific increase in proliferation in the far distant cerebral cortex (but not in the spinal cord or in the lateral ganglionic eminence), which in turn led to site-specific alterations in the cortical neuronal layers at P7. The increase in proliferation was caused by an increase in Wnt-signaling, mediated by, at least in part, altered hindbrain choroid plexus expression levels and the ensuing increased CSF protein levels of the Wnt-signaling modulators Wnt4 and Tgm2.

This work revealed for the first time, the choroid plexus as a potential modulator of Wnt-signaling in the developing brain. It also highlighted that the hindbrain choroid plexus, being the first to appear, can alter the behavior of progenitor cells at the opposite end of the ventricular system prior to the differentiation of the other choroid plexuses. This period is also notable as the ventricular system is still an enclosed cavity, not connected with the fluid in the subarachnoid space and does not yet have any directional flow, making it more possible for molecules secreted from the fourth ventricular choroid plexus to reach the forebrain and influence the behavior of the neural stem cells (**Figure 4**). In support of this, in the above study we also found that the increase in proliferation and Wnt-signaling was no longer present at E16, when the influence of the hindbrain choroid plexus would be much reduced due to the now much larger (unaffected) lateral ventricular choroid plexuses in closer proximity to the cortical neural stem cells (Johansson et al., 2013).

This work also showed that not all regions in the CNS responded to the altered CSF in the same way (or at all). We suggest that select tissues are prepared for certain signaling molecules, by the expression of not only receptors but also by the expression of modulators and inhibitors of the different signaling pathways. Thus, neurogenesis can be seen as a reciprocal process between the choroid plexus and the neural stem cells mediated via the CSF (**Figure 4**).

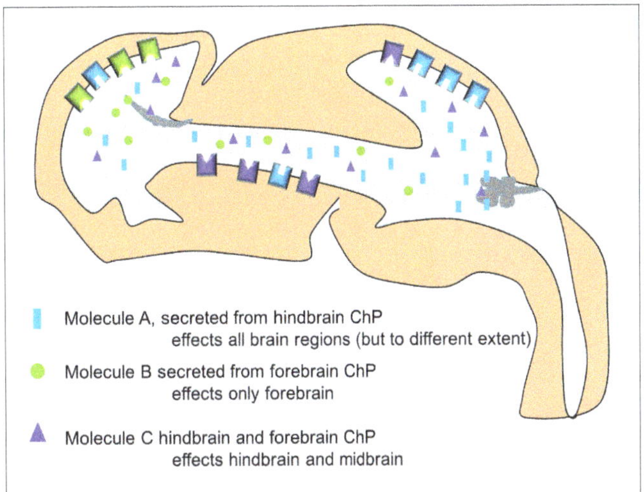

FIGURE 4 | Simplified schematic drawing of how choroid plexus mediated changes in CSF composition differentially alters the behavior of the neural stem cells along the neuroaxis via differences in their ability to respond (here exemplified by the presence and density of receptors).

CONCLUSIONS AND FUTURE DIRECTIONS

In conclusion, there is substantial evidence that there is indeed a role played by the choroid plexus-CSF-signaling axis in the modulation of developmental neurogenesis. However, much more remains to be discovered. The specific mechanisms by which the choroid plexuses modulate brain development both in terms of the choroid plexuses as whole organs as well as specific aspects of their functions (e.g., transfer of blood-borne molecules or secretion of a particular molecule) needs to be investigated. Further detailed studies of choroid plexus impact on different brain regions and developmental time-points would increase our understanding of the whole process of brain development. Understanding the role of the choroid plexus-CSF signaling axis and its impact on brain development can also lead to novel routes and mechanisms for treatment approaches for a multitude of developmental disorders and in the long-run also for application to adult neurodegeneration and brain injuries.

REFERENCES

Baruch, K., Deczkowska, A., David, E., Castellano, J. M., Miller, O., Kertser, A., et al. (2014). Aging-induced type I interferon response at the choroid plexus negatively affects brain function. *Science* 346, 89–93. doi: 10.1126/science.1252945

Beschorner, R., Waidelich, J., Trautmann, K., Psaras, T., and Schittenhelm, J. (2013). Notch receptors in human choroid plexus tumors. *Histol. Histopathol.* 28, 1055–1063.

Bill, B. R., Balciunas, D., McCarra, J. A., Young, E. D., Xiong, T., Spahn, A. M., et al. (2008). Development and notch signaling requirements of the zebrafish choroid plexus. *PLoS ONE* 3:e3114. doi: 10.1371/journal.pone.0003114

Braun, S. M., and Jessberger, S. (2014). Adult neurogenesis: mechanisms and functional significance. *Development* 141, 1983–1986. doi: 10.1242/dev.104596

Brightman, M. W., and Reese, T. S. (1969). Junctions between intimately apposed cell membranes in the vertebrate brain. *J. Cell Biol.* 40, 648–677. doi: 10.1083/jcb.40.3.648

Catala, M. (1998). Embryonic and fetal development of structures associated with the cerebro-spinal fluid in man and other species. Part I: the ventricular system, meninges and choroid plexuses. *Arch. Anat. Cytol. Pathol.* 46, 153–169.

Dang, L., Fan, X., Chaudhry, A., Wang, M., Gaiano, N., and Eberhart, C. G. (2006). Notch3 signaling initiates choroid plexus tumor formation. *Oncogene* 25, 487–491. doi: 10.1038/sj.onc.1209074

Desmond, M. E., and Jacobson, A. G. (1977). Embryonic brain enlargement requires cerebrospinal fluid pressure. *Dev. Biol.* 57, 188–198. doi: 10.1016/0012-1606(77)90364-5

Dziegielewska, K. M., Ek, J., Habgood, M. D., and Saunders, N. R. (2001). Development of the choroid plexus. *Microsc. Res. Tech.* 52, 5–20. doi: 10.1002/1097-0029(20010101)52:1<5::AID-JEMT3>3.0.CO;2-J

Dziegielewska, K. M., Evans, C. A., Lai, P. C., Lorscheider, F. L., Malinowska, D. H., Mollgard, K., et al. (1981). Proteins in cerebrospinal fluid and plasma of fetal rats during development. *Dev. Biol.* 83, 193–200. doi: 10.1016/S0012-1606(81)80024-3

Ek, C. J., Habgood, M. D., Dziegielewska, K. M., and Saunders, N. R. (2003). Structural characteristics and barrier properties of the choroid plexuses in developing brain of the opossum (Monodelphis Domestica). *J. Comp. Neurol.* 460, 451–464. doi: 10.1002/cne.10661

Ek, C. J., Wong, A., Liddelow, S. A., Johansson, P. A., Dziegielewska, K. M., and Saunders, N. R. (2010). Efflux mechanisms at the developing brain barriers: ABC-transporters in the fetal and postnatal rat. *Toxicol. Lett.* 197, 51–59. doi: 10.1016/j.toxlet.2010.04.025

Falcao, A. M., Marques, F., Novais, A., Sousa, N., Palha, J. A., and Sousa, J. C. (2012). The path from the choroid plexus to the subventricular zone: go with the flow! *Front. Cell. Neurosci.* 6:34. doi: 10.3389/fncel.2012.00034

Gato, A., Moro, J. A., Alonso, M. I., Bueno, D., De La Mano, A., and Martin, C. (2005). Embryonic cerebrospinal fluid regulates neuroepithelial survival, proliferation, and neurogenesis in chick embryos. *Anat. Rec. A Discov. Mol. Cell. Evol. Biol.* 284, 475–484. doi: 10.1002/ar.a.20185

Guldbrandsen, A., Vethe, H., Farag, Y., Oveland, E., Garberg, H., Berle, M., et al. (2014). In-depth characterization of the cerebrospinal fluid proteome displayed through the CSF Proteome Resource (CSF-PR). *Mol. Cell. Proteomics.* doi: 10.1074/mcp.M114.038554. [Epub ahead of print].

Hebert, J. M., Mishina, Y., and McConnell, S. K. (2002). BMP signaling is required locally to pattern the dorsal telencephalic midline. *Neuron* 35, 1029–1041. doi: 10.1016/S0896-6273(02)00900-5

Huang, X., Ketova, T., Fleming, J. T., Wang, H., Dey, S. K., Litingtung, Y., et al. (2009). Sonic hedgehog signaling regulates a novel epithelial progenitor domain of the hindbrain choroid plexus. *Development* 136, 2535–2543. doi: 10.1242/dev.033795

Huang, X., Liu, J., Ketova, T., Fleming, J. T., Grover, V. K., Cooper, M. K., et al. (2010). Transventricular delivery of Sonic hedgehog is essential to cerebellar ventricular zone development. *Proc. Natl. Acad. Sci. U.S.A.* 107, 8422–8427. doi: 10.1073/pnas.0911838107

Hunter, N. L., and Dymecki, S. M. (2007). Molecularly and temporally separable lineages form the hindbrain roof plate and contribute differentially to the choroid plexus. *Development* 134, 3449–3460. doi: 10.1242/dev.003095

Imayoshi, I., Shimogori, T., Ohtsuka, T., and Kageyama, R. (2008). Hes genes and neurogenin regulate non-neural versus neural fate specification in the dorsal telencephalic midline. *Development* 135, 2531–2541. doi: 10.1242/dev.021535

Johansson, P., Dziegielewska, K., and Saunders, N. (2008b). Low levels of Na, K-ATPase and carbonic anhydrase II during choroid plexus development suggest limited involvement in early CSF secretion. *Neurosci. Lett.* 442, 77–80. doi: 10.1016/j.neulet.2008.06.068

Johansson, P. A., Cappello, S., and Gotz, M. (2010). Stem cells niches during development–lessons from the cerebral cortex. *Curr. Opin. Neurobiol.* 20, 400–407. doi: 10.1016/j.conb.2010.04.003

Johansson, P. A., Dziegielewska, K. M., Ek, C. J., Habgood, M. D., Liddelow, S. A., Potter, A. M., et al. (2006). Blood-CSF barrier function in the rat embryo. *Eur. J. Neurosci.* 24, 65–76. doi: 10.1111/j.1460-9568.2006.04904.x

Johansson, P. A., Dziegielewska, K. M., Ek, C. J., Habgood, M. D., Mollgard, K., Potter, A., et al. (2005). Aquaporin-1 in the choroid plexuses of developing mammalian brain. *Cell Tissue Res.* 322, 353–364. doi: 10.1007/s00441-005-1120-x

Johansson, P. A., Dziegielewska, K. M., Liddelow, S. A., and Saunders, N. R. (2008a). The blood-CSF barrier explained: when development is not immaturity. *Bioessays* 30, 237–248. doi: 10.1002/bies.20718

Johansson, P. A., Irmler, M., Acampora, D., Beckers, J., Simeone, A., and Gotz, M. (2013). The transcription factor Otx2 regulates choroid plexus development and function. *Development* 140, 1055–1066. doi: 10.1242/dev.090860

Kratzer, I., Liddelow, S. A., Saunders, N. R., Dziegielewska, K. M., Strazielle, N., and Ghersi-Egea, J. F. (2013). Developmental changes in the transcriptome of the rat choroid plexus in relation to neuroprotection. *Fluids Barriers CNS* 10:25. doi: 10.1186/2045-8118-10-25

Lehtinen, M. K., Zappaterra, M. W., Chen, X., Yang, Y. J., Hill, A. D., Lun, M., et al. (2011). The cerebrospinal fluid provides a proliferative niche for neural progenitor cells. *Neuron* 69, 893–905. doi: 10.1016/j.neuron.2011.01.023

Liddelow, S. A., Dziegielewska, K. M., Ek, C. J., Habgood, M. D., Bauer, H., Bauer, H. C., et al. (2013). Mechanisms that determine the internal environment of the developing brain: a transcriptomic, functional and ultrastructural approach. *PLoS ONE* 8:e65629. doi: 10.1371/journal.pone.0065629

Liddelow, S. A., Dziegielewska, K. M., Ek, C. J., Johansson, P. A., Potter, A. M., and Saunders, N. R. (2009). Cellular transfer of macromolecules across the developing choroid plexus of Monodelphis domestica. *Eur. J. Neurosci.* 29, 253–266. doi: 10.1111/j.1460-9568.2008.06571.x

Liddelow, S. A., Dziegielewska, K. M., Møllgård, K., Phoenix, T. N., Temple, S., Vandeberg, J. L., et al. (2011b). SPARC/osteonectin, an endogenous mechanism for targeting albumin to the blood-cerebrospinal fluid interface during brain development. *Eur. J. Neurosci.* 34, 1062–1073. doi: 10.1111/j.1460-9568.2011.07821.x

Liddelow, S. A., Dziegielewska, K. M., Vandeberg, J. L., Noor, N. M., Potter, A. M., and Saunders, N. R. (2011a). Modification of protein transfer across blood/cerebrospinal fluid barrier in response to altered plasma protein composition during development. *Eur. J. Neurosci.* 33, 391–400. doi: 10.1111/j.1460-9568.2010.07509.x

Liddelow, S. A., Dziegielewska, K. M., Vandeberg, J. L., and Saunders, N. R. (2010). Development of the lateral ventricular choroid plexus in a marsupial,

Monodelphis domestica. *Cerebrospinal Fluid Res.* 7:16. doi: 10.1186/1743-8454-7-16

Lindeman, G. J., Dagnino, L., Gaubatz, S., Xu, Y., Bronson, R. T., Warren, H. B., et al. (1998). A specific, nonproliferative role for E2F-5 in choroid plexus function revealed by gene targeting. *Genes Dev.* 12, 1092–1098. doi: 10.1101/gad.12.8.1092

Mairet-Coello, G., Tury, A., and Dicicco-Bloom, E. (2009). Insulin-like growth factor-1 promotes G(1)/S cell cycle progression through bidirectional regulation of cyclins and cyclin-dependent kinase inhibitors via the phosphatidylinositol 3-kinase/Akt pathway in developing rat cerebral cortex. *J. Neurosci.* 29, 775–788. doi: 10.1523/JNEUROSCI.1700-08.2009

Marques, F., Sousa, J. C., Coppola, G., Gao, F., Puga, R., Brentani, H., et al. (2011). Transcriptome signature of the adult mouse choroid plexus. *Fluids Barriers CNS* 8:10. doi: 10.1186/2045-8118-8-10

Martin, C., Bueno, D., Alonso, M. I., Moro, J. A., Callejo, S., Parada, C., et al. (2006). FGF2 plays a key role in embryonic cerebrospinal fluid trophic properties over chick embryo neuroepithelial stem cells. *Dev. Biol.* 297, 402–416. doi: 10.1016/j.ydbio.2006.05.010

Miyan, J. A., Zendah, M., Mashayekhi, F., and Owen-Lynch, P. J. (2006). Cerebrospinal fluid supports viability and proliferation of cortical cells *in vitro*, mirroring *in vivo* development. *Cerebrospinal Fluid Res.* 3:2. doi: 10.1186/1743-8454-3-2

Møllgård, K., Milinowska, D. H., and Saunders, N. R. (1976). Lack of correlation between tight junction morphology and permeability properties in developing choroid plexus. *Nature* 264, 293–294. doi: 10.1038/264293a0

Møllgård, K., and Saunders, N. R. (1975). Complex tight junctions of epithelial and of endothelial cells in early foetal brain. *J. Neurocytol.* 4, 453–468. doi: 10.1007/BF01261375

Nielsen, C. M., and Dymecki, S. M. (2010). Sonic hedgehog is required for vascular outgrowth in the hindbrain choroid plexus. *Dev. Biol.* 340, 430–437. doi: 10.1016/j.ydbio.2010.01.032

Redshaw, N., Wheeler, G., Hajihosseini, M. K., and Dalmay, T. (2009). microRNA-449 is a putative regulator of choroid plexus development and function. *Brain Res.* 1250, 20–26. doi: 10.1016/j.brainres.2008.11.020

Silva-Vargas, V., Crouch, E. E., and Doetsch, F. (2013). Adult neural stem cells and their niche: a dynamic duo during homeostasis, regeneration, and aging. *Curr. Opin. Neurobiol.* 23, 935–942. doi: 10.1016/j.conb.2013.09.004

Swetloff, A., and Ferretti, P. (2005). Changes in E2F5 intracellular localization in mouse and human choroid plexus epithelium with development. *Int. J. Dev. Biol.* 49, 859–865. doi: 10.1387/ijdb.051996as

Taverna, E., Gotz, M., and Huttner, W. B. (2014). The cell biology of neurogenesis: toward an understanding of the development and evolution of the neocortex. *Annu. Rev. Cell Dev. Biol.* 30, 465–502. doi: 10.1146/annurev-cellbio-101011-155801

Von Frowein, J., Wizenmann, A., and Gotz, M. (2006). The transcription factors Emx1 and Emx2 suppress choroid plexus development and promote neuroepithelial cell fate. *Dev. Biol.* 296, 239–252. doi: 10.1016/j.ydbio.2006.04.461

Wilting, J., and Christ, B. (1989). An experimental and ultrastructural study on the development of the avian choroid plexus. *Cell Tissue Res.* 255, 487–494. doi: 10.1007/BF00218783

Wolburg, H., and Paulus, W. (2010). Choroid plexus: biology and pathology. *Acta Neuropathol.* 119, 75–88. doi: 10.1007/s00401-009-0627-8

Zappaterra, M. D., Lisgo, S. N., Lindsay, S., Gygi, S. P., Walsh, C. A., and Ballif, B. A. (2007). A comparative proteomic analysis of human and rat embryonic cerebrospinal fluid. *J. Proteome Res.* 6, 3537–3548. doi: 10.1021/pr070247w

17

The *Drosophila* surface glia transcriptome: evolutionary conserved blood-brain barrier processes

Michael K. DeSalvo[1], Samantha J. Hindle[1], Zeid M. Rusan[1], Souvinh Orng[1], Mark Eddison[2], Kyle Halliwill[3] and Roland J. Bainton[1]*

[1] Department of Anesthesia and Perioperative Care, University of California San Francisco, San Francisco, CA, USA
[2] Janelia Farm Research Campus, The Howard Hughes Medical Institute, Ashburn, VA, USA
[3] Pharmaceutical Sciences and Pharmacogenomics, University of California San Francisco, San Francisco, CA, USA

***Correspondence:**
Roland J. Bainton, Department of Anesthesia and Perioperative Care, University of California San Francisco, Genentech Hall, Room S312C, 600 16th Street, San Francisco, CA 94158, USA
e-mail: baintonr@anesthesia.ucsf.edu

Central nervous system (CNS) function is dependent on the stringent regulation of metabolites, drugs, cells, and pathogens exposed to the CNS space. Cellular blood-brain barrier (BBB) structures are highly specific checkpoints governing entry and exit of all small molecules to and from the brain interstitial space, but the precise mechanisms that regulate the BBB are not well understood. In addition, the BBB has long been a challenging obstacle to the pharmacologic treatment of CNS diseases; thus model systems that can parse the functions of the BBB are highly desirable. In this study, we sought to define the transcriptome of the adult *Drosophila melanogaster* BBB by isolating the BBB surface glia with fluorescence activated cell sorting (FACS) and profiling their gene expression with microarrays. By comparing the transcriptome of these surface glia to that of all brain glia, brain neurons, and whole brains, we present a catalog of transcripts that are selectively enriched at the *Drosophila* BBB. We found that the fly surface glia show high expression of many ATP-binding cassette (ABC) and solute carrier (SLC) transporters, cell adhesion molecules, metabolic enzymes, signaling molecules, and components of xenobiotic metabolism pathways. Using gene sequence-based alignments, we compare the *Drosophila* and Murine BBB transcriptomes and discover many shared chemoprotective and small molecule control pathways, thus affirming the relevance of invertebrate models for studying evolutionary conserved BBB properties. The *Drosophila* BBB transcriptome is valuable to vertebrate and insect biologists alike as a resource for studying proteins underlying diffusion barrier development and maintenance, glial biology, and regulation of drug transport at tissue barriers.

Keywords: blood-brain barrier, transcriptome, surface glia, Affymetrix array

INTRODUCTION

Endothelial cells constituting the capillaries of the vertebrate central nervous system (CNS) have special properties that enable a potent blood-brain barrier (BBB). The BBB preserves CNS homeostasis by preventing the entry of harmful molecules and facilitating the passage of essential molecules such as metabolites. While the brain vascular endothelial cells are the anatomic BBB, all members of the neurovascular unit (NVU—endothelial cells, pericytes, astrocytes, extracellular matrix, and neurons) are thought to contribute to the development and maintenance of BBB processes (Janzer and Raff, 1987; Sobue et al., 1999; Armulik et al., 2010; Daneman et al., 2010b). That being said, the barrier functions of the BBB are largely provided by vascular endothelial machinery: intercellular protein complexes, active efflux transporters, and carrier-mediated transporters (Zlokovic, 2008). In particular, the formation of tight junction (TJ) complexes between endothelial cells renders paracellular fluid flux impossible (Hirase et al., 1997; Saitou et al., 2000; Nitta et al., 2003). Also, endothelial cell expression of ABCB1 (i.e., MDR1/P-glycoprotein), an ATP-binding cassette (ABC) transporter found at the luminal surface, is responsible for the efflux of unwanted substrates back into the blood (Cordon-Cardo et al., 1989; Loscher and Potschka, 2005), and expression of SLC2A1 (i.e., GLUT1), a solute carrier (SLC) transporter found at both surfaces, shuttles glucose between the blood and the brain (Boado and Pardridge, 1990; Pardridge et al., 1990). Characterizing the entire repertoire of genes underlying BBB physiology is of paramount importance given that (1) little is known about the regulatory mechanisms that grant the BBB its properties, (2) the etiologies of numerous CNS diseases that include BBB dysfunctions (Daneman, 2012), and (3) CNS disease treatments that depend on efficient delivery of therapeutics across the BBB (Pardridge, 2005).

Genomic approaches to characterizing cellular BBB structures have yielded important resources for understanding the BBB. Enerson and Drewes (Enerson and Drewes, 2006) isolated blood microvessels, which contained endothelial cells, pericytes, extracellular matrix, and remnant astrocytic end feet, from rat brains and used serial analysis of gene expression to produce the first profile of a vertebrate BBB transcriptome. Daneman et al.

(2010a) used fluorescence activated cell sorting (FACS) to purify brain vascular endothelial cells from mice and used Affymetrix GeneChips to survey the transcriptome of the endothelial BBB component. Both of these studies identified known BBB transcripts, but more importantly, they also identified novel transcripts enriched at the BBB. Indeed, the BBB genes involved in CNS disease progression are not known in most cases (Daneman, 2012). In addition, strategies for delivering pharmaceuticals to the CNS have often centered on disrupting previously identified BBB drug efflux transporters such as ABCB1, but these direct strategies have been met with limited success (de Vries et al., 2007; Wu et al., 2011; Lin et al., 2013). Thus, in-depth exploration of the genes that regulate the integrated chemical protection physiologies present at the BBB is needed for overcoming BBB-related challenges.

A major limitation to studying the hundreds of BBB genes in vertebrates is that obtaining mutants is both time consuming and costly. For this reason, we have focused on using the *Drosophila* BBB as a model for the study of BBB function. Previous studies have shown that the insect BBB is analogous to the vertebrate BBB (Stork et al., 2008; Mayer et al., 2009; DeSalvo et al., 2011). The *Drosophila* CNS is similarly protected by a BBB with one main noteworthy difference: insects have an open circulatory system where molecules are dissolved in a fluid called hemolymph that bathes organs, instead of being distributed in a vascular system. For this reason, the insect BBB encapsulates the CNS (Stork et al., 2008). Resembling the multiple cell type architecture of the vertebrate NVU, the insect BBB is composed of two glial subtypes collectively known as surface glia—the apical perineurial glia (PG) and basal subperineurial glia (SPG) (Stork et al., 2008) (**Figure 1**). In addition, endothelial cells of the vertebrate NVU are surrounded by an extracellular matrix in which pericytes are embedded, and in the insect glial BBB, a similar matrix termed the neural lamella is apical to the PG (Stork et al., 2008). Moreover, cellular junctions precluding small molecule diffusion between cells are paramount to BBB function. The insect equivalent of the vertebrate TJ is the septate junction (SJ), consisting of similar molecular components, present between the SPG to prevent paracellular molecule diffusion (Wu and Beitel, 2004). Finally, the ABC drug efflux transporter Mdr65 is expressed in the SPG and is involved in chemical protection of the CNS, analogous to the function of its vertebrate homolog ABCB1 (Mayer et al., 2009). Fundamental CNS homeostasis requirements imposed across animal phyla suggest that numerous conserved BBB physiologies will likely be discovered in *Drosophila*.

We present here a transcriptome of the *Drosophila* BBB surface glia. We assess the relative enrichment of genes expressed at the BBB by comparing the surface glia transcriptome to that of all brain glia, brain neurons, and whole brains. By way of example we show that many genes found in the highly purified transcriptome are both highly expressed and enriched in the surface glia. We use gene set enrichment analyses to validate our surface glia transcriptome and show that the *Drosophila* surface glia possess many cellular processes and molecular functions also resident at the vertebrate BBB. Furthermore, we demonstrate that our data can be used to find many novel genes expressed in the surface glia. Lastly, we use BLAST to identify genes expressed in both invertebrate and vertebrate BBBs, pointing to likely evolutionary conserved mechanisms of BBB function that can now be tested using the *Drosophila* model system. Together with the vast and readily available molecular genetic tools for *Drosophila*, our data provide a wealthy resource for rapidly screening through a large group of conserved BBB proteins for phenotypes of interest.

MATERIALS AND METHODS

FLY GENETICS

The following GAL4/UAS-GFP reporter lines were used to facilitate FACS of different CNS cell types: (1) *9-137*-GAL4 (a P-element insertion line found in a screen of a large P-GAL4 collection (Ulrike Heberlein, Janelia Farm Research Campus, VA) that drives expression in the surface glia), crossed to pJFRC2, a previously published *UAS-mCD8-GFP* line (Pfeiffer et al., 2010)

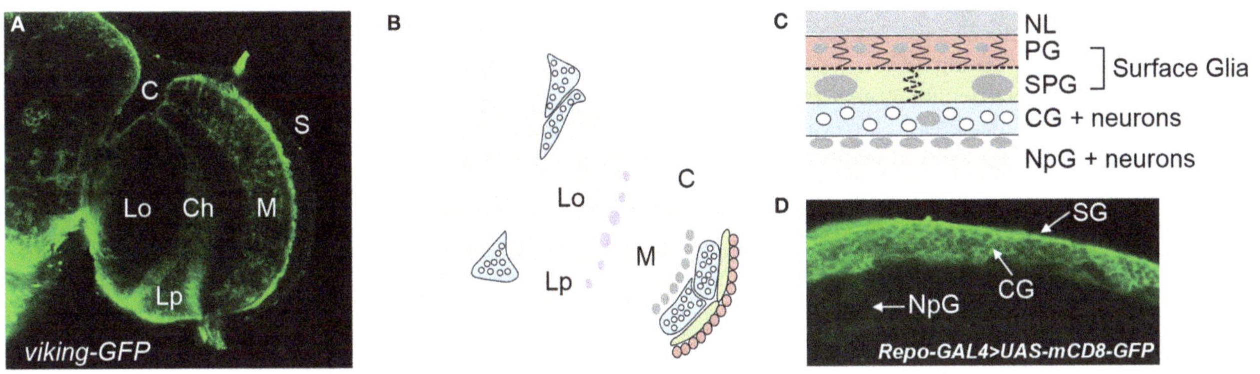

FIGURE 1 | Types of glia in the adult brain of *Drosophila*. (A) Different regions of the optic lobe of an adult brain as visualized by a GFP-fusion protein of the pan-glial gene, *viking*. Glia are located at the brain surface (S) and the cortex (C), in addition to the medulla (M), lobula (Lo), and lobular plate (Lp) neuropils. The chiasm (Ch) is a glial region dividing the different neuropils. **(B)** A schematic of the optic lobe illustrating the different glial subtypes. Perineurial glia (PG) are seen in red, subperineurial glia (SPG) in green, and cortex glia (CG) in blue. The white circles within each cortex glia are neuronal cell bodies. Nuclei of neuropil glia (NpG) are in gray at the surface of the medulla neuropil. Nuclei of chiasm glia are in purple. **(C)** A cross section of the brain surface moving from the neural lamella (NL) to the neuropil. **(D)** Different glial subtypes at the brain surface as visualized by *UAS-mCD8-GFP* under control of the pan-glial driver *repo*-GAL4.

available from the Bloomington Stock Center; (2) *repo*-GFP, a recombinant line of *repo*-GAL4 and *UAS-mCD8-GFP* that drives expression in all glia (Marc Freeman, UMass, MA); and (3) *elav*-GFP, a recombinant line of *elav*-GAL4 and *UAS-mCD8-GFP* that drives expression in all neurons. Whole brain controls were of wildtype Canton-S. For anatomic characterization of *9-137*-GAL4, we crossed this line to nuclear-localized GFP (*UAS-StingerGFP*) (Barolo et al., 2000) in addition to pJFRC2. FlyTrap lines are available from http://flytrap.med.yale.edu/ using genotype IDs stated in **Figure 5**.

WHOLE BRAIN IMAGING

Whole brain confocal images were acquired using previously reported methods (Mayer et al., 2009; DeSalvo et al., 2011; Pinsonneault et al., 2011). Briefly, flies were injected with 12.5 mg/ml 70 kDa Dextran Texas Red® (Invitrogen, D1864) and left to recover overnight. Dextran labeling of the brains allows for demarcation of the surface glia barrier. Fly heads were fixed *in situ* for 15 min with 3.7% paraformaldehyde prior to brain dissection. Fixed brains were then incubated for 1 h at room temperature in a blocking buffer (PBS containing 5% goat serum and 4% Tween® 20), and then probed with rabbit anti-GFP antibody (Abcam ab6556, 1:1000 dilution) overnight at 4°C. Brains were washed three times for 30 min in 1× PBS and incubated with FITC-conjugated goat anti-rabbit antibody (Jackson Immuno Research Laboratories, 1:100 dilution) for 45 min at room temperature. Brains were washed three times for 45 min in PBS and mounted in Dakocytomation Fluorescent Mounting Medium. Brains were visualized on a Zeiss LSM510 confocal microscope at 40× magnification.

TISSUE PROCESSING AND FACS

Brains were dissected under Schneider's media (SM) containing 1% BSA (filter sterilized) and transferred directly to a tube containing ice-cold 500 μL SM/BSA. Each tube contained 10–15 brains. Brains were washed with 1 mL SM/BSA and re-suspended in 220 uL SM/BSA. Collagenase A (Roche No. 10103586001) and DNase I were added to final concentrations of 2 mg/mL and 20 units, respectively. Brains were dissociated at 37°C in a Thermomixer according to the following conditions: 1000 rpm for 20 min (*elav*/neurons), 500 rpm for 20 min (*repo*/all glia), and 500 rpm for 5 min (*9-137*/surface glia). EDTA (pH 7) was added to a final concentration of 5 mM to inactivate the collagenase. Dissociated tissue was filtered through 100 μm filter (70 μm for neurons) and immediately sorted using a 100 μm nozzle on a BD FACSAria at the Laboratory for Cell Analysis at UCSF. Except whilst in the Thermomixer and the FACS machine, brains/cells were kept on ice.

FACS sorting was performed according to the following gating procedure: (1) an initial SSC-A/FSC-A gate to minimize debris; (2) a FSC-W/FSC-A gate to minimize doublets and large cellular aggregates; and (3) a PE-A/FITC-A gate to choose only GFP-positive cells. GFP-positive cells from multiple tubes were sorted into a single tube containing a small volume of sheath fluid. These cells were sorted again to increase purity, and during this sort, the initial scatter gate was modified to capture neurons and glia according to their unique scatter properties (see **Figure 3**). At this step, cells were sorted directly into ice-cold RNA lysis buffer (Ambion RNAqueous Micro Kit). When possible, re-sorted cells were analyzed again to determine their final purity levels. Of the five replicates for *elav*, an average of 9705 cells were sorted at an average purity of 95%; *repo*, 8849 cells at 96% purity; and *9-137*, 6093 cells at 93% purity.

MICROARRAY DATA ACQUISITION AND ANALYSIS

Each replicate for the microarray analysis represented sorted cells originating from different growth bottles and processed on different days. Five total replicates were run for each of the following genotypes: wildtype whole brain, and sorted GFP-positive cells from *repo* (all glia), *elav* (neurons), and *9-137* (surface glia). RNA was isolated using Ambion RNAqueous Micro columns and amplified using NuGEN's Ovation FFPE WTA System. Amplified RNA was processed and hybridized to Affymetrix *Drosophila* Genome 2.0 GeneChips at the Gladstone Institutes Genomics Core facility. All microarray data analysis was performed using R/Bioconductor packages (Gentleman et al., 2004). CEL files were read and raw data normalized using RMA in the affy package (Irizarry et al., 2003; Gautier et al., 2004). Prior to statistical analysis, probes were filtered if the Present sum was less than 4 for all genotypes; in other words, a probe needed to be expressed in at least one genotype to be included. This metric was shown to significantly reduce false positives (McClintick and Edenberg, 2006). 7090 probes were filtered according to this criterion. The remaining probes were used for statistical analyses in the limma package (Smyth, 2004). Pairwise comparisons were performed for all possible combinations, and fold changes and standard errors were estimated by fitting a linear model for each gene. Empirical Bayes smoothing to the standard errors was applied and differentially expressed genes were chosen according to an FDR-adjusted $P < 0.05$. Lists of differentially expressed genes were trimmed to ensure that genes were indeed expressed in the enriched genotype (expression > 100 AND Present sum ≥ 4). Gene set enrichment analyses of the differentially expressed genes were performed using default settings in DAVID Bioinformatics (Huang et al., 2009a,b). Significantly enriched gene sets were identified using a Benjamini-adjusted $P < 0.05$.

BLAST ANALYSIS

Using Ensembl Biomart (Kinsella et al., 2011), RefSeq protein IDs were retrieved for 144 known mouse BBB proteins according to Daneman (2012) and Zlokovic (2008). We chose to ignore proteins listed by Daneman (2012) that were up-regulated in the mouse BBB during disease. A fasta file containing all protein sequences was generated using Batch Entrez (http://www.ncbi.nlm.nih.gov/sites/batchentrez), and these sequences were compared to a BLAST-able database containing all *Drosophila* proteins using the BLAST+ command line (blastp with a E-value cutoff of 10^{-5}). The blast2table perl script was used to parse the output file showing only the top HSP for each BLAST hit. We then linked the RefSeq protein ID for each fly BLAST hit to its corresponding Affymetrix probe IDs, which allowed us to annotate each BLAST hit with its expression and enrichment values in the surface glia transcriptome. Positive expression in the surface glia was assessed by having a Present sum ≥4 AND an expression level ≥100. Surface glia enrichment was assessed by having a positive enrichment relative to neurons OR whole brain.

RESULTS

ISOLATION OF SURFACE GLIA RNA

To purify the BBB surface glia from adult *Drosophila* brains, we used a GAL4/UAS genetic approach (Brand and Perrimon, 1993) to fluorescently label the surface glia. To do this, we first identified the *9-137* enhancer trap line, which drives GAL4 expression specifically in the surface glia. When crossed to UAS-GFP reporter lines, the *9-137*-GAL4 results in specific GFP labeling of the PG and SPG (**Figure 2**), allowing the specific isolation of surface glia to a purity of >90% using FACS (**Figure 3**). We used a similar protocol to isolate neurons and a more inclusive population of glia. All brain glial subtypes (**Figure 1**), including surface glia, were isolated from flies expressing *UAS-mCD8-GFP* under the control of the pan-glial driver *repo*-GAL4 (Xiong et al., 1994); neurons were specifically isolated using the pan-neuronal driver *elav*-GAL4 (Campos et al., 1987; Robinow and White, 1988). Total RNA from five replicate samples for each of surface glia, all glia, neurons, and whole brains were amplified and hybridized to Affymetrix *Drosophila* Genome 2.0 GeneChips for downstream transcriptomic analysis. All microarray data is deposited in Gene Expression Omnibus (GSE45344), and the master matrix of filtered normalized data used as input for statistical analyses is found in Table S1. While we chose to focus on the surface glia-enriched transcriptome in this study, the comprehensive data set generated here is valuable for other avenues of research. For example, the data may provide broad insight into glial biology when analyzed for gene enrichment of additional glial subtypes such as the adult cortex and neuropil glia (**Figure 1**).

THE SURFACE GLIA TRANSCRIPTOME

To gain insight into the genes required for specialized BBB functions in *Drosophila*, we first looked at transcript abundance in the surface glia. The microarray data were normalized using RMA in the R/Bioconductor package affy (Irizarry et al., 2003; Gautier et al., 2004). **Table 1** reports the 50 most abundant transcripts in the surface glia together with their ratiometric enrichments relative to whole brain, neurons, and all glia. We acknowledge that Affymetrix expression signals are not perfect reflections of gene expression levels since signal values are the result of several factors both biological and technical. However, this list does appear to reveal specialized gene expression in the surface glia. For example, extracellular matrix collagens (*vkg* and *Cg25C*) are both highly expressed and highly enriched, and a SLC5 sodium-iodide symporter (*CG5687*) is the most enriched gene among the top 50 most abundant surface glia transcripts. Therefore, the data in **Table 1** suggest that Affymetrix signal abundance for the surface glia samples is somewhat indicative of surface glia functional requirements.

To further investigate the specialized functions of the BBB, we determined the differentially expressed genes in surface glia by performing pairwise comparisons to whole brain, neurons, and all glia using limma software (Smyth, 2004). Table S2 contains differentially expressed genes for all pairwise comparisons performed in limma. **Table 2** reports the top 50 enriched surface glia genes for each comparison. Relative to whole brain, there are 1010 genes up-regulated (i.e., enriched) and 3899 genes down-regulated in the surface glia. Relative to neurons, there are 1183 genes up-regulated and 2979 genes down-regulated in surface glia. Relative to all glia, there are 543 genes up-regulated and 568 genes down-regulated in surface glia. Expression fold changes are greatest in the surface glia-neuron comparison (max = 729, mean = 15.6, median = 3.7), followed by the surface glia-brain comparison (max = 247, mean = 6.0, median = 2.9) and the surface glia-all glia comparison (max = 35, mean = 4.5, median = 3.5). This enrichment trend can in part be explained by the amount of surface glia RNA in each comparison sample. Neuronal samples contain

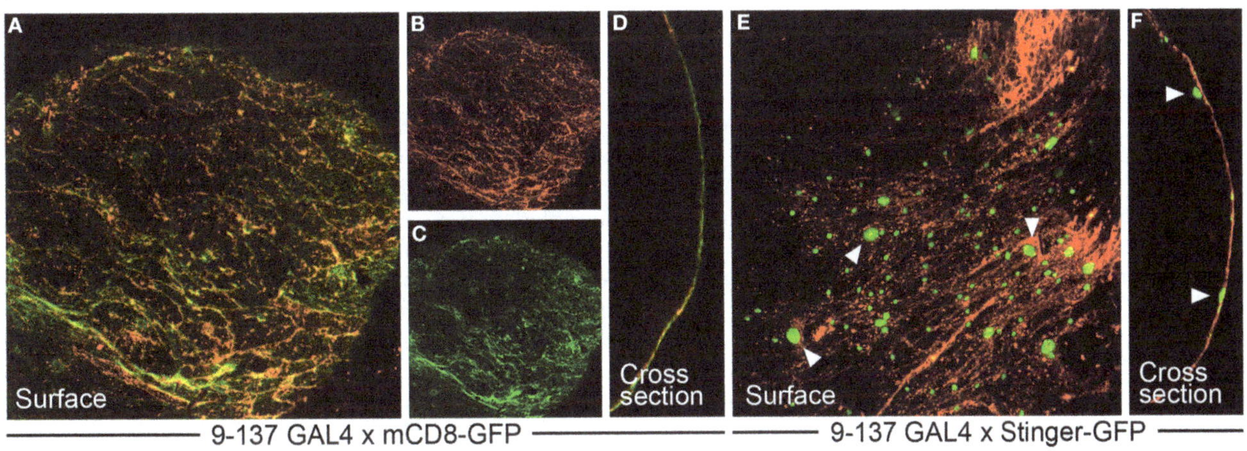

FIGURE 2 | The *9-137* P-GAL4 line specifically drives expression in the surface glia layer. (A–D) *9-137*-GAL4 crossed to mCD8-GFP (membrane-bound) shows hallmarks of surface glia expression. **(A–C)** GFP expression at the surface colocalizes with dextran, which marks the boundaries of the PG cells in a characteristic flagstone pattern. **(D)** The cross-section image shows complete overlap between dextran and GFP. **(E,F)** *9-137*-GAL4 crossed to Stinger-GFP (nuclear-localized) demarcates small PG and large SPG nuclei. Arrowheads mark representative large SPG nuclei. **(F)** The cross-section image shows PG nuclei embedded in the dextran layer with SPG nuclei positioned below the dextran/PG layer.

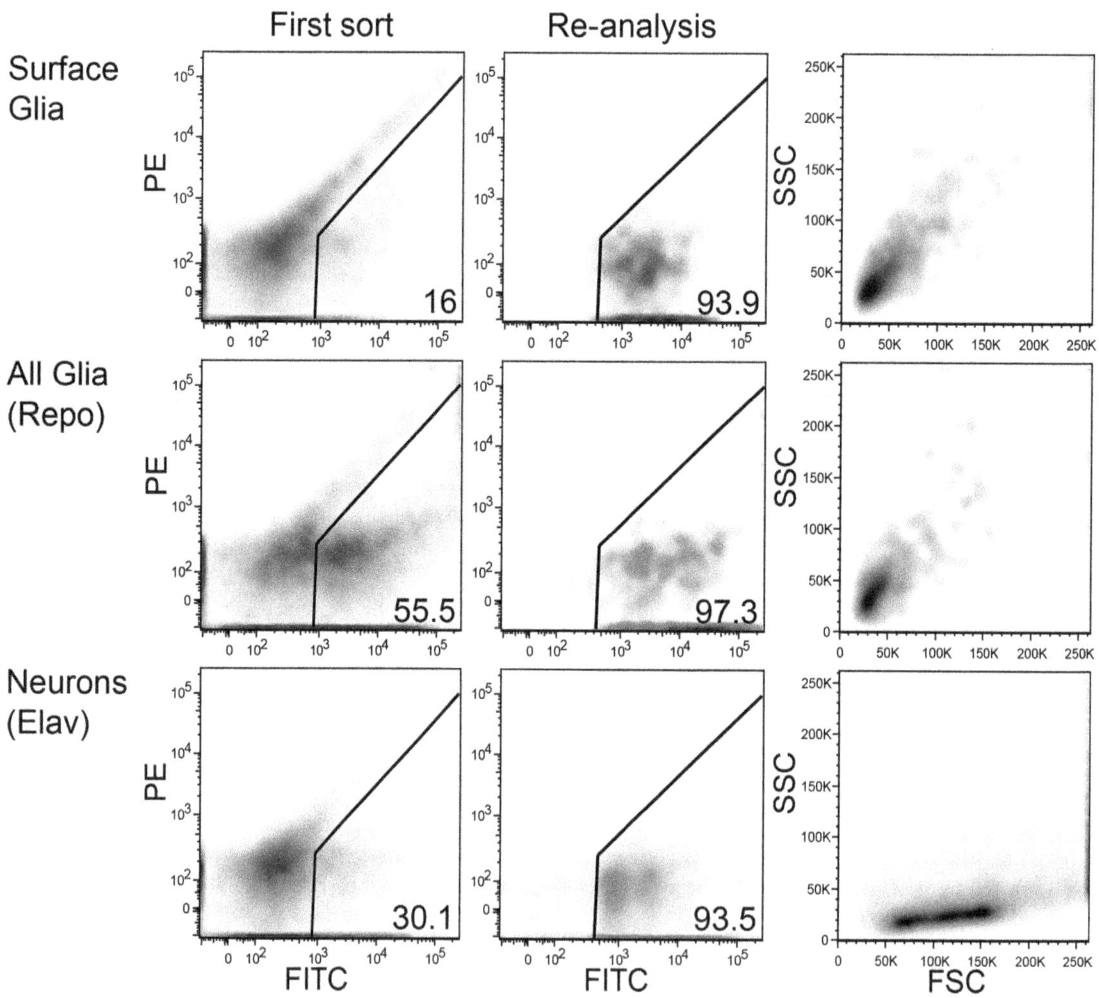

FIGURE 3 | Representative FACS density plots of sorted neurons and glia from adult *Drosophila* brains. Left panels show red (PE) vs. green (FITC) fluorescence of dissociated brain cells. A population of autofluorescent particles extends diagonally across each plot. The GFP-positive gate lies to the right of the autofluorescence axis. The middle panels also show red vs. green fluorescence, but these plots demonstrate the high purity of sorted GFP-positive cells. The re-sorting of GFP-positive cells leads to high levels of purity. Right panels show side (SSC) and forward (FSC) scatter for the highly pure sorted cells in the middle panels. Interestingly, neurons (bottom) and glia (top and middle) have unique, nearly exclusive scatter properties.

no surface glia, brain samples contain a small proportion of surface glia, and all glia samples contain a substantial proportion of surface glia mixed with other glial subtypes. Thus, as expected, the number of differentially expressed genes and their fold changes is maximal in the surface glia-neuron comparison reflecting sample cell-type homogeneity and likely functional specialization.

VALIDATING THE SURFACE GLIA TRANSCRIPTOME AS A BBB GENE PROFILE

To infer specialized molecular pathways present in the surface glia from their transcriptome, we performed gene set enrichment analyses using DAVID Bioinformatics (Huang et al., 2009a,b). **Table 3** lists selected enriched Gene Ontology (GO) categories, KEGG pathways, Interpro domains, and PIR superfamilies among genes enriched in surface glia relative to brain, neurons, and all glia (for all results see Table S3). The DAVID Bioinformatics results support the view of the surface glia being the primary component of the *Drosophila* BBB.

Consistent with the surface glia being a chemical protection interface, we see numerous enriched categories associated with drug metabolism, cell adhesion, and transport (**Table 3**). Selected genes in these categories are listed in **Table 4** and reveal striking signatures of chemical protection physiology. For example, there are numerous cytochrome P450 (CYP), glutathione S-transferase (GST), and UDP-glucuronosyltransferase (UGT) enzymes enriched in the surface glia. These enrichment results account for all phases of drug metabolism. Phase I reactions include oxidation reactions by CYPs; phase II reactions include conjugation reactions, such as glucoronidation by UGTs and glutathionylation by GSTs; and phase III reactions involve excretion of drug metabolites by transporters (Sheweita, 2000; Homolya et al., 2003). These excretory transporters are often ABC transporters. Notable ABC transporters involved in drug

Table 1 | The 50 highest expressed genes in the surface glia (SG) transcriptome.

Probe	Symbol	Signal	SG/B	SG/N	SG/AG	Function
1639180_at	*Arc1*	17, 218 ± 1568	1.52	10.67	9.74	Nucleic acid/zinc ion binding
1627489_a_at	*CG10433*	16, 152 ± 1251	1.59	54.99	1.41	Defense response
1639614_s_at	*RpL41*	15, 533 ± 1949	0.77	1.35	1.20	Cytosolic large ribosomal subunit
1639145_s_at	*Atpα*	15, 084 ± 1190	1.10	1.17	0.99	Na,K ATPase alpha subunit
1633109_at	*CR42862*	14, 265 ± 4275	1.04	1.06	1.07	Non-protein-coding gene
1639694_s_at	*Arc1*	13, 937 ± 2103	1.64	35.22	25.58	Nucleic acid/zinc ion binding
1625719_at	*Atpalpha*	13, 363 ± 1697	0.89	0.90	0.86	Na,K ATPase alpha subunit
1637526_s_at	*Gγ30A*	13, 201 ± 2297	0.93	0.72	0.75	GPCR signaling
1639229_at	*vkg*	12, 278 ± 3159	8.89	161.51	1.96	Collagen
1630150_s_at	*Cg25C*	12, 239 ± 2512	6.78	396.13	2.28	Collagen
1636548_at	*blw*	11, 894 ± 2063	1.10	1.21	0.90	Mitochondrial ATP synthase α-subunit
1629065_s_at	*Vha26*	11, 814 ± 678	1.35	1.16	1.13	V-ATPase E subunit
1632873_at	*MtnA*	11, 230 ± 3013	0.89	30.51	1.34	Metal ion binding
1632683_s_at	*copiaGIP*	11, 090 ± 1461	1.36	1.82	1.32	Transposable element
1630946_at	*Vha16*	11, 017 ± 694	0.90	1.16	1.09	V-ATPase C subunit
1632248_s_at	*CycG*	10, 855 ± 795	1.48	1.11	1.14	Cell cycle
1630941_s_at	*sesB*	10, 802 ± 1476	0.86	1.10	1.02	ATP transport
1629152_at	*CG31451*	10, 674 ± 1916	0.61	0.77	0.83	
1625370_s_at	*gem*	10, 661 ± 1147	2.35	20.23	2.02	Transcription factor
1636186_s_at	*Fer2LCH*	10, 528 ± 640	1.12	1.17	1.13	Ferritin
1637525_s_at	*Mpcp*	10, 468 ± 1136	1.18	0.99	0.97	Phosphate transport
1628694_a_at	*14-3-3ε*	10, 365 ± 565	0.93	0.97	1.08	Protein binding
1625633_a_at	*Argk*	10, 229 ± 1768	0.94	1.34	1.06	Arginine kinase
1633443_s_at	*CG2082*	10, 203 ± 664	2.01	1.78	1.40	Protein binding
1630452_at	*HDC20239*	9739 ± 2567	0.91	2.49	1.24	
1624564_s_at	*RpS14a*	9683 ± 681	1.22	1.22	1.22	Cytosolic small ribosomal subunit
1634961_s_at	*Vha68-2*	9288 ± 926	9.48	182.70	2.86	V-ATPase A subunit
1634989_at	*Acon*	9255 ± 1106	1.59	1.66	1.38	Aconitate hydratase
1640729_s_at	*nrv3*	9244 ± 2404	0.70	1.00	1.15	Na:K-exchanging ATPase complex
1638351_s_at	*Ef1alpha48D*	9206 ± 663	1.67	3.18	1.21	Translation elongation
1623073_s_at	*ctp*	9178 ± 894	0.99	0.88	1.04	Microtubule motor activity
1625672_s_at	*CT33405*	9074 ± 1, 941	0.76	0.92	0.96	
1637393_at	*Vmat*	8981 ± 1797	1.61	1.37	0.96	Monoamine transport
1632117_s_at	*Vha16*	8927 ± 552	0.88	1.10	1.16	V-ATPase C subunit
1625638_a_at	*Hex-A*	8835 ± 1331	2.20	2.25	1.57	Hexokinase
1633034_s_at	*Fer1HCH*	8817 ± 959	1.10	1.19	1.12	Ferritin
1639761_s_at	*Gγ1*	8677 ± 1394	0.80	0.83	0.86	GPCR signaling
1627732_s_at	*CG30415*	8626 ± 913	0.91	1.03	0.91	
1626163_s_at	*Act5C*	8621 ± 1612	0.91	1.18	1.14	Actin
1637059_s_at	*DnaJ-1*	8620 ± 1366	1.38	0.92	1.42	Heat shock protein
1625131_s_at	*Vha55*	8560 ± 862	1.18	1.05	1.00	V-ATPase B subunit
1639596_at	*CG7781*	8555 ± 2131	1.09	1.37	1.58	
1635449_s_at	*Dip-B*	8518 ± 814	11.56	42.13	1.99	Aminopeptidase
1637164_at	*Tctp*	8470 ± 465	1.38	1.62	1.33	Guanyl-nucleotide exchange factor
1625997_s_at	*GH03753*	8393 ± 3436	0.70	2.24	1.26	Transposable element
1631168_at	*CG5687*	8333 ± 963	19.50	432.04	4.80	Sodium:iodide symporter
1639597_at	*Obp44a*	8311 ± 3564	0.39	6.50	0.96	Odorant binding
1633606_s_at	*CG8229*	8224 ± 1617	0.83	0.87	0.84	
1628814_s_at	*CG9894*	8224 ± 2175	0.78	0.79	0.98	
1629659_s_at	*CG5119*	8188 ± 2028	1.19	1.35	1.25	Nucleotide binding

Signals (with standard deviations) represent the average of five replicate normalized expression values. Enrichments in SG relative to brain (B), neurons (N), and all glia (AG) are simple ratios and do not reflect statistically significant differences.

Table 2 | The 50 most enriched surface glia genes according to three separate comparisons.

Surface glia/brain			Surface glia/neurons			Surface glia/all glia		
Probe	**Symbol**	**FC**	**Probe**	**Symbol**	**FC**	**Probe**	**Symbol**	**FC**
1629317_at	*Nplp3*	247	1641566_s_at	*Indy*	729	1625042_at	*CG31288*	35
1629827_s_at	*Hsp70Ba*	144	1639660_s_at	*CG10550*	563	1639694_s_at	*Arc1*	34
1636747_at	*CG8051*	117	1629317_at	*Nplp3*	453	1623624_at	*CG14869*	22
1636947_at	*bbg*	116	1631168_at	*CG5687*	436	1638964_at	*CG7800*	19
1623624_at	*CG14869*	93	1630150_s_at	*Cg25C*	398	1623788_at	*CG7461*	16
1625042_at	*CG31288*	68	1635210_a_at	*Ppn*	367	1639180_at	*Arc1*	16
1633428_at	*prc*	67	1631925_at	*Mdr65*	299	1635522_a_at	*santa-maria*	14
1631380_s_at	*LanB1*	66	1636835_at	*CG16700*	292	1628075_at	*olf186-M*	14
1624982_s_at	*CG5080*	55	1634767_at	*CG6126*	275	1628779_a_at	*svp*	14
1630142_at	*sog*	46	1641320_s_at	*CG3168*	241	1631535_at	*Vinc*	13
1641490_s_at	*Tsp*	46	1636274_at	*wgn*	225	1640065_at	*GstE7*	13
1628235_at	*CG7203*	42	1633674_at	*cv-d*	216	1632021_at	*Cyp6a20*	13
1632317_at	*CG3036*	41	1639229_at	*vkg*	215	1638661_at	*yip7*	13
1626839_s_at	*blot*	40	1640509_s_at	*lama*	213	1640303_a_at	*pst*	13
1639424_at	*CG6910*	38	1634961_s_at	*Vha68-2*	203	1630633_at	*CG13130*	12
1634620_a_at	*stl*	38	1636947_at	*bbg*	203	1627073_a_at	*CG10126*	12
1628075_at	*olf186-M*	37	1635183_at	*Spn43Ab*	180	1624543_s_at	–	12
1635210_a_at	*Ppn*	36	1630380_at	*CG3837*	154	1636947_at	*bbg*	12
1630233_at	*CG5399*	36	1624839_at	*h*	152	1629062_at	*CG13252*	12
1640509_s_at	*lama*	35	1633639_at	*Cyp28d1*	152	1626271_at	*CG9634*	12
1625116_at	*trol*	35	1636747_at	*CG8051*	148	1624744_a_at	*nuf*	12
1641566_s_at	*Indy*	34	1627773_a_at	*Jheh2*	146	1638226_at	*CG10562*	11
1629256_a_at	*CG31547*	34	1626839_s_at	*blot*	142	1625476_a_at	*CG1674*	11
1638661_at	*yip7*	33	1631569_s_at	*Gp150*	139	1625477_a_at	*CG4797*	11
1634767_at	*CG6126*	33	1623624_at	*CG14869*	135	1628235_at	*CG7203*	11
1625477_a_at	*CG4797*	33	1623200_at	*fng*	133	1636149_at	*CG31705*	11
1628739_at	*Vmat*	32	1624982_s_at	*CG5080*	129	1637481_at	*Tollo*	11
1624156_at	*Ugt86Da*	31	1633112_at	*moody*	127	1631948_s_at	*Clk*	10
1623364_at	*CG4250*	29	1625477_a_at	*CG4797*	116	1638132_at	*CG10184*	10
1626645_at	*CG8596*	28	1631646_at	*spri*	116	1637281_at	–	10
1639660_s_at	*CG10550*	28	1639424_at	*CG6910*	104	1636274_at	*wgn*	10
1623655_at	*Yp2*	27	1629009_at	*Cyp28a5*	100	1629009_at	*Cyp28a5*	10
1640912_s_at	*scaf*	26	1628465_a_at	*CG34417*	97	1626319_a_at	*IM10*	10
1633674_at	*cv-d*	25	1640912_s_at	*scaf*	96	1633254_at	*CG7787*	10
1628052_at	*Cyp6a17*	25	1636653_at	*nec*	94	1640922_a_at	*Hnf4*	9
1632160_s_at	*CG15279*	24	1631380_s_at	*LanB1*	94	1640896_at	*CG4462*	9
1640896_at	*CG4462*	24	1634063_a_at	*stumps*	93	1636747_at	*CG8051*	9
1635770_at	*CG31097*	23	1638964_at	*CG7800*	90	1634237_at	*nimC3*	9
1627000_s_at	*CG6231*	23	1623364_at	*CG4250*	88	1624156_at	*Ugt86Da*	9
1626724_at	*CG32687*	23	1637359_at	*Lsd-2*	86	1624839_at	*h*	9
1623019_a_at	*Unc-89*	23	1632500_at	*CG10226*	85	1627315_s_at	*Pld*	9
1625041_at	*Oatp74D*	21	1632980_at	*CG3902*	85	1633765_at	–	9
1636268_at	*CG10570*	21	1632744_a_at	*if*	83	1625185_at	*CAH2*	9
1629271_at	*CG10444*	21	1632317_at	*CG3036*	83	1631227_at	*CG5793*	9
1638956_at	*Fas2*	20	1632839_a_at	*CG8312*	81	1637089_at	*Syb*	9
1631168_at	*CG5687*	20	1640303_a_at	*pst*	79	1630286_at	*AnnIX*	9
1629062_at	*CG13252*	20	1632021_at	*Cyp6a20*	78	1632160_s_at	*CG15279*	9
1625857_at	*CG8451*	20	1629886_s_at	*for*	78	1641566_s_at	*Indy*	9
1631359_s_at	*Vha100-2*	19	1638063_at	*CG34417*	74	1635770_at	*CG31097*	8
1634036_at	*CG8788*	19	1636149_at	*CG31705*	73	1640703_at	*CG30460*	8

Fold changes (FC) are limma-estimated, and all genes are statistically significant according to an FDR-adjusted $P < 0.05$.

Table 3 | Selected results from gene set enrichment analyses performed using DAVID Bioinformatics on differentially expressed genes enriched in surface glia (SG) relative to brain (B), neurons (N), and all glia (AG).

Enriched term	Category	SG/B		SG/N		SG/AG	
		N	P (adj)	N	P (adj)	N	P (adj)
DRUG METABOLISM							
dme00040:Pentose and glucuronate interconversions	KEGG pathway			12	4.6E-02		
dme00980:Metabolism of xenobiotics by cytochrome P450	KEGG pathway			20	1.6E-03		
GO:0004364 glutathione transferase activity	GO MF			11	3.2E-02		
CELL ADHESION MOLECULES							
GO:0005912 adherens junction	GO CC	14	1.1E-04	14	1.1E-03		
GO:0007155 cell adhesion	GO BP	22	2.8E-02	30	8.5E-04	21	4.5E-03
TRANSPORTERS							
GO:0015293 symporter activity	GO MF	16	2.4E-02	19	8.4E-03	14	1.4E-02
GO:0015849 organic acid transport	GO BP			12	4.7E-02		
IPR001140:ABC transporter, transmembrane region	Interpro domain	8	5.0E-02				
IPR011701:Major facilitator superfamily MFS-1	Interpro domain	20	1.6E-02	21	2.8E-02	16	1.9E-02
Transport	SP_PIR keyword			49	1.0E-02	31	1.8E-02
BASEMENT MEMBRANE/ECM							
GO:0005605 basal lamina	GO CC	5	1.4E-03	5	3.3E-03		
GO:0031012 extracellular matrix	GO CC	18	5.5E-07	19	2.4E-06	11	4.1E-03
METABOLISM							
dme00071:Fatty acid metabolism	KEGG pathway	11	1.2E-02	14	2.3E-03	9	2.2E-02
GO:0016052 carbohydrate catabolic process	GO BP			23	4.1E-06		
MISCELLANEOUS							
GO:0001666 response to hypoxia	GO BP	7	3.0E-02				
GO:0005811 lipid particle	GO CC	39	6.2E-06	73	2.4E-21	23	1.9E-02
GO:0006952 defense response	GO BP	22	2.8E-02	26	2.3E-02		
GO:0022626 cytosolic ribosome	GO CC			31	1.2E-09		
GO:0045185 maintenance of protein location	GO BP	12	1.5E-03				
IPR015897:CHK kinase-like	Interpro domain			14	3.7E-02	10	4.2E-02
PIRSF036514:alpha-crystallin-related small heat shock protein	PIR superfamily	6	6.7E-03				

GO MF, Gene ontology molecular function; BP, biological process; and CC, cellular component. P-values are Benjamini-adjusted.

metabolism and efflux include members of the B and C class, such as ABCB1 and MRP1-4 (ABCC1-4). Our results show three B class ABC transporters to be highly enriched in the surface glia (*Mdr65*, *Mdr49*, and *CG10226*). These three transporters are all highly homologous to vertebrate ABCB1, and we have previously shown that Mdr65 has a conserved function in drug efflux at the apical surface of the *Drosophila* BBB (Mayer et al., 2009). Other enriched transporters in the surface glia include numerous SLC transporters, reflecting the function of the surface glia as a metabolic barrier similar to the vertebrate vascular endothelial BBB component.

In compliance with the BBB functioning as a diffusion barrier, numerous genes constituting SJs are enriched in the surface glia, including the components *Fasciclin 2* (*Fas2*), *lethal (2) giant larvae* (*l(2)gl*), *Neuroglian* (*Nrg*), and *nervana 2* (*nrv2*) (**Table 4**). Also enriched is Moody, a GPCR involved in a signaling pathway that regulates SJ formation (Bainton et al., 2005). Interestingly, the innexin gap junction genes *ogre (inx1)* and *inx2* are enriched in the surface glia and *Drosophila inx1* and *inx2* have recently been linked to coordination of neural stem cell proliferation in response to the metabolic status of the animal (Spéder and Brand, 2014). Thus, the surface glia transcriptome may provide insight into higher order BBB processes. Overall, gene set enrichment analyses of the surface glia transcriptome confirms that the surface glia possess characteristics of BBB physiology.

Although the expression and large enrichment of genes listed in **Table 4**, especially *moody* and *Mdr65*, indicate that our cell isolation techniques are of high purity, we wanted to further validate our approach. Therefore, we searched the literature for genes known to be expressed and functional in the surface glia. We selected 29 genes represented by 36 probe IDs (listed in **Table 5**). We primarily focused on genes where mutations and/or RNAi-mediated knockdown lead to BBB leakiness indicating that the expressed genes function to maintain BBB integrity. If our surface glia transcriptome is valid, we would expect these 29 genes to be present in our data. To decide whether a gene is expressed, we look at two values: (1) the average normalized expression level of five replicate samples and (2) the sum of five replicate sample Present calls for the gene's probe(s). While there are no standards for calling a gene expressed based on Affymetrix data, we set a threshold of a Present sum ≥ 4 and/or an expression level >100. For example, *moody* and *Mdr65*, two genes enriched

Table 4 | Differentially expressed genes enriched in surface glia (SG) relative to brain (B), neurons (N), and all glia (AG) involved in characteristic BBB structures (the basal lamina) and physiologies (drug metabolism, cellular junctions, and transport).

Probe	Symbol	SG/B	SG/N	SG/AG	Function
BASAL LAMINA/ECM					
1630150_s_at	*Cg25C*	7.01	398.29	2.37	Collagen
1635210_a_at	*Ppn*	35.65	366.65	2.57	Structural constituent
1639229_at	*vkg*	8.88	215.02		Collagen
1623624_at	*CG14869*	93.06	135.34	21.93	Basal lamina/ECM
1633428_at	*prc*	67.36	67.61		Collagen-like
1641324_at	*LanA*	18.52	24.42		Laminin
1632666_at	*LanB2*	7.09	16.07		Laminin
DRUG METABOLISM					
1633639_at	*Cyp28d1*		151.51		Cytochrome P450
1629009_at	*Cyp28a5*		100.38	9.68	Cytochrome P450
1632021_at	*Cyp6a20*	10.84	78.07	12.72	Cytochrome P450
1624156_at	*Ugt86Da*	30.74	72.63	9.26	UDP-glucuronosyltransferase
1635727_a_at	*Cyp4g15*		42.62	3.45	Cytochrome P450
1623957_s_at	*GstS1*		38.55		Glutathione S-transferase
1640065_at	*GstE7*	13.84	20.65	12.98	Glutathione S-transferase
1628345_at	*Cyp6a9*	7.11	18.98		Cytochrome P450
1639944_at	*Cyp9f2*		18.69	3.83	Cytochrome P450
1628052_at	*Cyp6a17*	24.54	13.35		Cytochrome P450
1641191_s_at	*Ugt36Bc*	4.54	12.01	5.16	UDP-glucuronosyltransferase
1637129_at	*GstE3*	6.17	11.89	4.84	Glutathione S-transferase
1637309_a_at	*Cyp12e1*	1.89	10.52	4.23	Cytochrome P450
1641481_at	*Ugt86Dd*	4.24	6.63	2.65	UDP-glucuronosyltransferase
1628353_at	*GstD1*	2.01	5.56	2.24	Glutathione S-transferase
1632070_at	*Ugt58Fa*	2.68	4.63	2.04	UDP-glucuronosyltransferase
1639381_at	*Cyp6a19*	4.72	4.31	1.98	Cytochrome P450
SEPTATE JUNCTIONS					
1633112_at	*moody*		127.46		GPCR signaling
1624774_a_at	*Fas2*	4.68	11.58	3.60	Homophilic adhesion
1627491_at	*G-iα65A*		11.23		GPCR signaling
1637410_s_at	*l(2)gl*	3.77	10.09	6.20	Linker
1627651_a_at	*loco*	6.76	8.69		GPCR signaling
1636146_at	*Nrg*		5.63	5.40	Heterophilic adhesion
1625215_s_at	*nrv2*		3.45		Na,K-ATPase
TRANSPORT					
1641566_s_at	*Indy*	34.46	729.03	8.52	SLC13—Na-dep. sulfate/carboxylate transport
1631168_at	*CG5687*	20.28	435.65	5.21	SLC5—sodium:iodide symport
1631925_at	*Mdr65*	7.59	298.68	2.97	MDR/ABC-B
1636835_at	*CG16700*	9.23	292.19	2.56	SLC36—H^+-coupled amino acid transport
1634767_at	*CG6126*	33.08	275.36	2.48	SLC22—organic anion transport
1641320_s_at	*CG3168*	4.16	241.14	5.92	Putative sugar transport
1636747_at	*CG8051*	117.32	147.84	9.34	SLC16—monocarboxylate transport
1626839_s_at	*blot*	39.99	141.76	6.01	Neurotransmitter transport
1625477_a_at	*CG4797*	32.57	116.05	11.00	SLC2—sugar transport
1637359_at	*Lsd-2*	2.96	85.98	3.05	Lipid transport
1632500_at	*CG10226*	7.86	85.48	4.97	MDR/ABC-B
1628739_at	*Vmat*	32.04	41.26		SLC18—monoamine transport
1628659_at	*Mdr49*	12.52	33.67		MDR/ABC-B
1629271_at	*CG10444*	20.73	22.65	3.06	SLC5—sodium:iodide symport

Enrichment values are limma-estimated fold changes, and all genes are significant according to an FDR-adjusted $P < 0.05$.

Table 5 | Gene expressed in surface glia at any stage of development according to the literature.

Probe	Symbol	Stage	Glia	SG signal	P	SG/B	SG/N	SG/AG	Pheno	References
1628276_s_at	*Bsg*	A	sg	7831 ± 851	5	8.12	5.78	2.23		Curtin et al., 2007; Edwards and Meinertzhagen, 2010
1627454_a_at	*cora*	E	spg	7100 ± 887	5	1.74			X	Stork et al., 2008
1631925_at	*Mdr65*	A	spg	6078 ± 1406	5	7.59	298.68	2.97	X	Mayer et al., 2009
1640457_s_at	*Bsg*	A	sg	5866 ± 1154	5	−1.57	2.51	3.29		Curtin et al., 2007; Edwards and Meinertzhagen, 2010
1641566_s_at	*Indy*	A	pg	5716 ± 1370	5	34.46	729.03	8.52	X	DeSalvo et al., 2011
1632465_s_at	*CG6424*	A	pg	4878 ± 1002	5					DeSalvo et al., 2011
1625215_s_at	*nrv2*	EL	spg	3026 ± 667	5		3.45		X	Stork et al., 2008
1636146_at	*Nrg*	EL	spg	2645 ± 914	5		5.63	5.40	X	Stork et al., 2008; Hatan et al., 2011
1633112_at	*moody*	A	spg	2412 ± 824	5		127.46		X	Bainton et al., 2005; Schwabe et al., 2005
1624021_a_at	*dlg1*	L	spg	2241 ± 1521	5	−2.60	−2.48		X	Unhavaithaya and Orr-Weaver, 2012
1627651_a_at	*loco*	A	sg	2165 ± 1139	5	6.76	8.69		X	Schwabe et al., 2005; Kaplow et al., 2008
1629844_s_at	*rap*	L	sg	1290 ± 653	5		−2.26			Kaplow et al., 2008
1637463_a_at	*Nrg*	EL	spg	1099 ± 868	5		4.52		X	Stork et al., 2008; Hatan et al., 2011
1627114_at	*CG3793*	A	spg	1095 ± 379	5				X	DeSalvo et al., 2011
1626001_at	*Nrg*	EL	spg	991 ± 700	3				X	Stork et al., 2008; Hatan et al., 2011
1628336_a_at	*Lac*	E	sg	839 ± 296	5				X	Strigini et al., 2006
1623571_a_at	*CG9328*	A	pg	738 ± 537	4	−2.97			X	DeSalvo et al., 2011
1627491_at	*G-iα65A*	E	spg	697 ± 824	4		11.23		X	Schwabe et al., 2005
1628262_a_at	*CG1322*	E	sg	459 ± 604	5					Layden et al., 2006
1628135_s_at	*pck*	E	spg	421 ± 391	4				X	Stork et al., 2008
1641247_at	*Ranbp21*	A	pg	356 ± 413	5				X	DeSalvo et al., 2011
1632164_at	*scrib*	L	spg	336 ± 314	3		−5.91			Hatan et al., 2011
1635984_at	*Neu3*	A	spg	225 ± 49	1					DeSalvo et al., 2011
1639459_a_at	*Nrx-IV*	EL	spg	213 ± 168	4				X	Baumgartner et al., 1996; Schwabe et al., 2005; Strigini et al., 2006; Hatan et al., 2011
1639402_a_at	*scrib*	L	spg	191 ± 119	3					Hatan et al., 2011
1637017_at	*Cont*	E	spg	167 ± 181	4	−4.35			X	Stork et al., 2008
1631573_a_at	*wunen*	E	spg	166 ± 138	4	−3.31			X	Ile et al., 2012
1639768_at	*coiled*	EL	spg	152 ± 210	3	−5.87	−10.20		X	Hijazi et al., 2011; Syed et al., 2011
1633904_at	*scrib*	L	spg	151 ± 122	2	−3.60	−4.07			Hatan et al., 2011
1623874_at	*CG14215*	A	pg	150 ± 127	4				X	DeSalvo et al., 2011
1625358_s_at	*vari*	A	pg	144 ± 88	2	−2.05			X	DeSalvo et al., 2011
1629115_s_at	*scrib*	L	spg	96 ± 75	3	−3.80	−7.27			Hatan et al., 2011
1627649_at	*Neu3*	A	spg	43 ± 16	0	−3.29				DeSalvo et al., 2011
1637014_at	*sinu*	E	spg	30 ± 15	1	−19.50	−22.60	−8.78	X	Stork et al., 2008
1624994_at	*dup*	L	spg	19 ± 5	2					Unhavaithaya and Orr-Weaver, 2012
1624203_s_at	*Gli*	A	spg	8 ± 3	1	−2.18			X	DeSalvo et al., 2011

We found 29 genes for which 36 probes are listed here—genes are often represented by multiple probes (e.g., Nrg). For "Stage," E, embryo; L, larvae; and A, adult. The "Glia" column specifies which glia layer the gene is expressed in—sg, both surface glia layers; spg, subperineurial glia; and pg, perineurial glia. Signals (with standard deviations) represent the average of five replicate normalized expression values. P = the P sum, or the number of replicates (max = 5) for which the probe was called present. Enrichment values are limma-estimated fold changes significant at an FDR-adjusted $P < 0.05$. An X in the "Pheno" column denotes that disrupting expression or function of the gene produces a BBB phenotype—usually leakage of large MW dextrans into the brain.

in the surface glia, have average normalized expression levels of 2412 and 6078 units, respectively. Both genes also have Present call sums of 5, meaning they were called Present in all 5 replicates of sorted surface glia samples. According to this metric, most of the genes in **Table 5** can be classified as being expressed in our samples of surface glia. However, our microarray methods did not recognize expression of the following known surface glia genes (Present sum < 4 AND expression < 100): *sinuous (sinu)*, *double parked* (*dup*), and *Gliotactin* (*Gli*). In addition, it is not clear via Affymetrix GeneChips data whether the following genes are expressed in surface glia (Present sum < 4 OR expression < 100): *Neu3*, *scrib*, *vari*, and *coiled* (*cold*). However, preliminary data from deep sequencing of the surface glia transcriptome indicate that the above undetected genes are expressed in the BBB glia, and that *dup*, *Gli*, *Neu3*, *scrib*, and *vari* are also enriched in the BBB glia (data not shown). This suggests that although we can be reasonably confident in the genes present in our surface glia microarray, we need to be cautious in our interpretation of the absent calls, as these could be false negatives.

Next, we tested whether the 29 surface glia genes, as a group, have greater expression levels and Present sums compared to all other genes on the microarray. With respect to gene expression level, a two-sample Kolmogorov-Smirnov test revealed a significant difference in the distribution of expression values for known surface glia genes and all other genes on the microarray ($D = 0.3442$, $p = 0.0004$). This difference can be seen graphically in **Figure 4**: a density plot (**Figure 4A**) and a cumulative frequency plot (**Figure 4B**) of log2 surface glia expression for both groups

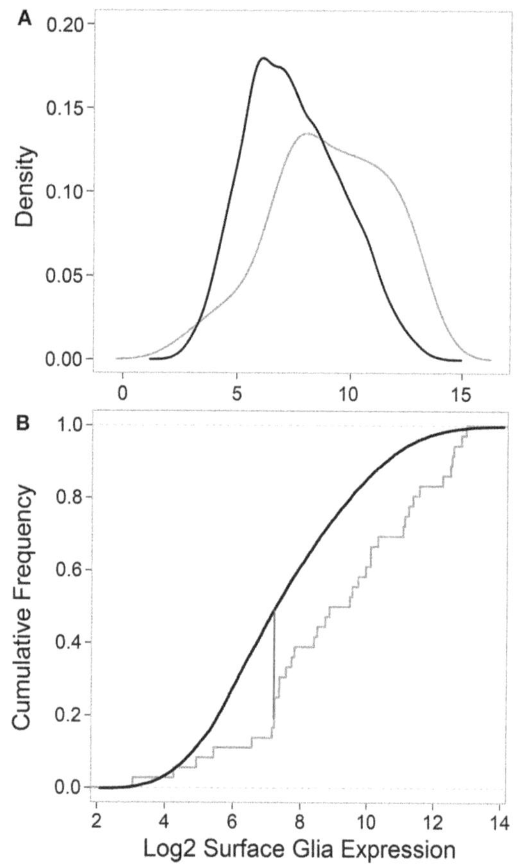

FIGURE 4 | Comparing data for known surface glia genes to all other probes on the microarray validates the surface glia transcriptome. **(A)** Kernal density estimates based on surface glia log2 gene expression for known surface glia genes (gray) and all other probes on the microarray (black). The distribution of data for known surface glia genes is significantly greater than that for all other probes on the microarray (Two-sample Kolmogorov-Smirnov test, $D = 0.3435$, $P = 0.0004$). **(B)** A cumulative frequency plot of the same data also illustrates the significant difference in distributions between known surface glia genes and all other probes on the microarray. The red line corresponds to the D-statistic, the point of greatest separation between the curves. At this point, 81.6% of known surface glia genes have higher expression levels, which is in stark contrast to 51.7% for all other probes on the microarray.

of genes showing that, by and large, known surface glia genes have greater expression values than all other genes on the microarray. With respect to Present sum data, we used a hypergeometric test to determine whether the distribution of Present sums in known surface glia genes was significantly different (and greater) than that for all other genes on the microarray. According to our stringent standard of requiring a Present sum ≥ 4 to call a probe expressed, we find that 24 of 36 (67%) probes representing known surface glia genes have a Present sum ≥ 4. Comparing this to 4488 of 11645 (39%) of the remaining probes on the array, the hypergeometric test indeed finds a significant difference between these distributions ($p = 0.0002$). Even if we loosen our criteria and allow a Present sum ≥ 3, there is still a significant difference (29 of 36 [81%] for known surface glia genes and 6063 of 11645 [52%] for all other probes—$p = 9.5 \times 10^{-5}$). Overall, we find that our microarray data shows positive expression for known surface glia genes leading us to conclude that the surface glia transcriptome is highly quantitative and accurate.

Central to validating our cell isolation and transcriptomic techniques is showing that genes identified as enriched in the surface glia are indeed expressed in these cell layers. To demonstrate surface glia-localized expression, we searched the FlyTrap GFP Protein Trap database (http://flytrap.med.yale.edu/) (Morin et al., 2001; Kelso et al., 2004; Buszczak et al., 2007; Quinones-Coello et al., 2007) for protein and enhancer traps available for surface glia-enriched genes. As a control, we also included one gene (*Vha55*) that, based on our transcriptome, was roughly equally expressed in neurons, glia, and surface glia. We also searched the Bloomington Stock Collection for transgenic lines containing GFP-fusion proteins for any surface glia-enriched genes, and found one for *hairy* (*h*). Lastly, we targeted the expression of VMAT using polyclonal antibodies specific to the glia-specific isoform of VMAT (DVMAT-B) previously found to store histamine in the *Drosophila* visual system (Romero-Calderon et al., 2008). Microarray data for all genes in **Figure 5** are listed in Table S4. The images in **Figure 5** indeed demonstrate that surface glia-enriched genes identified in the microarray data are expressed in these cell layers. However, surface glia enrichment does not equate to specific expression in the surface glia. Many surface glia-enriched genes are also expressed in other glial subtypes. For example, the first gene shown in **Figure 5** is *viking* (*vkg*), which encodes a collagen IV protein, and is enriched 9-fold relative to whole brain and 215-fold relative to neurons. The GFP protein trap for *vkg* shows pan-glial expression (see also **Figure 1** for another image of the *vkg* protein trap), which is consistent with a previous study (Freeman et al., 2003). Interestingly, the *vkg* protein trap also allows for visualization of the neural lamella, and its enrichment in surface glia suggests deposition of the neural lamella by the surface glia.

Surface glia-localized expression can be assessed using both brain surface and cross-section confocal images (**Figure 5**). Co-localization with injected 70 kDa dextran helps to differentiate the PG from the SPG since dextran demarcates the PG layer (DeSalvo et al., 2011). Expression in the surface glia can be identified by any of the following characteristics: (1) surface images show a "flagstone" pattern of cell junctions characteristic of the PG, e.g., *Vha55*, *I'm not dead yet* (*Indy*), and *l(2)08717*; (2)

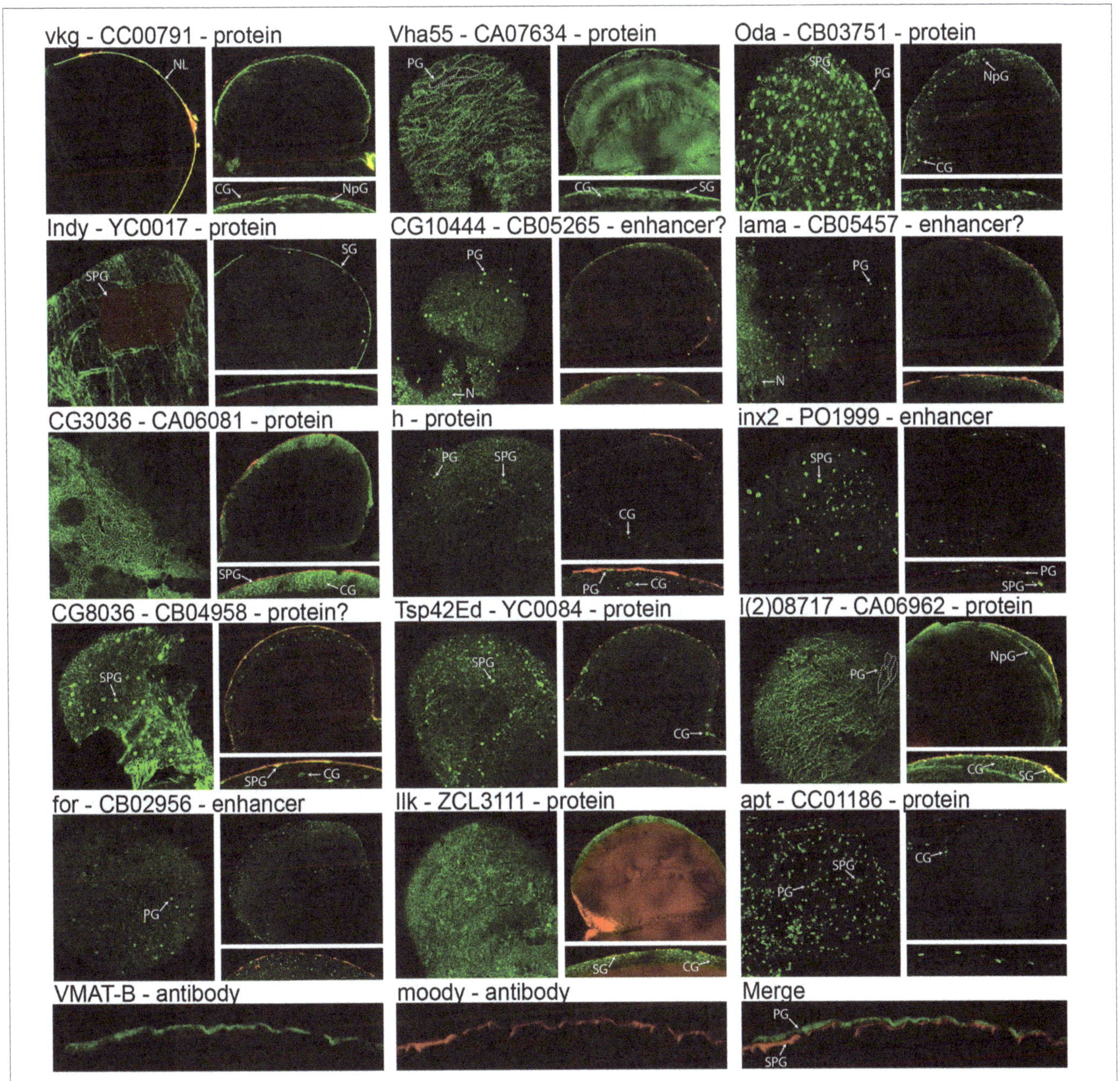

FIGURE 5 | Expression and localization of surface glia-enriched genes. Gene symbols are followed by the FlyTrap database ID number and whether the GFP exon results in a GFP-fusion protein (Protein), likely results in a GFP-fusion protein (Protein?), is controlled by nearby enhancers (Enhancer), or is likely controlled by nearby enhancers (Enhancer?). With the exception of *vkg*, each FlyTrap line has a surface image followed by a cross section image and a zoomed-in image of the surface glia layer in cross section. For *vkg*, instead of a surface image, we present a cross-section showing the GFP-positive neural lamella. Localization to the surface glia layer can be assessed using surface images that show membrane GFP at the boundaries of perineurial glia (PG) [see dotted lines in *Vha55* and *l(2)08717*] or subperineurial glia (SPG) (see shaded cell in *Indy*). In cross section images of membrane GFP, localization to the surface glia can be determined because injection with 70 kDa rhodamine dextran demarcates the PG layer (no dextran was used for *Vha55*, *Oda*, *apt*, and VMAT-B). For nuclear GFP, surface images reveal small PG nuclei and large SPG nuclei. In cross section, these nuclei are within the dextran layer (PG-localized) or slightly below (SPG-localized). Many surface glia-enriched genes are also expressed in other glial subtypes, such as cortex glia (CG) and neuropil glia (NpG), and in rare cases we found that surface glia-enriched genes were also expressed in neurons (N). VMAT-B expression is visualized with polyclonal antibodies (green) and localized by co-staining with antibodies to the SPG-specific Moody protein (red).

surface images show the SJ boundaries characteristic of the SPG, e.g., *Indy*; (3) surface and cross-section images show numerous, small PG nuclei, e.g., *Ornithine decarboxylase antizyme* (*Oda*), *CG10444*, *innexin 2* (*inx2*), *lamina ancestor* (*lama*), *foraging* (*for*), and *apontic* (*apt*); and (4) surface and cross-section images show sparse, large SPG nuclei, e.g., *Oda*, *CG8036*, *h*, *inx2*, and *apt*. Furthermore, many of the images (e.g., *Vha55*, *Indy*, *CG3036*, and *CG8036*) show a pattern of GFP expression similar to that seen when staining adult brains with antibodies to the Moody protein (Schwabe et al., 2005; Mayer et al., 2009). This pattern resembles a mosaic of small circular cell junctions, which is due to either (1) contact between the basal surface of the SPG and the underlying cortex glia, or (2) expression in both the SPG and cortex glia. Indeed, many of the surface glia-enriched genes are also expressed in the cortex glia. Membrane-bound GFP expression in cortex glia is seen in *CG3036*, *CG8036*, *l(2)08717*, and *Integrin-linked kinase* (*Ilk*). Nuclear-GFP expression in cortex glia is seen in *Oda*, *h*, *Tetraspanin 42Ed* (*Tsp42Ed*), and *apt*.

Regarding expression of the glia-specific DVMAT-B, we co-stained adult brains with Moody and DVMAT-B antibodies. Moody is specifically expressed in the SPG (Bainton et al., 2005; Mayer et al., 2009), and the results show DVMAT-B expression apical and non-overlapping with Moody, thus pinpointing DVMAT-B to the PG layer (**Figure 5**). Of the 16 surface glia-enriched genes shown in **Figure 5**, we found that *Vmat* and *Indy* were the only surface glia-specific genes in the adult brain. Furthermore, we also found that one of the protein traps (*Ilk* GFP) caused the BBB to be leaky, indicated by the large accumulation of 70 kDa dextran in the brains. *Ilk* is expressed in surface and cortex glia. In this case, GFP fusion likely disrupts protein function leading to BBB leakiness. In addition to showing that surface glia-enriched genes are indeed expressed in these cell types, we also found that our control gene *Vha55* had a more global expression pattern in the brain. This is consistent with our transcriptome, further confirming the validity of our cell isolation and transcriptomic methods. Thus, these data provide a suitable starting point for an investigator interested in elucidating gene function in surface glia-localized processes.

While little is known about the fly surface glia, there is a wealth of knowledge on neuronal physiology where many proteins and processes are highly conserved among metazoans (Venter et al., 1988; Anderson and Greenberg, 2001). Thus, we can further validate our cell isolation and transcriptomic methods by analyzing neuronal genes and pathways. As anticipated, overrepresented gene set enrichment categories related to neuronal physiology are seen for genes enriched in whole brains, neurons, and all glia samples relative to those of the surface glia (**Table 6**). Neurons are 3-fold more numerous than glia in the fly brain (Pfrieger and Barres, 1995), thus, it was to be expected that the genes enriched in our whole brain and neuron samples largely function in synaptic transmission, axonogenesis, vesicle-mediated transport, regulation of neurotransmitter levels, and neurotransmitter receptor activity. Genes enriched in all glia relative to the surface glia include those involved in axon guidance, neuron development, and synapse formation. These functions are consistent with the activities of the abundant cortex and neuropil glia, which are more intimately involved in neuronal development and function (Edwards and Meinertzhagen, 2010).

ADULT BBB TRANSCRIPTOME POINTS TO GENES REQUIRED THROUGHOUT DEVELOPMENT FOR BBB FUNCTION

Having shown that our adult BBB transcriptome is a reliable resource, we were now well positioned to ask how the adult BBB profile compares to that of the embryo. We used data from the Berkeley *Drosophila* Genome Project (BDGP) *in situ* database (http://insitu.fruitfly.org/cgi-bin/ex/insitu.pl) to obtain gene expression patterns in the embryonic CNS. The BDGP *in situ* database classifies *in situ* gene expression patterns during embryonic development according to a controlled vocabulary

Table 6 | Selected results from gene set enrichment analyses performed using DAVID Bioinfomatics on differentially expressed genes enriched in brain (B), neurons (N), and all glia (AG) relative to surface glia (SG).

Enriched term	Category	SG/B		SG/N		SG/AG	
		N	P (adj)	N	P (adj)	N	P (adj)
GO:0001505 regulation of neurotransmitter levels	GO BP	55	8.0E-07	32	2.2E-02		
GO:0007268 synaptic transmission	GO BP	90	6.7E-10	61	3.8E-06		
GO:0007409 axonogenesis	GO BP	80	1.3E-05	76	9.1E-12	17	1.4E-02
GO:0007411 axon guidance	GO BP	58	8.4E-05	57	2.2E-10	13	2.8E-02
GO:0007610 behavior	GO BP	129	2.5E-02	106	1.1E-04		
GO:0007611 learning or memory	GO BP	32	2.4E-02	26	8.0E-03		
GO:0008038 neuron recognition	GO BP			23	1.1E-04		
GO:0008355 olfactory learning	GO BP			18	2.2E-02		
GO:0016192 vesicle-mediated transport	GO BP	136	1.8E-05	85	4.2E-02		
GO:0016319 mushroom body development	GO BP			20	5.2E-03		
GO:0019933 cAMP-mediated signaling	GO BP	11	3.3E-02	11	1.6E-03		
GO:0030594 neurotransmitter receptor activity	GO MF	32	3.7E-02	29	3.9E-04		
GO:0031644 regulation of neurological system process	GO BP			9	2.4E-02		
GO:0034702 ion channel complex	GO CC	27	5.3E-03	26	6.2E-06	9	1.0E-02
GO:0045202 synapse	GO CC	65	6.4E-08	53	3.7E-09		
GO:0048512 circadian behavior	GO BP	22	1.5E-03	17	4.3E-03		
GO:0048666 neuron development	GO BP	131	2.9E-07	114	1.0E-12	26	2.9E-03

GO BP, Gene ontology biological process; MF, molecular function; and CC, cellular component. P-values are Benjamini-adjusted.

that corresponds to specific anatomic structures (Tomancak et al., 2002, 2007). The BDGP vocabulary includes gene expression in the lateral cord surface glia and central brain surface glia for embryos in stages 13–16. We asked whether surface glia-enriched genes in the adult brain are more likely to have embryonic surface glia *in situ* staining compared to non-surface glia-enriched genes. Indeed, we found that genes enriched in adult surface glia relative to whole brain are more likely to contain embryonic surface glia *in situ* staining (Chi-squared test with Yates' continuity correction: $X^2 = 4.76$, $df = 1$, p-value $= 0.0291$, odds ratio $= 2.12$). We also obtained a significant result for genes enriched in surface glia relative to neurons ($X^2 = 7.32$, $df = 1$, p-value $= 0.0068$, odds ratio $= 2.26$). The results point to 18 genes that are expressed in surface glia during all stages of development and adulthood (*in situ* images can be found on the BDGP website). These genes include: (1) six known glial genes (*G-iα65A*, *Mdr65*, *Glutamine synthetase 2*, *repo*, *moody*, and *nrv2*) with previously published *in situ* images (Xiong et al., 1994; Auld et al., 1995; Freeman et al., 2003; Schwabe et al., 2005); (2) six annotated genes that to our knowledge were not known to be expressed in surface glia throughout development (*babos*, *Minichromosome maintenance 5*, *Hsp27*, *Major Facilitator Superfamily Transporter 3*, *pericardin*, and *mutagen-sensitive 209*); and (3) six non-annotated genes (*CG10702*, *CG11164*, *CG3168*, *CG4829*, *CG5080*, and *CG6126*). These findings already highlight a good starting point for furthering our knowledge of embryonic BBB formation, maintenance and function. Together with profiling of the embryonic BBB, our adult BBB transcriptome would provide a valuable resource to gain further insight into BBB dynamics during development.

NEURONAL PHYSIOLOGY GENES IDENTIFIED IN THE MICROARRAY DATA

Interestingly, we observed some SJ components [e.g., *sinuous* (*sinu*), *scribbled* (*scrib*), *varicose* (*vari*), *Contactin* (*Cont*), and *discs large 1* (*dlg1*)] were enriched in brain and neurons relative to surface glia (Table S2). Assuming these genes are mainly involved in SJ formation, this observation suggests the existence of SJs amongst cells of the adult brain besides the surface glia. Although neuropil glia in the adult CNS ensheath axons (Edwards and Meinertzhagen, 2010), very little has been published on SJs among cells other than the surface glia. It seems likely that other cells form SJs given that this has been found in the peripheral nervous system (Banerjee and Bhat, 2008). Furthermore, enrichment of SJ genes in neurons points to neuron-localized expression of these genes. In the embryonic and larval peripheral nervous system, axons are ensheathed by inner and outer glial membranes involving the expression of SJ proteins Neurexin IV (Nrx-IV), Cont, and Nrg (Banerjee et al., 2006). All three of these proteins are expressed in the glial cells, while Nrg is also expressed by the neurons. Similarly, Nrx-IV is expressed by neurons in the larval CNS where it mediates glial wrapping but is independent of SJ formation (Stork et al., 2008). Given these results, it seems likely that neurons of the adult CNS express SJ components thereby mediating axon insulation by ensheathing glia. This is consistent with axo-glial SJs at the nodes of Ranvier of myelinated axons in the vertebrate nervous system (Bhat et al., 2001; Bhat, 2003).

BBB GENES CONSERVED BETWEEN DROSOPHILA AND VERTEBRATES

Using BLAST, we compared the fly and mouse BBB transcriptomes to assess what BBB genes are conserved across evolution. We took a focused approach by targeting known molecular components of the vertebrate BBB covered in reviews by Zlokovic (2008) and Daneman (2012). These proteins are central to the BBB's role as a diffusion barrier (TJs), chemoprotective interface (drug transporters), and conduit for metabolite passage between the blood and brain (SLC transporters). In short, we retrieved sequences for 144 known proteins expressed at the mouse BBB and searched for BLAST homologs ($E < 10^{-5}$) in the fly genome. Fly BLAST hits were then annotated with our surface glia transcriptome data to determine which fly homologs are expressed and/or enriched at the BBB.

TIGHT AND ADHERENS JUNCTION PROTEINS

Of the 16 TJ components targeted in our comparative analysis, nine have fly homologs expressed in the surface glia, six of which have homologs enriched in the surface glia (**Table 7**). According to our methods, the fly genome does not contain true homologs for seven TJ proteins: claudin 3, claudin 5, claudin 12, occludin, immunoglobulin superfamily member 5, peripheral myelin protein 22, and lipolysis stimulated lipoprotein receptor. The importance of some of these proteins to TJ formation is well documented (Hirase et al., 1997; Saitou et al., 2000; Nitta et al., 2003), and the absence of true fly homologs perhaps highlights the differing composition of cell-cell junctions between flies and vertebrates (Wu and Beitel, 2004). We note that claudin-like proteins have been characterized in *Drosophila* (i.e., Sinu, Megatrachea, and Kune-kune), and they are involved in SJ formation (Behr et al., 2003; Wu et al., 2004; Nelson et al., 2010); however, their level of homology with vertebrate claudins is less than the significance level chosen in our BLAST analysis.

The calcium/calmodulin-dependent serine protein kinase (MAGUK family) protein (CASK—same symbol in mouse and fly) is the only highly conserved TJ protein ($E = 0$) co-expressed at both the fly and mouse BBBs. Other strong BLAST hits ($E < 10^{-40}$) exist for: membrane associated guanylate kinase, WW and PDZ domain containing 1 (MAGI1); multiple PDZ domain protein (MPDZ); and TJ proteins 1 and 2 (TJP1 and TJP2), which are nearly equally homologous to fly PYD. Interestingly, CASK, MAGI1, TJP1, and TJP2 are all membrane-associated proteins containing guanylate kinase and PDZ domains. MPDZ also contains PDZ domains. These proteins help link transmembrane proteins to the cytoskeleton and bind signaling complexes together (PDZ domain) (Ranganathan and Ross, 1997), and function in signaling themselves (guanylate kinase domain). Our results thus point to strong evolutionary conservation of such proteins at the BBB.

With the exception of PYD, most of the fly homologs of mouse TJ proteins, while expressed in the surface glia, are not specifically enriched. Most of the enriched fly homologs are weakly homologous ($E > 10^{-30}$); for example, PPN, FAS2, and CG7981 are highly enriched in the surface glia but are weakly homologous ($E > 10^{-10}$) to mouse JAM-A. However, with respect to adherens junction proteins, there are various highly conserved proteins ($E = 0$) co-expressed at the fly and mouse BBBs, which

Table 7 | Fly genes homologous to known junctional components expressed at the mouse BBB.

Mouse prot	No. exp.	Best hit	E	SG exp.	SG/B	SG/N	No. enr.	Fly prot	E	SG exp.	SG/B	SG/N
Adherens junctions												
CDH5 (VE-cadherin)	4	CADN	2.E-44	1863		−2.4	0					
CTNNA1 (α-catenin)	3	α-CAT	0	924		−3.7	1	VINC	4.E-13	2475	11.8	29.9
CTNNB1 (β-catenin)	1	ARM	0	3511		−1.9	0					
JUP (γ-catenin)	1	ARM	0	3511		−1.9	0					
PECAM1	1	CG42330	1.E-07	518	−4.9	−1.9	0					
Tight junctions												
CASK	37	CASK	0	2260	−2.5	−2.3	5	FOR	2.E-21	697	10.9	77.9
								Unc-89	1.E-29	952	22.5	20.6
								PHKγ	3.E-50	1931	−2.8	2.3
								Lk6	3.E-35	1352	−2.3	2.2
								Par-1	1.E-37	1182	−2.2	1.7
CGNL1 (JACOP)	1	ZIP	6.E-21	2240			0					
ESAM	1	CG42368	4.E-06	271			0					
F11R (JAM-A)	11	ROBO	1.E-10	901	−6.1		4	PPN	7.E-06	3397	35.7	366.7
								CG7981	7.E-06	8162	34.5	37.4
								FAS2	6.E-07	4442	20.3	11.6
								NRG	4.E-07	2645		5.6
MAGI1	15	Magi	4.E-92	297			2	CG33967	3.E-17	997	2.3	6.3
								GRIP	2.E-09	325	10.0	4.5
MARVELD2 (TRIC)	1	Su(Tpl)	4.E-11	1811			0					
MPDZ (MUPP1)	11	Patj	2.E-68	810			1	PYD	2.E-07	3927	5.6	−6.9
TJP1 (ZO1)	3	PYD	6.E-94	3927	5.6	−6.9	1	PYD	6.E-94	3927	5.6	−6.9
TJP2 (ZO2)	4	PYD	2.E-92	3927	5.6	−6.9	1	PYD	2.E-92	3927	5.6	−6.9

The left side of the table lists the number of homologs expressed in the surface glia (SG) followed by the best BLAST hit and its SG expression and enrichments relative to brain (B) and neurons (N). The right side lists all homologs enriched in the surface glia. No significant BLAST hits for Cldn5, Cldn12, Cldn3, Ocln, Igsf5, Pmp22, and Lsr.

include α-Catenin, and β- and γ-Catenin (equally homologous to fly Armadillo). A high BLAST hit ($E = 2 \times 10^{-44}$) also exists for VE-cadherin. These results indicate that adherens junction proteins are conserved throughout evolution and function at the BBB in both flies and mice.

Overall, strong conservation between TJ proteins is absent, but we do see conservation between junctional adaptor proteins and adherens junction proteins. These trends were found previously (Knust and Bossinger, 2002) and are not surprising given the ultrastructural differences between the TJ and SJ. In vertebrates, the TJ is apical to the adherens junction, but in *Drosophila* the SJ is basal to the adherens junction. Some of the fly homologs to TJ proteins are localized at a comparable site termed the marginal zone or subapical region (Knust and Bossinger, 2002; Wu and Beitel, 2004), similarly, some of the mouse homologs to SJ proteins are localized at a comparable site termed the basal region (Wu and Beitel, 2004). In conclusion, our results point to the *Drosophila* BBB and SJ complex being a relevant model for the role of adaptor proteins and adherens junction proteins in regulating the diffusion barrier at the BBB.

TRANSPORTERS

Besides junctional proteins, the best-studied components of the BBB are the diverse array of ABC and SLC transporters. BLAST hits expressed and enriched at the fly BBB to our targeted set of extensively studied, functionally important mouse BBB transporters (**Table 8**) reveal striking sequence conservation. For example, mouse BBB transporters that have highly conserved homologs ($E < 10^{-90}$) expressed at the fly BBB include: GLUT1, CAT1, LAT1, EAAT1, ABCB1A, BCRP, MRP1, and MRP5. Furthermore, the same homologs for LAT1, ABCB1A, BCRP, MRP1, and MRP5 are not only expressed but also enriched at the fly BBB, and they are among a group of highly conserved homologs enriched at the fly BBB (e.g., there are three fly proteins enriched at the BBB with high homology to ABCB1A). These results point to strong selective pressure for the conservation of BBB-localized transport of glucose, amino acids, and the numerous ABC transporter substrates, thus indicating that across species it is these proteins that are essential for the function of a selective barrier.

Interestingly, we also see that the best BLAST hit is often not the most BBB-enriched homolog. For example, fly GLUT1 is the most homologous fly protein to mouse GLUT1 ($E = 10^{-124}$). Fly GLUT1 is expressed at the BBB (surface glia expression = 711), but it is enriched in neurons. However, six other less homologous BLAST hits are highly enriched in surface glia. CG3168 and CG4797 are both annotated as putative sugar transporters with weak homology to GLUT1 ($E = 6 \times 10^{-9}$ and 2×10^{-15}, respectively), but they are enriched 214- and 116-fold in surface glia relative to neurons, respectively. We obtained similar results for MCT1 and LRP1, thus indicating that neurons and surface glia in the adult fly brain might use different transporters to transport

Table 8 | Fly genes homologous to known transporters expressed at the mouse BBB (for notes on table format, see Table 7).

Mouse prot	No. exp.	Best hit	E	SG exp.	SG/B	SG/N	No. enr.	Fly prot	E	SG exp.	SG/B	SG/N
Abcb1a (Mdr1a/Pgp)	4	MDR49	0	1485	12.5	33.7	3	Mdr65	0	6078	7.6	298.7
								CG10226	0	3133	7.9	85.5
								MDR49	0	1485	12.5	33.7
Abcc1 (Mrp1)*	4	CG5789	0	218	5.7	17.1	4	CG5789	0	218	5.7	17.1
								SUR	2.E-54	111	5.2	4.3
								CG11897	0	2090	5.0	2.8
								MRP	0	2618	3.1	
Abcc5 (Mrp5)**	4	MRP	0	2618	3.1		4	CG5789	1.E-166	218	5.7	17.1
								SUR	7.E-52	111	5.2	4.3
								CG11897	1.E-180	2090	5.0	2.8
								MRP	0	2618	3.1	
Abcg2 (Bcrp)	6	W	2.E-76	171	9.9	−2.2	3	CG31689	5.E-52	184	2.3	8.8
								CG3164	1.E-51	610		5.2
								W	2.E-76	171	9.9	−2.2
Atp1a2	8	ATPα	0	15084			2	CG42321	4.E-11	6251	1.5	
								CG31729	2.E-06	1040	2.2	
Lrp1	13	CG8909	0	450	−19.2	−5.4	8	LPR1	1.E-143	3632	15.2	43.2
								CG7981	1.E-44	8162	34.5	37.4
								SLOW	3.E-06	769	12.8	27.1
								SHF	1.E-14	1102	7.6	13.6
								DI	5.E-11	299	4.7	12.1
								N	1.E-14	362		4.7
								MGL	0	1900	2.0	1.9
								CUE	1.E-23	2734	2.3	
Slc1a1 (EAAT3)***	2	EAAT1	2.E-92	2260			0					
Slc1a2 (Eaat2)	2	EAAT2	2.E-90	820	−5.9	−4.9	0					
Slc2a1 (Glut1)	8	GLUT1	1.E-124	711	−3.6	−4.0	6	CG3168	6.E-09	4663	4.2	241.1
								CG4797	2.E-15	5031	32.6	116.1
								CG4607	4.E-25	1021	16.6	59.3
								CG30035	1.E-28	6887	8.1	54.2
								CG6231	2.E-08	1911	23.1	23.8
								ORCT	1.E-05	428	2.2	11.2
Slc4a2	2	CG8177	0	4468			0					
Slc7a1 (Cat1)	5	CG13248	1.E-111	370			2	Jhl-21	6.E-07	1628		9.9
								CG9413	2.E-06	4326	2.1	2.7
Slc7a3 (Cat3)	1	CG13248	1.E-101	370			0					
Slc7a5 (LAT1)	5	Jhl-21	1.E-115	1628		9.9	2	Jhl-21	1.E-115	1628		9.9
								CG9413	7.E-82	4326	2.1	2.7
Slc9a1 (Nhe1)	2	NHE1	1.E-45	132	−2.2		0					
Slc16a1 (MCT1)	6	CG3409	1.E-29	1177		−2.4	3	CG8051	4.E-09	1472	117.3	147.8
								KAR	2.E-15	3132	13.7	9.4
								CG13907	2.E-24	4225	3.8	3.9
Slc19a1 (RFC1)	1	CG6574	1.E-51	253	2.6	2.8	1	CG6574	1.E-51	253	2.6	2.8
Slc22a8 (OAT3)	6	ORCT	1.E-60	428	2.2	11.2	6	CG6126	4.E-58	5224	33.1	275.4
								CG3168	5.E-15	4663	4.2	241.1
								CG6231	1.E-26	1911	23.1	23.8
								ORCT2	2.E-57	1166	18.2	12.4
								CG4630	1.E-46	651	8.3	12.2
								ORCT	1.E-60	428	2.2	11.2
Slc38a1 (SNAT1)****	1	CG13743	7.E-15	291	−9.5	−8.6	0					
Slc39a10	4	FOI	5.E-63	1643	2.4	1.8	2	CATSUP	1.E-20	430	2.6	2.6
								FOI	5.E-63	1643	2.4	1.8
Slco1c1 (OATP-F)*****	1	OATP74D	1.E-63	2041	21.4	64.0	1	Oatp74D	1.E-63	2041	21.4	64.0

Significant BLAST hits that are not expressed in surface glia: Slc19a2, Slc19a3, Slc30a1, and Tfrc.

**Nearly identical results for Abcc4 (Mrp4);*

***Nearly identical results for Abcc6 (Mrp6);*

****Nearly identical results for Slc1a3 (Eaat1);*

*****Nearly identical results for Slc38a3 (SNAT3) and Slc38a5 (SNAT5);*

******Nearly identical results for Slco1a4 (Oatp2) and Slco2b1 (OATP-B).*

sugar, monocarboxylates, and lipoproteins, and may allow differential regulation over substrate entry into the brain vs. neuronal uptake.

Overall, we see that the fly and mouse BBBs contain highly homologous transporters, which highlights the importance of these transporters in chemical protection and the transport of metabolites at the BBB regardless of the cell type that expresses them. Our previous investigations on the efflux transporter Mdr65 (Mayer et al., 2009), a fly homolog of ABCB1A, taken together with the elucidation of many more highly homologous BBB transporters in the present study, points to the *Drosophila* surface glia BBB as a relevant model for studying evolutionary conserved BBB-localized transport properties despite the fact that it is of glial rather than endothelial origin.

OTHER NOTABLE GENES CO-EXPRESSED AT THE BBB

Noteworthy results among eight additional mouse BBB genes and their fly homologs (**Table 9**) include the co-enrichment of carbonic anhydrases at the mouse and fly BBBs, which indicates a conserved BBB physiology focused on brain carbon dioxide and bicarbonate homeostasis. We also see very high homology between mouse and fly gamma-glutamyltranspeptidase (GGT1) protein sequences. In vertebrates, GGT1 is expressed at the luminal surface of the BBB where it functions in both amino acid transport and the regulation of glutathione levels (and thus the detoxification processes involving GSTs) (Courtay et al., 1992; Hawkins et al., 2006). An alternative explanation might be that the surface glia express GGT1 similar to astroctyes, where they function to facilitate glutathione synthesis in neurons (Valdovinos-Flores and Gonsebatt, 2012). Another striking result in **Table 9** is the conservation of insulin signaling at the mouse and fly BBBs. The *Drosophila* insulin receptor (InR) is the best BLAST hit to both mouse INSR and IGF1R ($E = 0$ for both). Our data suggest that *InR* is expressed in surface glia at low levels; however, another BLAST hit to mouse INSR, CG3837 ($E = 3 \times 10^{-75}$), is highly enriched in the surface glia. CG3837 was recently identified as a secreted decoy of the insulin receptor (SDR) (Okamoto et al., 2013). SDR acts as an antagonist of insulin signaling and its secretion into the hemolymph by the surface glia of larvae controls body growth; SDR mutants have an abnormally rapid growth rate resulting in larger adult body size. FlyAtlas (Chintapalli et al., 2007) data indicate that *InR* is nearly equally expressed in all tissues, whereas CG3837/*SDR* expression is more restricted, with the highest expression in the CNS. Our microarray data and the data in (Okamoto et al., 2013)

Table 9 | Fly genes homologous to known genes expressed at the mouse BBB (for notes on table format, see Table 7).

Mouse prot	No. exp.	Best hit	E	SG exp.	SG/B	SG/N	No. enr.	Fly prot	E	SG exp.	SG/B	SG/N
Bsg	4	ROBO	4.E-10	901	−6.1		1	CG31605	2.E-09	7831	8.1	5.8
Car4	4	CAH2	2.E-26	860	10.0		3	CAH1	8.E-19	799	−2.4	3.6
								CG11284	7.E-18	1756	5.6	2.5
								CAH2	2.E-26	860	10.0	
Ggt1	2	CG4829	1.E-103	1132	−3.6	2.6	1	CG4829	1.E-103	1132	−3.6	2.6
Igf1r	37	INR	0	135			8	CG3837	3.E-78	2097	5.7	153.9
								HTL	2.E-53	422	3.0	19.9
								CG10702	2.E-56	635	3.6	16.5
								FPS85D	2.E-46	1257	14.1	9.7
								PVR	4.E-36	944	5.5	6.1
								PHKγ	1.E-11	1931	−2.8	2.3
								Par-1	1.E-09	1182	−2.2	1.7
								HOP	7.E-40	2470	2.0	−3.3
Insr (IR)	41	INR	0	135			9	CG3837	3.E-75	2097	5.7	153.9
								FOR	3.E-09	697	10.9	77.9
								HTL	1.E-53	422	3.0	19.9
								CG10702	7.E-72	635	3.6	16.5
								Fps85D	7.E-48	1257	14.1	9.7
								PVR	2.E-35	944	5.5	6.1
								PHKγ	9.E-13	1931	−2.8	2.3
								Par-1	1.E-10	1182	−2.2	1.7
								HOP	9.E-37	2470	2.0	−3.3
Kdr (Flk-1)	32	HTL	4.E-68	422	3.0	19.9	7	for	2.E-11	697	10.9	77.9
								UNC-89	2.E-10	952	22.5	20.6
								HTL	4.E-68	422	3.0	19.9
								FPS85D	3.E-31	1257	14.1	9.7
								PVR	1.E-51	944	5.5	6.1
								SGG	5.E-10	6594	1.7	−1.6
Lef1	2	PAN	2.E-51	6202		−1.8	0					
Ptch1	1	PTR	2.E-12	1241	10.1	9.4	1	PTR	2.E-12	1241	10.1	9.4

suggest that this high CNS expression of CG3837/*SDR* is specifically located in the surface glia (6-fold enriched relative to brain and 154-fold enriched relative to neurons). As *Drosophila* adult body size is predetermined in the larval stages, the maintained expression of CG3837/SDR in the adult surface glia suggests the possibility of novel roles for the adult BBB in insulin regulated physiologies independent of body size control.

Lastly, we note that the surface glia also express homologs of the vertebrate BBB proteins LEF1 and PTCH1. LEF1 is a Wnt-responsive transcription factor (Liebner et al., 2008; Stenman et al., 2008; Daneman et al., 2009), and PTCH1 is a mediator of sonic hedgehog signaling (Alvarez et al., 2011). This final set of genes again illustrates that the *Drosophila* surface glia can be used to model evolutionary conserved BBB-localized signaling and regulatory proteins. Overall, our surface glia transcriptome will continue to provide an evolutionary comparative framework as more essential BBB proteins are identified in vertebrates.

DISCUSSION

Here we have described techniques for the isolation and transcriptome characterization of the adult brain *Drosophila* surface glia. We have shown that our techniques are of high quality yielding a quantitative transcriptomic portrait of the surface glia constituting the BBB. While organ-specific transcriptomes exist for *Drosophila* (Wang et al., 2004; Chintapalli et al., 2007), cell-type-specific data sets have been slower to emerge (Salmand et al., 2011; Berger et al., 2012; Bryantsev and Cripps, 2012; Siddiqui et al., 2012). Ultimately, cell-type-specific transcriptomes will enable us to discern how different cells interact to produce the emergent physiologic properties of a tissue or organ. In our case, we have sampled the two outermost cell layers of the *Drosophila* CNS, and our results confirm that this surface glia layer indeed possesses the hallmarks of a potent chemical protection interface equivalent to the vertebrate brain vascular endothelial BBB component.

That being said, the *Drosophila* model for vertebrate BBB physiology can and should be refined. First, the surface glia transcriptome contains two glial subtypes, the PG and SPG, thus having separate transcriptomes for these cell layers will increase the resolution at which to assign the conserved gene expression patterns discussed in this report. Second, the cortex glia that lie directly underneath the SPG are well positioned to influence BBB properties similar to astrocyte end feet positioning in the vertebrate CNS. Obtaining a transcriptome for these glia will likely add to our understanding of how conserved BBB properties are manifested in the *Drosophila* equivalent of the vertebrate NVU. We have shown that such refinements are feasible by our methodologies, and most importantly, that they are necessary to further research into the mechanisms of development, maintenance, and regulation of conserved BBB properties.

Failure to efficiently circumvent the BBB for the treatment of neurological diseases highlights the complex homeostatic mechanisms that exist at the BBB. Without a model system for which many of the interacting biological processes can be assessed *in vivo*, there will be little progress into understanding BBB development, maintenance, and regulation. The surface glia BBB of *Drosophila* is exactly the model system that is needed. Pharmacokinetics can be measured *in vivo*, hypotheses can be tested with forward and reverse genetics, different cell populations can be manipulated simultaneously, and small molecule modifiers of BBB homeostasis can be found with high-throughput screens. Previously, it was known that the *Drosophila* BBB possesses a few characteristics of the vertebrate BBB; for example, cellular junctions similar to vertebrate TJs (Juang and Carlson, 1994; Schwabe et al., 2005; Stork et al., 2008), a single drug efflux transporter similar to vertebrate ABCB1A (Mayer et al., 2009), and lipoprotein transport (Brankatschk and Eaton, 2010). Now, our characterization of the surface glia transcriptome indicates that numerous processes/structures are evolutionarily conserved between flies and vertebrates. These include: drug efflux (i.e., many B and C class ABC transporters), adherens junctions, insulin signaling, and the basal lamina. The results alone for SLC transporters are staggering. The fly and mouse BBBs co-express highly homologous SLC transporters involved in the transport of amino acids, bicarbonate, organic anions, monocarboxylates, folates, glucose, and zinc. Preliminary deep sequencing of the surface glia transcriptome suggests that about 50% more SLC transporters than revealed by GeneChips are conserved in fly and vertebrate BBBs (data not shown). With this foundation of conserved BBB gene expression patterns, we can begin to perform *in vivo*, translatable experiments in the *Drosophila* BBB model system at a scale unattainable to vertebrate researchers.

INTERESTING GENES FOR FUTURE STUDY

In addition to various surface glia enriched genes, our investigation revealed two surface glia-specific genes, *Vmat* and *Indy*. Using immunostaining, we showed that DVMAT-B specifically localized to the PG layer of the BBB. DVMAT-B has been shown to localize to the fenestrated glia of the *Drosophila* visual system, where it is thought to function in histamine storage (Romero-Calderon et al., 2008). The fenestrated glia are thought to be the visual system equivalent of PG cells (DeSalvo et al., 2011). Relatively little is known about the contribution of the PG cells to BBB functions; however, the PG-localized expression of DVMAT-B may suggest a role for PG cells in the storage of monoamines, and may function to isolate peripheral and CNS effects of monoamines. *Indy*, the other surface glia-specific gene we identified, encodes a sodium-independent dicarboxylate cotransporter (homologous to mammalian NaDC1, NaDC3, and NaCT) and, like its mammalian counterparts, has been shown to transport intermediates of the Krebs cycle (Rogina et al., 2000; Inoue et al., 2002; Knauf et al., 2002, 2006). Intermediates of the Krebs cycle also have signaling roles, and can act through various G-protein coupled receptors with potential roles in regulating blood pressure and as a hypoxia sensor (Sadagopan et al., 2007; Sapieha et al., 2008). NaDC3 has also been postulated as a glutathione transporter, with implications in oxidative stress regulation (Lash, 2005; Li et al., 2012). NaDC3 and NaCT have been shown to be expressed in neurons and astrocytic glia (Lamp et al., 2011). We have previously shown that *Drosophila* Indy is expressed in both the SPG and the PG layers (DeSalvo et al., 2011), though the polarity of its expression is currently not known. Due to its high similarity to the mammalian SLC13 transporters, its surface glia expression may suggest a role for Indy as a metabolic regulator or sensor of oxidative stress in the BBB. Furthermore, the transcriptional repressor hairy has been suggested as a metabolic switch protein in *Drosophila*, with its upregulation causing hypoxia resistance (Zhou et al., 2008). We found *hairy* to be significantly enriched in the adult surface glia, further suggesting an important metabolic role for the BBB.

We also discovered a leaky BBB phenotype caused by a protein trap in the surface glia-enriched gene *Integrin linked kinase* (*Ilk*). Mammalian integrin linked kinase is involved in transducing signals from the extracellular matrix, through integrins, to initiate downstream intracellular signaling cascades (reviewed in Wu and Dedhar, 2001). Integrin signaling is required to maintain BBB integrity in mammalian endothelial cells; disrupting this critical link between the ECM and intracellular targets led to disruption of TJs and resulted in BBB leakiness (Osada et al., 2011). Our results, therefore, suggest there might be a conserved role in the *Drosophila* BBB for integrin/Ilk signaling from the ECM/basal lamina to regulate BBB integrity. As the role for integrin/Ilk signaling in maintaining BBB integrity has also been linked to collagen composition in the ECM (Gould et al., 2005; Vahedi et al., 2007), it might be of interest to investigate the role of the PG cells, which we have shown to express the collagen IV gene *Vkg*, in neural lamella (basal lamina) composition and SPG septate junction integrity, and the response of PG cells during conditions that perturb BBB function.

Overall, our surface glia transcriptome has identified a number of interesting, conserved genes present in the adult *Drosophila* BBB. We are now well poised to interrogate the interactions between the BBB, underlying neurons and glia, and hemolymph-facing neural lamella to understand the possible feedback mechanisms that occur between the CNS and the whole organism.

ACKNOWLEDGMENTS

We thank Rich Daneman and all members of his lab at UCSF for fruitful lab meeting discussions regarding all techniques and analyses described here. Charlie Kim and Sharon Bergquist are thanked for their help in developing the brain dissociation protocols, and Sarah Elmes is thanked for her help developing FACS isolation methods. This research was supported by NIH GRANTs R01GM081863 and R21NS082856, and NIEHS R21 ES021412 (P.I. Roland J. Bainton). Also the UCSF Department of Anesthesia and Perioperative Care and the Sandler foundation.

REFERENCES

Alvarez, J. I., Dodelet-Devillers, A., Kebir, H., Ifergan, I., Fabre, P. J., Terouz, S., et al. (2011). The Hedgehog pathway promotes blood-brain barrier integrity and CNS immune quiescence. *Science* 334, 1727–1731. doi: 10.1126/science.1206936

Anderson, P. A., and Greenberg, R. M. (2001). Phylogeny of ion channels: clues to structure and function. *Comp. Biochem. Physiol. B Biochem. Mol. Biol.* 129, 17–28. doi: 10.1016/S1096-4959(01)00376-1

Armulik, A., Genove, G., Mae, M., Nisancioglu, M. H., Wallgard, E., Niaudet, C., et al. (2010). Pericytes regulate the blood-brain barrier. *Nature* 468, 557–561. doi: 10.1038/nature09522

Auld, V. J., Fetter, R. D., Broadie, K., and Goodman, C. S. (1995). Gliotactin, a novel transmembrane protein on peripheral glia, is required to form the blood-nerve barrier in Drosophila. *Cell* 81, 757–767. doi: 10.1016/0092-8674(95)90537-5

Bainton, R. J., Tsai, L. T., Schwabe, T., DeSalvo, M., Gaul, U., and Heberlein, U. (2005). moody encodes two GPCRs that regulate cocaine behaviors and blood-brain barrier permeability in Drosophila. *Cell* 123, 145–156. doi: 10.1016/j.cell.2005.07.029

Banerjee, S., and Bhat, M. A. (2008). Glial ensheathment of peripheral axons in Drosophila. *J. Neurosci. Res.* 86, 1189–1198. doi: 10.1002/jnr.21574

Banerjee, S., Pillai, A. M., Paik, R., Li, J., and Bhat, M. A. (2006). Axonal ensheathment and septate junction formation in the peripheral nervous system of Drosophila. *J. Neurosci.* 26, 3319–3329. doi: 10.1523/JNEUROSCI.5383-05.2006

Barolo, S., Carver, L. A., and Posakony, J. W. (2000). GFP and beta-galactosidase transformation vectors for promoter/enhancer analysis in Drosophila. *Biotechniques* 29, 726, 728, 730, 732.

Baumgartner, S., Littleton, J. T., Broadie, K., Bhat, M. A., Harbecke, R., Lengyel, J. A., et al. (1996). A Drosophila neurexin is required for septate junction and blood-nerve barrier formation and function. *Cell* 87, 1059–1068. doi: 10.1016/S0092-8674(00)81800-0

Behr, M., Riedel, D., and Schuh, R. (2003). The claudin-like megatrachea is essential in septate junctions for the epithelial barrier function in Drosophila. *Dev. Cell* 5, 611–620. doi: 10.1016/S1534-5807(03)00275-2

Berger, C., Harzer, H., Burkard, T. R., Steinmann, J., van der Horst, S., Laurenson, A. S., et al. (2012). FACS purification and transcriptome analysis of drosophila neural stem cells reveals a role for Klumpfuss in self-renewal. *Cell Rep.* 2, 407–418. doi: 10.1016/j.celrep.2012.07.008

Bhat, M. A. (2003). Molecular organization of axo-glial junctions. *Curr. Opin. Neurobiol.* 13, 552–559. doi: 10.1016/j.conb.2003.09.004

Bhat, M. A., Rios, J. C., Lu, Y., Garcia-Fresco, G. P., Ching, W., St. Martin, M., et al. (2001). Axon-glia interactions and the domain organization of myelinated axons requires neurexin IV/Caspr/Paranodin. *Neuron* 30, 369–383. doi: 10.1016/S0896-6273(01)00294-X

Boado, R. J., and Pardridge, W. M. (1990). The brain-type glucose transporter mRNA is specifically expressed at the blood-brain barrier. *Biochem. Biophys. Res. Commun.* 166, 174–179. doi: 10.1016/0006-291X(90)91927-K

Brand, A. H., and Perrimon, N. (1993). Targeted gene expression as a means of altering cell fates and generating dominant phenotypes. *Development* 118, 401–415

Brankatschk, M., and Eaton, S. (2010). Lipoprotein particles cross the blood-brain barrier in Drosophila. *J. Neurosci.* 30, 10441–10447. doi: 10.1523/JNEUROSCI.5943-09.2010

Bryantsev, A. L., and Cripps, R. M. (2012). Purification of cardiac cells from Drosophila embryos. *Methods* 56, 44–49. doi: 10.1016/j.ymeth.2011.11.004

Buszczak, M., Paterno, S., Lighthouse, D., Bachman, J., Planck, J., Owen, S., et al. (2007). The carnegie protein trap library: a versatile tool for Drosophila developmental studies. *Genetics* 175, 1505–1531. doi: 10.1534/genetics.106.065961

Campos, A. R., Rosen, D. R., Robinow, S. N., and White, K. (1987). Molecular analysis of the locus elav in *Drosophila melanogaster*: a gene whose embryonic expression is neural specific. *EMBO J.* 6, 425–431.

Chintapalli, V. R., Wang, J., and Dow, J. A. (2007). Using FlyAtlas to identify better *Drosophila melanogaster* models of human disease. *Nat. Genet.* 39, 715–720. doi: 10.1038/ng2049

Cordon-Cardo, C., O'Brien, J. P., Casals, D., Rittman-Grauer, L., Biedler, J. L., Melamed, M. R., et al. (1989). Multidrug-resistance gene (P-glycoprotein) is expressed by endothelial cells at blood-brain barrier sites. *Proc. Natl. Acad. Sci. U.S.A.* 86, 695–698. doi: 10.1073/pnas.86.2.695

Courtay, C., Oster, T., Michelet, F., Visvikis, A., Diederich, M., Wellman, M., et al. (1992). Gamma-glutamyltransferase: nucleotide sequence of the human pancreatic cDNA. Evidence for a ubiquitous gamma-glutamyltransferase polypeptide in human tissues. *Biochem. Pharmacol.* 43, 2527–2533. doi: 10.1016/0006-2952(92)90140-E

Curtin, K. D., Wyman, R. J., and Meinertzhagen, I. A. (2007). Basigin/EMMPRIN/CD147 mediates neuron-glia interactions in the optic lamina of Drosophila. *Glia* 55, 1542–1553. doi: 10.1002/glia.20568

Daneman, R. (2012). The blood-brain barrier in health and disease. *Ann. Neurol.* 72, 648–672. doi: 10.1002/ana.23648

Daneman, R., Agalliu, D., Zhou, L., Kuhnert, F., Kuo, C. J., and Barres, B. A. (2009). Wnt/beta-catenin signaling is required for CNS, but not non-CNS, angiogenesis. *Proc. Natl. Acad. Sci. U.S.A.* 106, 641–646. doi: 10.1073/pnas.0805165106

Daneman, R., Zhou, L., Agalliu, D., Cahoy, J. D., Kaushal, A., and Barres, B. A. (2010a). The mouse blood-brain barrier transcriptome: a new resource for understanding the development and function of brain endothelial cells. *PLoS ONE* 5:e13741. doi: 10.1371/journal.pone.0013741

Daneman, R., Zhou, L., Kebede, A. A., and Barres, B. A. (2010b). Pericytes are required for blood-brain barrier integrity during embryogenesis. *Nature* 468, 562–566. doi: 10.1038/nature09513

DeSalvo, M., Mayer, N., Mayer, F., and Bainton, R. J. (2011). Physiologic and anatomic characterization of the brain surface glia barrier of Drosophila. *Glia* 59, 1322–1340. doi: 10.1002/glia.21147

de Vries, N. A., Zhao, J., Kroon, E., Buckle, T., Beijnen, J. H., and van Tellingen, O. (2007). P-glycoprotein and breast cancer resistance protein: two dominant transporters working together in limiting the brain penetration of topotecan. *Clin. Cancer Res.* 13, 6440–6449. doi: 10.1158/1078-0432.CCR-07-1335

Edwards, T. N., and Meinertzhagen, I. A. (2010). The functional organisation of glia in the adult brain of Drosophila and other insects. *Prog Neurobiol* 90, 471–497. doi: 10.1016/j.pneurobio.2010.01.001

Enerson, B. E., and Drewes, L. R. (2006). The rat blood-brain barrier transcriptome. *J. Cereb. Blood Flow Metab.* 26, 959–973. doi: 10.1038/sj.jcbfm.9600249

Freeman, M. R., Delrow, J., Kim, J., Johnson, E., and Doe, C. Q. (2003). Unwrapping glial biology: Gcm target genes regulating glial development, diversification, and function. *Neuron* 38, 567–580. doi: 10.1016/S0896-6273(03)00289-7

Pfrieger, F. W., and Barres, B. A. (1995). What the fly's glia tell the fly's brain. *Cell* 83, 671–674. doi: 10.1016/0092-8674(95)90178-7

Gautier, L., Cope, L., Bolstad, B. M., and Irizarry, R. A. (2004). affy–analysis of Affymetrix GeneChip data at the probe level. *Bioinformatics* 20, 307–315. doi: 10.1093/bioinformatics/btg405

Gentleman, R. C., Carey, V. J., Bates, D. M., Bolstad, B., Dettling, M., Dudoit, S., et al. (2004). Bioconductor: open software development for computational biology and bioinformatics. *Genome Biol.* 5, R80. doi: 10.1186/gb-2004-5-10-r80

Gould, D. B., Phalan, F. C., Breedveld, G. J., van Mil, S. E., Smith, R. S., Schimenti, J. C., et al. (2005). Mutations in Col4a1 cause perinatal cerebral hemorrhage and porencephaly. *Science* 308, 1167–1171. doi: 10.1126/science.1109418

Hatan, M., Shinder, V., Israeli, D., Schnorrer, F., and Volk, T. (2011). The Drosophila blood brain barrier is maintained by GPCR-dependent dynamic actin structures. *J. Cell Biol.* 192, 307–319. doi: 10.1083/jcb.201007095

Hawkins, R. A., O'Kane, R. L., Simpson, I. A., and Vina, J. R. (2006). Structure of the blood-brain barrier and its role in the transport of amino acids. *J. Nutr.* 136(1 Suppl):218S–226S.

Hijazi, A., Haenlin, M., Waltzer, L., and Roch, F. (2011). The Ly6 protein coiled is required for septate junction and blood brain barrier organisation in Drosophila. *PLoS ONE* 6:e17763. doi: 10.1371/journal.pone.0017763

Hirase, T., Staddon, J. M., Saitou, M., Ando-Akatsuka, Y., Itoh, M., Furuse, M., et al. (1997). Occludin as a possible determinant of tight junction permeability in endothelial cells. *J Cell Sci* 110(Pt 14):1603–1613.

Homolya, L., Varadi, A., and Sarkadi, B. (2003). Multidrug resistance-associated proteins: Export pumps for conjugates with glutathione, glucuronate or sulfate. *Biofactors* 17, 103–114. doi: 10.1002/biof.5520170111

Huang, D. W., Sherman, B. T., and Lempicki, R. A. (2009a). Bioinformatics enrichment tools: paths toward the comprehensive functional analysis of large gene lists. *Nucleic Acids Res.* 37, 1–13. doi: 10.1093/nar/gkn923

Huang, D. W., Sherman, B. T., and Lempicki, R. A. (2009b). Systematic and integrative analysis of large gene lists using DAVID bioinformatics resources. *Nat. Protoc.* 4, 44–57. doi: 10.1038/nprot.2008.211

Ile, K. E., Tripathy, R., Goldfinger, V., and Renault, A. D. (2012). Wunen, a Drosophila lipid phosphate phosphatase, is required for septate junction-mediated barrier function. *Development* 139, 2535–2546. doi: 10.1242/dev.077289

Inoue, K., Fei, Y. J., Huang, W., Zhuang, L., Chen, Z., and Ganapathy, V. (2002). Functional identity of *Drosophila melanogaster* Indy as a cation-indeendent, electroneutral transporter for tricarboxylic acid-cycle intermediates. *Biochem. J.* 367(Pt 2):313–319. doi: 10.1042/BJ20021132

Irizarry, R. A., Bolstad, B. M., Collin, F., Cope, L. M., Hobbs, B., and Speed, T. P. (2003). Summaries of affymetrix genechip probe level data. *Nucleic Acids Res.* 31:e15. doi: 10.1093/nar/gng015

Janzer, R. C., and Raff, M. C. (1987). Astrocytes induce blood-brain barrier properties in endothelial cells. *Nature* 325, 253–257. doi: 10.1038/325253a0

Juang, J. L., and Carlson, S. D. (1994). Analog of vertebrate anionic sites in blood-brain interface of larval Drosophila. *Cell Tissue Res.* 277, 87–95. doi: 10.1007/BF00303084

Kaplow, M. E., Korayem, A. H., and Venkatesh, T. R. (2008). Regulation of glia number in Drosophila by Rap/Fzr, an activator of the anaphase-promoting complex, and Loco, an RGS protein. *Genetics* 178, 2003–2016. doi: 10.1534/genetics.107.086397

Kelso, R. J., Buszczak, M., Quinones, A. T., Castiblanco, C., Mazzalupo, S., and Cooley, L. (2004). Flytrap, a database documenting a GFP protein-trap insertion screen in *Drosophila melanogaster*. *Nucleic Acids Res.* 32(Database issue):D418–D420. doi: 10.1093/nar/gkh014

Kinsella, R. J., Kahari, A., Haider, S., Zamora, J., Proctor, G., Spudich, G., et al. (2011). Ensembl BioMarts: a hub for data retrieval across taxonomic space. *Database (Oxford)* 2011:bar030. doi: 10.1093/database/bar030

Knauf, F., Mohebbi, N., Teichert, C., Herold, D., Rogina, B., Helfand, S., et al. (2006). The life-extending gene Indy encodes an exchanger for krebs-cycle intermediates. *Biochem. J.* 397, 25–29. doi: 10.1042/BJ20060409

Knauf, F., Rogina, B., Jiang, Z., Aronson, P. S., and Helfand, S. L. (2002). Functional characterization and immunolocalization of the transporter encoded by the life-extending gene Indy. *Proc. Natl. Acad. Sci. U.S.A.* 99, 14315–14319. doi: 10.1073/pnas.222531899

Knust, E., and Bossinger, O. (2002). Composition and formation of intercellular junctions in epithelial cells. *Science* 298, 1955–1959. doi: 10.1126/science.1072161

Lamp, J., Keyser, B., Koeller, D. M., Ullrich, K., Braulke, T., and Muhlhausen, C. (2011). Glutaric aciduria type 1 metabolites impair the succinate transport from astrocytic to neuronal cells. *J. Biol. Chem.* 286, 17777–17784. doi: 10.1074/jbc.M111.232744

Lash, L. H. (2005). Role of glutathione transport processes in kidney function. *Toxicol. Appl. Pharmacol.* 204, 329–342. doi: 10.1016/j.taap.2004.10.004

Layden, M. J., Odden, J. P., Schmid, A., Garces, A., Thor, S., and Doe, C. Q. (2006). Zfh1, a somatic motor neuron transcription factor, regulates axon exit from the CNS. *Dev. Biol.* 291, 253–263. doi: 10.1016/j.ydbio.2005.12.009

Li, B., Lee, M. S., Lee, R. S., Donaldson, P. J., and Lim, J. C. (2012). Characterization of glutathione uptake, synthesis, and efflux pathways in the epithelium and endothelium of the rat cornea. *Cornea* 31, 1304–1312. doi: 10.1097/ICO.0b013e31823f76bd

Liebner, S., Corada, M., Bangsow, T., Babbage, J., Taddei, A., Czupalla, C. J., et al. (2008). Wnt/beta-catenin signaling controls development of the blood-brain barrier. *J. Cell Biol.* 183, 409–417. doi: 10.1083/jcb.200806024

Lin, F., Marchetti, S., Pluim, D., Iusuf, D., Mazzanti, R., Schellens, J. H., et al. (2013). Abcc4 together with Abcb1 and Abcg2 form a robust cooperative drug efflux system that restricts the brain entry of camptothecin analogs. *Clin. Cancer Res.* 19, 2084–2095. doi: 10.1158/1078-0432.CCR-12-3105

Loscher, W., and Potschka, H. (2005). Blood-brain barrier active efflux transporters: ATP-binding cassette gene family. *NeuroRx* 2, 86–98. doi: 10.1602/neurorx.2.1.86

Mayer, F., Mayer, N., Chinn, L., Pinsonneault, R. L., Kroetz, D., and Bainton, R. J. (2009). Evolutionary conservation of vertebrate blood-brain barrier chemoprotective mechanisms in Drosophila. *J. Neurosci.* 29, 3538–3550. doi: 10.1523/JNEUROSCI.5564-08.2009

McClintick, J. N., and Edenberg, H. J. (2006). Effects of filtering by Present call on analysis of microarray experiments. *BMC Bioinformatics* 7:49. doi: 10.1186/1471-2105-7-49

Morin, X., Daneman, R., Zavortink, M., and Chia, W. (2001). A protein trap strategy to detect GFP-tagged proteins expressed from their endogenous loci in Drosophila. *Proc. Natl. Acad. Sci. U.S.A.* 98, 15050–15055. doi: 10.1073/pnas.261408198

Nelson, K. S., Furuse, M., and Beitel, G. J. (2010). The Drosophila Claudin Kune-kune is required for septate junction organization and tracheal tube size control. *Genetics* 185, 831–839. doi: 10.1534/genetics.110.114959

Nitta, T., Hata, M., Gotoh, S., Seo, Y., Sasaki, H., Hashimoto, N., et al. (2003). Size-selective loosening of the blood-brain barrier in claudin-5-deficient mice. *J. Cell Biol.* 161, 653–660. doi: 10.1083/jcb.200302070

Okamoto, N., Nakamori, R., Murai, T., Yamauchi, Y., Masuda, A., and Nishimura, T. (2013). A secreted decoy of InR antagonizes insulin/IGF signaling to restrict body growth in Drosophila. *Genes Dev.* 27, 87–97. doi: 10.1101/gad.204479.112

Osada, T., Gu, Y.-T., Kanazawa, M., Tsubota, Y., Hawkins, B. T., Spatz, M., et al. (2011). Inter-endothelial claudin-5 expression depends upon cerebral endothelial cell matrix adhesion by b1-integrins. *J. Cereb. Blood Flow Metab.* 31, 1972–1985. doi: 10.1038/jcbfm.2011.99

Pardridge, W. M. (2005). The blood-brain barrier: bottleneck in brain drug development. *NeuroRx* 2, 3–14. doi: 10.1602/neurorx.2.1.3

Pardridge, W. M., Boado, R. J., and Farrell, C. R. (1990). Brain-type glucose transporter (GLUT-1) is selectively localized to the blood-brain barrier. Studies with quantitative western blotting and *in situ* hybridization. *J. Biol. Chem.* 265, 18035–18040.

Pfeiffer, B. D., Ngo, T. T., Hibbard, K. L., Murphy, C., Jenett, A., Truman, J. W., et al. (2010). Refinement of tools for targeted gene expression in Drosophila. *Genetics* 186, 735–755. doi: 10.1534/genetics.110.119917

Pinsonneault, R. L., Mayer, N., Mayer, F., Tegegn, N., and Bainton, R. J. (2011). Novel Models for studying the blood-brain and blood-eye barriers in Drosophila. *Methods Mol. Biol.* 686, 357–369. doi: 10.1007/978-1-60761-938-3_17

Quinones-Coello, A. T., Petrella, L. N., Ayers, K., Melillo, A., Mazzalupo, S., Hudson, A. M., et al. (2007). Exploring strategies for protein trapping in Drosophila. *Genetics* 175, 1089–1104. doi: 10.1534/genetics.106.065995

Ranganathan, R., and Ross, E. M. (1997). PDZ domain proteins: scaffolds for signaling complexes. *Curr. Biol.* 7, R770–R773. doi: 10.1016/S0960-9822(06)00401-5

Robinow, S., and White, K. (1988). The locus elav of *Drosophila melanogaster* is expressed in neurons at all developmental stages. *Dev. Biol.* 126, 294–303. doi: 10.1016/0012-1606(88)90139-X

Rogina, B., Reenan, R. A., Nilsen, S. P., and Helfand, S. L. (2000). Extended life-span conferred by cotransporter gene mutations in Drosophila. *Science* 290, 2137–2140. doi: 10.1126/science.290.5499.2137

Romero-Calderon, R., Uhlenbrock, G., Borycz, J., Simon, A. F., Grygoruk, A., Yee, S. K., et al. (2008). A glial variant of the vesicular monoamine transporter is required to store histamine in the Drosophila visual system. *PLoS Genet.* 4:e1000245. doi: 10.1371/journal.pgen.1000245

Sadagopan, N., Li, W., Roberds, S. L., Major, T., Preston, G. M., Yu, Y., et al. (2007). Circulating succinate is elevated in rodent models of hypertension and metabolic disease. *Am. J. Hypertens.* 20, 1209–1215. doi: 10.1016/j.amjhyper.2007.05.010

Saitou, M., Furuse, M., Sasaki, H., Schulzke, J. D., Fromm, M., Takano, H., et al. (2000). Complex phenotype of mice lacking occludin, a component of tight junction strands. *Mol. Biol. Cell* 11, 4131–4142. doi: 10.1091/mbc.11.12.4131

Salmand, P. A., Iche-Torres, M., and Perrin, L. (2011). Tissue-specific cell sorting from Drosophila embryos: application to gene expression analysis. *Fly (Austin)* 5, 261–265. doi: 10.4161/fly.5.3.16509

Sapieha, P., Sirinyan, M., Hamel, D., Zaniolo, K., Joyal, J. S., Cho, J. H., et al. (2008). The succinate receptor GPR91 in neurons has a major rle in retinal angiogenesis. *Nat. Med.* 14, 1067–1076. doi: 10.1038/nm.1873

Schwabe, T., Bainton, R. J., Fetter, R. D., Heberlein, U., and Gaul, U. (2005). GPCR signaling is required for blood-brain barrier formation in drosophila. *Cell* 123, 133–144. doi: 10.1016/j.cell.2005.08.037

Sheweita, S. A. (2000). Drug-metabolizing enzymes: mechanisms and functions. *Curr. Drug Metab.* 1, 107–132. doi: 10.2174/1389200003339117

Siddiqui, N. U., Li, X., Luo, H., Karaiskakis, A., Hou, H., Kislinger, T., et al. (2012). Genome-wide analysis of the maternal-to-zygotic transition in Drosophila primordial germ cells. *Genome Biol.* 13, R11-2012-13-2-r11. doi: 10.1186/gb-2012-13-2-r11

Smyth, G. K. (2004). Linear models and empirical Bayes methods for assessing differential expression in microarray experiments. *Stat. Appl. Genet. Mol. Biol.* 3, 1–25. doi: 10.2202/1544-6115.1027

Sobue, K., Yamamoto, N., Yoneda, K., Hodgson, M. E., Yamashiro, K., Tsuruoka, N., et al. (1999). Induction of blood-brain barrier properties in immortalized bovine brain endothelial cells by astrocytic factors. *Neurosci. Res.* 35, 155–164. doi: 10.1016/S0168-0102(99)00079-6

Spéder, P., and Brand, A. H. (2014). Gap junction proteins in the blood-brain barrier control nutrient-dependent reactivation of Drosophila neural stem cells. *Dev Cell* 30, 309–321. doi: 10.1016/j.devcel.2014.05.021

Stenman, J. M., Rajagopal, J., Carroll, T. J., Ishibashi, M., McMahon, J., and McMahon, A. P. (2008). Canonical Wnt signaling regulates organ-specific assembly and differentiation of CNS vasculature. *Science* 322, 1247–1250. doi: 10.1126/science.1164594

Stork, T., Engelen, D., Krudewig, A., Silies, M., Bainton, R. J., and Klambt, C. (2008). Organization and function of the blood-brain barrier in Drosophila. *J. Neurosci.* 28, 587–597. doi: 10.1523/JNEUROSCI.4367-07.2008

Strigini, M., Cantera, R., Morin, X., Bastiani, M. J., Bate, M., and Karagogeos, D. (2006). The IgLON protein Lachesin is required for the blood-brain barrier in Drosophila. *Mol. Cell. Neurosci.* 32, 91–101. doi: 10.1016/j.mcn.2006.03.001

Syed, M. H., Krudewig, A., Engelen, D., Stork, T., and Klambt, C. (2011). The CD59 family member Leaky/Coiled is required for the establishment of the blood-brain barrier in Drosophila. *J. Neurosci.* 31, 7876–7885. doi: 10.1523/JNEUROSCI.0766-11.2011

Tomancak, P., Beaton, A., Weiszmann, R., Kwan, E., Shu, S., Lewis, S. E., et al. (2002). Systematic determination of patterns of gene expression during Drosophila embryogenesis. *Genome Biol.* 3:RESEARCH0088. doi: 10.1186/gb-2002-3-12-research0088

Tomancak, P., Berman, B. P., Beaton, A., Weiszmann, R., Kwan, E., Hartenstein, V., et al. (2007). Global analysis of patterns of gene expression during Drosophila embryogenesis. *Genome Biol.* 8, R145. doi: 10.1186/gb-2007-8-7-r145

Unhavaithaya, Y., and Orr-Weaver, T. L. (2012). Polyploidization of glia in neural development links tissue growth to blood-brain barrier integrity. *Genes Dev.* 26, 31–36. doi: 10.1101/gad.177436.111

Vahedi, K., Kubis, N., Boukobza, M., Arnoult, M., Massin, P., Tournier-Lasserve, E., et al. (2007). COL4A1 mutation in a patient with sporadic, recurrent intracerebral hemorrhage. *Stroke* 38, 1461–1464. doi: 10.1161/STROKEAHA.106.475194

Valdovinos-Flores, C., and Gonsebatt, M. E. (2012). The role of amino acid transporters in GSH synthesis in the blood-brain barrier and central nervous system. *Neurochem. Int.* 61, 405–414. doi: 10.1016/j.neuint.2012.05.019

Venter, J. C., di Porzio, U., Robinson, D. A., Shreeve, S. M., Lai, J., Kerlavage, A. R., et al. (1988). Evolution of neurotransmitter receptor systems. *Prog. Neurobiol.* 30, 105–169. doi: 10.1016/0301-0082(88)90004-4

Wang, J., Kean, L., Yang, J., Allan, A. K., Davies, S. A., Herzyk, P., et al. (2004). Function-informed transcriptome analysis of Drosophila renal tubule. *Genome Biol.* 5:R69. doi: 10.1186/gb-2004-5-9-r69

Wu, C., and Dedhar, S. (2001). Integrin-linked kinase (ILK) and its interactors: a new paradigm for the coupling of extracellular matrix to actin cytoskeleton and signaling complexes. *J. Cell Biol.* 155, 505–510. doi: 10.1083/jcb.200108077

Wu, V. M., and Beitel, G. J. (2004). A junctional problem of apical proportions: epithelial tube-size control by septate junctions in the Drosophila tracheal system. *Curr. Opin. Cell Biol.* 16, 493–499. doi: 10.1016/j.ceb.2004.07.008

Wu, V. M., Schulte, J., Hirschi, A., Tepass, U., and Beitel, G. J. (2004). Sinuous is a Drosophila claudin required for septate junction organization and epithelial tube size control. *J. Cell Biol.* 164, 313–323. doi: 10.1083/jcb.200309134

Wu, W., Dnyanmote, A. V., and Nigam, S. K. (2011). Remote communication through solute carriers and ATP binding cassette drug transporter pathways: an update on the remote sensing and signaling hypothesis. *Mol. Pharmacol.* 79, 795–805. doi: 10.1124/mol.110.070607

Xiong, W. C., Okano, H., Patel, N. H., Blendy, J. A., and Montell, C. (1994). repo encodes a glial-specific homeo domain protein required in the Drosophila nervous system. *Genes Dev.* 8, 981–994. doi: 10.1101/gad.8.8.981

Zhou, D., Xue, J., Lai, J. C., Schork, N. J., White, K. P., and Haddad, G. G. (2008). Mechanisms underlying hypoxia tolerance in *Drosophila melanogaster*: hairy as a metabolic switch. *PLoS Genet.* 4:e1000221. doi: 10.1371/journal.pgen.1000221

Zlokovic, B. V. (2008). The blood-brain barrier in health and chronic neurodegenerative disorders. *Neuron* 57, 178–201. doi: 10.1016/j.neuron.2008.01.003

Permissions

All chapters in this book were first published by Frontiers; hereby published with permission under the Creative Commons Attribution License or equivalent. Every chapter published in this book has been scrutinized by our experts. Their significance has been extensively debated. The topics covered herein carry significant findings which will fuel the growth of the discipline. They may even be implemented as practical applications or may be referred to as a beginning point for another development.

The contributors of this book come from diverse backgrounds, making this book a truly international effort. This book will bring forth new frontiers with its revolutionizing research information and detailed analysis of the nascent developments around the world.

We would like to thank all the contributing authors for lending their expertise to make the book truly unique. They have played a crucial role in the development of this book. Without their invaluable contributions this book wouldn't have been possible. They have made vital efforts to compile up to date information on the varied aspects of this subject to make this book a valuable addition to the collection of many professionals and students.

This book was conceptualized with the vision of imparting up-to-date information and advanced data in this field. To ensure the same, a matchless editorial board was set up. Every individual on the board went through rigorous rounds of assessment to prove their worth. After which they invested a large part of their time researching and compiling the most relevant data for our readers.

The editorial board has been involved in producing this book since its inception. They have spent rigorous hours researching and exploring the diverse topics which have resulted in the successful publishing of this book. They have passed on their knowledge of decades through this book. To expedite this challenging task, the publisher supported the team at every step. A small team of assistant editors was also appointed to further simplify the editing procedure and attain best results for the readers.

Apart from the editorial board, the designing team has also invested a significant amount of their time in understanding the subject and creating the most relevant covers. They scrutinized every image to scout for the most suitable representation of the subject and create an appropriate cover for the book.

The publishing team has been an ardent support to the editorial, designing and production team. Their endless efforts to recruit the best for this project, has resulted in the accomplishment of this book. They are a veteran in the field of academics and their pool of knowledge is as vast as their experience in printing. Their expertise and guidance has proved useful at every step. Their uncompromising quality standards have made this book an exceptional effort. Their encouragement from time to time has been an inspiration for everyone.

The publisher and the editorial board hope that this book will prove to be a valuable piece of knowledge for researchers, students, practitioners and scholars across the globe.

List of Contributors

Ingrid Kratzer, Sophorn Chip and Zinaida S. Vexler
Department of Neurology, University of California San Francisco, San Francisco, CA, USA

Nathalie Strazielle
Brain-i, Lyon, France
Oncoflam Team, Lyon Neuroscience Research Center, INSERM, U1028, CNRS, UMR5292, Université Lyon 1, Lyon, France

Jean-François Ghersi-Egea
Oncoflam Team, Lyon Neuroscience Research Center, INSERM, U1028, CNRS, UMR5292, Université Lyon 1, Lyon, France
BIP Platform, Lyon Neuroscience Research Center, INSERM, U1028, CNRS, UMR5292, Université Lyon 1, Lyon, France

Helen B. Stolp
Division of Biomedical Engineering and Health Sciences, Department of Perinatal Imaging and Health, King's College London, London, UK

Zoltán Molnár
Department of Physiology, Anatomy and Genetics, University of Oxford, Oxford, UK

Jean-Jacques Dreifuss
Department of Neuroscience, University of Geneva, Geneva, Switzerland

Pia A. Johansson
Institute for Stem Cell Research, Helmholtz Center Munich, Munich, Germany

Hans-Christian Bauer
Institute of Tendon and Bone Regeneration, Paracelsus Medical University, Salzburg, Austria
Spinal Cord Injury and Tissue Regeneration Center, Paracelsus Medical University, Salzburg, Austria

Brent Roy Bill
Semel Institute for Neuroscience and Human Behavior, University of California Los Angeles, Los Angeles, CA, USA

Chaithanyarani Parupalli and Bensheng Ju
Chemical Biology and Therapeutics, St. Jude Children's Research Hospital, Memphis, TN, USA

Stefanie Limmer, Astrid Weiler, Anne Volkenhoff, Felix Babatz and Christian Klämbt
Institut für Neuro-und Verhaltensbiologie, Universität Münster, Münster, Germany

Vladimir Korzh
Agency for Science, Technology and Research of Singapore, Institute of Molecular and Cell Biology, Singapore, Singapore
National University of Singapore, Department of Biological Sciences, Singapore, Singapore

Sophie Whish, Katarzyna M. Dziegielewska, Natassya M. Noor, Mark D. Habgood and Norman R. Saunders
Department of Pharmacology and Therapeutics, University of Melbourne, Parkville, VIC, Australia

Kjeld Møllgård
Department of Cellular and Molecular Medicine, Institute of Cellular and Molecular Medicine, University of Copenhagen, Copenhagen, Denmark

Shane A. Liddelow
Department of Pharmacology and Therapeutics, University of Melbourne, Parkville, VIC, Australia
Department of Neurobiology, Stanford University, Palo Alto, CA, USA

Samantha J. Richardson
School of Medical Sciences, RMIT University, Bundoora, VIC, Australia

Hannah E. Henson
Chemical Biology and Therapeutics, St. Jude Children's Research Hospital, Memphis, TN, USA
Integrated Program in Biomedical Sciences, College of Graduate Health Sciences, University of Tennessee Health Science Center, Memphis, TN, USA

Michael R. Taylor
Chemical Biology and Therapeutics, St. Jude Children's Research Hospital, Memphis, TN, USA
Pharmaceutical Sciences Division, School of Pharmacy, University of Wisconsin Madison, Madison, WI, USA

Mariella Errede, Francesco Girolamo, Marco Rizzi, Mirella Bertossi, Luisa Roncali and Daniela Virgintino
Department of Basic Medical Sciences, Neurosciences and Sensory Organs, University of Bari School of Medicine, Bari, Italy

Samantha J. Richardson, Roshen C. Wijayagunaratne and Damian G. D'Souza
School of Medical Sciences, RMIT University, Bundoora, VIC, Australia

Veerle M. Darras and Stijn L. J. Van Herck
Laboratory of Comparative Endocrinology, Biology Department, KU Leuven, Leuven, Belgium

Julien Pansiot and Donatella Bettati
INSERM U1141, Robert Debre's Hospital, Paris, France
Université Paris Diderot, Sorbonne Paris Cité, UMRS 1141-PROTECT, Paris, France
PremUP, Paris, France

Raffaella Moretti
INSERM U1141, Robert Debre's Hospital, Paris, France
Université Paris Diderot, Sorbonne Paris Cité, UMRS 1141-PROTECT, Paris, France
PremUP, Paris, France
S. Maria della Misericordia Hospital, Università degli Studi di Udine, Udine, Italy

Giuseppe Damante
S. Maria della Misericordia Hospital, Università degli Studi di Udine, Udine, Italy

Jean François Ghersi-Egea
Lyon Neurosciences Research Center, INSERM U1028, CNRS UMR5292–Lyon University, Lyon, France

Nathalie Strazielle
Lyon Neurosciences Research Center, INSERM U1028, CNRS UMR5292–Lyon University, Lyon, France
Brain-i, Lyon, France

Bobbi Fleiss and Pierre Gressens
INSERM U1141, Robert Debre's Hospital, Paris, France
Université Paris Diderot, Sorbonne Paris Cité, UMRS 1141-PROTECT, Paris, France
PremUP, Paris, France
Department of Division of Imaging Sciences and Biomedical Engineering, Centre for the Developing Brain, St. Thomas' Hospital, London, UK

Luigi Titomanlio
INSERM U1141, Robert Debre's Hospital, Paris, France
Université Paris Diderot, Sorbonne Paris Cité, UMRS 1141-PROTECT, Paris, France
PremUP, Paris, France
Pediatric Emergency Department, APHP, Robert Debré Hospital, Paris, France

Melanie A. Huntley
Department of Bioinformatics and Computational Biology, Genentech Inc., South San Francisco, CA, USA

Nga Bien-Ly and Ryan J. Watts
Department of Neuroscience, Genentech Inc., South San Francisco, CA, USA

Richard Daneman
Department of Pharmacology, University of California, San Diego, La Jolla, CA, USA

Samantha J. Hindle and Roland J. Bainton
Department of Anesthesia and Perioperative Care, University of California, San Francisco, San Francisco, CA, USA

David Bueno, Maryam Parvas, Ismaïl Hermelo and Jordi Garcia-Fernàndez
Department of Genetics, Faculty of Biological Sciences, University of Barcelona, Barcelona, Spain

Hans-Christian Bauer
Institute of Tendon and Bone Regeneration, Paracelsus Medical University-Spinal Cord Injury and Tissue Regeneration Center Salzburg, Salzburg, Austria
Department of Traumatology and Sports Injuries, Paracelsus Medical University, Salzburg, Austria
Austrian Cluster for Tissue Regeneration, Vienna, Austria

Andreas Traweger
Institute of Tendon and Bone Regeneration, Paracelsus Medical University-Spinal Cord Injury and Tissue Regeneration Center Salzburg, Salzburg, Austria
Austrian Cluster for Tissue Regeneration, Vienna, Austria

István A. Krizbai
Biological Research Centre, Institute of Biophysics, Hungarian Academy of Sciences, Szeged, Hungary
Institute of Life Sciences, Vasile Goldis Western University of Arad, Arad, Romania

Hannelore Bauer
Department of Organismic Biology, University of Salzburg, Salzburg, Austria

Pia A. Johansson
Institute for Stem Cell Research, Helmholtz Center Munich, German Research Center for Environmental Health, Munich, Germany

Michael K. DeSalvo, Samantha J. Hindle, Zeid M. Rusan, Souvinh Orng and Roland J. Bainton
Department of Anesthesia and Perioperative Care, University of California San Francisco, San Francisco, CA, USA

Mark Eddison
Janelia Farm Research Campus, The Howard Hughes Medical Institute, Ashburn, VA, USA

Index

www.ingramcontent.com/pod-product-compliance
Lightning Source LLC
LaVergne TN
LVHW082144200926
848484LV00008B/2103
9798887404936